The ESC Textbook of Cardiovascular Nursing

ESC SERIES PUBLICATIONS PAGE

The ESC Textbook of Cardiovascular Medicine (Third Edition)
Edited by A. John Camm, Thomas F. Lüscher, Gerald Maurer, and Patrick W. Serruys

The ESC Textbook of Intensive and Acute Cardiovascular Care (Third Edition)
Edited by Marco Tubaro, Pascal Vranckx, Eric Bonnefoy-Cudraz, Susanna Price, and Christiaan Vrints

The ESC Textbook of Cardiovascular Imaging (Third Edition)
Edited by José Luis Zamorano, Jeroen J. Bax, Juhani Knuuti, Patrizio Lancellotti, Fausto J. Pinto, Bogdan A. Popescu, and Udo Sechtem

The ESC Textbook of Preventive Cardiology
Edited by Stephan Gielen, Guy De Backer, Massimo Piepoli, and David Wood

The EHRA Book of Pacemaker, ICD, and CRT Troubleshooting: Case-Based Learning with Multiple Choice Questions
Edited by Haran Burri, Carsten Israel, and Jean-Claude Deharo

The EACVI Echo Handbook
Edited by Patrizio Lancellotti and Bernard Cosyns

The ESC Handbook of Preventive Cardiology: Putting Prevention into Practice
Edited by Catriona Jennings, Ian Graham, and Stephan Gielen

The EACVI Textbook of Echocardiography (Second Edition)
Edited by Patrizio Lancellotti, José Luis Zamorano, Gilbert Habib, and Luigi Badano

The EHRA Book of Interventional Electrophysiology: Case-Based Learning with Multiple Choice Questions
Edited by Hein Heidbuchel, Mattias Duytschaever, and Haran Burri

The ESC Textbook of Vascular Biology
Edited by Robert Krams and Magnus Bäck

The ESC Textbook of Cardiovascular Development
Edited by José Maria Pérez-Pomares and Robert Kelly

The EACVI Textbook of Cardiovascular Magnetic Resonance
Edited by Massimo Lombardi, Sven Plein, Steffen Petersen, Chiara Bucciarelli-Ducci, Emanuela Valsangiacomo Buechel, Cristina Basso, and Victor Ferrari

The ESC Textbook of Sports Cardiology
Edited by Antonio Pelliccia, Hein Heidbuchel, Domenico Corrado, Mats Borjesson, and Sanjay Sharma

The ESC Handbook of Cardiac Rehabilitation: A Practical Clinical Guide
Edited by Ana Abreu, Jean-Paul Schmid, and Massimo Piepoli

The ESC Textbook of Cardiovascular Nursing

EDITED BY

Catriona Jennings

Honorary Professor and Director of Nursing and Interdisciplinary Relations, National Institute for Prevention and Cardiovascular Health, National University of Ireland, Galway, Republic of Ireland

Felicity Astin

Professor of Nursing, School of Human and Health Sciences, University of Huddersfield and Calderdale and Huddersfield NHS Foundation Trust, Huddersfield, UK

Donna Fitzsimons

Professor of Nursing, Head of School of Nursing & Midwifery Queen's University Belfast, Belfast, UK

Ekaterini Lambrinou

Professor in Medical Nursing and Specialties and Gerontology Department of Nursing, School of Health Sciences, Cyprus University of Technology, Limassol, Cyprus

Lis Neubeck

Professor of Cardiovascular Nursing, School of Health and Social Care, Edinburgh Napier University, Edinburgh, UK

David R. Thompson

Professor of Nursing, School of Nursing and Midwifery, Queen's University Belfast, Belfast, UK

OXFORD
UNIVERSITY PRESS

ACNAP
Association of Cardiovascular Nursing & Allied Professions

ESC
European Society of Cardiology

OXFORD
UNIVERSITY PRESS

Great Clarendon Street, Oxford, OX2 6DP,
United Kingdom

Oxford University Press is a department of the University of Oxford.
It furthers the University's objective of excellence in research, scholarship,
and education by publishing worldwide. Oxford is a registered trade mark of
Oxford University Press in the UK and in certain other countries

Impression: 1

Published in the United States of America by Oxford University Press
198 Madison Avenue, New York, NY 10016, United States of America

British Library Cataloguing in Publication Data
Data available

Library of Congress Control Number: 2021945003

ISBN 978–0–19–884931–5

DOI: 10.1093/med/9780198849315.001.0001

Printed in Great Britain by
Bell & Bain Ltd., Glasgow

Foreword

The ESC Textbook of Cardiovascular Nursing is an important resource for cardiovascular nurses at all stages of their career. It is the work of leading experts in cardiovascular care and is divided into three sections. The first section, 'The centrality of nursing within cardiovascular care', comprises three chapters: 'The epidemiology of cardiovascular disease', 'Delivering high-quality cardiovascular care', and 'Key considerations for continuing professional development and specialization'. This section describes the public health needs of the population with cardiovascular problems and how best to prepare nurses to meet the challenges of delivering evidence-based cardiovascular care.

The second section, 'Holistic nursing care: assessment, intervention, and evaluation', comprises nine chapters. The first chapter is called 'Anatomy and physiology of the healthy heart' and provides an overview of how the healthy heart functions. This is followed by 'Nursing assessment and care planning in the context of cardiovascular care'. Together, these two chapters provide an important foundation on which to develop the condition-specific content that follows about the management and care of patients presenting with common cardiovascular conditions. These chapters are entitled 'Care of the patient with coronary heart disease', 'Care of the patient with cardiac arrhythmias', 'Care of the patient with valvular heart disease', 'Care of the patient with inherited cardiac conditions and congenital heart diseases', and 'Care of the patient with heart failure'. Many cardiovascular conditions are long term and so the patient plays an important role in managing their heart health. The next chapter, 'Cardiovascular prevention and rehabilitation', provides a comprehensive overview which offers both online and hard copy resources and references, which could well serve as a standalone guide to cardiovascular risk reduction and health promotion. 'Pharmacology for cardiovascular nurses' is an exceptionally well-organized and well-written chapter and provides readers with a logical, easy-to-follow approach to understand cardiac medications.

The textbook concludes with a section entitled 'Professional considerations for nurses working in cardiovascular care' which includes three chapters. An important part of the nurse's role is as an educator, but few have had the opportunity to access training in this field. The chapter entitled 'Patient education and communication' addresses this gap. The chapters that follow consider some of the challenges that nurses face as well as a snapshot of what the future may hold for the professions: 'Addressing the current challenges for the delivery of holistic care' and 'Looking forward: the future of cardiovascular care'.

The authors' commitment to evidence-informed practice makes this textbook of great value to all nurses who care for cardiac patients. Most of the authors are themselves researchers and they cite the latest evidence as well as current clinical practice guidelines and advocate for a 'patient-centred care approach' for all cardiac patients and their families.

The ESC Textbook of Cardiovascular Nursing is practical for both graduate and postgraduate nursing programmes that provide courses on cardiovascular care. It should be essential reading for nurses who work in inpatient and/or outpatient cardiovascular settings. Its value extends to hospital wards and nursing units, including intensive care units as well as the community setting.

Catriona Jennings, editor-in-chief, is Honorary Professor at the National University of Ireland, Galway, and an internationally recognized clinician, educator, and scientist with many years of experience in the prevention of cardiovascular disease. Among her accomplishments are the EUROACTION trials and the EUROASPIRE surveys that promote interdisciplinary models of preventive care. She is also one of the founders of the Masters of Science, Postgraduate Diploma in Preventive Cardiology and the clinical Preventive Cardiology programme, both developed at Imperial College London. Professor Jennings's extensive background in nursing practice and research is amply evident throughout this excellent textbook.

Felicity Astin, co-editor, is a clinical academic nurse and Professor of Nursing at the University of Huddersfield and holds a joint appointment with Calderdale and Huddersfield NHS Foundation Trust. She led the development and publication of the original Core Curriculum for the Continuing Professional Development of Nurses in Europe, supported by the expertise of the Association of

Cardiovascular Nursing and Allied Professions (ACNAP) Education Committee. The Core Curriculum has been translated into several languages and provided the impetus for this textbook. Professor Astin's applied research focuses upon person-centred care in cardiology practice to examine patients' experiences of the care they receive and use the findings to drive improvement in healthcare provision.

Donna Fitzsimons, co-editor, is Professor of Nursing and is currently Head of the School of Nursing and Midwifery and a member of the Senate at Queen's University Belfast. She holds several significant leadership roles at the European Society of Cardiology (ESC), was the first nurse elected to the ESC Board (2014–2020), and contributed to the Clinical Practice Guidelines in the same period. She pioneered the launch of the ESC Patient Forum between 2018 and 2020 and is committed to the involvement of patients, carers, and the wider interdisciplinary team as a means to enhance patient experience and outcomes. Professor Fitzsimons's research is widely cited and has guided patient care and professional development for several decades.

Ekaterini Lambrinou, co-editor, is Associate Professor and first elected academic staff in the Department of Nursing at the Cyprus University of Technology, Limassol, Cyprus. Her research and cardiovascular nursing mainly focus on the care of patients with heart failure. She has actively contributed to ESC Guidelines and position statements. She is a regular contributor to the activities of ACNAP and the Heart Failure Association of the ESC.

Lis Neubeck, co-editor, is Professor of Cardiovascular Health in the School of Health and Social Care at Edinburgh Napier University. She is Honorary Professor of Sydney Nursing School, Charles Perkins Centre, University of Sydney in Australia where she lived before her appointment in Edinburgh. Her research focuses on innovative solutions to secondary prevention of cardiovascular disease, identification and management of atrial fibrillation, and technologies to improve access to healthcare. Professor Neubeck has been awarded several grants for her research, for which she has been widely acknowledged and honoured. She is the current President of the ESC ACNAP.

David R. Thompson, co-editor, is Professor of Nursing at Queen's University Belfast. He is Honorary Professor in the Department of Psychiatry, University of Melbourne, Australia; Adjunct Professor in the School of Public Health, Monash University, Melbourne, Australia; Honorary Professor in the School of Nursing and Midwifery, University of Queensland, Brisbane, Australia; and Distinguished Professor in the School of Nursing at Anhui Medical University, Hefei, China. In addition, he is a founding editor of the *European Journal of Cardiovascular Nursing*. Professor Thompson's research focuses on understanding the experiences, concerns, and needs of patients, their partners, and family. His prolific publications on cardiac care, specifically cardiac rehabilitation and psychosocial responses to illness, have guided the care of cardiac patients for several decades.

This distinguished group of scientists, educators, and clinicians have produced a fresh, state-of-the-art textbook. As a fellow of the ESC and the American Heart Association, I have worked with these esteemed colleagues for more than three decades. Their textbook is a boon to all those in the nursing profession who care for patients with heart disease. I recommend it without reservation.

Erika Sivarajan Froelicher, MA, MPH, PhD, FAAN
Emeritus Professor
Department of Physiological Nursing,
School of Nursing, and
Department of Epidemiology and Statistics,
School of Medicine
University of California San Francisco
San Francisco, CA, USA

Letter to nurses from the ESC Patient Forum

'It is more important to know what sort of person has a disease than to know what sort of disease a person has.'

William Osler

Dear Nurses,

While the aphorism by William Osler may still have some resonance, this textbook demonstrates that in the twenty-first century it is possible to know both the person and the disease, and through positive therapeutic relationships that respect the patient perspective to better achieve the outcomes that matter to patients.

This textbook combines the objective clinical details with the recognition of the importance of patient participation in care and understanding the emotional impact of cardiovascular disease on patients. Knowledge and understanding save lives and make a real difference to the quality of life of those whom you care for.

Recognizing that we, your patients, are persons and what defines us is so much more than our illness, is fundamental for our care. We wish to be listened to, treated as individuals with feelings, and given the opportunity to have a voice in the decisions about our treatment and care.

Being a patient is also being weak and vulnerable. You go with us through some of the darkest hours and most intimate moments in our lives. In this situation, a positive personal encounter can turn a potentially frightening experience into a compassionate interaction.

We are thankful for the much-needed human touch, the reassurance, and the humanity nurses provide while we are surrounded by beeping and flashing monitors or anxiously awaiting a medical procedure.

We hope that you will inquire about our hopes and expectations and explain what we should expect in the following days and weeks and how our lives will change.

We count on you, with care and understanding, to help us to believe we can confidently take on the challenges ahead, that everything is going to be all right, that *we* will be all right.

We need our nurses to always be alert and develop special little antennas that help you notice even our smallest handicaps, our pain, our fears because in respect of your unenviable workload and the stressful environment we might not dare to say something.

Nurses, we count on your scientific knowledge incorporated in this book, and we rely on you to help us—with kindness, compassion, and empathy.

You are our hand-holders and comforters, reassurance providers, listeners, and translators and our appreciation and thanks for your dedication, support, and efforts is endless.

Your ESC Patient Forum

Preface

We are proud to present this textbook on cardiovascular care to you on behalf of the European Society of Cardiology (ESC) Association of Cardiovascular Nursing and Allied Professionals (ACNAP). The team of editors and authors of this textbook are experienced practitioners who wish to dedicate this textbook to all those individual patients and families who we have cared for throughout our own careers and who have helped to teach us what we know today. We realize that the care of patients with cardiovascular disease is becoming increasingly specialized and that there is a need for resources to better educate and support staff new to the area. This textbook is just one of those resources developed by ACNAP. We hope it inspires you to ask questions, search for answers, and become the best cardiovascular nurse you can be. There is now a strong body of evidence confirming that educating the nursing workforce internationally increases patient safety and saves lives. As a cardiovascular nurse, we understand that you will be committed to that objective, and we further hope that the learning within this textbook will help you to work more closely with us to help fulfil the ESC mission, which is to reduce the burden of cardiovascular disease across the world.

This textbook builds on our Core Curriculum for the Continuing Professional Development of Nurses Working in Cardiovascular Care and provides in-depth learning for nurses specializing in caring for patients with coronary heart disease, cardiac arrhythmias, valvular heart disease, inherited cardiac conditions and congenital heart diseases, and heart failure. The pathology of these conditions is described as well as the normal anatomy and physiology of the heart. While tailoring nursing assessment and interventions to the care of patients with heart disease, it emphasizes high-quality holistic care taking account of the needs of patients with complex comorbidities, as well as their families. The imperative of prevention and rehabilitation in terms of both primary and secondary prevention is confirmed as well as educational, behavioural, and therapeutic interventions. The epidemiology of cardiovascular disease is covered including disease burden and inequalities across European regions. Chapters devoted to patient education and communication and to pharmacology are also included. The textbook concludes with a chapter which looks into the future challenges and opportunities for nurses and the evolution of nursing in cardiovascular care.

This textbook is designed for registered nurses working in a cardiology setting, to be used alongside a variety of teaching and learning approaches, including problem and team-based learning using clinical cases to facilitate how to apply theory in practice, and guided reflective practice to encourage learners to develop new knowledge and ways to practise that arise from thinking about their own or other observed practice. Cross-referencing is used to encourage learners to make links and to explore all parts of the textbook that are relevant to their learning. The textbook is not aimed at advanced nurse practitioners who would expect more advanced educational content; nevertheless, they may find it to be a useful educational tool. It is just one innovative element within the suite of ACNAP resources developed over recent years that are available at https://www.escardio.org/Sub-specialty-communities/Association-of-Cardiovascular-Nursing-&-Allied-Professions. We encourage you to join the ACNAP international community of nurses, where you can be part of a vibrant community of nurses of all kinds who are dedicated to driving up the quality of cardiovascular care, and you can benefit from connecting with them and becoming an active part of this community.

Since the creation of coronary care units in the 1960s, the evolution of cardiac surgery, and the development of interventional cardiology, which includes close monitoring and management of patients by nurses supported by modern technology, our profession has had an increasingly important role in cardiovascular care requiring extended skills, specialization, and autonomy. These clinical nurse specialist roles have contributed to the delivery of holistic and person-centred cardiovascular care. Importantly, nurses, whose fundamental premise is the delivery of holistic care, are in a prime position to contribute to reducing health inequalities, improving health literacy, and playing an important role in preventing disease. However, the expectation of what nurses can and should do in the context of cardiovascular care varies significantly across Europe and indeed globally. This variation is a function of several factors including the culture of healthcare and the standing of nurses within it; the education and preparation of nurses for both general and specialist care; the healthcare system of each country; and the availability of physicians and specially trained nurses and the nature of interdisciplinary working.

In 1980, Professor Paul Hugenholtz, first Fellow, Founder, and early President of the ESC, acknowledged the importance of building on the potential of nurses and actively encouraged this professional group to get involved in the ESC. Attie Immink, a nurse from the Netherlands, took the initiative by bringing nursing sessions into the ESC Congress and finally establishing the ESC Working Group on Cardiovascular Nursing in 1991.This small group of specialist nurses, mainly from Northern Europe, had ambitious goals to put nursing research on the European map. The group held their first scientific conference in the spring of 2000 in Glasgow, UK, and established the *European Journal of Cardiovascular Nursing* in 2002, which has subsequently grown to become a leading nursing journal globally. In 2006, the Working Group was transformed into the ESC Council on Cardiovascular Nursing and Allied Professions, and in 2018, the Council became the seventh Association of the ESC—the ACNAP.

ACNAP has conducted two surveys of nursing education principally among its membership and attendees at EuroHeartCare conferences, the first between 2009 and 2011 and the second in 2018. Both have identified a huge variation in the availability and content of specialist cardiovascular education and training for nurses across Europe. In the most recent survey[1] of 876 European nurses, while most reported being educated to bachelor level, a significant minority of 46% had reached masters or doctorate level, possibly reflecting the study population of conference attendees and those holding membership with a professional association. Despite this, many reported feeling unable to fulfil their clinical roles to optimal levels. These perceptions were particularly evident in relation to acute care and cardiovascular risk factor management with respondents expressing a need for education and training opportunities either as face-to-face courses or via blended or e-learning modes. This textbook is just one part of that armoury that we hope will help you join with us in the fight against heart disease.

An important priority for improving the quality of care for patients with cardiovascular disease, which is the largest cause of premature mortality worldwide, is to build on the potential of the nursing workforce. In order for nurses to fulfil this potential, there is a need for standardization in the education and preparation of nurses for specialization. The ACNAP strategic plan builds on its commitment to further nursing science in Europe, but also looks beyond this goal to address both education and clinical practice issues. Education is supported through the annual scientific EuroHeartCare Congress which reaches out to nurses and allied professionals across Europe and other countries worldwide, and also with the ACNAP Core Curriculum which was launched in 2015. Curricula for nursing education vary enormously across European countries, but these curricula define the essential content for cardiovascular nursing. In addition, issues around health policy, regulation, and assessment of competencies mean that nurses are prevented from practising to the full extent of their education and training. In some countries, nursing lacks the formal and recognized medical specialty training that physicians undergo where roles are clearly defined. If nurses are to meaningfully contribute to meeting the ESC mission of reducing the burden of cardiovascular diseases in Europe and, further, to reducing premature mortality from non-communicable diseases to levels recommended by the World Health Organization, these training issues must be addressed.

The ACNAP Core Curriculum, which exists alongside the ESC Core Curriculum for the Cardiologist, serves as a template for structure, content, and educational philosophy in national academic institutions, especially in those countries where this is missing. Like the cardiology core curriculum, it also requires the development of specialist curricula within the field of cardiovascular medicine. ACNAP, in collaboration with the Heart Failure Association and the European Association of Percutaneous Cardiovascular Interventions, has already published nursing curricula. In addition, ACNAP has worked with the Preventive Cardiovascular Nurses Association to develop a Certificate Programme in Cardiovascular Preventive Care.

Given the large global burden of cardiovascular diseases, and ageing populations with comorbidities and complex care needs, nurses, who represent the largest healthcare workforce worldwide, are well placed to advocate for and deliver evidence-based care and to make an important contribution to the delivery of high-quality cardiovascular care across the different healthcare economies in Europe and beyond. In order to fulfil the real potential of our international workforce, we need to ensure that nurses entering into specialization, following their basic nursing education, receive appropriate training for specialization which is of an equal standard across Europe. Despite all the considerable progress in cardiovascular care over recent decades, there is still much to be done and we hope that this textbook supplies you with the knowledge and inspiration to help you play your part in beating the world's biggest killer.

A word of sincere thanks and acknowledgement is due to the authors—expert clinicians, researchers, and educationalists from all over the world and, in some cases, who represent nursing leadership groups which are partners of ACNAP internationally. In working with these bodies, ACNAP has been able to contribute to international leadership initiatives to promote cardiovascular nursing education and research and improve clinical practice. Our hope is that all these partners will find our ACNAP textbook useful in supporting the education and preparation of nurse specialists internationally.

Reference

1. Fitzsimons D, Carson M, Hansen T, Neubeck L, Tanas M, Hill L. The varied role, scope of practice and education of cardiovascular nurses in ESC-affiliated countries: An ACNAP survey. Eur J Cardiovasc Nurs. 2021;20(6):572–9.

Catriona Jennings
Felicity Astin
Donna Fitzsimons
Ekaterini Lambrinou
Lis Neubeck
David R. Thompson

Contents

Symbols and abbreviations

AAS	acute aortic syndrome
ABG	arterial blood gas
ABPM	ambulatory blood pressure monitoring
ACE	angiotensin-converting enzyme
ACNAP	Association of Cardiovascular Nursing and Allied Professions
ACS	acute coronary syndrome(s)
ADP	adenosine diphosphate
ADR	adverse drug reaction
AF	atrial fibrillation
AHA	American Heart Association
AI	artificial intelligence
AMI	acute myocardial infarction
ANP	advanced nurse practitioner
APN	advanced practice nurse
ARB	angiotensin II receptor blocker
AV	atrioventricular
AVSD	atrioventricular septal defect
BACPR	British Association for Cardiovascular Prevention and Rehabilitation
BMI	body mass index
BNP	B-type natriuretic peptide
bpm	beats per minute
CABG	coronary artery bypass graft
CAD	coronary artery disease
CCS	chronic coronary syndrome(s)
CCTGA	congenitally corrected transposition of the great arteries
CHD	congenital heart disease
CI	confidence interval
CNS	clinical nurse specialist
COVID-19	coronavirus disease 2019
CPVT	catecholaminergic polymorphic ventricular tachycardia
CRT	cardiac resynchronization therapy
CRT-D	cardiac resynchronization therapy device
CS	cardiogenic shock
cTn	cardiac troponin
CVD	cardiovascular disease
CVH	cardiovascular health
CVPR	cardiovascular prevention and rehabilitation
DALY	disability-adjusted life year
DBP	diastolic blood pressure
DCM	dilated cardiomyopathy
DOAC	direct oral anticoagulant
ECG	electrocardiography/electrocardiogram
ECMO	extracorporeal membrane oxygenation
EDS	Ehlers–Danlos syndrome
EDV	end-diastolic volume
ESC	European Society of Cardiology
EU	European Union
FS	frailty syndrome
FTAAD	familial thoracic aortic aneurysm and dissection
GBD	Global Burden of Disease
GCNLF	Global Cardiovascular Nursing Leadership Forum
GTN	glyceryl trinitrate
HbA1c	glycated haemoglobin
HBPM	home blood pressure monitoring
HCM	hypertrophic cardiomyopathy
HDL-C	high-density lipoprotein cholesterol
HDL-C	high-density lipoprotein
HFmrEF	heart failure with a mid-range ejection fraction
HFpEF	heart failure with a preserved ejection fraction
HFrEF	heart failure with a reduced ejection fraction
HSBC	Health Behaviour in School-age Children
hs-TnT	high-sensitivity troponin T
ICC	inherited cardiac condition
ICCU	intensive cardiac care unit
ICD	implantable cardioverter defibrillator
ICN	International Council of Nurses
ICVH	ideal cardiovascular health
IHI	Institute for Healthcare Improvement
INR	international normalized ratio
IVR	idioventricular rhythm
LDL	low-density lipoprotein
LDL-C	low-density lipoprotein cholesterol
LMWH	low-molecular-weight heparin
LQTS	long QT syndrome
LV	left ventricle/ventricular
LVEF	left ventricular ejection fraction
LVNC	left ventricular non-compaction
LVOTO	left ventricular outflow tract obstruction
MAP	mean arterial pressure
MCS	mechanical circulatory support
MEA	mean electrical axis
MFRR	multifactor risk reduction
MI	myocardial infarction
MINOCA	myocardial infarction with non-obstructive coronary arteries

MONICA	Multinational MONItoring of Trends and Determinants of CArdiovascular Disease
NACP	National Cardiac Audit Programme
NICE	National Institute for Health and Care Excellence
NOAC	non-vitamin K antagonist oral anticoagulant
NRT	nicotine replacement therapy
NSTE	non-ST-segment elevation
NSTEMI	non-ST-segment elevation myocardial infarction
NYHA	New York Heart Association
OARS	Open-ended questions, Affirmation, Reflective listening, Summarizing
OGTT	oral glucose tolerance test
PCI	percutaneous coronary intervention
PCSK9	proprotein convertase subtilisin/kexin type 9
PDA	patent ductus arteriosus
PDSA	Plan–Do–Study–Act
PPCI	primary percutaneous coronary intervention
PPCM	peripartum cardiomyopathy
PREM	patient-reported experience measure
PRO	patient-related outcome
PROM	patient-reported outcome measure
QI	quality improvement
RAAS	renin–angiotensin–aldosterone system
RCM	restrictive cardiomyopathy
RCT	randomized controlled trial
RV	right ventricle/ventricular
S1	first heart sound
S2	second heart sound
S3	third heart sound
S4	fourth heart sound
SA	sinoatrial
SBP	systolic blood pressure
SCAI	Society for Cardiovascular Angiography and Interventions
SCD	sudden cardiac death
SCORE	Systematic Coronary Risk Evaluation
SMART	Specific, Measurable, Achievable, Realistic, Timely
STEMI	ST-segment elevation myocardial infarction
SVT	supraventricular tachycardia
TAVI	transcatheter aortic valve implantation
TCS	temporary circulatory support
TGA	transposition of the great arteries
TOF	tetralogy of Fallot
TWI	T-wave inversion
UFH	unfractionated heparin
UK	United Kingdom
URL	upper reference limit
US	United States
VAD	ventricular assist device
VA-ECMO	venoarterial extracorporeal membrane oxygenation
VKA	vitamin K antagonist
VSD	ventricular septal defect
VT	ventricular tachycardia
WHO	World Health Organization

Contributors

Neil Angus, RN, MN BN (Hons),
PG Cert (Professional & Higher Education) FHEA
Senior Lecturer
University of the Highlands and Islands, Inverness, UK

Felicity Astin, RN, BSc (Hons), PG Cert (Education), MSc, PhD, FHEA
Professor of Nursing
University of Huddersfield and Calderdale and Huddersfield NHS Foundation Trust
Huddersfield, UK

Alison Atrey, BSc, PG Dip, Ad PG Dip, SRD, PhD
Honorary Clinical Fellow
National University of Ireland
Ireland, Galway

Abigail Barrowcliff MPharm IPP PG(Dip) Pharm
Advanced Clinical Pharmacist - Cardiovascular Services
Leeds Teaching Hospitals NHS Trust
Leeds, UK

Kathy Berra, MSN, NP, BC, MSN, NP-BC, FAANP, FPCNA, FAHA, FAAN
Co-Director, The LifeCare Company
Stanford Prevention Research Center (Ret)
Stanford University School of Medicine (Ret)
Stanford, CA, US

Howard T. Blanchard, DNP, MEd, RN, ACNS-BC, CEN
Clinical Nurse Specialist
Massachusetts General Hospital, Boston, MA, US

Britt Borregaard, RN, MPQM, PhD
Associate Professor
Odense University Hospital, Odense, Denmark

Tootie Bueser, RN, MSc, PhD
Director for Nursing & Midwifery, South East Genomic Medicine Alliance
Guy's & St Thomas' Hospital NHS Foundation Trust
London, UK

Diane L. Carroll, PhD, RN, FAAN, FAHA, FESC
Nurse Researcher, Munn Center
Nursing Research
Massachusetts General Hospital, Boston, MA, USA

Rosie Cervera-Jackson, RN, MA (Oxon), MSt, DipHe
Practice Educator Royal Brompton Hospital
London, UK

Tara Conboy, RGN, BSc, MScN, MScPC, FIPC
Occupational Health Advisor
Medmark Occupational Health, Dublin, Ireland

Susan Connolly, MB BCh BAO, PhD, FRCP Edin
Consultant Cardiologist
Western Health and Social Care Trust, Enniskillen, UK

Margaret Cupples, MD, FRCGP
Emeritus Professor
Queen's University Belfast, Belfast, UK

Guy De Backer, MD, PhD
Emeritus Professor
Ghent University, Ghent, Belgium

Lisa Dullaghan, MSc, RN
Interim Assistant Director Nursing—Safe & Effective Care
South Eastern Health & Social Care Trust, Belfast, UK

Nina Fålun, RN, ICN, MSc
Clinical Nurse Specialist
Haukeland University Hospital
Bergen, Norway
Senior lecturer
Western Norway University of Applied Sciences
Bergen, Norway

Donna Fitzsimons, BSc, PhD
Professor and Head of School of Nursing & Midwifery,
Queen's University Belfast, Northern Ireland

Robyn Gallagher, RN, BA, MN, PhD
Professor of Nursing
The University of Sydney, Sydney, Australia

Irene Gibson, RGN, MA, PG Dip, FNIPC
Director of Programmes and Innovation at the National Institute for Cardiovascular Health (NIPC)
Galway, Ireland

Ian Graham, MB, BCh, BA, BAO, FRCPI, FESC, FTCD
Professor of Cardiovascular Medicine
Trinity College Dublin, Dublin, Ireland

Tina B. Hansen, PhD
Associate Professor
Zealand University Hospital, Denmark

Emma Harris, BSc, PhD
Research Fellow in Patient Education and Communication
University of Huddersfield, Huddersfield, UK

Laura L. Hayman, PhD, MSN, FAAN, FAHA, FPCNA
Professor of Nursing
UMass Boston and UMass Medical School, Boston, MA, US

Jeroen Hendriks, RN, MSc, PhD
Professor of Cardiovascular Nursing
Flinders University and Royal Adelaide Hospital, Adelaide, Australia

Loreena Hill, BSc, MSc, PhD
Lecturer (Teaching & Research)
Queen's University Belfast, Belfast, UK

Jodie Ingles, GradDipGenCouns, PhD, MPH
Head, Clinical Genomics Laboratory and Cardiac Genetic Counsellor
Centre for Population Genomics, Garvan Institute of Medical Research, and UNSW Sydney, Sydney, Australia
Centenary Institute, The University of Sydney, Sydney, Australia
Department of Cardiology, Royal Prince Alfred Hospital, Sydney, Australia

Shirley Ingram, RGN, MSc
Advanced Nurse Practitioner
Registered Nurse Prescriber
Department of Cardiology
Tallaght University Hospital
Dublin, Ireland

Tiny Jaarsma, RN, PhD
Professor
Linköping University, Linköping, Sweden

Catriona Jennings, BA (Hons), PhD, PG Cert ULT, FESC, FPCNA, FIPC
Honorary Professor of Nursing and Interdisciplinary Relations
National University of Ireland—Galway, Galway, Ireland

Ian D. Jones, RN, PhD, PGCLT
Professor of Cardiovascular Nursing
Liverpool John Moores University, Liverpool, UK

Jennifer Jones, PhD, MSc, PGCertEd, MCSP, HPC, FIPC
Associate Professor
National University of Ireland, Galway and Director of Training and Education
National Institute for Prevention and Cardiovascular Health
Galway, Ireland

Jan Keenan, RN, DipN (London), PGDip Ed, MSc
Non-Medical Prescribing Lead, Oxford university Hospitals, and Visiting Fellow, Oxford Brookes University

Mary Kerins, RGN, SCM, Cert CCU, Dip Cardiac Rehabilitation, MSc
Manager of Cardiac Rehabilitation Services
St James's Hospital, Dublin, Ireland

Rani Khatib, DPharm (PhD), FRPharmS
Consultant Cardiology Pharmacist and Honorary Senior Lecturer
Leeds Teaching Hospitals NHS Trust and University of Leeds, Leeds, UK

Selina Kikkenborg Berg, RN. Ph.d. FESC. FAHA
Professor of Cardiology
The Heart Center
Copenhagen University Hospital Rigshospitalet, Denmark

Eleni Kletsiou, RN, MSc, PhD
University General Hospital Attikon, Athens, Greece

Sue Koob, MPA
CEO
Preventive Cardiovascular Nurses Association, Madison, WI, US

Martha Kyriakou, RN, BSc, MSc, PhD
Nurse
Nicosia General Hospital, Nicosia; and Cyprus University of Technology, Limassol, Cyprus

Ekaterini Lambrinou, RN, BSc, MSc, PhD, FESC, FHFA
Professor in Medical Nursing & Specialties and Gerontology Nursing
Director, MSc in Advanced Acute and Intensive Cardiology Care
Department of Nursing, School of Health Sciences, Cyprus University of Technology

Sandra B. Lauck, PhD
Clinical Associate Professor and Clinician Scientist
University of British Columbia, Vancouver, BC, CA

Ricardo Leal, BSc, MSc
Charge Nurse,
Royal Brompton Hospital - Adult Intensive Care,
London, UK

Geraldine Lee, BSc, PhD
Reader in Advanced Clinical Practice
Kings College London, London, UK

María Teresa Lira, MScN, CV Specialist, FPCNA
Executive Coordinator of Research Unit
Hospital Clínico Fuerza Aérea de Chile Santiago, Chile

Ana Ljubas, Msc, FESC
Assistant Director for Nursing, Head Nurse
University Hospital Centre Zagreb, Zagreb, Croatia

Gabrielle McKee, BA (Mod), PhD
Associate Professor
Trinity College Dublin, Dublin, Ireland

Pascal McKeown, MD, FRCP, FESC
Head of School and Dean of Education
School of Medicine, Dentistry & Biomedical Sciences
Queen's University Belfast, Whitla Medical Building
Lisburn Road, Belfast

Philip Moons, PhD, RN, FESC, FAHA, FAAN
Professor of Healthcare and Nursing Science
KU Leuven, Leuven, Belgium; University of Gothenburg, Gothenburg, Sweden; and University of Cape Town, Cape Town, South Africa

Lis Neubeck, BA (Hons), PhD, FESC
Professor of Cardiovascular Nursing
Edinburgh Napier University, Edinburgh, UK

Tone M. Norekvål, RN, MSc, PhD, FESC, FAHA
Professor of Nursing
Haukeland University Hospital, Bergen; and University of Bergen; and Western Norway University of Applied Sciences, Bergen, Norway

Valentino Oriolo, MSc, FESC
Cardiac ACP
Department of Emergency UHBW Associate Senior Lecturer CVS Pharmacology
UWE Education Chair, EAPCI
Education Committee, ACNAP
Supervision and Assessment Lead, AIM, HEE

Andreas Protopapas, RN, BSc, MMedSc, PhD
Lecturer in Nursing
European University Cyprus, Nicosia, Cyprus

Trine B. Rasmussen, PhD
Associate Professor/Senior Researcher
University of Copenhagen/Herlev and Gentofte University Hospital, Copenhagen, Denmark

Todd Ruppar, RN, PhD, FAHA, FAAN
John L. and Helen Kellogg Professor of Nursing
Rush University, Chicago, IL, US

Julie Sanders, RN, BSc (Hon), MSc, PhD, FESC
Director Clinical Research
St Bartholomew's Hospital
Barts Health NHS Trust and Honorary Clinical Professor of Cardiovascular Nursing, The Wiliam Harvey Research Institute, Queen Mary University of London
London, UK

Chantal F. Ski, PhD
Professor and Director of the Integrated Care Academy
University of Suffolk, Ipswich, UK

Anna Stromberg, PhD
Professor
Linköping University; and Linköping University Hospital, Linköping, SE

David R. Thompson, RN, BSc, MA, PhD, MBA, FRCN, FAAN, FESC, MAE
Professor of Nursing
Queen's University Belfast, Belfast, UK

Jo Tillman, RGN, BSc, MSc
Senior Nurse/Matron
Royal Brompton Hospital, Guys and St Thomas' NHS Foundation Trust, London, UK

Izabella Uchmanowicz, RN, PhD, FESC, FHFA
Professor
Wroclaw Medical University, Wroclaw, Poland

Ercole Vellone, PhD, RN, FESC, FAAN
Associate Professor of Nursing
University of Rome Tor Vergata, Rome, Italy

Franki Wilson, MPharm, PGDip
Advanced Clinical Pharmacist
Leeds Teaching Hospitals, Leeds, UK

Alison Woolley, RN, ANP, MSc
Lead Nurse for Pre-Operative Cardiac Surgery
St George's University Hospital NHS Foundation Trust, London, UK

Section 1: The centrality of nursing within cardiovascular care

1 The epidemiology of cardiovascular disease

GUY DE BACKER, IAN GRAHAM, MARÍA TERESA LIRA, LAURA L. HAYMAN, AND IZABELLA UCHMANOWICZ

CHAPTER CONTENTS

KEY MESSAGES

- Cardiovascular disease (CVD) remains a major cause of total mortality in Europe, accounting for 45% of all deaths in Europe as a whole and 37% of total mortality in the European Union.
- Results from the European Society of Cardiology Atlas of Cardiology demonstrate important inequalities, with CVD deaths accounting for more than 50% of all deaths in some countries compared with less than 30% in others.
- Disability-adjusted life years may be among the most appropriate quantitative indicators of how effective preventive and therapeutic strategies are in reducing the CVD burden.
- Another indicator of the burden of CVD morbidity is the hospitalization rate for cardiovascular conditions which is 30% higher in men than in women, in particular for acute myocardial infarction admissions.
- Global risk calculation has been considered the best tool for comprehensive cardiovascular primary prevention, to deal with the risk of developing atherosclerotic CVD.
- To prevent death and morbidity from CVD, the guidelines highlight the importance of identifying asymptomatic patients who would be candidates for more intensive, evidence-based medical interventions that reduce CVD risk.
- In recent years, challenges in cardiovascular risk estimation efforts have included how to estimate it in different vulnerable groups more accurately, such as children and adolescents, young adults, older adults, and immigrants, and how other factors, such as social status or literacy, may influence expected outcomes.

- The nurse or nurse specialist is uniquely well placed to play a pivotal role in risk estimation and management through her or his knowledge of the science of risk estimation, its practical application, and her or his role as counsellor and advisor through the nurse's unique relationship with patients, families, and communities for holistic assessment and shared decision-making.
- Regardless of the strategy, prevention of CVD should be coordinated and implemented at many levels, from international roadmaps and guidelines to national and regional policies and standard operating procedures of individual healthcare centres and other business entities.
- Prevention of CVD should take a multidisciplinary, multifactorial, and societal approach including strategies to improve health literacy, empowerment, self-care management, and environmental adaptations.

Introduction

In this chapter, we will cover the available epidemiological data for cardiovascular disease (CVD). The chapter starts with a description of the health burden caused by CVD in Europe using different data sources. A brief historical background is given of CVD followed by a description of the burden of CVD mortality and morbidity. The prevalence of CVD, which refers to the number of people who are currently living with CVD in the population, and economic burden of CVD are also discussed. Next, risk factors for CVD are described focusing on atherosclerosis and certain genetic conditions (e.g. familial hypercholesterolaemia). CVD risk estimation is highlighted along with an overview of clinical practices. The preventive role of nurses is intimately linked to estimating the patient's risk for CVD and working with the health team and the patient in their shared decision-making. Additionally, there is a detailed description of several risk estimation equations and the important role of risk modifiers and biomarkers. Challenges in cardiovascular risk estimation efforts have included not only how to address it in different regions or countries, but also how to estimate it in different vulnerable groups more accurately, such as children and adolescents, young adults, older adults, and immigrants, and how other factors, such as social status or literacy, may influence expected outcomes. Finally, there is a section on an explanation of the CVD epidemic and consequences for the future. Prevention of CVD should take a multidisciplinary, multifactorial, and societal approach including strategies to improve health literacy, empowerment, self-care management, and environmental adaptations.

The burden of cardiovascular disease across Europe

The purpose of this section is to describe the health burden caused by CVD to society in Europe using different data sources. Reports from authorities dealing with the burden of CVD are available particularly from the European Society of Cardiology (ESC),[1] the European Heart Network,[2] the World Health Organization (WHO),[3] and the Global Burden of Disease (GBD) study group.[4]

Comparisons of these results are not always possible because the data are not harmonized from the outset; results are also presented for sets of different countries, for example, all or some of the 53 member states of the WHO's European Region, of the 28 European Union (EU) member states, and of the 56 ESC member countries. Mortality statistics are mainly based on official data with limitations regarding the quality of the data, including cause of death certification. Results on morbidity from the GBD study have been estimated by modelling surveillance data and results from surveys and from hospital records, all of which also have limitations in terms of validity and precision. Clearly, standardization across Europe of definitions, data collection methods, and validation procedures is required, with an emphasis on real data to reduce the need for estimates and modelling.

Historical background

The epidemic of CVD is a dramatic story in its own right. It started with alarming rises in CVD mortality rates in Western countries after the Second World War, resulting in a warning by the Executive Board of the WHO in 1969: 'Mankind's greatest epidemic: coronary heart disease has reached enormous proportions striking more and more at younger subjects. It will result in coming years in the greatest epidemic mankind has faced unless we are able to reverse the trend by concentrated research into its cause and prevention.' In the absence of precise and valid statistics it was difficult to understand the epidemic. This was the background of the world's largest epidemiological study ever conducted of heart disease, stroke, risk factors, and population trends: the Multinational MONItoring of Trends and Determinants of CArdiovascular Disease (MONICA) Project[5]. During the 1980s and 1990s, the attack rates of acute myocardial infarction (AMI) were registered in communities across four continents during a 10-year period using a standardized protocol. In people aged 35–64 years, large differences in attack rates of AMI were observed as well as large differences in changes

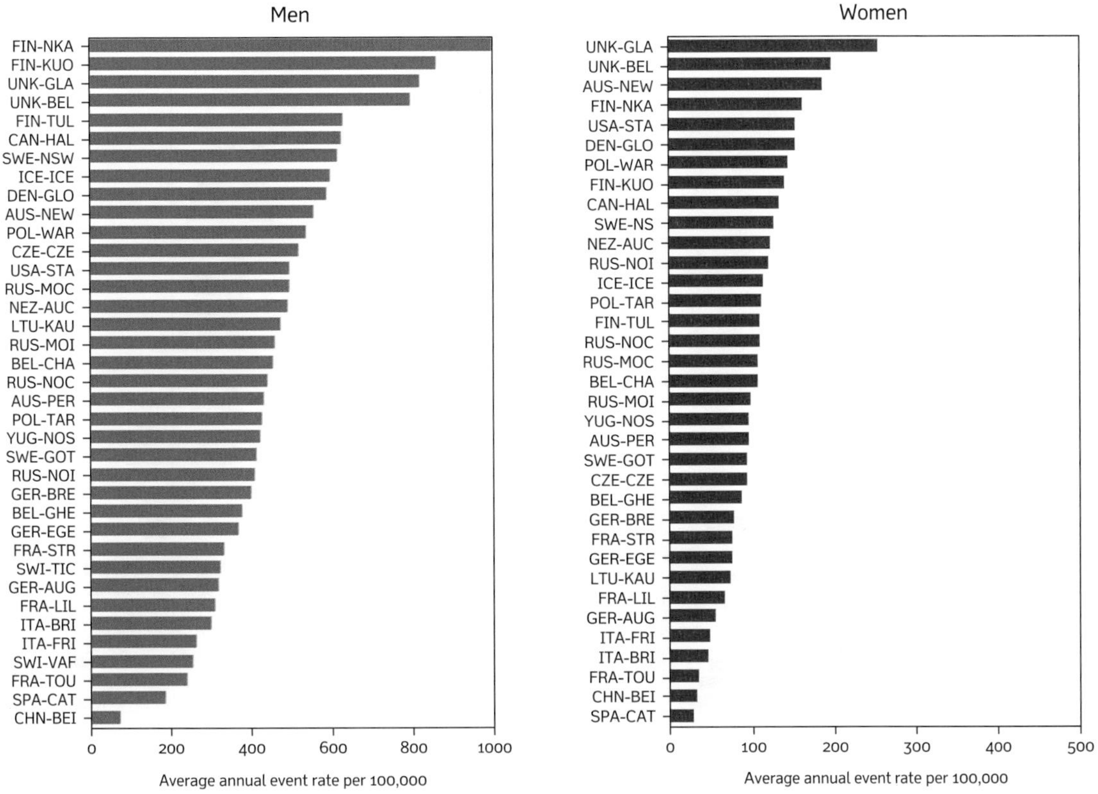

Fig. 1.1 Average annual age-standardized event rates of AMI per 100,000, for men and women aged 35–64 years, based on observations during the first 3 years of registration in the mid-1980s (see reference[5] for the precise years and the identification of the communities).

Source data from Tunstall-Pedoe H. MONICA. Monograph and multimedia sourcebook: world's largest study of heart disease, stroke, risk factors, and population trends 1979–2002. Geneva: World Health Organization; 2003.

of these attack rates over time; this is illustrated in ➤ Fig. 1.1 and ➤ Fig. 1.2.

These results and others clearly illustrate the dynamics of the epidemic of CVD in the last decades of the twentieth century, confirming the trends seen in official mortality statistics and illustrating large differences between communities and over time. The results also showed that temporal changes in attack rates of AMI varied by region within countries, for instance, in Belgium, where a significant difference in attack rate of AMI and in temporal change was observed between the populations of Ghent and Charleroi, two cities 100 km apart in which the same healthcare system is operational (see ➤ Fig. 1.1 and ➤ Fig. 1.2 comparing BEL-GHE with BEL-CHA). The overall conclusion of the MONICA Project was that changes in cardiovascular risk factors explain partly the variation in population trends in coronary heart disease[6] and that changes in coronary care and secondary prevention were strongly linked with declining coronary endpoints.[7]

Cardiovascular disease mortality

CVD is still a major cause of total mortality in Europe, accounting for 45% of all deaths in Europe as a whole (40% in men and 49% in women) and 37% of total mortality in the EU (34% in men and 40% in women).[2] Results from the ESC Atlas of Cardiology demonstrate important inequalities, with CVD deaths accounting for more than 50% of all deaths in some countries compared with less than 30% in others.[1] Although the annual number of deaths from CVD has declined in some high-income Western European countries between 1990 and 2013, globally in Europe more and more people are dying from CVD. This is mainly due to the demographic growth and the ageing of

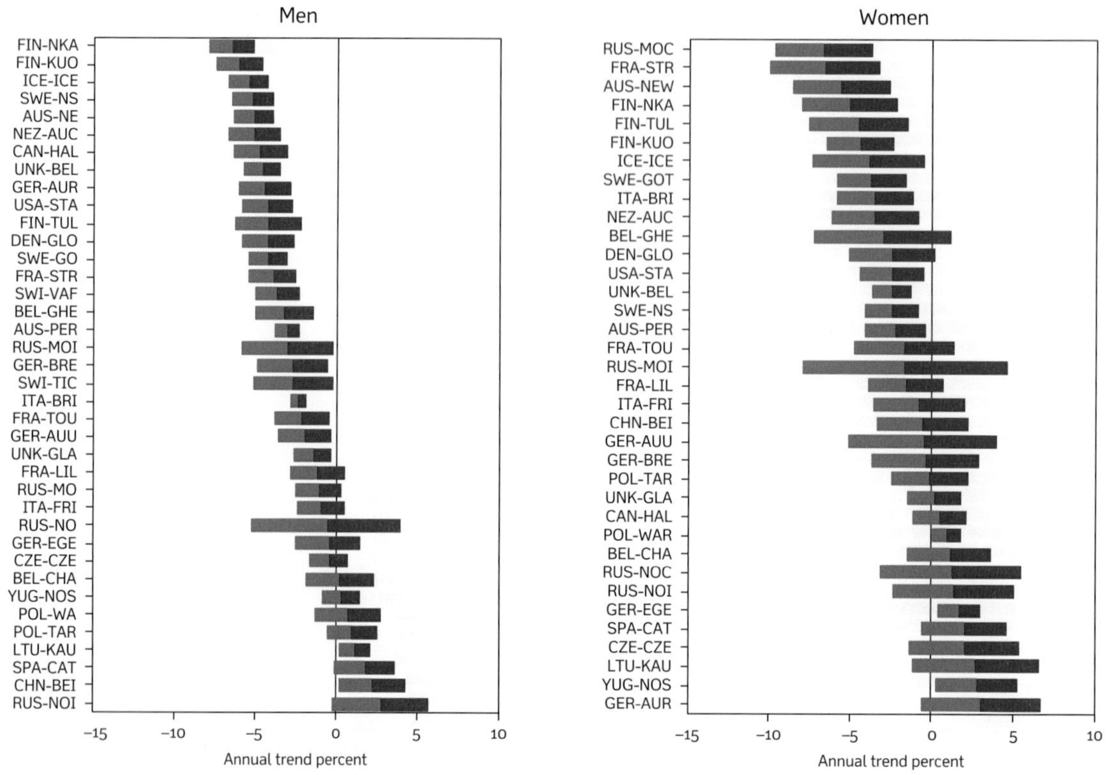

Fig. 1.2 Average annual change from the mid-1980s to the mid-1990s in age-standardized attack rates of AMI in per cent, for men and women aged 35–64 years at baseline. The horizontal bars represent the annual trend in per cent and the 95% confidence intervals. Declining trends are shown to the left of the zero line, increasing trends to the right (see reference (5) for the precise years and the identification of the communities).

Source data from Tunstall-Pedoe H. MONICA. Monograph and multimedia sourcebook: world's largest study of heart disease, stroke, risk factors, and population trends 1979–2002. Geneva: World Health Organization; 2003.

populations—more women than men ultimately die from CVD, particularly from stroke, and this also has to do with their longer life expectancy. These results should warn us that the burden of CVD will remain a major challenge as the European population grows and ages.

The rise in the absolute number of people dying from CVD is in sharp contrast with the significant decline that has been observed in age-adjusted CVD mortality rates in many European countries. This steep decline in age-adjusted CVD mortality rates had already started from the early 1970s onwards in some high-income countries in Europe; a similar but delayed pattern is now observed from the beginning of this century in other mainly Central and Eastern European countries. However, recent statistics suggest that the decline in CVD mortality among adults in some countries in past decades is now plateauing, especially in young adults.[8–11]

In 2014, age-standardized mortality rates from coronary heart disease across ESC member countries were 214 and 384 per 100,000 in women and men, respectively. The variation between countries is huge with rates greater than 500 and greater than 800 per 100,000 in women and men, respectively, in Belarus, Kyrgyzstan, Republic of Moldova, the Russian Federation, and Ukraine compared with less than 60 and less than 120 per 100,000 in women and men, respectively, in France, Luxembourg, the Netherlands, Portugal, and Spain.[1] Age-standardized mortality rates for stroke are less different between the sexes but large differences are also present between countries.

Temporal changes between 1985 and 2014 in 38 ESC member countries reveal a decline in the age-standardized mortality rate for CVD from 374 to 209 deaths per 100,000 in women and from 586 to 339 per 100,000 in men. This decline was observed in both high-income and

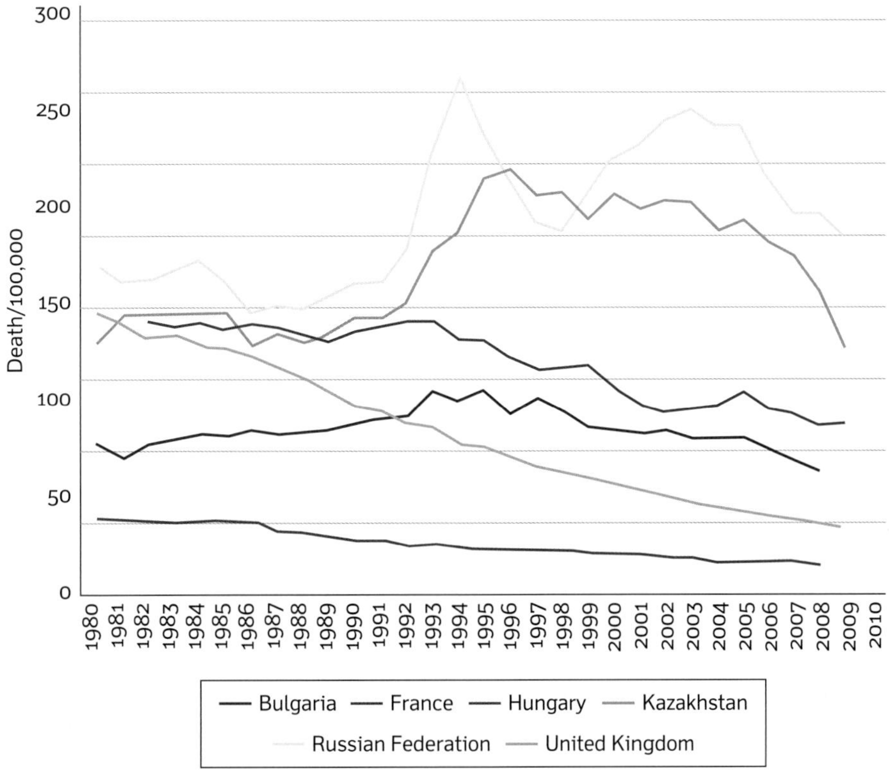

Fig. 1.3 Time trends in coronary heart disease mortality, men under 65 years.

middle-income countries but large differences existed at the national level.[1]

In summary, CVD and coronary heart disease mortality peaked in Western Europe in the 1960s. From then on, the gradient changed from South–North to West–East, with Eastern Europe peaking in the 1980s and 1990s. In ➤ Fig. 1.3 and ➤ Fig. 1.4, time trends in coronary heart disease mortality are presented for men and women, respectively, aged less than 65 years from 1980 to 2010 in a few selected countries. It should be appreciated that showing coronary heart disease mortality in people younger than 65 years may be misleading because an apparent decline may reflect a transfer of events to older ages, and the total burden of CVD may still increase. Furthermore, as outlined later, a reducing CVD case fatality rate may conceal the true disease burden, as more people live with CVD as a chronic disease.

The causes of declines in coronary heart disease mortality have been explored by Simon Capewell through a technique known as IMPACT modelling.[12] In general, over half of the observed declines relate to changes in major risk factors, notably smoking, elevated blood pressure and cholesterol (mainly reflecting diet), and under half to treatments; in ➤ Fig. 1.5, the percentages of the decrease in deaths from coronary heart disease attributed to treatments and to risk factor changes are presented based on studies using the IMPACT model and others.[13]

Premature cardiovascular disease mortality

Although around two-thirds of all CVD deaths in Europe occur in people aged over 75, approximately 1.3 million people die annually of CVD before that age, which can be considered as premature mortality. This is a serious burden to society not only at the level of the individual patient but also from a socioeconomic perspective. It is also assumed that a large proportion of these premature CVD deaths can be prevented by lifestyle adaptations and an optimal control of CVD risk factors.

In Europe, these premature CVD deaths are responsible for 35% of all deaths before the age of 75 years; in some high-income countries, cancer has now taken over the lead as a cause of premature mortality. In contrast to CVD

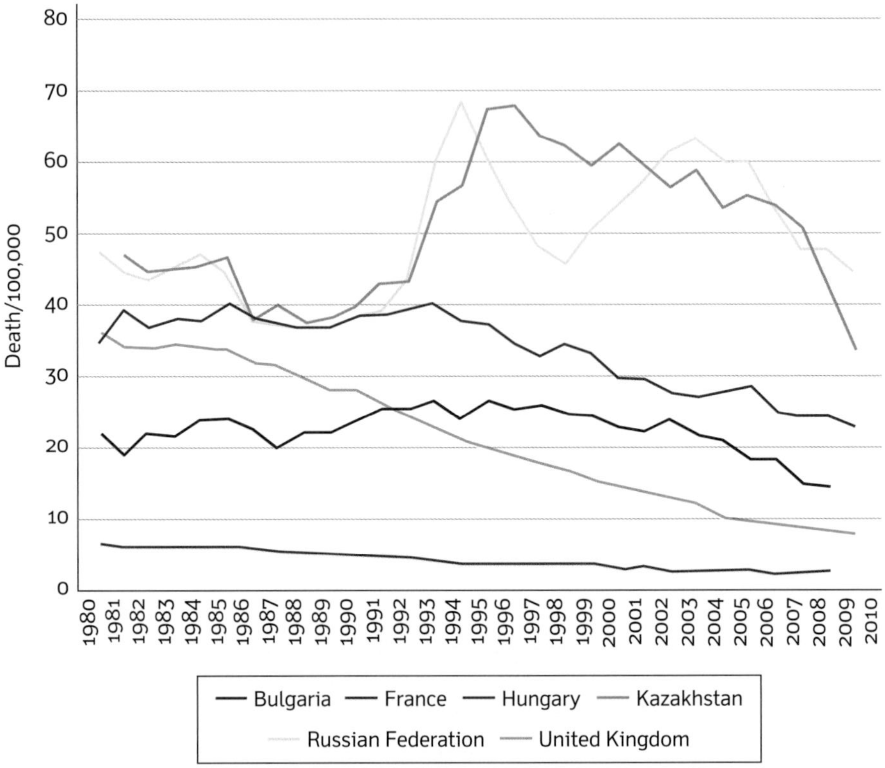

Fig. 1.4 Time trends in coronary heart disease mortality, women under 65 years.

mortality at all ages, less women than men died prematurely from CVD in the ESC member countries.[1]

Morbidity

Given the significant decline of the case fatality due to CVD, the most recent CVD mortality statistics no longer reflect the real burden of disease in absolute number. Statistics on the morbidity of CVD are, however, less available or less comparable between countries because of differences in defining and ascertaining morbidity. Some results are presented here on the incidence and the prevalence of CVD, on disability-adjusted life years (DALYs) lost due to CVD, and on hospitalizations for CVD.

Incidence

The incidence of CVD gives the number of new cases that occur within a given time period, such as 1 year. Estimates from the GBD database show that in 2015 the annual incidence of CVD was more than 11 million new cases in Europe as a whole,[2] 5.4 million in men and 5.8 million in women. One-half of all new cases was due to ischaemic heart disease, slightly more in men than in women; stroke accounted for 14% of all new cases, somewhat more in women than in men. In the EU, the annual incidence of CVD in 2015 was estimated at 6 million new cases.

Results from the ESC Atlas of Cardiology[2] reveal that CVD in ESC member countries increased from 1990 to 2015 in high- and middle-income countries, respectively, by 11% and 22% in women and by 17% and 26% in men.

Prevalence

The prevalence of CVD refers to the number of people who are currently living with CVD in the population. Based on GBD data, it was estimated that, in 2015, 85 million people out of the 831 million inhabitants in the 53 countries of the WHO's European region lived with CVD; of these 85 million, almost 49 million lived in the EU.[14] According to GBD data, there were approximately 83.5 million people living with CVD in the ESC member countries in 2015.[1]

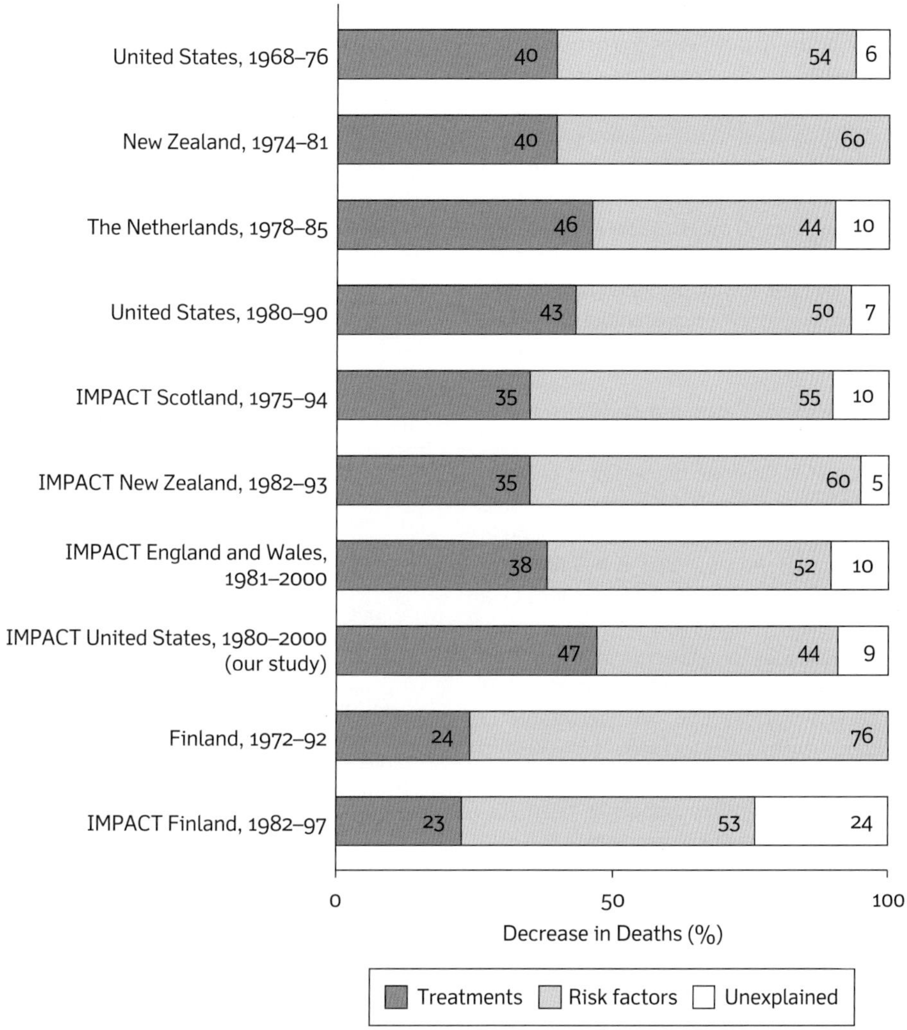

Fig. 1.5 Illustration of IMPACT modelling estimates of the proportionate causes of declines in coronary heart disease mortality. Percentages of the decrease in deaths from coronary heart disease attributed to treatments and risk factor changes. See original study for references.[12]

Age-standardized prevalence rates of CVD were higher in men compared to women and were higher in Central and Eastern Europe compared with Northern, Western, and Southern Europe.

Over the past 25 years, the absolute number of patients with CVD increased in Europe by 34% in men and by 29% in women; in the EU, the respective rise was 32% in men and 26% in women.

The age-standardized prevalence rates decreased slightly over the same time period in Europe: with a relative reduction of 9% in men and 5% in women with, however, large differences between countries such as −16.6% in men in Germany compared to +4% in men in Belarus.[2]

Disability-adjusted life years lost due to CVD

DALYs may be among the most appropriate quantitative indicators of how effective preventive and therapeutic strategies are in reducing the CVD burden. A DALY can be thought of as one lost year of 'healthy' life. DALYs lost due to CVD encompass both premature CVD deaths and physical and psychosocial disabilities caused by living with

CVD. The sum of DALYs lost due to CVD can be thought of as an indicator of the gap between the actual health status of a population and the optimal health situation where all people live to an advanced age in good health, free of CVD.

According to GBD data,[4] in 2015, DALYs lost due to CVD in women and men across ESC member states accounted for a total of 8 million and 36 million years lost, respectively, which corresponded to 22% and 24% of all DALYs lost. In Europe as a whole, it was estimated that 64 million DALYs were lost due to CVD, representing 23% of all DALYs; in the EU, that figure was 26 million, representing 19% of all DALYs.[2]

The rates of DALYs from CVD are generally higher in Central and Eastern Europe than in Northern, Southern, and Western Europe.[2] To illustrate the variation between countries, results of crude rates of WHO estimates for the number of DALYs lost due to CVD per 1000 population in a few European countries are presented in ➤ Table 1.1.[15] In both sexes, the numbers differ between countries by a factor of four to five.

Between 1990 and 2015, a reduction in mean age-standardized rates of DALYs from CVD per 100,000 lost to CVD was observed across ESC member states in both women (from 5759 to 3451) and men (from 9764 to 6326). There was also in 2015 a clear difference in age-standardized rates of DALYs from ischaemic heart disease per 100,000 lost to ischaemic heart disease between high-income ESC member countries (1004 and 2407 in women and men, respectively) compared with middle-income ESC member countries (2715 and 5977 in women and men, respectively). Broadly speaking, there is a West–East gradient, as with CVD mortality.

Hospitalizations

Another indicator of the burden of CVD morbidity is the hospitalization rate for cardiovascular conditions. The WHO European Hospital Mortality database for 31 European countries provides admission rates for CVD per 1000 population.[16]

The admission rate was 30% higher in men than in women, in particular for AMI admissions. Between countries, significant differences in admission rates existed but no geographical pattern appeared; these differences may reflect both differences in the severity of CVD burden and in the access to healthcare systems. As an illustration, results of hospitalization admission rates are given in ➤ Table 1.2 for CVD, AMI, and heart failure for the years 2011 or 2012 in some European countries.

Table 1.1 Estimated DALYs lost due to CVD per 1000 population in some European countries, 2012

Country	All, n/1000	Men, n/1000	Women, n/1000
France	40	44	36
Switzerland	41	44	37
UK	46	53	39
Sweden	55	60	50
Belgium	51	56	46
Italy	54	57	51
Finland	63	76	51
Germany	67	72	62
Czech Republic	85	94	76
Poland	90	106	74
Croatia	95	102	87
Romania	125	139	111
Latvia	153	177	134
Bulgaria	167	187	149
Russian Federation	181	217	150
Ukraine	194	214	177

Source data from World Health Organization. Health Statistics and Information Systems. http://www.who.int/healthinfo/global_burden_disease.

Economic burden of cardiovascular disease

The burden of CVD can also be expressed in economic terms. The estimated cost to the EU economy is €210 billion per year; around 53% (€111 billion) is due to healthcare costs, 26% (€54 billion) to productivity losses, and 21% (€45 billion) to the informal care of people with CVD[2] (http://www.ehnheart.org/cvd-statistics/cvd-statistics-2017.html). Approximately 28% of the overall costs of CVD is related to coronary heart disease and 20% to stroke. The costs of CVD are responsible for 8% of the total healthcare expenditure in Europe, varying

Table 1.2 Hospital inpatient admission rates per 1000 population for CVD, AMI, and heart failure, 2011–2012, by country

Country	CVD, *n*/1000	AMI, *n*/1000	Heart failure, *n*/1000
Ireland	14.0	1.9	1.4
Spain	14.5	1.6	2.2
UK	14.7	1.8	1.3
The Netherlands	19.5	2.4	1.8
Switzerland	21.5	3.2	2.0
France	23.9	1.6	3.3
Czech Republic	30.7	2.6	3.9
Hungary	35.5	2.4	3.7
Austria	40.0	2.5	2.9
Germany	40.3	3.8	4.6
Lithuania	45.4	4.1	4.6

Source data from World Health Organization. Health Statistics and Information Systems. http://www.who.int/healthinfo/global_burden_disease.

from 3% to 19% between countries. In 2015, the costs per capita were €218,000 in Europe as a whole varying from €48,000 to €365,000 between countries.[2]

Summary

- Statistics from different databases show that CVD remains a major cause of death, accounting for 45% of all deaths in Europe and 37% of total mortality in the EU.
- There still exist important inequalities in CVD mortality with deaths from AMI and stroke being on average higher in Central and Eastern Europe compared to Northern, Southern, and Western European countries.
- Age-adjusted CVD mortality rates started to decline in the 1970s in some high-income countries in Europe and have also been falling since the beginning of this century in middle-income European countries. This decline is, however, plateauing in young adults in some countries of the world.
- The CVD burden remains a major challenge when absolute numbers are considered: the annual incidence is estimated at 11 million new cases of CVD in Europe and 6 million new cases in the EU. In 2015, more than 85 million people were living with CVD in Europe.
- Although mean age-standardized rates of DALYs from CVD have been reduced across ESC member states, CVD was responsible for 8 and 36 million years lost in women and men, respectively, in 2015, accounting for 22% and 24% of all DALYs lost.
- Regarding costs to the EU economy, it is estimated that CVD costs approximately €210 billion per year.

Cardiovascular risk across the lifespan

Introduction

From an early era, mankind has been searching for ways of predicting the future. In the health arena, the focus has been on identifying risk factors for the development of future avoidable health-threatening events. A risk factor is something that is likely to increase the chances that a particular event will occur,[17] thus increasing the likelihood of developing a disease. This term was coined in 1961 by Dr Thomas R. Dawber of the Framingham Heart Study which led to the identification of the major CVD risk factors, most of which are modifiable, suggesting the possibility of intervention for prevention.[18]

The atherosclerosis associated with CVD starts in early childhood and develops slowly, but at a variable rate, over many years. While age is sometimes considered as a risk factor, it is really just a measure of exposure time. Starting with a variable genetic predisposition, the rate of progression is then modified by the intensity of lifestyle, environmental, and biochemical risk factors. This forms the basis of preventive strategies.

While certain genetic conditions such as familial hypercholesterolaemia may be associated with aggressive CVD, in most people, the rate of increase in low-density lipoprotein cholesterol and blood pressure may be determined by multiple mutations or polymorphisms which, individually, have a small effect. These may have a very modest effect on 5-year risk but, because they operate from birth, their effect on true lifetime risk may have been underappreciated. This has been supported by Mendelian randomization studies[19] which provide evidence that low-density lipoprotein cholesterol and raised blood pressure are (1) truly causal and (2) that their rate of rise is genetically determined, although of course modified by conventional risk factors over the years. As will be noted in the later section on the future of risk estimation, this raises the possibility of identifying young people and families in whom lifestyle measures to reduce risk are particularly important.

Cardiovascular disease risk estimation: overview and use in clinical practice

The role of risk estimation

The integrated approach to estimating the cardiovascular risk of an individual is based on the concept that classic risk factors (age, sex, abnormal lipids, smoking, hypertension, diabetes) have a combined effect on cardiovascular risk which may be stronger than the isolated effect of each one of them. The INTERHEART study[20] found that in different regions of the world these factors (including also abdominal obesity, psychosocial factors, consumption of fruits, vegetables, alcohol, and regular physical activity) accounted for 90.4% of the population-attributable risk for myocardial infarction, and the risk increased exponentially when they clustered. However, the incidence of coronary heart disease, atherosclerotic CVD, and the burden of risk of each risk factor (attributable risk) differ significantly among populations.[21,22] The preventive role of nurses is intimately linked to knowing the attributable risk of these factors, estimating the patient's risk of developing CVD or dying from it (using an appropriate tool), and working with the health team and the patient in their shared decision-making on how to adopt measures to mitigate the effect of modifiable cardiovascular risk factors.[23–25]

Absolute, total, or global cardiovascular risk is defined as the probability of developing coronary disease or other CVD in a determined period of time, generally 5–10 years. Based on the weight of each risk factor in a given population, the sum of all these in an arithmetic equation aims to estimate an individual's risk of suffering a cardiovascular event as low, intermediate, or high.[26] Correct risk stratification is crucial for adequate risk management to improve outcomes. It supports guideline recommendations about treatment priorities, initiation or adjustment of medication, lifestyle modification, and resource allocation and aims to avoid over- or undertreatment in individuals with low or high risk respectively.[26–29]

Relative risk compares the possibility of suffering a cardiovascular event in a person with risk factors compared to one without.[30] At individual level, risk models help to educate and motivate people to introduce lifestyle changes and to improve their treatment adherence to achieve risk reduction,[23,28,31] including those whose short-term risk is low or moderate, mainly due to their young age.[32,33] Nurses can help people understand the effect of a particular risk behaviour by reviewing the relative risk of that factor; that is, how its modification can impact the future risk of suffering a cardiovascular event. For example, a woman aged 65 years with normal total cholesterol and systolic blood pressure but who smokes, can reduce her chance of a fatal cardiovascular event by 40–50% in the next 10 years if she stops smoking. There are several examples of nurse-delivered cardiovascular risk management, tailored to risk estimation and raising awareness strategies, as nurses are increasingly undertaking this task worldwide.[30,31,34,35]

Risk estimation equations

One of the first risk estimation tools was the Framingham equation[36] that includes risk factors, previously identified as objectively, strongly, and independently related to coronary heart disease, using logistic and parametric regression models. These risk factors were measured at a baseline examination of a healthy cohort who were followed up for 10 years or more, with ascertainment of cardiovascular events. From these data, a baseline risk was derived and then beta-coefficients (in effect multipliers) calculated using Cox or Weibull methods to estimate the effects of rising levels of individual risk factors. This model is the baseline for the majority of the risk stratification instruments developed worldwide, such as the European risk charts[37], the Systematic COronary Risk Evaluation (SCORE) project (38) the revised WHO CVD risk charts[39], the American College of Cardiology/American Heart Association 2013 pooled cohort risk equations[40] and, more recently, the SCORE2 and SCORE2-OP risk charts.[41,42]

It is nowadays usual to model stroke and coronary heart disease risks separately because the proportions may vary (proportionately more strokes in low-risk countries) and regional differences in risk are also shown between the sexes. The effect of age should be allowed to vary; absolute risk increases with age but relative risk reduces and the use of a constant beta-coefficient may overestimate risk in older people.

Over the past three decades, many risk algorithms have been developed or adapted, after realizing that the initial instruments may under- or overestimate risk when applied to a different population.[43–45] In 2008, Beswick et al. identified more than a hundred prognostic models for cardiovascular primary prevention.[46] Therefore, in order to use risk equations, they need to be properly adapted, according to specific epidemiological data, and their predictive value must be validated accordingly. External validation is an essential step in the development of risk prediction models. This process evaluates and demonstrates the applicability and transportability of this model from the original cohort from whom it was constructed (derivation cohort) so they could be reliably used in a different cohort.[47] Validation requires a cohort with enough statistical power and evaluates two main attributes of the equation: *calibration*, the ability to predict the risk of suffering an event by comparing the observed versus predicted events, and *discrimination*, the ability to identify individuals according to their risk (high–intermediate–low) of developing an event in a certain period of time. According to findings, recalibration methods are defined and reclassification of individuals may be performed.[48–50]

➤ Table 1.3 summarizes the key points of the validation process. In internal validation, the model is tested against a random subsample of the cohort from which the model was derived but this may be more a test of the mathematics than of the actual performance. An external validation is clearly preferable, in which the model is tested against a well-defined different cohort.

Although the importance of validation of risk instruments is strongly advised, it is frequently not performed. Collins et al. conducted a systematic review of articles, which describes the evaluation of 120 prediction models.[51] They evidenced poorly reported key details such as calibration, inappropriate designs, and lack of acknowledgement of missing data—all crucial performance measures of prediction models. Explicit guidelines for the validation of these instruments have not yet been developed, and it is apparent that no tool is perfect. Nevertheless, understanding the multivariate properties of these stratification models and appreciating their inherent limitations could improve a more accurate recognition of patients, especially on both sides of the spectrum: high and low risk.[52–54]

Even though CVD risk estimation is recommended due to the conviction that it can play an important role in therapeutic decisions of individuals and populations when used properly, recent studies have found that in Europe risk assessment is not always performed to guide clinical practice.[55] Risk equations have little value if they are not used by clinicians on a daily basis.[56] Lack of time, disdain of prediction rules, and multiplicity of risk models with unclear knowledge of the best choice are some of the reasons to not routinely apply risk prediction tools.[26]

Table 1.3 Definitions of CVD risk score terminology

Discrimination	The ability to identify who will and who will not develop CVD *Components of discrimination* 1. Sensitivity: percentage of individuals who developed CVD and were identified correctly 2. Specificity: percentage who did *not* develop CVD and were identified correctly 3. Area under the curve (AUC): a way of expressing the maximum achievable sensitivity and specificity 4. Positive predictive value: percentage above a certain score (cut-point) who actually develop CVD 5. Negative predictive value: percentage below a certain score (cut-point) who remain disease free
Calibration	Goodness of fit; the extent to which predicted and actual cases coincide
Net Reclassification Index	The percentage of individuals who move to a higher or lower risk category when a new risk factor is added to the equation

The 2021 European guidelines on CVD prevention in clinical practice address some of these points.[28] The guidelines review the advantages and limitations of risk charts, compare usefulness of lifetime versus 10-year cardiovascular risk estimation tools, and thoroughly analyse the role of other factors not included in the standard tools (modifiers and biomarkers).

Certain people are at high or very high risk and do not require a risk scoring system but rather immediate attention to all risk factors. These include people with known CVD, most diabetics, and patients with moderate to severe chronic kidney disease. Risk scoring systems such as SCORE2 and SCORE2-OP are for use specifically in people who are apparently healthy, that is, in a primary prevention setting. ➤ **Table 1.4** summarizes the current European recommendations on risk assessment.[28]

A recent report (2019) from the European Association of Preventive Cardiology in collaboration with the Acute Cardiovascular Care Association and the Association of Cardiovascular Nursing and Allied Professions about risk prediction tools in CVD prevention has been released.[26] It presents a summary of available tools, aiming to aid the clinicians 'to choose the right tool for the right patient', highlighting aspects to consider for different populations (i.e. younger or older adults, ethnic minorities, immigrants, and geographic regions), taking into account several considerations for selecting prediction tools. It also recommends the use of prediction algorithms for different patient categories, at the U-Prevent website (https://u-prevent.com/). It should be noted that some of the algorithms on this website require further validation studies.

The role of risk modifiers and biomarkers in CVD risk estimation

Despite the broad spectrum of available instruments and the recommendation for more specific use, it is widely acknowledged that risk algorithms have their own limitations.[26,29] Most of the score models are based on observations from many years ago, and epidemiological data have been shown to be very dynamic with rising or falling incidences of CVD compared with baseline data.[29] Moreover, cardiovascular risk factor profiles also vary, leading to changes in their attributable

Table 1.4 Recommendations for CVD risk assessment

Recommendations	Class[a]	Level[b]
Systematic global CVD risk assessment is recommended in individuals with any major vascular risk factor (i.e. family history of premature CVD, FH, CVD risk factors such as smoking, arterial hypertension, DM, raised lipid level, obesity, or comorbidities increasing CVD risk).	I	C
Systematic or opportunistic CV risk assessment in the general population in men >40 years of age and in women >50 years of age or postmenopausal with no known ASCVD risk factors may be considered.	IIb	C
In those individuals who have undergone CVD risk assessment in the context of opportunistic screening, a repetition of screening after 5 years (or sooner if risk was close to treatment thresholds) may be considered.	IIb	C
Opportunistic screening of BP in adults at risk for the development of hypertension, such as those who are overweight or with a known family history of hypertension, should be considered	IIa	B
Systematic CVD risk assessment in men <40 years of age and women <50 years of age with no known CV risk factors is not recommended.	III	C

ASCVD = atherosclerotic cardiovascular disease; BP = blood pressure; CV = cardiovascular; CVD = cardiovascular disease; DM = diabetes mellitus; FH = familial hypercholesterolaemia.
[a] Class of recommendation.
[b] Level of evidence.

risk, affecting their weight in risk equations.[57,58] Such secular changes can be dealt with by recalibration using updated mortality and risk factor information. Recalibration is also possible for non-fatal events but is methodologically much more challenging. HeartScore, the electronic version of SCORE, contains recalibrated charts for many European countries (https:// www.heartscore.org/).

In the continuous search to refine the predictive ability of risk stratification instruments, several studies have been conducted[59] to include in these tools other factors that have demonstrated a strong and independent association with the chance of developing CVD, such as elevated high-sensitivity C-reactive protein (hsCRP), low ankle–brachial index, elevated apolipoprotein B, and family history of premature atherosclerotic CVD.[60] However, their addition to the models have not resulted in improvement in their discrimination, probably because they have been measured with methods that are useful but not sufficient (area under the ROC curve, c-statistic) or the lack of understanding, for example, of the complex genetic basis of CVD.[56,59–62]

Several investigators have been testing new methods that may reclassify risk when adding other risk markers to a prediction model, such as the net reclassification index developed by Pencina et al.,[63] but their utility is still to be demonstrated.[58,59,62] In practice, adding more factors to a risk equation may only make it more complex (limiting also its use in countries with limited resources). Instead, they propose to take them into account as complementary information to assist clinical judgement, especially in those individuals at intermediate risk or near a threshold of risk stratification between two categories.[29,56,60,62]

Cardiovascular risk modifiers, including biomarkers, are comorbid conditions or markers not routinely screened but with the potential of providing additional prognostic guidance.[29,60] The most recommended additional factors that improve or modify risk estimation, and whose assessment is feasible in daily practice, are physical activity, socioeconomic status, social isolation or lack of social support, family history of premature CVD, body mass index and central obesity, coronary artery calcium score, other lipids as triglycerides or apolipoprotein B, ankle–brachial blood pressure index, and carotid ultrasonography.[28,29,60] In comparative studies of markers of subclinical atherosclerosis, the coronary artery calcium score has shown the best reclassification ability in intermediate risk, even at extreme ages (≤45 years, ≥75 years).[28,29,60]

Regardless of the risk group classification, and the use of modifiers to refine risk stratification, nurses must be aware of the importance of taking a detailed personal and family history.[64] Moreover, medical history is the first factor to determine the most suitable risk assessment tool.[26] Monitoring and appropriately treating severe isolated risk factors as dyslipidaemia, diabetes, or hypertension and encouraging lifestyle changes in the presence of inactivity, smoking, obesity, or unhealthy eating habits such as salt and saturated fat intake, must be the core of nurse-led management. Also, routine reassessment of cardiovascular risk factors, and cardiovascular risk stratification, will ensure optimal risk factor management across the lifespan.[65]

In summary, global risk calculation has been considered, for almost two decades, the best tool for comprehensive cardiovascular primary prevention, aiding in the establishment of health priorities, to deal with the risk of developing atherosclerotic CVD.[27,37,43] Recent reports and guidelines from several interdisciplinary task forces, including nursing,[26,27] continue to identify as a crucial component of effective action the identification of individuals at high risk of suffering a cardiovascular event. To prevent death and morbidity from CVD, the guidelines highlight the importance of identifying asymptomatic patients who would be candidates for more intensive, evidence-based medical interventions that reduce CVD risk. This remains a major public health challenge as a significant number of events occur in the apparently healthy population, and young individuals with severe isolated risk factors are usually classified as being at intermediate risk using standard risk equations.[29]

Nurses must be aware of epidemiological considerations, including the burden of risk factors and the particular incidence of CVD in their target population, as well as select the appropriate risk estimation tool, reviewing their validation process to judge and estimate how useful a certain model is for their own clinical practice and considering additional valuable data enabling individual tailored risk management.

Finally, it is important to highlight that not only primary prevention of CVD requires risk estimation to guide evidence-based management. Patients with other cardiovascular-specific pathologies or risk factors, not always included in the estimation equations, may benefit from the use of specific risk tools. For example, for patients with diabetes, there is the ADVANCE risk engine[66] or the DIAL model[67]; for patients with a vascular disease history, the SMART (which is in the process of recalibration)[68] and SMART-REACH models[69] are available; for patients with coronary artery disease the EUROASPIRE risk model estimates 2-year risk of recurrent CVD[70] and for patients with heart failure, the MAGGIC risk calculator[71] or the Seattle heart failure model[72] are proposed. The U-Prevent website, recommended by current guidelines,[26] includes these and other algorithms for different patient categories.

Cardiovascular risk estimation in special populations

Introduction

In recent years, challenges in cardiovascular risk estimation efforts have included not only how to address it in different regions or countries, but also how to estimate it in different vulnerable groups more accurately, such as children and adolescents, young adults, older adults, and immigrants, and how other factors, such as social status or literacy, may influence expected outcomes.

Also, some comorbidities are relevant for CVD management, either because they share risk factors or because some processes or treatments inherent to the pathology increase the cardiovascular risk. Some examples are chronic kidney disease,[73] inflammatory arthritis,[35] cancer treatments,[28,74] especially breast cancer patients who receive highly cardiotoxic treatments leading to heart failure incidence rates of up to 30%[75] and an increased CVD mortality risk exceeding their breast cancer mortality risk,[76] and HIV patients with increased survival, due to more effective and widespread treatment,[77] in whom a recent meta-analysis found a twofold higher AMI risk association with chronic HIV infection.[78]

Cardiovascular risk in children and adolescents

Valid and reliable instruments for prediction of adult-onset CVD based on estimation of risk in childhood and adolescence do not exist. During the past 40 years, however, substantial research attention has focused on factors that contribute to the development and progression of atherosclerotic and hypertensive processes in early life. Results of this research have informed guidelines for assessment and management of established risk factors for CVD with emphasis on promoting cardiovascular health in childhood and adolescence and reducing risk for incident CVD in adulthood.[79]

Evidence supporting the importance of prevention and management of established risk factors for CVD beginning early in life emanates from basic, clinical, and population-based studies. Autopsy studies have demonstrated that atherosclerotic processes begin in childhood and are associated with the presence of potentially modifiable and non-modifiable risk factors including smoking, obesity, dyslipidaemia, and elevated blood pressure.[80,81] Tracking of these risk factors from childhood to adulthood has been observed in studies conducted in the US and globally.[82-84] Data from several studies including the Cardiovascular Risk in Young Finns Study link the presence of cardiovascular risk factors in adolescence with indicators of subclinical atherosclerosis in adulthood (e.g. carotid artery intima–media thickness).[85] In contrast, longitudinal studies have demonstrated that preservation of low levels of cardiovascular risk is associated with less subclinical atherosclerosis in adulthood.[86–87] Finally, the prevalence of potentially modifiable risk factors in childhood and adolescence, as documented in population-based studies conducted globally, underscore the importance of prevention beginning early in the life course.[88,89] Risk factors of particular concern are the prevalence and trends of overweight and obesity, a recognized risk factor for type 2 diabetes mellitus and CVD.

The WHO collaborative, cross-sectional Health Behaviour in School-age Children (HBSC) survey has provided data (estimates) of health behaviours and well-being as well as socioenvironmental factors in children and adolescents in Europe since 1983.[90] Based on self-reported height and weight, recent HBSC data, consistent with reports from the GBD study, indicate that the prevalence of overweight and obesity among 11-, 13-, and 15-year-olds is high but varies between countries and the sexes.[91,92] In all three age groups, the reported prevalence was higher in Southern Europe than in Northern Europe. In the GBD study, 24% and 23% of boys and girls, respectively, were either overweight or obese in developed/high-income countries.[92] The prevalence of overweight and obesity in children and adolescents in developing/low- and middle-income countries also increased substantially from approximately 8% in 1980 to 13% in 2013 for boys and girls.[92] Since obesity clusters with other established risk factors for CVD in childhood and adolescence, healthcare providers are advised to assess and monitor blood pressure, lipid profile, and insulin resistance in children and adolescents who present with obesity.[79]

Central to preventing overweight and obesity and promoting cardiovascular health across the life course are lifestyle behaviours, particularly patterns of physical activity and dietary intake. Methodological limitations notwithstanding, data from the WHO and findings from epidemiological studies conducted in Europe provide insight and have been used to guide and inform recommendations for clinical and public health practice, multilevel policies, as well as future research.[93,94] A recent report from the 2013/2014 HBSC study focused on 29 European countries emphasizes the importance of factors that operate beyond the individual level in acquisition and maintenance of physically active lifestyles.[95] While WHO and other evidence-based guidelines recommend at least 60 minutes/day of moderate- to vigorous-intensity physical activity for children and adolescents aged 5–17 years, global data support the findings of Weinberg and colleagues and point to the importance of social and environmental determinants of health behaviours and health.[95] In this recent report from HBSC, substantial variation in activity was observed within countries including within Europe. For example, 40% of 11-year-olds in Finland met WHO guidelines while only 13% of their counterparts in Italy met the recommendations for 60 minutes/day of moderate- to vigorous-intensity physical activity. Relatedly, 76% of Danish 15-year-olds but only 30% of their Albanian counterparts participated in vigorous physical activity outside the school environment for two or more hours per week.[95] Taken together and consistent with studies conducted in the US,[96] the findings from this study point to the importance of macro-level factors that operate beyond the level of the individual as key determinants of health behaviours and health. While additional research is needed to explicate the pathways and mechanisms through which these macro-level factors interact with individual characteristics to influence health behaviours and health in children and adolescents, healthcare providers, child health advocates, and other stakeholders are advised to consider these factors in assessing and managing health behaviours and in developing and implementing preventive interventions for children and adolescents.

Establishing and maintaining healthy patterns of dietary intake across the life course are also influenced by macro-level factors, referred to as contexts (e.g. families, schools, communities) in socioecological models of health and development.[97] In the 2016 HBSC comprehensive report, inequalities in eating behaviours were documented and attributed to differences in contextual characteristics: children and adolescents from less affluent families were generally more likely to self-report a 'poorer' diet as well as other health behaviours than their more affluent counterparts.[91] Specifically, breakfast and fruit consumption as well as daily evening meals were more common in children and adolescents from higher-affluence families. Daily soft drink consumption, primarily sugar-sweetened beverages, was associated with lower affluence in most countries and regions but was more common among higher-affluence groups in Albania, Armenia, Estonia, the Republic of Moldova, and Romania. A well-established major contributor to overweight and obesity, the reported average daily consumption across all HBSC countries and regions for 13-year-old boys and girls was 21% and 16%, respectively. Consistent with global data, healthy eating behaviours became less common during the school-age/adolescent transition (11–15 years of age). Of note, and well documented globally, time spent being physically active declined during the school-age/adolescent transition particularly among girls. While 30% of 11-year-old boys met the requirement of 60 minutes/day of moderate- to vigorous-intensity physical activity, this decreased to 21% at age 15. A similar trend was observed for girls: 21% of 11-year-old girls met this daily requirement for physical activity while only 11% of 15-year-olds met the requirement.[91]

Adding to the importance of adolescence as a critical time for cardiovascular health promotion and preventive interventions are data on tobacco use, the leading cause of preventable death globally. While estimates for early initiation and weekly smoking have declined since the 2009/2010 HBSC survey, both remain high in some countries and regions.[91] The 'average' reported estimates across countries of 15-year-olds who smoke at least once per week was 12% and 11% for boys and girls, respectively. In contrast, in Croatia, 25% and 21% of 15-year-old boys and girls, respectively, reported smoking at least once a week. Of note, and consistent with US data, the prevalence of weekly smoking increased significantly with age (from 11 to 15 years of age) in most of the WHO European Region and was also associated with other adverse health behaviours including high levels of alcohol consumption and unhealthy eating habits.[91]

While the HBSC survey provides self-report estimates of health behaviours, patterns and trends over time as well as between and within-country differences in social determinants of health are important considerations. *Investing in Children: The European Child and*

Adolescent Health Strategy 2015–2020 reminds us of these important sociodemographic differences in determinants of health and encourages monitoring and surveillance of health behaviours and indicators of health over time and with efforts focused on obtaining high-quality data.[98]

The guiding principles of this document for European countries that are developing and/or revising child and adolescent health strategies are particularly noteworthy and include adopting a life-course and evidence-informed approach, promoting strong partnerships and intersectoral collaboration, and adopting a rights-based approach.[98]

Since CVD is the major cause of morbidity and premature mortality in most of the European countries, a life-course approach to individual/clinical and population-based primary prevention is particularly noteworthy. This guiding principle is based on the recognition that adult health and disease are rooted in health and experiences in previous stages of the life course and it systematically reflects economic, social, environmental, biomedical, behavioural, and other relevant factors that influence health. Targeted efforts to disrupt negative intergenerational cycles that are created by or contribute to health inequities are also emphasized.[98] *Investing in Children* outlines efforts designed to enhance the lifestyle behaviours central to cardiovascular health across the life course with particular emphasis on policies that support primordial prevention, preventing the development of established risk factors by developing and maintaining healthy lifestyle behaviours.[99] Successful adoption and implementation of such policies requires continuing emphasis on evidence-based multisectoral approaches. For example, the WHO European physical activity strategy for 2016–2025 contains priority policies including (but not limited to) adopting national guidelines tailored to the promotion of physical activity among adolescents, improving urban planning and transport infrastructure to promote active transport, creating environments to support physical activity for children and adolescents (free outdoor sport, safe walking and cycling routes), ensuring school curricula include a strong physical education component, and ensuring adolescents with lower affluence or disabilities have easy access to physical activity opportunities.[100]

Taken together, the prevalence and trends in CVD-related lifestyle behaviours in children and adolescents in Europe demonstrate some progress towards achieving established goals (e.g. reducing tobacco use). A major challenge to the health of current and future generations of Europeans is the prevalence and projected trends of overweight/obesity. A major risk factor for CVD in adults, obesity tracks from adolescence to adulthood with approximately 80% of obese adolescents retaining this chronic condition into adulthood. Patterns of physical activity and dietary intake are key components of maintaining energy balance and preventing overweight early in life and across the life course. Clearly, available data support the urgent need for implementation of evidence-based, multidisciplinary, multisectoral preventive interventions, as suggested in *Investing in Children*.[98] This document emphasizes investing in both individual as well as population-based approaches to prevent and manage overweight/obesity. Investing focused on individuals as well as population-based/public health approaches to prevent and manage overweight/obesity. Nurses and nurse practitioners working within multidisciplinary teams are well prepared and positioned in healthcare and community settings to assess and manage overweight/obesity as part of an integrated profile approach to cardiovascular health promotion and risk reduction for children and adolescents.[79] As the largest healthcare discipline globally and advocates for the health of the public, nurses and organized nursing societies must participate in targeted country- and region-specific activities designed to allocate resources and increase capacity for life-course ideal cardiovascular health for all peoples of the world.

Risk estimation in young adults (<50 years)

Absolute risk may not be accurate for younger populations as age is a relevant predictor of 10-year risk. Individuals under the age of 50 years will always tend to be classified with low absolute risk even in the presence of a very unfavourable risk factor profile or severely intense isolated factors, with a higher risk of early CVD onset and high risk across their remaining lifespan.[26,28,56,101] Some suggested strategies to address this are the use of relative risk charts or 'risk age', lifetime risk calculators, or CVD-free life years.[26,28,56,102]

For example, a 40-year-old man who smokes, has a total cholesterol level of 300 mg/dL (8 mmol/L), and a systolic blood pressure of 160 mmHg has a 3% absolute risk of presenting with a fatal cardiovascular event in the next 10 years. Compared with a 40-year-old man who does not smoke, has a normal total cholesterol level, and normal systolic blood pressure (whose estimate risk is 0%), his relative risk is three times higher than this second individual, of the same sex and age.

Also, the 40-year-old man with a 3% risk has the same risk as a 60-year-old man who does not smoke, has a normal total cholesterol level, and normal systolic blood pressure (3%). This comparison has been referred to as 'vascular age'.[101] In this example, the 40-year-old man with the described burden of risk has the same probability of dying of a cardiovascular event as the healthy 60-year-old man. Communicating lifestyle changes and the importance of adherence to treatment can reduce his relative risk; if he fails to modify his burden of risk factors, he may lose 20 years of CVD-free life.

Lifetime risk calculators aim to estimate the risk of an individual developing CVD at some point in their lifetime.[54,103] These estimations provide a more comprehensive assessment of the overall burden, because they also take into account competing risks (i.e. death from cancer).[102] Increases in life expectancy have also been taken into account for the need of longer-term risk prediction tools (i.e. 30-year risk).[104] However, these models also have some limitations. The main concerns are that their analyses have been restricted to risk factors measured at a single age (not considering dynamic changes of risk factor levels or treatment) and mainly in predominant populations.[102] In addition, the lack of cut-off points to define risk levels and guidelines for management using these scales have been pointed out.[101]

There are some modifiers of cardiovascular risk that are more prevalent in younger populations that need to be taken into account, such as substance abuse. Reports from the US national health survey two decades ago evidenced that regular cocaine use was associated with an increased likelihood of non-fatal myocardial infarction in people aged 18–45 years; 25% of these events were attributable to frequent use.[105] Cocaine produces acute effects such as electrocardiographic abnormalities, acute hypertension, arrhythmia, stroke, and AMI, due to coronary artery spasm resulting from adrenergic system stimulation, and long-term use induces cardiomyopathy, endothelial injury, and vascular fibrosis.[106,107]

In summary, risk estimation in younger adults needs more research[56] and nursing plays an important role in gathering evidence. Medical and family history (i.e. familial hypercholesterolaemia), lifestyle, behaviours, and modifiers must be thoroughly analysed. Estimation of the impact of risk factors, through relative risk, lifetime risk, or other similar approaches, is recommended. The information obtained regarding a predicted risk must translate into meaningful actions and sharing it with the patient raises awareness, increases self-motivation, and enables shared decision-making when setting realistic goals.[26]

Risk estimation in older people

Age is a measure of exposure time rather than being a risk factor as such, and older people with even modest risk factor levels may be at high risk with the possibility of overmedication. Several specific considerations apply to CVD risk estimation in older people. These have been addressed in the 2021 ESC Guidelines on CVD prevention in clinical practice[28] and the SCORE2-OP algorithm was specifically developed to estimate 10-year fatal and non-fatal CVD events adjusted for competing risk in apparently healthy people aged >=70 yrs[42].

Risk estimation in ethnic minorities and immigrants

Migration between countries is increasingly growing, especially in Europe, Asia, and North America.[108] According to the European Commission, 22.3 million non-EU citizens were living in the EU on 1 January 2018, representing 4.4% of the EU population; the main regions of origin are India, China, North Africa, and Pakistan.[109]

Ethnic differences in the prevalence of cardiovascular risk factors are well documented in the literature: genetic background, lifestyle, environmental factors, cultural and religious habits, awareness, and the way people perceive and cope with illness and disease influence cardiovascular health.[26,108,110] Therefore, the profile of burden of risk differs among immigrant populations.[111] For example, South Asians have a higher prevalence of diabetes and hypertension whereas white populations have a higher prevalence of smoking and obesity. On the other hand, Chinese and South Americans have a lower overall CVD risk.[28,108,112]

However, evidence suggests that CVD risk profiles change after a residence time, with ethnic-specific temporal trends declination in cardiovascular health over time, or with significative differences when compared with second-generation (born in host country) individuals.[28,108,110,112] This has been explained by the phenomenon of acculturation, that is, a process of 'adaptation and exchange of behavior patterns to the principal culture in the new country'. Nevertheless, its true effect remains uncertain and may be confounded by secular trends in the health of immigrants.[110]

Despite the high rates of immigration in recent times, data regarding risk factor burden, how nativity and length of residence influence changes in cardiovascular health, and cardiovascular event incidence among immigrants are scarce and vary in quality.[28,112] What has been demonstrated is that current risk estimation tools do not provide adequate estimations of CVD risk in ethnic minorities[28]; validated instruments underestimate[113] or overestimate[114] risk in patients from certain ethnic minority groups. For example, the multi-ethnic HEalthy LIfe in an Urban Setting (HELIUS) study from Amsterdam using SCORE found that ethnic minorities had a greater estimated risk of fatal CVD: however, further research is needed to assess if this translates into ethnic differences in CVD incidence.[111] Current guidelines recommend that ethnicity-specific CVD risk equations should be developed.

The future in cardiovascular disease estimation

As reviewed in the present chapter, all risk estimation systems have limitations and ongoing research is needed. In 2020, the Board of the ESC approved the establishment of a Cardiovascular Risk Collaboration based in the European Heart Health Institute in Brussels. This has a very ambitious work programme. The most immediate task was the development of the updated SCORE2 and SCORE2-OP risk models. These new charts and calculators estimate the risk of total (fatal plus non-fatal) CVD in low-, medium-, high-, and very high-risk regions of Europe and have been published recently.[41,42].

Recent publications[19] raise the possibility of a new approach to risk estimation starting in childhood. Mendelian randomization studies are analogous to randomized control trials in that the polymorphisms that determine cardiovascular risk are randomly distributed, making comparison with those who do not have the polymorphisms unlikely to be biased.

The polymorphisms that determine the rate of rise in blood cholesterol and blood pressure have a small effect on 5-year risk but a large and generally unappreciated effect on true lifetime risk, because they operate from birth throughout life. This may imply that the rate of rise in blood pressure or blood cholesterol in the early years of life estimates true lifetime risk, whereas the estimated 'lifetime' risk in current risk systems is based on cohorts that start at about age 40 years. In future, rather than considering 10-year risk, we may consider risk in terms of mmol/years of exposure to cholesterol or mmHg/years of exposure to blood pressure. This approach has the possibility of approaching the 'holy grail' of risk estimation—individualized risk estimates in early life. Even without genetic testing, an increase in low-density lipoprotein cholesterol and blood pressure (even within conventional 'normal' levels) may signify a young person in whom vigorous lifestyle advice may be wise, with periodic risk checks.

The role of the nurse

The nurse or nurse specialist is uniquely well placed to play a pivotal role in risk estimation and management through her or his knowledge of the science of risk estimation, its practical application, and her or his role as counsellor and advisor through the nurse's unique relationship with patients, families, and communities for holistic assessment and shared decision-making. Nurses may also have, or develop, unique skills in simple and accessible communications. Their role as facilitator/coordinator of the actions of the multidisciplinary prevention care team, mentors and role modelling of future nurses, and evidence-based practice protocols and standard operating procedures play a crucial part in the goal of achieving better cardiovascular health.[115]

Finally, experience has shown that nurses are particularly effective in participating in clinical audits of risk factor management such as the SUrvey of Risk Factors (SURF).[116] Indeed, SURF may be an example of the use of international research data to improve patient outcomes through promoting better risk factor control. In a similar way, international endeavours such as the Global Cardiovascular Nursing Leadership Forum (GCNLF)[117] may help nurses to engage with and support cardiovascular prevention worldwide through research, education, policy advice, and advocacy.

Explanation of the cardiovascular disease epidemic and consequences for the future

As described previously, CVD constitutes a serious health and economic burden, which is likely to increase further due to population ageing. As demonstrated earlier, the incidence of CVD seems, to a large degree, to be determined by environmental modifiable factors, especially those related to lifestyle, and, hence, it might be controllable. This puts particular emphasis on the prevention of CVD.[118]

Prevention of chronic conditions, such as CVD, can be discussed in at least two contexts. First, one can distinguish between primordial, primary, secondary, and tertiary prevention. These terms refer to preventing the penetration of risk factors into the population (primordial prevention); intervening before the illness occurred, thorough control of its existing risk factors (primary prevention); screening to identify the condition at its earliest stages, before the onset of signs and symptoms (secondary prevention); and managing the disease after it had been diagnosed, to slow down or stop its progression and to identify potential complications as early as possible (tertiary prevention).[119] Second, as outlined by Rose in 1985,[120] the risk of each chronic disease can be monitored and controlled at either individual or population level. Hence, this author proposed two approaches, the 'high-risk' strategy and the 'population' strategy. The former is aimed at identifying high-risk susceptible individuals and providing them with an individualized intervention, whereas the idea behind the latter is to control the determinants of the disease's incidence in the whole population.[120] While those two approaches have their pros and cons (➤ **Table 1.5**)[120] and were criticized by some authors in the context of CVD prevention,[121] they are complementary to one another and, as shown later in this section, can be easily implemented as the components of both primordial/primary and secondary prevention; although they are applicable to tertiary prevention too, this issue is out of the scope of the present chapter and as such, is not discussed.

Regardless of the strategy, prevention of CVD should be coordinated and implemented at many levels, from international roadmaps and guidelines to national and regional policies and standard operating procedures of individual healthcare centres and other business entities. This continuum should start from existing white papers on CVD prevention, such as the World Heart Federation roadmaps[122] and the 2021 European guidelines on CVD prevention.[28] These documents should be incorporated into national health policies to guide and facilitate the two above-mentioned strategies of the primary and secondary prevention of CVD. Examples of primordial/primary and secondary preventive measures of CVD within the framework of the 'population' and 'high-risk' strategy are shown in ➤ **Table 1.6**. As denoted in the table, all these activities should involve nurses, utilizing their knowledge and experience as initiators, advisors, or direct providers.

To summarize, the aim of CVD prevention is to avoid penetration of its risk factors (e.g. overweight, inappropriate diet, inadequate physical activity, and smoking) into the population, to control the risk factors that already exist within the population, and to identify patients with early, asymptomatic stages of the disease. While the activities from the scope of primordial prevention should be undertaken at a population level, primary and secondary prevention are of utmost importance in the case of high-risk groups, for example, in obese people, smokers, and individuals with a family history of CVD. Prevention of CVD should take a multidisciplinary, multifactorial, and societal approach including strategies to improve health literacy, empowerment, self-care management, and environmental adaptations at the workplace and in the milieu.

Table 1.5 Pros and cons of the 'population' and 'high-risk' strategy

	'Population' strategy	'High-risk' strategy
Pros	Radical Large potential for population Behaviourally appropriate	Intervention appropriate to an individual Subject motivation Physician motivation Cost-effective use of resources Favourable benefit-to-risk ratio
Cons	Small benefit to an individual Poor motivation of a subject Poor motivation of a physician Worrisome benefit-to-risk ratio	Difficulties and cost of screening Palliative and temporary—not radical Limited potential for individual and population Behaviourally inappropriate

Reproduced from Rose, G., Sick Individuals and Sick Populations, International Journal of Epidemiology, Volume 14, Issue 1, March 1985, Pages 32–38, https://doi.org/10.1093/ije/14.1.32 with permission from Oxford University Press.

Table 1.6 Examples of primordial/primary and secondary preventive measures of CVD that could be implemented within the framework of the 'population' and 'high-risk' strategy. Role of nurses defined as an initiator (I), advisor (A), and provider (P)

	Primordial/primary prevention	Secondary prevention
'Population' strategy	(I, A) Legal initiatives aimed at elimination/ attenuation of established risk factors of CVD (e.g. higher taxes for tobacco products, ban for vending machines with sweets and sodas in schools, etc.) (I, A) Legal initiatives aimed at the promotion of a healthy lifestyle (e.g. an act increasing the number of compulsory physical education classes in school curricula) (I, A, P) Administrative initiatives promoting a healthy lifestyle (e.g. national and regional programmes promoting physical activity and balanced diet) (I, P) Health education programmes (risk factors of CVD, healthy lifestyle) (I, A, P) Social media campaigns promoting a healthy lifestyle	(I, A) National and local screening programmes (I, A) Legal initiatives enforcing participation in mass screening programmes (e.g. a law increasing compulsory health insurance rate for those who permanently ignore personalized invitations for screening) (I, A, P) Health education programmes (early symptoms of CVD, available screening tests, and programmes) (I, A, P) Social media campaigns promoting participation in mass screening
'High-risk' strategy	(P) Identification of people at risk (within the scope of the activities mentioned above and/ or during everyday practice) (P) Individual education and counselling (P) Tailored interventions	(P) Identification of people at risk (within the scope of the activities mentioned above and/ or primary prevention and/or during everyday practice) (P) Individual education and counselling (P) Tailored follow-up programme

References

1. Timmis A, Townsend N, Gale C, Grobbee R, Maniadakis N, Flather M, et al. European Society of Cardiology: cardiovascular disease statistics 2017. Eur Heart J. 2018;39(7):508–79.
2. Wilkins E, Wilson L, Wickramasinghe K, Bhatnagar P. European Cardiovascular Disease Statistics 2017. Brussels: European Heart Network; 2017.
3. World Health Organization. WHO Mortality Database. http://www.who.int/healthinfo/mortality_data/en/.
4. Roth GA, Johnson C, Abajobir A, Abd-Allah F, Abera SF, Abyu G, et al. Global, regional, and national burden of cardiovascular diseases for 10 causes, 1990 to 2015. J Am Coll Cardiol. 2017;70(1):1–25.
5. Tunstall-Pedoe H. MONICA. Monograph and Multimedia Sourcebook: World's Largest Study of Heart Disease, Stroke, Risk Factors, and Population Trends 1979–2002. Geneva: World Health Organization; 2003.
6. Kuulasmaa K, Tunstall-Pedoe H, Dobson A, Fortmann S, Sans S, Tolonen H, et al. Estimation of contribution of changes in classic risk factors to trends in coronary-event rates across the WHO MONICA Project populations. Lancet. 2000;355(9205):675–87.
7. Tunstall-Pedoe H, Vanuzzo D, Hobbs M, Mähönen M, Cepaitis Z, Kuulasmaa K, et al. Estimation of contribution of changes in coronary care to improving survival, event rates, and coronary heart disease mortality across the WHO MONICA Project populations. Lancet. 2000;355(9205):688–700.
8. Briffa T, Nedkoff L, Peeters A, Tonkin A, Hung J, Ridout SC, et al. Discordant age and sex-specific trends in the incidence of a first coronary heart disease event in Western Australia from 1996 to 2007. Heart. 2011;97(5):400–404.
9. Ford ES, Capewell S. Coronary heart disease mortality among young adults in the U.S. from 1980 through 2002: concealed leveling of mortality rates. J Am Coll Cardiol. 2007;50(22):2128–32.
10. Wilmot KA, O'Flaherty M, Capewell S, Ford ES, Vaccarino V. Coronary heart disease mortality declines in the United States from 1979 through 2011: evidence for stagnation in young adults, especially women. Circulation. 2015;132(11):997–1002.

11. Mensah GA, Wei GS, Sorlie PD, Fine LJ, Rosenberg Y, Kaufmann PG, et al. Decline in cardiovascular mortality: possible causes and implications. Circ Res. 2017;120(2):366–80.
12. Ford ES, Capewell S. Proportion of the decline in cardiovascular mortality disease due to prevention versus treatment: public health versus clinical care. Annu Rev Public Health. 2011;32:5–22.
13. Ford E, Bloack PB. Explaining the decrease in US deaths from coronary artery disease: 1980–2000. N Engl J Med. 2007;356(23):2388–98.
14. European Heart Network. Annual report 2018. AIMS Math. 2019;4(1):166–69.
15. World Health Organization. Health statistics and information systems: global burden of disease. http://www.who.int/healthinfo/global_burden_disease/.
16. World Health Organization. Euro hospital mortality database. http://data.euro.who.int/hmdb/index.php.
17. Shiel W. Webster's New World Medical Dictionary. Hoboken, NJ: Wiley Publishing; 2008.
18. Dawber TR, Kannel WB, Revotskie N, Stokes J, Kagan A, Gordon T. Some factors associated with the development of coronary heart disease: six years' follow-up experience in the Framingham study. Am J Public Health. 1959;49(10):1349–56.
19. Ference BA, Bhatt DL, Catapano AL, Packard CJ, Graham I, Kaptoge S, et al. Association of genetic variants related to combined exposure to lower low-density lipoproteins and lower systolic blood pressure with lifetime risk of cardiovascular disease. JAMA. 2019;322(14):1381–91.
20. Yusuf PS, Hawken S, Ôunpuu S, Dans T, Avezum A, Lanas F, et al. Effect of potentially modifiable risk factors associated with myocardial infarction in 52 countries (the INTERHEART study): case-control study. Lancet. 2004;364(9438):937–52.
21. Roth GA, Huffman MD, Moran AE, Feigin V, Mensah GA, Naghavi M, et al. Global and regional patterns in cardiovascular mortality from 1990 to 2013. Circulation. 2015;132(17):1667–78.
22. Pirani N, Khiavi F. Population attributable fraction for cardiovascular diseases risk factors in selected countries: a comparative study. Mater Sociomed. 2017;29(1):35–39.
23. Jegan NRA, Kürwitz SA, Kramer LK, Heinzel-Gutenbrunner M, Adarkwah CC, Popert U, et al. The effect of a new lifetime-cardiovascular-risk display on patients' motivation to participate in shared decision-making. BMC Fam Pract. 2018;19(1):84.
24. Mishra R Monica. Determinants of cardiovascular disease and sequential decision-making for treatment among women: a Heckman's approach. SSM Popul Health. 2019;7:100365.
25. Lin GA, Fagerlin A. Shared decision making state of the science. Circ Cardiovasc Qual Outcomes. 2014;7(2):328–34.
26. Rossello X, Dorresteijn JA, Janssen A, Lambrinou E, Scherrenberg M, Bonnefoy-Cudraz E, et al. Risk prediction tools in cardiovascular disease prevention: a report from the ESC Prevention of CVD Programme led by the European Association of Preventive Cardiology (EAPC) in collaboration with the Acute Cardiovascular Care Association (ACCA) and the Association of Cardiovascular Nursing and Allied Professions (ACNAP). Eur J Prev Cardiol. 2019;26(14):1534–44.
27. Arnett DK, Blumenthal RS, Albert MA, Buroker AB, Goldberger ZD, Hahn EJ, et al. 2019 ACC/AHA Guideline on the primary prevention of cardiovascular disease: a report of the American College of Cardiology/American Heart Association Task Force on Clinical Practice Guidelines. Circulation. 2019;140(11):e596–646.
28. Visseren F, Mach F, Smulders YM, Carballo D, Koskinas KC, Bäck M, et al. on behalf of the Task Force for Cardiovascular Disease Prevention in Clinical Practice with Representatives of the European Society of Cardiology and 12 Medical Societies. With the special contribution of the European Association of Preventive Cardiology (EAPC). 2021 ESC Guidelines on cardiovascular disease prevention in clinical practice. *Eur Heart J* 2021; doi:10.1093/eurheartj/ehab484.
29. De Backer GG. Risk scoring in primary prevention of atherosclerotic cardiovascular disease: strengths and limitations. Eur J Prev Cardiol. 2019;26(14):1531–33.
30. Hart L, Little A. Interpreting measures of risk: translating evidence into practice. Nurse Pract. 2017;42(2):50–55.
31. Studziński K, Tomasik T, Krzysztoń J, Jóźwiak J, Windak A. Effect of using cardiovascular risk scoring in routine risk assessment in primary prevention of cardiovascular disease: an overview of systematic reviews. BMC Cardiovasc Disord. 2019;19(1):11.
32. Braun LT. Cardiovascular disease: strategies for risk assessment and modification. J Cardiovasc Nurs. 2006;21(6):S20–42.
33. Bucholz EM, Gooding HC, de Ferranti SD. Awareness of cardiovascular risk factors in U.S. young adults aged 18–39 years. Am J Prev Med. 2018;54(4):e67–77.
34. Voogdt-Pruis HR, Beusmans GHMI, Gorgels APM, Kester ADM, Van Ree JW. Effectiveness of nurse-delivered cardiovascular risk management in primary care: a randomised trial. Br J Gen Pract. 2010;60(570):40–46.
35. Primdahl J, Ferreira RJO, Garcia-Diaz S, Ndosi M, Palmer D, van Eijk-Hustings Y. Nurses' role in cardiovascular risk assessment and management in people with inflammatory arthritis: a European perspective. Musculoskeletal Care. 2016;14(3):133–51.

36. Dawber TR, Meadors GF, Moore FE. Epidemiological approaches to heart disease: the Framingham Study. Am J Public Health. 1951;41(3):279–86.
37. Wood D, De Backer G, Faergeman O, Graham I, Mancia G, Pyörälä K. Prevention of coronary heart disease in clinical practice. Recommendations of the Second Joint Task Force of European and other Societies on Coronary Prevention. Eur Heart J. 1998;19(10):1434–503.
38. Conroy RM, Pyörälä K, Fitzgerald AP, Sans S, Menotti A, De Backer G, et al. Estimation of ten-year risk of fatal cardiovascular disease in Europe: the SCORE Project. Eur Heart J. 2003;24(11):987–1003.
39. Kaptoge S, Pennells L, De Bacquer D, Cooney MT, Kavousi M, Stevens G, et al. World Health Organization cardiovascular disease risk charts: revised models to estimate risk in 21 global regions. Lancet Glob Health. 2019;7(10):e1332–45.
40. Goff DC, Lloyd-Jones DM, Bennett G, Coady S, D'Agostino RB, Gibbons R, et al. 2013 ACC/AHA guideline on the assessment of cardiovascular risk: a report of the American College of Cardiology/American Heart Association task force on practice guidelines. Circulation. 2014;63(25 Part B):2935–59.
41. SCORE2 working group and ESC Cardiovascular risk collaboration. SCORE2 risk prediction algorithms: new models to estimate 10-year risk of cardiovascular disease in Europe. Eur Heart J 2021;42:2439_2454.
42. SCORE2-OP working group and ESC Cardiovascular risk collaboration. SCORE2-OP risk prediction algorithms: estimating incident cardiovascular event risk in older persons in four geographical risk regions. Eur Heart J 2021;42:2455_2467.
43. Wood D. Asymptomatic individuals–risk stratification in the prevention of coronary heart disease. Br Med Bull. 2001;59(1):3–16.
44. Menotti A, Lanti M, Puddu PE, Kromhout D. Coronary heart disease incidence in northern and southern European populations: a reanalysis of the seven countries study for a European coronary risk chart. Heart. 2000;84(3):238–44.
45. Hippisley-Cox J, Coupland C, Vinogradova Y, Robson J, May M, Brindle P. Derivation and validation of QRISK, a new cardiovascular disease risk score for the United Kingdom: prospective open cohort study. BMJ. 2007;335(7611):136.
46. Beswick A, Brindle P, Fahey T, Ebrahim. S. A Systematic Review of Risk Scoring Methods and Clinical Decision Aids Used in the Primary Prevention of Coronary Heart Disease. London: Royal College of General Practitioners; 2008.
47. Collins GS, Altman DG. An independent and external validation of QRISK2 cardiovascular disease risk score: a prospective open cohort study. BMJ. 2009;339:b2584.
48. Damen JA, Pajouheshnia R, Heus P, Moons KGM, Reitsma JB, Scholten RJPM, et al. Performance of the Framingham risk models and pooled cohort equations for predicting 10-year risk of cardiovascular disease: a systematic review and meta-analysis. BMC Med. 2019;17(1):109.
49. Marrugat J, Subirana I, Comín E, Cabezas C, Vila J, Elosua R, et al. Validity of an adaptation of the Framingham cardiovascular risk function: the VERIFICA study. J Epidemiol Community Health. 2007;61(1):40–47.
50. Pennells L, Kaptoge S, Wood A, Sweeting M, Zhao X, White I, et al. Equalization of four cardiovascular risk algorithms after systematic recalibration: individual-participant meta-analysis of 86 prospective studies. Eur Heart J. 2019;40(7):621–31.
51. Collins GS, De Groot JA, Dutton S, Omar O, Shanyinde M, Tajar A, et al. External validation of multivariable prediction models: a systematic review of methodological conduct and reporting. BMC Med Res Methodol. 2014;14(1):40.
52. Ban J-W, Stevens R, Perera R. Predictors for independent external validation of cardiovascular risk clinical prediction rules: Cox proportional hazards regression analyses. Diagnostic Progn Res. 2018;2(1):3.
53. Debray TPA, Vergouwe Y, Koffijberg H, Nieboer D, Steyerberg EW, Moons KGM. A new framework to enhance the interpretation of external validation studies of clinical prediction models. J Clin Epidemiol. 2015;68(3):279–89.
54. Rahman MS, Ambler G, Choodari-Oskooei B, Omar RZ. Review and evaluation of performance measures for survival prediction models in external validation settings. BMC Med Res Methodol. 2017;17(1):60.
55. Mossakowska TJ, Saunders CL, Corbett J, MacLure C, Winpenny EM, Dujso E, et al. Current and future cardiovascular disease risk assessment in the European Union: an international comparative study. Eur J Public Health. 2018;28(4):748–54.
56. Cooney MT, Dudina AL, Graham IM. Value and limitations of existing scores for the assessment of cardiovascular risk: a review for clinicians. J Am Coll Cardiol. 2009;54(14):1209–27.
57. Georgiev B, Gothchev N, Trendafilova E, Baytcheva V, Gotchev D. Changes over time in cardiovascular risk profile of high-risk individuals. J Hypertens. 2017;35:e273.
58. Lee JJ, Pedley A, Hoffmann U, Massaro JM, Fox CS. Association of changes in abdominal fat quantity and quality with incident cardiovascular disease risk factors. J Am Coll Cardiol. 2016;68(14):1509–21.
59. Niiranen TJ, Vasan RS. Epidemiology of cardiovascular disease: recent novel outlooks on risk factors and clinical approaches. Expert Rev Cardiovasc Ther. 2016;14(7):855–69.
60. Arps K, Blumenthal RS, Martin SS. New aspects of the risk assessment guidelines: practical highlights, scientific evidence and future goals. American College of Cardiology. 2018. https://www.acc.org/

latest-in-cardiology/articles/2018/11/14/07/10/new-aspects-of-the-risk-assessment-guidelines.
61. Knowles JW, Ashley EA. Cardiovascular disease: the rise of the genetic risk score. PLoS Med. 2018;15(3):e1002546.
62. Lin JS, Evans CV, Johnson E, Redmond N, Coppola EL, Smith N. Nontraditional risk factors in cardiovascular disease risk assessment: updated evidence report and systematic review for the US preventive services task force. JAMA. 2018;320(3):281–97.
63. Pencina MJ, Steyerberg EW, D'Agostino RB. Net reclassification index at event rate: properties and relationships. Stat Med. 2017;36(28):4455–67.
64. Moonesinghe R, Yang Q, Zhang Z, Khoury MJ. Prevalence and cardiovascular health impact of family history of premature heart disease in the United States: analysis of the National Health and Nutrition Examination Survey, 2007–2014. J Am Heart Assoc. 2019;8(14):e012364.
65. Lobelo F, Rohm Young D, Sallis R, Garber MD, Billinger SA, Duperly J, et al. Routine assessment and promotion of physical activity in healthcare settings: a scientific statement from the American Heart Association. Circulation. 2018;137(18):e495–522.
66. Kengne AP. The ADVANCE cardiovascular risk model and current strategies for cardiovascular disease risk evaluation in people with diabetes. Cardiovasc J Afr. 2013;24(9–10):376–81.
67. Berkelmans GFN, Gudbjörnsdottir S, Visseren FLJ, Wild SH, Franzen S, Chalmers J, et al. Prediction of individual life-years gained without cardiovascular events from lipid, blood pressure, glucose, and aspirin treatment based on data of more than 500 000 patients with type 2 diabetes mellitus. Eur Heart J. 2019;40(34):2899–906.
68. Dorresteijn JAN, Visseren FLJ, Wassink AMJ, Gondrie MJA, Steyerberg EW, Ridker PM, et al. Development and validation of a prediction rule for recurrent vascular events based on a cohort study of patients with arterial disease: the SMART risk score. Heart. 2013;99(12):866–72.
69. Kaasenbrood L, Bhatt DL, Dorresteijn JAN, Wilson PWF, D'Agostino RB, Massaro JM, et al. Estimated life expectancy without recurrent cardiovascular events in patients with vascular disease: the SMART-REACH model. J Am Heart Assoc. 2018;7(16):e009217.
70. Rajan R, Al Jarallah M. New prognostic risk calculator for heart failure. Oman Med J. 2018;33(3):266.
71. Levy WC, Mozaffarian D, Linker DT, Sutradhar SC, Anker SD, Cropp AB, et al. The Seattle Heart Failure Model: prediction of survival in heart failure. Circulation. 2006;113(11):1424–33.
72. De Bacquer D, Ueda P, Reiner Z, De Sutter J, De Smedt D, Lovic D, et al. Prediction of recurrent event in patients with coronary heart disease: the EUROASPIRE Risk Model. EurJ Prev Cardiol 2020;. doi: 10.1093/eurjpc/zwaa128.
73. Gansevoort RT, Correa-Rotter R, Hemmelgarn BR, Jafar TH, Heerspink HJL, Mann JF, et al. Chronic kidney disease and cardiovascular risk: epidemiology, mechanisms, and prevention. Lancet. 2013;382(9889):339–52.
74. Coviello JS. Cardiovascular and cancer risk: the role of cardio-oncology. J Adv Pract Oncol. 2018;9(2):160–76.
75. Zamorano JL, Lancellotti P, Rodriguez Muñoz D, Aboyans V, Asteggiano R, Galderisi M, et al. 2016 ESC Position Paper on cancer treatments and cardiovascular toxicity developed under the auspices of the ESC Committee for Practice Guidelines. Eur Heart J. 2016;37(36):2768–801.
76. Gulati M, Mulvagh SL. The connection between the breast and heart in a woman: breast cancer and cardiovascular disease. Clin Cardiol. 2018;41(2):253–57.
77. Fontela C, Castilla J, Juanbeltz R, Martínez-Baz I, Rivero M, O'Leary A, et al. Comorbidities and cardiovascular risk factors in an aged cohort of HIV-infected patients on antiretroviral treatment in a Spanish hospital in 2016. Postgrad Med. 2018;130(3):317–24.
78. Rao SG, Galaviz KI, Gay HC, Wei J, Armstrong WS, Del Rio C, et al. Factors associated with excess myocardial infarction risk in HIV-infected adults: a systematic review and meta-analysis. J Acquir Immune Defic Syndr. 2019;81(2):224–30.
79. Expert Panel on Integrated Guidelines for Cardiovascular Health and Risk Reduction in Children and Adolescents. Expert Panel on Integrated Guidelines for Cardiovascular Health and Risk Reduction in Children and Adolescents: summary report. Pediatrics. 2011;128(Suppl 5):S213.
80. Berenson GS, Srinivasan SR, Bao W, Newman WP, Tracy RE, Wattigney WA. Association between multiple cardiovascular risk factors and atherosclerosis in children and young adults. N Engl J Med. 1998;338(23):1650–56.
81. McGill HC, McMahan CA, Zieske AW, Sloop GD, Walcott JV, Troxclair DA, et al. Associations of coronary heart disease risk factors with the intermediate lesion of atherosclerosis in youth. The Pathobiological Determinants of Atherosclerosis in Youth (PDAY) Research Group. Arterioscler Thromb Vasc Biol. 2000;20(8):1998–2004.
82. Bao W, Srinivasan SR, Wattigney WA, Bao W, Berenson GS. Usefulness of childhood low-density lipoprotein cholesterol level in predicting adult dyslipidemia and other cardiovascular risks: the Bogalusa Heart Study. Arch Intern Med. 1996;156(12):1315–20.
83. Chen X, Wang Y. Tracking of blood pressure from childhood to adulthood: a systematic review and meta-regression analysis. Circulation. 2008;117(25):3171–80.

84. Juhola J, Magnussen CG, Viikari JSA, Kähönen M, Hutri-Kähönen N, Jula A, et al. Tracking of serum lipid levels, blood pressure, and body mass index from childhood to adulthood: the Cardiovascular Risk in Young Finns Study. J Pediatr. 2011;159(4):584–90.
85. Raitakari OT, Juonala M, Kähönen M, Taittonen L, Laitinen T, Mäki-Torkko N, et al. Cardiovascular risk factors in childhood and carotid artery intima-media thickness in adulthood: the Cardiovascular Risk in Young Finns Study. JAMA. 2003;290(17):2277–83.
86. Aatola H, Koivistoinen T, Hutri-Kähönen N, Juonala M, Mikkilä V, Lehtimäki T, et al. Lifetime fruit and vegetable consumption and arterial pulse wave velocity in adulthood: the Cardiovascular Risk in Young Finns Study. Circulation. 2010;122(24):2521–28.
87. Chen W, Srinivasan SR, Li S, Xu J, Berenson GS. Metabolic syndrome variables at low levels in childhood are beneficially associated with adulthood cardiovascular risk: the Bogalusa Heart Study. Diabetes Care. 2005;28(1):126–31.
88. Laitinen T, Pahkala K, Magnussen CG, Viikari JSA, Oikonen M, Taittonen L, et al. Ideal cardiovascular health in childhood and cardiometabolic outcomes in adulthood: the Cardiovascular Risk in Young Finns Study. Circulation. 2012;125(16):1971–78.
89. Shay CM, Ning H, Daniels SR, Rooks CR, Gidding SS, Lloyd-Jones DM. Status of cardiovascular health in US adolescents: prevalence estimates from the National Health and Nutrition Examination Surveys (NHANES) 2005–2010. Circulation. 2013;127(13):1369–76.
90. Currie C, Nic Gabhainn S, Godeau E, Samdal O, Ravens-Sieberer U, Morgan A, et al. The health behaviour in school-aged children: WHO collaborative cross-national (HBSC) study: origins, concept, history and development 1982–2008. Int J Public Health. 2009;54(2):131–39.
91. Inchley J, Currie D, Young T, Samdal O, Torsheim T, Augustson L, et al. Growing Up Unequal: Gender and Socioeconomic Differences in Young People's Health and Well-Being. Health Behaviour in School-Aged Children (HBSC) Study: International Report from the 2013/2014 Survey (Health Policy For Children And Adolescents, No. 7). Copenhagen: World Health Organization; 2016.
92. Ng M, Fleming T, Robinson M, Thomson B, Graetz N, Margono C, et al. Global, regional, and national prevalence of overweight and obesity in children and adults during 1980–2013: a systematic analysis for the Global Burden of Disease Study 2013. Lancet. 2014;384(9945):766–81.
93. World Health Organization. Health statistics and information systems. http://www.who.int/healthinfo.
94. Henriksson P, Henriksson H, Gracia-Marco L, Labayen I, Ortega FB, Huybrechts I, et al. Prevalence of ideal cardiovascular health in European adolescents: the HELENA study. Int J Cardiol. 2017;240:428–32.
95. Weinberg D, Stevens GWJM, Bucksch J, Inchley J, De Looze M. Do country-level environmental factors explain cross-national variation in adolescent physical activity? A multilevel study in 29 European countries. BMC Public Health. 2019;19(1):680.
96. Kumanyika SK, Obarzanek E, Stettler N, Bell R, Field AE, Fortmann SP, et al. Population-based prevention of obesity: the need for comprehensive promotion of healthful eating, physical activity, and energy balance: a scientific statement from American Heart Association Council on Epidemiology and Prevention, Interdisciplinary Commi. Circulation. 2008;118(4):428–64.
97. Hayman LL, Helden L, Chyun DA, Braun LT. A life course approach to cardiovascular disease prevention. Eur J Cardiovasc Nurs. 2011;26(4):S22–34.
98. World Health Organization. Investing in Children: The European Child and Adolescent Health Strategy, 2015–2020. Copenhagen: WHO European Region; 2014.
99. Weintraub WS, Daniels SR, Burke LE, Franklin BA, Goff DC, Hayman LL, et al. Value of primordial and primary prevention for cardiovascular disease: a policy statement from the American Heart Association. Circulation. 2011;124(6):967–90.
100. World Health Organization. WHO European Physical Activity Strategy for 2016–2025. Copenhagen: WHO European Region; 2015.
101. Cuende JI. Vascular age versus cardiovascular risk: clarifying concepts. Rev Esp Cardiol. 2016;69(3):243–46.
102. Berry JD, Dyer A, Cai X, Garside DB, Ning H, Thomas A, et al. Lifetime risks of cardiovascular disease. N Engl J Med. 2012;366(4):321–29.
103. Lloyd-Jones DM, Leip EP, Larson MG, D'Agostino RB, Beiser A, Wilson PWF, et al. Prediction of lifetime risk for cardiovascular disease by risk factor burden at 50 years of age. Circulation. 2006;113(6):791–98.
104. Pencina MJ, D'Agostino RB, Larson MG, Massaro JM, Vasan RS. Predicting the 30-year risk of cardiovascular disease: the Framingham Heart Study. Circulation. 2009;119(24):3078–84.
105. Qureshi AI, Fareed M, Suri K, Guterman LR, Hopkins LN. Cocaine use and the likelihood of nonfatal myocardial infarction and stroke: data from the Third National Health and Nutrition Examination Survey. Circulation. 2001;103(4):502–506.
106. Qureshi AL, Chaudhry SA, Suri MF. Cocaine use and the likelihood of cardiovascular and all-cause mortality: data from the Third National Health and Nutrition Examination Survey Mortality Follow-up Study. J Vasc Interv Neurol. 2014;7(1):76–82.

107. Kim ST, Park T. Acute and chronic effects of cocaine on cardiovascular health. Int J Mol Sci. 2019;20(3):584.
108. Chiu M, Maclagan LC, Tu JV, Shah BR. Temporal trends in cardiovascular disease risk factors among white, South Asian, Chinese and black groups in Ontario, Canada, 2001 to 2012: a population-based study. BMJ Open. 2015;5(8):e007232.
109. Eurostat European Commission. Migration and migrant population statistics. Ago. 2019. https://ec.europa.eu/eurostat/statistics-explained.
110. Gupta P, Gan ATL, Man REK, Fenwick EK, Tham YC, Sabanayagam C, et al. Risk of incident cardiovascular disease and cardiovascular risk factors in first and second-generation Indians: the Singapore Indian Eye Study. Sci Rep. 2018;8(1):14805.
111. Perini W, Snijder MB, Peters RJG, Kunst AE. Ethnic disparities in estimated cardiovascular disease risk in Amsterdam, the Netherlands: the HELIUS study. Netherlands Heart J. 2018;26(5):252–62.
112. Lê-Scherban F, Albrecht SS, Bertoni A, Kandula N, Mehta N, Diez Roux AV. Immigrant status and cardiovascular risk over time: results from the Multi-Ethnic Study of Atherosclerosis. Ann Epidemiol. 2016;26(6):429–35.
113. Lloyd-Jones DM, Braun LT, Ndumele CE, Smith SC, Sperling LS, Virani SS, et al. Use of risk assessment tools to guide decision-making in the primary prevention of atherosclerotic cardiovascular disease: a special report from the American Heart Association and American College of Cardiology. Circulation. 2019;139(25):e1162–77.
114. Rana JS, Tabada GH, Solomon MD, Lo JC, Jaffe MG, Sung SH, et al. Accuracy of the atherosclerotic cardiovascular risk equation in a large contemporary, multiethnic population. J Am Coll Cardiol. 2016;67(18):2118–30.
115. European Society of Cardiology. Strategic plan 2016–2020. 2016. https://www.escardio.org/static_file/Escardio/Web/About/Documents/ESC-Strategic-plan-2016-2020.pdf.
116. Zhao M, Cooney MT, Klipstein-Grobusch K, Vaartjes I, De Bacquer D, De Sutter J, et al. Simplifying the audit of risk factor recording and control: a report from an international study in 11 countries. Eur J Prev Cardiol. 2016;23(11):1202–10.
117. PCNA. Global Cardiovascular Nursing Leadership Forum. https://gcnlf.pcna.net/.
118. Kotseva K, De Bacquer D, De Backer G, Rydén L, Jennings C, Gyberg V, et al. Lifestyle and risk factor management in people at high risk of cardiovascular disease. A report from the European Society of Cardiology European Action on Secondary and Primary Prevention by Intervention to Reduce Events (EUROASPIRE) IV cross-sectional survey in 14 European regions. Eur J Prev Cardiol. 2016;23(18):2007–18.
119. Strasser T. Reflections on cardiovascular diseases. Interdiscip Sci Rev. 1978;3(3):225–30.
120. Rose G. Sick individuals and sick populations. Int J Epidemiol. 1985;14(1):32–38.
121. Sniderman AD, Thanassoulis G, Wilkins JT, Furberg CD, Pencina M. Sick individuals and sick populations by Geoffrey Rose: cardiovascular prevention updated. J Am Heart Assoc. 2018;7(19):e010049.
122. World Heart Federation. World Heart Federation roadmap for heart failure. 2016. https://www.world-heart-federation.org/cvd-roadmap.

2 Delivering high-quality cardiovascular care

LIS NEUBECK, MARÍA TERESA LIRA, ERCOLE VELLONE, DONNA FITZSIMONS, LISA DULLAGHAN, AND JULIE SANDERS

CHAPTER CONTENTS

KEY MESSAGES

- High-quality care should be safe, effective, timely, equitable, efficient, and people-centred.
- Nurses need to understand the fundamentals of high-quality professional practice.
- The use of patient-reported outcome measures and patient-reported experience measures helps to bring the patient voice into high-quality care.
- Measurement and audit are important tools to determine the quality of care.
- It is imperative that nurses develop cultural competence.
- Understanding the barriers to high-quality care can help to overcome them to ensure that patient well-being is preserved.

Definition and elements of high quality of care

The World Health Organization (WHO) considers the delivery of high-quality care to be a global imperative in the drive to achieve universal health coverage.[1] Several elements have been defined as core elements or domains of high-quality care. One of the first definitions was proposed by the Institute of Medicine in 2001,[2] including six domains: safe, effective, timely, efficient, equitable, and people-centred (➤ Table 2.1). The WHO recommends that healthcare workers embrace a teamwork philosophy, participate in quality measurement of patients' desired outcomes using data to demonstrate effectiveness and safety, and consider patients and/or communities as partners in the effective care process.[1]

Table 2.1 Core elements of high quality of care

Safe	Minimizes harm due to errors and preventable injuries
Effective	Based on the best evidenced scientific knowledge available
Timely	Coordinates a comprehensive flowchart of care to avoid delays
Equitable	Provides care independently of personal characteristics (i.e. ethnicity)
Efficient	Avoids waste of time, resources, or duplication of tests (lack registers)
People-centred	Works in partnership taking into account values, needs, and preferences

Source data from Institute of Medicine. 2001. Crossing the Quality Chasm: A New Health System for the 21st Century. Washington, DC: The National Academies Press. https://doi.org/10.17226/10027.

These components are widely shared by multiple organizations and have become the framework for the description and regulation of high-quality professional practice of nursing,[3] as well as for the definition of quality care metrics or instruments to measure clinical care and outcomes worldwide.[4]

Fundamentals of high-quality professional practice

Within every profession, the ultimate goal is to deliver a high-quality professional service, measured by metrics agreed by consensus, and frequently monitored by a professional body that has responsibility for ensuring practice meets standards. In the nursing profession, practice excellence has been defined as a 'dynamic process that integrates the best theoretical and practice knowledge (praxis) in each [patient/] client encounter'.[5] This incorporates elements of professionalism, best practice, and humanistic holistic care throughout the life-course continuum by developing meaningful relationships with patients and the health team.[6] These characteristics, in combination with values and attitudes such as honesty, empathy, initiative, curiosity, and innovation, are crucial to achieve a high quality of care,[7,8] especially in non-communicable diseases such as cardiovascular disease.[9]

Nursing workforce

Nurses constitute the largest group of health workforce members worldwide. Consequently, they have a central role in delivering high-quality care across the continuum, improving individual, family, and community health.[10] It was noted by the Joint Commission on Accreditation of Healthcare Organizations, that nearly every person's lifetime healthcare experience involves the contribution of nurses,[11] and this is particularly true in cardiovascular healthcare, which ranges from primordial prevention in infancy through to debilitating and life-limiting conditions, such as heart failure, and to palliative care. Nursing has been identified as a critical factor in determining the quality of care patients receive.[12] Nurses play a role in hospital with cardiovascular patients, monitoring to detect clinical changes or possible errors, avoiding failure to rescue, and performing multiple tasks which have positioned nurses at the front lines of quality improvement (QI).[4] Nurses are important providers of outpatient services such as cardiovascular prevention and rehabilitation, heart failure, and arrhythmia specialist services, and act as a safety net to support patients living independently.

Core elements of high-quality care in professional practice

Care must be safe

Safety is a critical issue for contemporary healthcare, and many consider that safety is an inextricable component for delivery of quality care.[13] It is a key component of the fundamentals of care.[13] Failures or gaps in basic or fundamental aspects of care not only cause distress and dissatisfaction but have been identified as threats with significant risks for patients. It is imperative to consider both unsafe practice, which in itself harms the patients,[13] but also the failure to act. The harm attached to *care left undone* has been highlighted as a significant problem in contemporary nursing.[14] The delivery of care that is safe, patient-centred, compassionate, effective, and efficient is the responsibility of all healthcare professionals.[15] However, of all members of the healthcare team, nurses have been identified as critically important in ensuring patient safety, making a key contribution through their ability to coordinate and integrate the multiple aspects of quality care.[15]

Safety is influenced by other factors that are also components of quality care such as leadership, evidence-based practice, evidence-based nurse-sensitive outcomes measures, teamwork composition, and collaborative work. There are other challenges that directly affect patient safety such as nurse staffing ratios, high staff turnover, and poor working conditions. An inadequate nursing staff ratio also compromises the safety of nurses as well, with a two- to threefold increased risk of needlestick injuries occurring when staff levels are reduced.[16] When there is an adequate skill mix of staff with a higher number of registered nurses, there are fewer adverse events including complications after abdominal aortic surgery and lower infection rates in paediatric cardiac intensive care.[16] A systematic review of nurse staffing found better patient–nurse ratios were associated with a decrease in the risk of in-hospital mortality (odds ratio 0.86, 95% confidence interval 0.79–0.94) and nurse-sensitive outcomes.[17] Individual nurses' satisfaction with their role and competencies (i.e. knowledge, skills, and attitudes) can also affect patient safety.[16] Patients also have higher levels of satisfaction with their care when it is perceived to be safe.[18] Some aspects of safe cardiovascular care are related to those common to non-communicable diseases, for example, minimizing risk of complications or re-hospitalization, dealing with low adherence or errors in medication, close monitoring in acute phases, and educating patients with special devices.[19]

Care must be effective and evidence based

Evidence-based practice is essential to provide the highest quality care, while controlling healthcare costs.[20] Evidence-based protocols enable standard high-quality care across different health systems globally.[1] Evidence-based nursing for patients with cardiovascular disease has been developing for more than a decade,[21] integrating robust evidence in clinical guidelines for the prevention and treatment of cardiovascular disease and leading the implementation of cardiovascular nursing interventions to enable collection of outcomes data in a standardized way.[21] Critical decision-making for clinical practice is inherent in the role of the professional nurse, and it relies on both clinical expertise, and the best possible evidence, usually collated in guidelines or recommendations.[16]

Implementation of evidence-based practice is linked to a higher education preparedness of nurses (e.g. degree-prepared) and the expansion of scope of practice to the full range of nursing competencies.[22] It has been demonstrated that higher advanced and/or specialist nursing qualifications as well as master's degrees in research and doctoral and postdoctoral programmes have a crucial role in developing nursing skills, such as research leadership.[10]

In an evidence-based healthcare environment, nurses need to be able to utilize and generate robust evidence.[23] To assess nurse effectiveness, nursing-sensitive indicators are mandatory in creating the evidence around what clinical interventions are most effective.[10] The main challenges to develop evidence-based nursing practice are a lack of agreement on the elements of care and the type and quality of nursing research. Systematic reviews have highlighted that nursing research literature remains descriptive, with a low impact on practising nurses, making them difficult to interpret and follow clear evidence-based clinical practice.[14] Also, there is a lack of evidence of patient-related outcomes (PROs) collected directly from patients themselves, and sparse poor-quality evidence for fundamental nursing care interventions, with studies that did not define primary outcomes, used inappropriate metrics, or conducted analysis with significant risk of bias.[14]

The absence of standardized definitions among the healthcare system leaders (managers, policymakers) and professionals (researchers, clinicians, educators, etc.) lead to differences in parameters and variables that affect measurement and aggregation of data to develop robust evidence.[24] However, several efforts have been made to generate standardized quality metrics to build an evidence base and knowledge, including in cardiovascular care. Nursing research aims to address a paradigm between medical science and clinical need, and social sciences.[25] Consequently, nursing evidence tends to take a more holistic vision of human health.

Providing high-quality care that is informed by the latest evidence

Recent decades have witnessed a complete transformation in terms of how cardiovascular care is delivered, with new advances in technology, drug treatments, and interventional techniques revolutionizing patient care and improving treatment outcomes. During that time, those practising within the speciality have been kept updated by a process of continuous professional development that is now recognized as necessary for all professionals. The fundamental premise underpinning this innovation is that high-quality patient care requires practitioners who are up to date with the latest evidence and are skilled in acquiring, evaluating, and applying this within a patient- and family-centred context.[26] For nurses and allied professionals, this has meant developing new skills in evidence-informed practice that are now a cornerstone of our professional knowledge base.

What are evidence-based care and evidence-informed care?

There are currently ever-increasing amounts of data and evidence available within the healthcare arena. The challenge for those working within cardiovascular care is to determine the validity of these data and evaluate their relevance to our practice setting. Traditionally, as healthcare practitioners, evidence is available from a variety of different sources and each has its own utility. When assessing a patient who is presenting with chest pain, for example, it is important to communicate effectively to reassure the patient and explain the process of making a differential diagnosis. The nurse will ask a series of questions regarding the nature, severity, and implications of the patient's pain to help elucidate whether it is cardiac in origin; while at the same time checking the patient's vital signs, electrocardiogram, and high-sensitivity troponin. Data from each of these qualitative and quantitative sources will be assimilated and each play their part in arriving at a more definitive conclusion. It is to be expected then that nursing science embraces data from both qualitative and quantitative perspectives, triangulating them to provide a more holistic understanding of the patient experience (see also Chapter 5).

In 2019, the WHO distinguished between evidence-based practice and evidence-informed practice on the basis that the latter includes clinical judgement, which is somewhat open to interpretation.[27] The JBI (formerly Joanna Briggs Institute) Model of Evidence-Based Healthcare offers a more comprehensive and globally applicable theory of how knowledge is generated and translated into practice and policy change (➤ **Fig. 2.1**).

Within the European Society of Cardiology (ESC), it is recognized that there is a need to arrive at an expert consensus on the available evidence and provide clear guidance for practitioners. In order to achieve this, the ESC has produced Clinical Practice Guidelines across many specific cardiovascular conditions and also provides regular updates on these to ensure the latest contemporary guidance is available.

How do we source the latest evidence?

Despite engaging in regular educational activities and professional development, it is difficult to keep on top of the very latest evidence within cardiovascular care. There are a wide variety of strategies that can be used to help in this endeavour, which can be accessed through membership of the Association of Cardiovascular Nursing and Allied Professions (ACNAP) (https://www.escardio.org/Sub-specialty-communities/Association-of-Cardiovascular-Nursing-&-Allied-Professions), including the *European Journal of Cardiovascular Nursing*, the clinical case gallery, ACNAP essentials4U, the annual congress, and a range of other research and evidence-based resources. There are also many useful research databases such as PubMed, MEDLINE, the Cochrane Library, and CINHAL that can be searched using keywords to identify the latest evidence in cardiovascular care.

What is the role of the ESC Guidelines?

The field of cardiovascular care has evolved at an unprecedented rate over recent decades with huge advances in diagnostics, interventional techniques, pharmacotherapy, and the evidence underpinning lifestyle change. It is never easy to weigh up the risks and benefits of particular treatment strategies and apply these to the specific preferences of an individual patient and/or their family members. In order to keep abreast of the most recent data, practitioners frequently turn to Clinical Practice Guidelines produced by the ESC. These Guidelines have been produced by the ESC since the mid-1990s and they represent one of the premier educational products of the Society. In order to develop consensus on the latest trials and research that is undertaken on an international basis, the ESC charges a group of recognized experts on specific topics to constitute a Task Force. Great care is taken to ensure the diversity and independence of this team that is usually led by two chairpersons. Every year these Task Forces of the ESC produce four or five Guidelines and a range of Position Papers and Consensus Documents. Each one takes a minimum of 2 years to develop and represents the ESC perspective on the best available evidence on which to inform the clinical practice of doctors, nurses, and allied professionals.

All of this work is governed by the Clinical Practice Guidelines Committee of the ESC which meets regularly to discuss priorities and implement strategies that maintain the highest levels of integrity and quality assurance within the ESC Guidelines. In the past decade, there has always been an ACNAP representative on this Committee

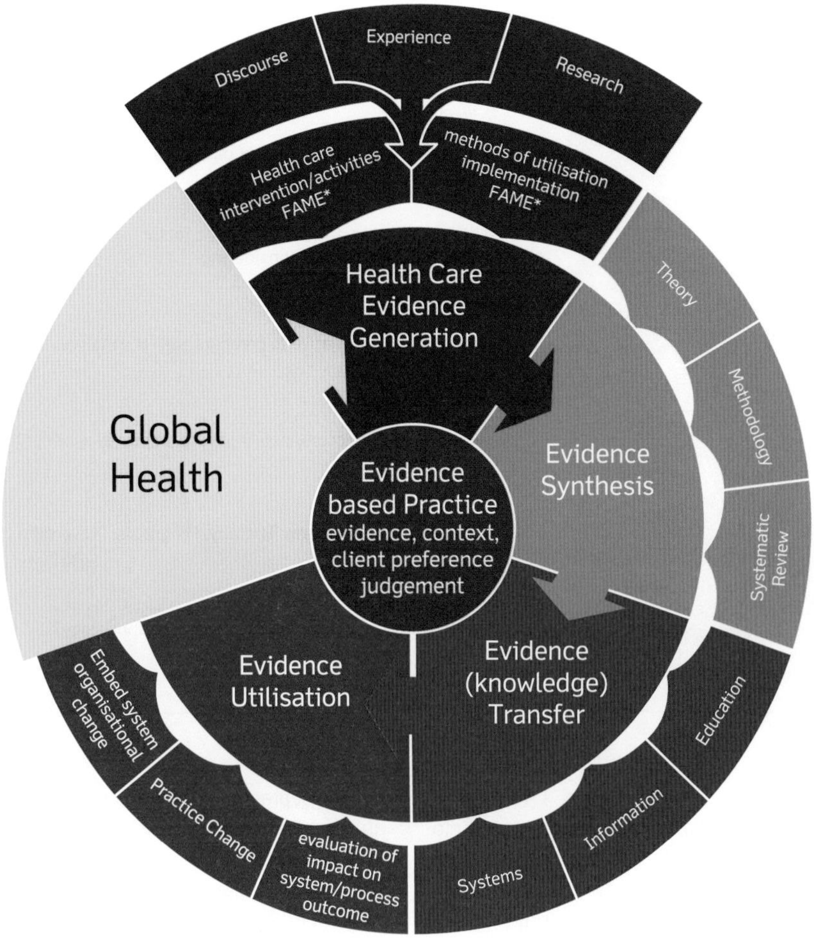

Fig. 2.1 The JBI Model of Evidence-Based Healthcare.

Reproduced from Jordan Z, Lockwood C, Munn Z, Aromataris E. The updated Joanna Briggs Institute Model of Evidence-Based Healthcare. Int J Evid Based Healthc. 2019 Mar;17(1):58–71. doi: 10.1097/XEB.0000000000000155 with permission from Wolters Kluwer.

to ensure the transfer of this important source of evidence into the professional domain of those practitioners who enjoy the majority of patient contact. As a result, it becomes the responsibility of nurses and allied professionals to familiarize themselves with this scientific content and develop strategies by which they can optimize its translation into practice. Given the diversity of educational preparation, roles, responsibilities, and autonomy that nurses and allied professions receive throughout Europe, it is a challenging objective and ACNAP is there to support members to navigate this.

The first stage in this journey is to develop an inquiring mind, that is clearly focused on one question:

Is this the best care, intervention, therapy, or procedure that we can offer this person (patient) to optimize his or her treatment experience and outcome?

What a simple question—but one that frequently has a very complicated answer! The 'PICOTS' model is frequently used to help refine the question you are asking (➤ Table 2.2).

To begin with, it is naïve to assume that within all the various healthcare infrastructures that exist throughout Europe nurses and allied professionals have the insight, courage, or autonomy to question traditional practice in this way, to challenge the status quo, and to advocate on behalf of the patient. This has been well recognized

Table 2.2 The PICO model for clinical questions

P	**P**atient, **P**opulation, or **P**roblem	How would I describe a group of patients similar to mine?
I	**I**ntervention, Prognostic Factor, or Exposure	Which main intervention, prognostic factor, or exposure am I considering?
C	**C**omparison or Intervention (if appropriate)	What is the main alternative to compare with the intervention?
O	**O**utcome you would like to measure or achieve	What can I hope to accomplish, measure, improve, or affect?
T	What **T**ype of question are you asking?	Diagmosis, Aetiology/Harm, Therapy, Prognosis, Prevention
S	What type of **S**tudy do you want to find	What would be the best study design/methodology?

within the Be Guideline Smart Initiative. Over recent years, ACNAP has developed a range of resources to help support nurses and allied professionals to become more effective in implementing evidence-informed care. These are available on the ESC ACNAP webpage (https://www.escardio.org/Sub-specialty-communities/Association-of-Cardiovascular-Nursing-&-Allied-Professions) and are updated regularly. They have been developed and supported by the National Societies of the ESC in conjunction with our industry partners. We would advise you to browse the various sources of information and support that exist online in order to update yourself with contemporary practice and work with your local colleagues and team members to enable their more widespread dissemination into practice.

How do we evaluate evidence?

There is a plethora of unreliable data available within the cardiovascular arena, some of which reach the status of 'fake news', but it is sometimes challenging to recognize it as such for professionals and patients alike. There are a wide range of critical appraisal tools available to help practitioners evaluate evidence and make informed decisions. The next critical element is having the skills to evaluate the quality of evidence before making changes to clinical practice. There are many methods of evaluating quality available to practitioners such as CASP, the Critical Appraisal Skills Programme (http://casp-uk.net/). These usually offer a checklist or series, but beyond this, it is important to understand if the research design was appropriate to the research question, if the data were collected appropriately, and if there are any potential issues of bias. Quantitative data should be robust, reproducible, and generalizable. Qualitative data should be trustworthy and authentic. Nurses need to understand that not all research is of the same calibre. To address this, the ESC uses classes of recommendations and levels of evidence to identify the strength of the evidence (➤ **Fig. 2.2**).

Care must be timely

Access to care at the right time is critical to ensure that cardiovascular conditions are well managed. In the acute setting, access to primary percutaneous intervention, or where that is not available, thrombolysis, can reduce the likelihood of myocardial damage, and therefore of subsequent heart failure or death (see Chapter 5 and Chapter 6 for tools to deliver timely care in emergency situations). Timely care is also important in ensuring patients have access to medications. Heart failure nurses

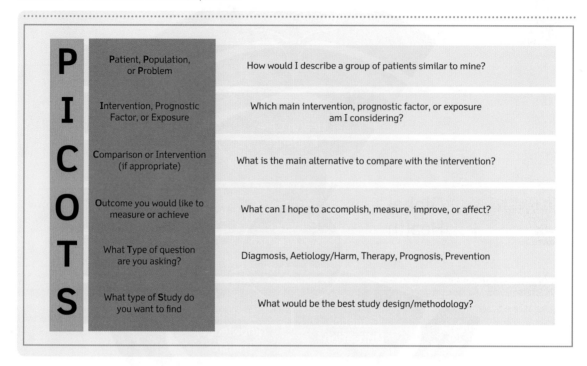

Classes of recommendations		
Classes of recommendations	**Definition**	**Suggested wording to use**
Class I	Evidence and or general agreement that a given treatment or procedure is beneficial, useful, effective	Is recommended/is indicated
Class II	Conflicting evidence and/or a divergence of opinion about the usefulness/efficacy of the procedure	
Class IIa	Weight of evidence/opinion is in favour of usefulness/efficacy	Should be considered
Class IIb	Usefulness/efficacy is less well-established by evidence/opinion	May be considered
Class III	Evidence or general agreement that the given treatment or procedures not useful/effective, and in some cases may be harmful	is not recommended

Level of evidence	
Level of evidence A	Data derived from multiple randomised clinical trials or meta-analysis
Level of evidence B	Data derived from single randomised clinical trials or large non-randomised trials
Level of evidence C	Consensus of opinion of the experts and/or small studies, retrospective studies, registries

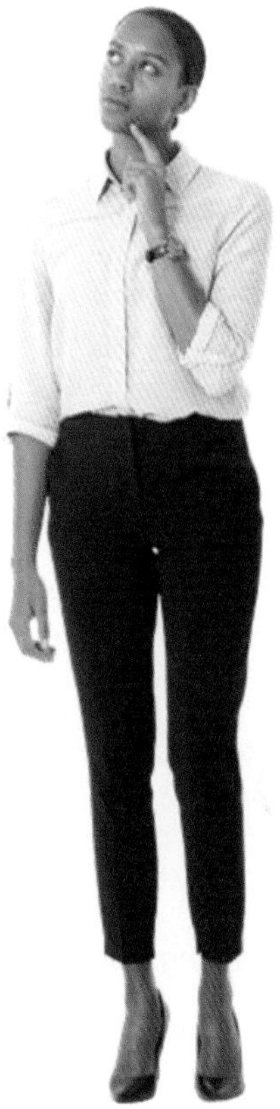

Fig. 2.2 Definitions of the ESC levels of evidence and classes of recommendation.

play a critical role in identifying early signs of worsening heart failure, and this has been demonstrated to prevent hospitalizations and death. Delays in treatment are also likely to raise anxiety, which has a strong relationship with adverse outcomes in cardiovascular patients. Cardiovascular prevention and rehabilitation attendance is known to decrease with any delays of recruitment to the service.[28]

Care must be equitable

Globalization and migration have generated a significant increase in ethnic, cultural, and linguistic diversity in many countries, challenging health services and providers to be able to respond accordingly. Understanding and addressing health needs requires cultural competence and is recognized as a major strategy to address health inequities and identified as a core requirement for effective patient-centred care. Therefore, nurses must recognize their crucial role in reducing inequalities.

Cultural competence is multifaceted and includes the ability to work and communicate effectively and appropriately with people from culturally diverse backgrounds. Furthermore, culturally competent systems are able to meet diverse social, cultural, and linguistic needs. Cultural competence components have not yet been fully defined. Cultural awareness, cultural knowledge, and cultural skills/behaviour have been recognized as key aspects as they have the greatest impact in health context. These components are relevant in the ability to communicate, perform physical assessments, and collect health data from culturally/ethnically diverse patients.

According to the US National Center for Cultural Competence, racial and ethnic minorities are disproportionately burdened by chronic illness and cardiovascular health disparities have been well documented, and continue to be a main concern. The goal of cultural competence education for health professionals is to achieve equitable, effective healthcare including diverse populations and has been highlighted as a core competency for leadership in cardiovascular nursing. Several groups have discussed and proposed universal standards of cultural competences for nurses, not only to guide clinical practice but also research, education, and administration, including the definition of culturally competent outcomes. Patient satisfaction, trust, health status, and adherence to treatment have been tested in proposed models but still further development is needed, becoming an important challenge for nursing, considering also that social expectations of nursing vary significantly from country to country.

Care must be efficient

Determining if healthcare is efficient is often viewed in terms of financial costs to the healthcare provider. Of course, the economic cost is important. However, to truly determine if healthcare is efficient, a range of measures need to be taken into account. Much of the literature focuses on how to evaluate efficiency, and there are a range of tools that can be used to do this. However, efficient care links closely to quality indicators.

Measuring quality

Unless the quality and safety of care is audited, improvements cannot be determined.[25] The WHO states that 'a core set of quality indicators is critically important for judging whether activities are producing higher quality of care leading to significant change in health outcomes'.[1] There are several definitions of an indicator, most of them agree that they should be measurable, valid, reliable, specific, related to performance or outcomes, enable comparisons (across populations, healthcare sectors, geographic locations), and should be established by consensus.[25] Standardized data sets promote transparency, provide feedback, and support clinical, administrative, and health policy decision-making. Therefore, definitions are crucial to operationalize concepts, set variables and parameters, and define or develop measurement tools.[10] Nursing metrics have been defined as process performance quality indicators that provide a framework to measure fundamental nursing care. However, nursing outcome measures have proven to be complex and non-specific, being responsible for a lack of basic information for healthcare providers in the past. The development of standardized metrics for nursing is essential, and caring is a fundamental nursing value and key indicator of nursing quality.[29] A user-friendly framework of indicators with systematic performance measurements of key patient-sensitive metrics and staff-sensitive metrics are an example of efforts to generate standardized data sets, to increase visibility of nursing's contribution.

To achieve the aims of increasing nurses' visibility, nurses are mandated to champion the development of better metrics, generating a routinely collected data set of relevant measures.[25] This will require the ability to articulate care with the often time-consuming process of collecting the necessary data.[14] The use of time-saving metrics technology, such as real-time indicators (i.e. patient falls, medication errors, infection rates, patient self-reported outcomes, workload measures, and employee injuries), aids in the process, but will need nurses to improve their capacity to understand, influence, and use new technologies and informatics, including remote care.

Developing nursing quality care metrics using evidence-based standards and agreed through consensus provides a plausible framework to generate evidence about the quality of nursing care, highlighting areas of good practice, those that require improvement, as well as enabling the sharing of process lessons. Results of these models' implementation have shown higher staff awareness of metrics and standards, improved patient care and documentation, generated better evidence, and achieved more accurate measurement across services.

However, there are still ongoing challenges related to quality measurement or outcome indicators that must be addressed by robust research, especially in complex care processes, such as those performed in interprofessional collaboration models. Most studied outcomes have been on observational or physiological measures, with very few collecting PROs. Shifts in the model of care implies also a shift in quality outcome measures. Patient-centred care, is focused on enhancing patients' satisfaction/experience and this should be measured accordingly. Despite its increasing importance, there is still lack of consensus regarding appropriate measurement of these data.[30]

Measuring quality in cardiology

Quality management in cardiology care has undergone a rapid evolution over the past three decades. Isolated efforts at simple quality measures have developed into national programmes dedicated towards the public reporting of healthcare performance on a range of cardiology quality metrics. There is clear evidence that healthcare is not always safe and can lead to poorer patient outcomes. To enhance safety and quality in cardiology care, clinical guidelines have been developed by international societies such as the ESC and the American Heart Association to guide healthcare professionals in specific treatments for cardiac conditions using current evidence. The use of guidelines should help with daily clinical decisions for treatment; however, there are still variations between different hospitals and regions.[31] Guidelines, although essential, are insufficient alone to determine if quality care is being delivered. Processes that assure, monitor, and continually improve quality must be built into the foundations of healthcare systems.[1]

At its core, quality management in cardiology care is designed to improve the quality of care delivered to cardiac patients and, in doing so, improve patient safety and outcomes such as patient experience, hospital readmission, and mortality.[32] Quality management is normally sought through a set of activities that are intended to ensure that services are safe and meet patient needs and requirements in a systematic and reliable manner. These methods lead to a level of quality control that should allow patients and service providers to have confidence in their healthcare services.[33] Cardiology nurses play a vital role in the quality management of cardiology services as they understand the needs of cardiac patients and are the healthcare professionals who most directly impact the cardiac patient's experience of care. Therefore, cardiology nurses need to develop quality management understanding and capability so they can contribute to and lead on quality initiatives that positively impact outcomes for cardiac patients.

The primary goal of quality management in healthcare is optimizing performance to improve patient outcomes. It is therefore important to consider the Institute for Healthcare Improvement (IHI) Triple Aim initiative which provides a framework for improving healthcare delivery outcomes. It is IHI's belief that QIs must be developed to simultaneously pursue the three dimensions of the IHI Triple Aim[34]:

- Improving the patient experience of care.
- Improving the health of populations.
- Reducing the per capita cost of healthcare.

Quality management—the Juran Trilogy (1986)

The Juran Trilogy, also known as the Quality Trilogy (➤ **Fig. 2.3**),[35] was developed by Dr Joseph Juran in 1986 as an approach to manage quality. It has become the basis for most quality management best practices worldwide and consists of three quality-related functions: planning, control, and improvement. Together these functions provide an active interrelated approach

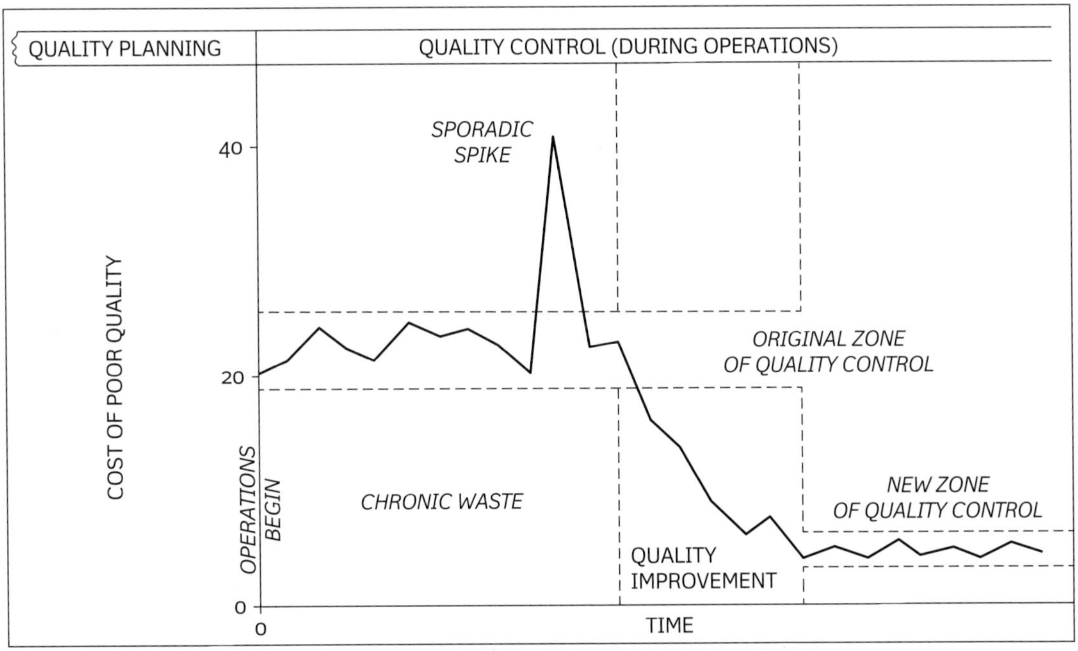

Fig. 2.3 The Quality Trilogy.

Reprodued from Defeo JA and Juran JM. Juran's Quality Handbook: The Complete Guide to Performance Excellence 6/e: McGraw Hill Professional; 2010 with permission from McGraw Hill.

for high-performance management and improved patient outcomes.

Quality planning

Quality planning begins with a comprehensive understanding of the patient's needs. In the planning stage, it is critical to define who the patient group are and find out their needs.[35] Areas of poor control of practice and gaps in care need to be identified and built in during the quality planning stage. Planning activities should be done with a multidisciplinary team, with all key stakeholders represented. It is important to take into account different stakeholder views and in particular engage with patients about what they feel matters. By working in partnership with patients, they can help to identify what the priority areas of focus should be and how to address them. Patient engagement in developing effective service delivery can benefit patients, both in their experience of care and the quality of the service they receive.[36] Once patients' needs are identified, the requirements for the change can be defined and designed.

During the planning phase, it is important to determine what data are needed to know the changed process is achieving the predicted improvement. For example, if a QI project is attempting to reduce the 30-day readmission rate for heart failure patients, then the number of patients discharged with a primary diagnosis of heart failure and the number of these patients readmitted within 30 days of discharge need to be captured. Control metrics which demonstrate improvement need to be considered at the quality planning stage and an infrastructure for the data requirements included in the design.

Quality control

Quality control is a key method for improving quality in healthcare through the measurement of performance and detection of emerging problems. Quality control is the continuous measurement of performance; ensuring that a process remains stable over time (in control) and that its performance remains within the upper and lower control limits. Quality control involves the measurement of key input, process, and outcome data and focuses on monitoring the system, detecting emerging problems (special causes), and taking steps to address them.[35]

Quality control consists of internal and external quality control; internal quality control involves metrics and indicators that assess individual practices and determine how teams are performing against local standards. These control metrics will include key nursing performance indicators for safety (early warning scores, omitted medication, falls risk, malnutrition screening), incidents, complaints, patient experience, and internal audit programmes. It is a registrant's responsibility to be knowledgeable of the internal quality control levels expected within their organization.

External quality control measures are designed to provide hospitals with performance data and highlight areas for improvement. External quality control within cardiology care has undergone significant change with the development of European and worldwide best practice guidance, global research studies, and national audit programmes that report on a number of quality measures. National registries, such as the SWEDEHEART Registry, were implemented to track patient outcomes and improve quality in cardiovascular care. The chosen measures are based on evidence-based guidelines for prevention and treatment of multiple conditions, including acute myocardial infarction, heart failure, and stroke.

One such national registry is the UK's National Cardiac Audit Programme (NACP); this programme highlights aspects of safety, clinical effectiveness, and outcomes for cardiac patients. The NACP has six subspecialty audits—Adult Cardiac Surgery, Adult Percutaneous Coronary Interventions, Cardiac Rhythm Management, Heart Failure, Congenital Heart Disease in Children and Adults, and Myocardial Ischaemia National Audit Project. The audit findings recognize areas of clinical excellence that can be adopted across the National Health Service, but also identify areas where care falls below expected standards. These standards are used to determine local and national QI aims for healthcare professionals, service managers, and commissioners.

The Myocardial Ischaemia National Audit Project (MINAP) is a domain within the NCAP that contains information about the care provided to patients who are admitted to hospital with acute coronary syndromes. Data are collected and analysed to illustrate the 'patient journey' from a call to the emergency services or their self-presentation at an emergency department, through diagnosis and treatment at hospital, to the prescription of preventive medications on discharge. Provision of care by staff practising in participating hospitals is expressed through clinically important quality control indicators.

Quality improvement

If you want better performance, you need a better design.

QI is the use of systematic tools and methods to continuously improve the quality of care and outcomes for patients.[37] While quality control focuses on identifying problems in patient care, it cannot move a system to a higher level of performance beyond the constraints of an existing system design. QI focuses on finding opportunities to improve quality by changing and redesigning systems.

QI provides the opportunity for system or process redesign that can lead to higher levels of performance. System redesign, testing of new ideas, and measurement are required to determine if the new ideas are leading to improvement.

There are many QI methodologies available, such as Lean, Six Sigma, Total Quality Management, and Model for Improvement. There is no one 'right' QI approach for all change, the characteristics of the current system must be considered when deciding which approach to QI will have the greatest application and impact.[38]

The IHI model for improvement is a QI methodology that provides a framework for designing, testing, and implementing changes.[34] The framework allows changes to be tested in a low-risk environment to determine efficacy before large-scale adoption. The model is designed to be flexible and comprehensive, rather than a rigid step-by-step approach that can inhibit innovation.

The model is based on three fundamental questions that define the endpoint (➤ **Fig. 2.4**):

- What are we trying to accomplish?
- How will we know that a change is an improvement?
- What changes can we make that will result in an improvement?

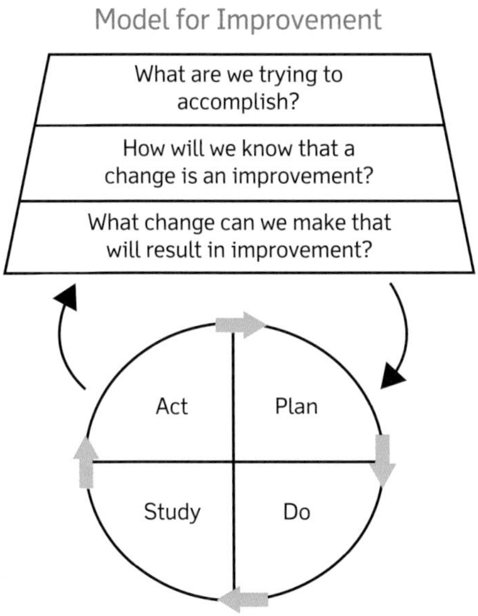

Fig. 2.4 IHI model for quality improvement.

Reproduced from Langley GL, Moen R, Nolan KM, Nolan TW, Norman CL, Provost LP. The Improvement Guide: A Practical Approach to Enhancing Organizational Performance (2nd edition). San Francisco: Jossey-Bass Publishers; 2009 with permission from John Wiley and Sons.

The Model for Improvement is an approach to continuous improvement where changes are tested in small rapid cycles that involve Plan–Do–Study–Act (PDSA) cycles. The PDSA cycle creates the structure for testing and implementing the change. Testing the change under a variety of conditions can demonstrate that the improvement can be sustained in the future. Implementation of the change should be managed as a series of PDSA cycles as these small-scale tests of change are central to iterative improvement.[39]

PDSA cycles form the foundation for implementation of a successful intervention and increase the chances of long-term success. The scale and spread approach in QI is where smaller incremental steps within services can grow and lead to larger, sustainable organizational change.[40]

Data over time—run charts and control (Shewhart) charts

QI requires change to occur; however, not all changes result in improvement. One of the fundamental tools of QI is to understand the variation in the process over time. This can be done using run charts and control (Shewhart) charts. A run chart is the simplest of charts and consists of a single line plotting data over time with a central median line (➤ **Fig. 2.5**).

Run charts provide a valuable tool at the beginning of a project, as they can reveal important information about a process before enough data have been collected to create a control chart. Run charts can be used for:

- Displaying data to monitor performance of one or more process/es.
- Determining if a change has resulted in improvement.
- Demonstrating whether the improved performance has been sustained.[41]

Control charts also plot a single line of data over time with a central median line but include upper and lower control limits. These limits are calculated based on the data being plotted and can demonstrate if the system is stable (within the control limits) or unstable (outside the control limits) (➤ **Fig. 2.6**).

Control charts are used to monitor the redesigned process to ensure it sustains the improved performance (with new upper and lower control limits), reduced variation, and improved results.

Data challenges

The importance of having access to robust, real-time data for quality management is recognized.[42] However, there can often be a lag in data being available and good

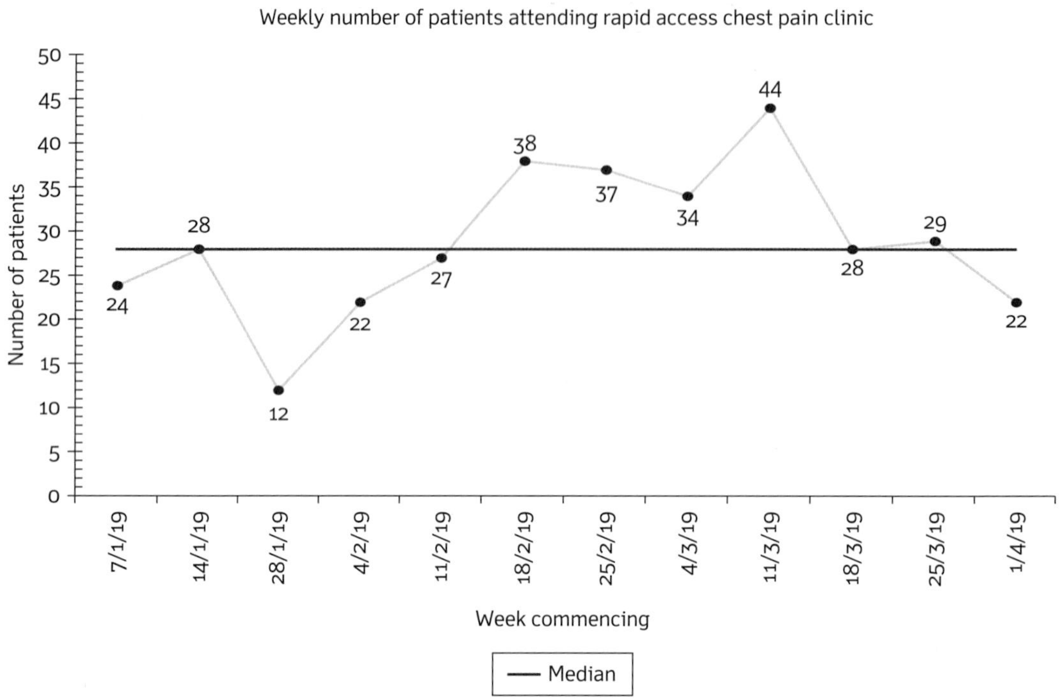

Fig. 2.5 Example of a run chart.

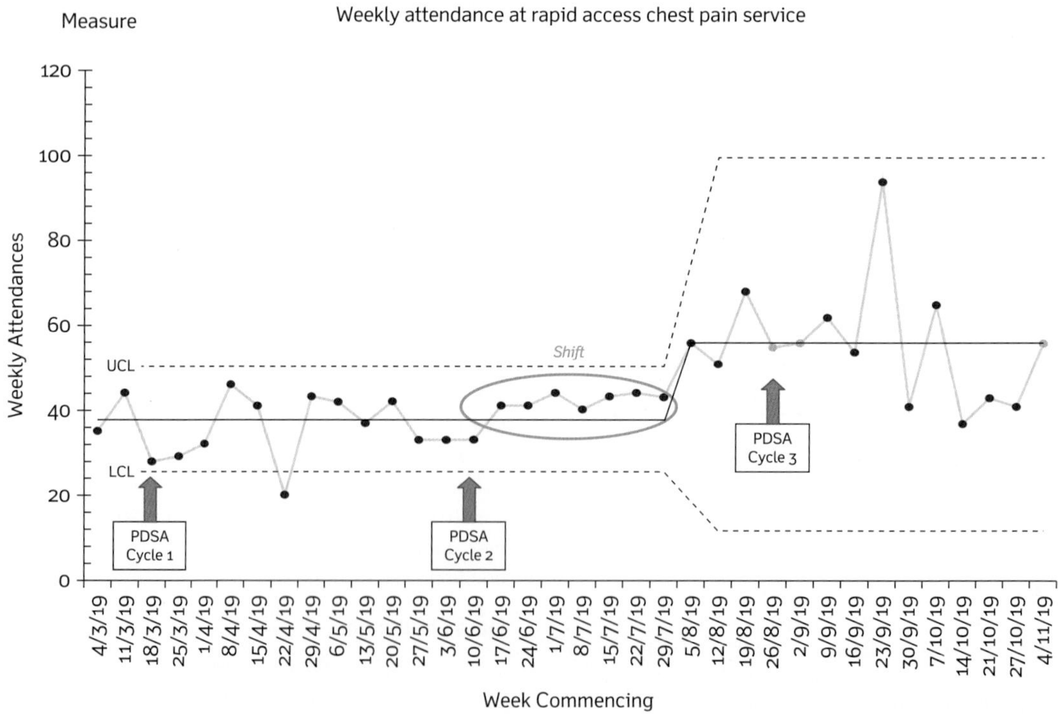

Fig. 2.6 Example of a control chart.

evidence being delivered; this is problematic for clinical leaders and policymakers who require this data to effectively drive improvements in cardiovascular care. Healthcare organizations need a modern approach to data management that supports a complete understanding of the patient's journey, with real-time access to healthcare metrics and data.

Additionally, healthcare data can be challenging to access; data can be hidden in information systems and the collections of data available often don't link together. The result is a delay in the adoption of new systems, inadequate responses to healthcare programmes, and poor engagement and experience. Cardiology nurses need to be aware of data available locally and be able to develop simple measures and data that provide reliable datasets to demonstrate improvement.

Embedding a culture for quality management

Quality management in healthcare requires long-term commitment and a shared determination to make a difference; it involves empowering staff to understand quality problems, develop effective solutions, and put them into practice.[42] Sustainable changes are more likely to result from an approach that involves team members in developing and implementing the change.[43] Healthcare will not reach its full potential until quality management becomes an intrinsic part of everyone's job, in all parts of the system.[44] This involves building will and capability and engaging healthcare professionals in participating, innovating, and leading QI at the frontline.

There are many successful examples where QI has been embedded in practice; one being the South Eastern Health and Social Care Trust in Belfast, Northern Ireland. In 2011, the Trust set out on a journey to create a culture of QI where all health and social care professionals felt supported to take part in transforming patient safety, care quality, and the patients experience. The Trust developed the 'Safety, Quality & Experience' (SQE) training programme that enables staff to deliver improvements in areas that matter to them and to patients. During the programme, participants learn QI methodology and put their new knowledge into practice with coaching and support from mentors, to deliver an improvement that will benefit patients. This has led to a range of SQE projects across all specialties, including cardiology projects to improve patient flow at the Rapid Access Chest Pain clinic and to increase patient awareness of novel anticoagulants prior to coronary angiography. The Trust has embedded a QI culture across a large-scale organization by engaging frontline practitioners in SQE. The success of the SQE training has quickly spread further afield, with other trusts now sending healthcare professionals to complete the programme and bring the learning back into their own organization.

Section Summary

Complex healthcare issues are best addressed by quality management approaches that engage frontline staff and embed collaborative interprofessional team working. Quality management requires the attention of all the stakeholders: patients, healthcare professionals, healthcare policymakers, patient advocates, and commissioners of care. Quality management in cardiology nursing remains an active area for innovation and improvement. More than ever before, the impact of QI efforts on patient outcomes will be crucial to improve cardiovascular health in the coming years. Cardiology nurses are the healthcare professionals who most directly impact the cardiac patient's experience of care and therefore need to be at the forefront of quality management initiatives that positively impact outcomes for patients.

Role of technology and informatics in quality of care

Technology plays an important part in assuring quality of care. Currently, the role of technology for care provision is now thought as essential to nursing care. The Topol review, conducted to provide independent advice on how technology will change the role of healthcare providers, emphasized three key points for incorporating digital healthcare[45]:

1. Patients need to be included as partners and informed about health technologies, with a particular focus on vulnerable/marginalized groups to ensure equitable access.
2. The healthcare workforce needs expertise and guidance to evaluate new technologies, using processes grounded in real-world evidence.
3. The gift of time: wherever possible, the adoption of new technologies should enable staff to gain more time to care, promoting deeper interaction with patients.

The integration of health information technology in clinical practice workflows has been developing quickly in the last decade and digital technologies have profoundly impacted every aspect of nursing care, from training (i.e. simulated skills) to patients' remote self-care. High-quality care requires the best use of innovative technological advances.

Electronic medical records and automated medication records reduce nurses' paperwork, improving direct patient care and safety.[16] Studies have reported 2.75 fewer hours per shift on medication administration (reallocated to patient care and training) with a 79% reduction in medication errors.[16] A recent systematic review explored the usefulness of electronic data for long-term monitoring of patients with cardiovascular chronic diseases, such as hypertension and heart failure.[46]

Nursing, as with other health professions, is constantly challenged with emerging advances and it is imperative to understand and influence the development and use of new technologies. Nursing training is often focused on issues relevant to clinical practice, with less interest from nurses in adopting technological interventions or being major players involved in the design of new technology tools.[13] Also, nurses are seldom involved in technological purchase decisions with poor results in the organization's investment.[16] To succeed in the implementation of new technology in the clinical setting, direct caregivers must be involved in the overall process. Therefore, nursing needs to move from a reactive approach to technological advances to an anticipating and influencing approach.[29]

Including technology and informatics in their initial education, being aware and exploring current developments, foreseeing their impacts, and working with information technology experts will help nurses to develop health informatics and digital tools and learn how technology can improve efficiency, promote safer practice, and increase engagement. Furthermore, all technology requires early and ongoing assessment over healthcare effects. High-quality research is essential to understand the nursing position, patients' perceptions, and outcomes when technology is utilized.

PROMs and PREMs in delivering high-quality and values-based healthcare

Given the global burden of cardiovascular disease and the need to increase the likelihood of desired health outcomes, values-based healthcare (which aims to increase the value that is derived from the resources available for a population) is important from both the patient and societal perspective.[47] This links specifically with the 'effective' and 'person-centred' quality care domains. Emphasis has previously been given to mortality outcome and, to a lesser extent, morbidity outcome. However, to optimize health outcomes, those important to patients must be prioritized and globally health ministers have stated the need to invest in measures that 'matter most to people'. Primarily, the focus has been on PROs but patient-reported experience measures (PREMs) have been gaining international recognition in relation to both quality of care and values-based healthcare.[48]

PROs are health outcomes directly reported by the patient without interpretation by others, measuring the patient's perception of the impact of their condition or treatment on their health. In contrast, PREMs measure quality of care in relation to the patient's experience while they were receiving care. This is often considered a quality indicator rather than a direct quality measure.[49] However, a consistent positive association between patient experience, safety, and clinical effectiveness has been found across a range of clinical specialities,[50] demonstrating patients are able to distinguish between safety, clinical effectiveness, and experience.[51] Thus, patient experience should be considered a core measurement in assessing healthcare outcomes in the delivery of high-quality care.[52]

Use of PROMs and PREMs in advancing high-quality care

PROs are predominately measured using patient-reported outcome measures (PROMs), usually in the form of a standardized questionnaire. PROMs can be used 'actively' at the patient level for shared decision-making or 'passively' at the aggregated level to inform clinical guidelines and commissioning, for performance assessment and benchmarking, and for research and QI.

While many clinical guidelines, including those from the ESC, do now refer to the need for PROM assessment, there is little evidence of extensive use at the individual patient level, despite its value in shared decision-making, personalized care, and values-based care. However, greater PRO use occurs at the aggregate level. For example, in England and the US, PROMs are used extensively for certain conditions, while in Sweden, PROs are included within their national quality registers with approximately 40% also including PREMs.[53] Likewise, in Denmark a national system for PROs reporting is currently being established. Patient experience is also a key objective in Pay For Performance (P4P) programmes in Australia, the US, and some European countries, aimed at reducing variation in quality of care and to develop strategic commissioning.[1]

To advance the consistent use of PROMs and PREMs in outcomes measurement, the International Consortium for Health Outcomes Measurement (ICHOM: https://www.ichom.org) has developed standardized measurement outcomes by clinical condition as agreed by a consortium of experts and patient representatives to focus on what matters most to patients. Of the available cardiovascular standard sets (atrial fibrillation, hypertension in low- and middle-income countries, heart failure, and coronary artery disease), all include PROs, while the hypertension in low- and middle-income countries standard set also includes patient experience. Likewise for research, the Core Outcome Measures in Effectiveness Trials (COMET: http://www.comet-initiative.org) initiative includes papers where core outcomes for research in specific clinical areas have been defined. For example, the core outcome datasets for coronary artery disease[54] and cardiac surgery[55] both include PROs.

PROM and PREM tools in cardiovascular care

PROM tools are generally either generic (applied to any patient or general population) or disease specific (applied to a particular condition or treatment) and both should be used in healthcare assessment as they provide complementary information. However, while there are a plethora of PROM instruments, not all are developed and validated adhering to robust psychometric principles, and surprisingly, only a small proportion include patient involvement to decide what outcomes to measure.[56] Selecting the right instrument can be challenging although databases such as COSMIN (COnsensus-based Standards for the selection of health Measurement Instruments: https://www.cosmin.nl) and PROMIS (Patient-Reported Outcomes Measurement Information System: http://www.healthmeasures.net/explore-measurement-systems/promis) can be useful.

In Europe and the UK, the EQ-5D has been the most widely used simple generic preference-based measure of health and is well received by patients,[57] although the SF-36 is also often the generic tool of choice both in and outside the US. ➤ Table 2.3 includes some examples of commonly used, well-validated cardiovascular disease-specific PROMs.

While ➤ Table 2.3 includes commonly used PROMs, other tools do exist. For example, the McNew questionnaire (myocardial infarction, coronary disease, and heart failure), symptoms of illness score (cardiac surgery), and more recently the ESC European Association of Preventive Cardiology-developed HeartQoL (core cardiac tool). Likewise, there are disease-specific PROMs for other cardiovascular conditions, for example, the Atrial Fibrillation Symptom Scale (AFSS), the Cardiff Cardiac Ablation patient-reported outcome measure (C-CAP), the Cambridge Pulmonary Hypertension Outcome Review (CAMPHOR), and the PROM-CR1, which is in development for cardiac rehabilitation. However, further development and validation work in these areas is needed.

Table 2.3 Examples of validated disease-specific questionnaires

Angina and coronary artery disease	Seattle Angina Questionnaire (SAQ)
Cardiomyopathy	Kansas City Cardiomyopathy Questionnaire (KCCQ)
Coronary revascularization (percutaneous coronary intervention and coronary artery bypass grafting)	Coronary Revascularisation Outcome Questionnaire (CROQ)
Heart failure	Minnesota Heart Failure Questionnaire (MHFQ) and KCCQ

PREMs can be either relational (patient experience of their relationships during treatment) or functional (experience of practical issues, such as facilities available) and both generic and disease-specific PREM tools exist. Like PROMs, there are a vast number of PREM tools with generic instruments accounting for just over two-thirds. Again, validity and reliability across all PREM tools has been shown to be highly variable but the Hospital Consumer Assessment of Healthcare Providers and System (HCAHPS), the Norwegian Patient Experience Questionnaire (NORPEQ), the Picker Patient Experience Questionnaire (PPE-15), and the Patient Experiences with In-patient Care (I-PAHC) instruments have been found to demonstrate the most evidence of validity and reliability for in-hospital PREMs.

The future: PROMs and PREMs core to delivering high-quality cardiovascular care

To deliver high-quality and values-based care, PROMs and PREMs need to be fully integrated into everyday clinical practice. A significant amount of work is needed for this to become commonplace, but there are four key areas worthy of focus. Firstly, appropriate and robustly developed and validated disease-specific tools, including involvement and/or co-production with patients, are needed in cardiovascular care areas where none exist, or where do they exist, fall short of the scientific required standard. To address this, the ESC led by ACNAP has recently created both a Patient Engagement Forum and a PROMs committee to focus on these areas. Secondly, and aligned to point one, greater robust evidence is needed on PROMs and PREMs. Thus, methodologically rigorous research is needed that aligns, where possible, to standardized core dataset recommendations and reports using CONSORT-PRO guidelines (reporting of PROs in randomized trials). Thirdly, there needs to be adoption of appropriate electronic technologies to support the routine introduction of PROMs and PREMs into clinical practice.[58] Finally, and most importantly, a widespread general culture shift in shared decision-making, and the value and inclusion of PROMs in this, is needed.

Care must be people-centred

A central element of ensuring that people remain at the core of our healthcare is ensuring a focus on patient-centred care. Although the terms patient-centred care and people-centred care are often used interchangeably, there are differences. Patient-centred care is often viewed as a central component of management of a non-communicable disease. Patient-centred care has been defined as 'Providing care that is respectful of and responsive to individual patient preferences, needs, and values and ensuring that patient values guide all clinical decisions'.[59] It is associated with improved effectiveness, health outcomes, and patient experiences especially in vulnerable cardiovascular populations such as older patients with a high burden of comorbidities.

Patient-centred care principles are intimately related to actual nursing challenges such as sharing decision-making, health literacy, language access, and cultural competence. Considering patient/family preferences, understanding that each person experiences a condition in a unique way with their own expectations, are directly related to nursing empathic competences and communication skills that will also enable patients to actively participate in their care (shared decision-making).

Empowering and enabling patients to participate in their own care and being involved in health strategy decisions is crucial in patients with long-term conditions such as cardiovascular disease. Self-care and self-management are particularly important in achieving desired outcomes. However, learning to share decisions with patients as partners in their own care requires a fully prepared, informed, and engaged patient and implies significant changes in the traditional paternalistic model of care. For example, in patients with anticoagulant treatment, it is important to develop culturally adapted, high-quality, comprehensive, up-to-date evidence education tools in a way that can make intellectual, emotional, and practical sense to the patient.

Patient- and family-centred care are two of the several multidimensional terms referring to innovative approaches to care. These models recommend that care is delivered and planned around the convenience of both the individual and their family members. The concepts of patient-centred care and family-centred care have gained increasing public prominence in recent years as an attempt to improve the quality of care and meet the needs of patients. In Australia, for example, patient-centred care has been practised for more than a decade, with the adoption of self-determination and autonomy as the pillars of this movement. As part of patient-centred care and family-centred care, patients are also situated in the front row, as they are increasingly asking the healthcare systems to participate in their care process.[60]

Patient-centred care and family-centred care are therefore identified as contemporary concepts, as opposed to the less acceptable old ways of healthcare delivery, when physicians chose to adopt a paternalistic approach, thus limiting the interventions and the inputs from patients and families. Patient-centred care and family-centred care identify similar approaches and philosophies of caring, but according to some sources, each of them can be conceived according to the context of care and the patients involved. For instance, in paediatrics, the concept of family-centred care can prevail, to emphasize the right and the responsibilities of the parents towards their children's well-being. However, in adulthood, the concept of family-centred care is more merged to that of patient-centred care, to emphasize also the role of patients in individual care decisions. Thus, it is common to find the terms patient- and family-centred care used interchangeably across the literature.[59]

Key concepts and benefits of patient- and family-centred care

Patient- and family-centred care principles are built upon the relationships and collaborations of its most important members, namely patients, families, physicians, nurses, and other professionals. The Institute for Patient- and Family-Centred Care (https://www.ipfcc.org/) and other groups reached agreement on the following principles of patient-centred care:

- Information sharing: the exchange of honest, objective, and unbiased information between families and providers.
- Respect and honouring differences: cultural diversity and family traditions, including knowledge, values,

beliefs, and cultural backgrounds are respected and honoured.

- Partnership and collaboration: patients and families collaborate with providers at all levels of healthcare, participating in decision-making at the level they choose.
- Negotiation: medical care plans are flexible and agreed upon by families and patients. Choices and decisions about their health are favoured and shared between team members.
- Care in the context of family and community: policies and systems are developed so that they are tailored to patients' and families' needs in all settings, including community-based services.

The aforementioned principles suggest the presence of two common ingredients that are essential to achieve patient- and family-centred care outcomes: being receptive and responsive to the needs of the individuals and their families, and supporting their participation in the care process.

Patient- and family-centred care: impact on outcomes

Considerable research has been conducted to explore the benefits of patient- and family-centred care models. Evidence indicates that they can improve several outcomes, related to patients, healthcare providers, and health systems. In patients, studies have found a positive relationship between patient- and family-centred care and satisfaction. In 2008, Wolf conducted a randomized controlled trial to examine the effect of patient-centred care during discharge from an acute surgical care setting, and found that participants in the patient-centred care group rated their satisfaction and quality of services more highly.[61] Similarly, in 2000, Counsell found increased satisfaction with care when patient-centred care was adopted from hospital admission to discharge.[62] Other studies have reported a decrease in hospital readmissions and use of healthcare services. Heart failure patients who were managed using a patient-centred approach during their hospital stay, were less likely to be readmitted with a recurrence within 30 days of discharge. Data from a randomized study showed that patient-centred care was associated with less annual visits for specialty care, less frequent hospitalizations, and reduced laboratory tests. A patient-centred care approach can also improve patient self-care. Furthermore, a systematic review found that the use of educational strategies for adult patients with heart failure improved self-care, quality of life, and knowledge, particularly when it was delivered by a multidisciplinary team.[63]

The benefits of patient- and family-centred care can also extend beyond patient outcomes, and may also encompass healthcare providers and health systems. For example, when staff incorporated patient-centred care practices, these were associated with lower turnover intentions, and higher quality of care. In addition, patient-centred care was negatively correlated with medical errors and near misses. These important benefits of patient- and family-centred care can have a number of implications for healthcare providers and health systems. For example, nurses can use patient- and family-centred care as an instrument to improve both the quality of care, and also the context in which they work and their well-being. Policymakers demonstrating interest in particular patient- and family-centred care models can promote, disseminate, and implement these initiatives in light of their evidence-based effectiveness.[64] Given the evidence for benefit of patient-centred care, it would seem logical that its adoption should be incorporated into clinical guidelines. However, a review and expert consensus from the ACNAP Science Committee evaluated a selection of ESC Guidelines and found that the inclusion of patient-centred care as a recommendation is low.[65]

Strategies for successful patient- and family-centred care

Patient- and family-centred care is now considered a central aspiration of most high-quality healthcare systems. Major effort has been made to enhance partnership and collaboration with patients and families. However, successful patient- and family-centred care goes beyond the improvement of these relationships. In 2009, a team from the Group Health Research Institute (Seattle, WA, US) oriented their research on people-centred care and developed a framework to help understand the areas for action, implementation, and improvement.[66] To promote the adoption of people-centred care, healthcare systems should orient their strategies through these three macro levels: (1) interpersonal, (2) clinical, and (3) structural levels of care (➤ Table 2.4).

Interpersonal level of care

Strategies to implement patient- and family-centred care begin with improving the interpersonal level of care. This context encompasses the relationship between healthcare providers and patients/families. It is essential to develop effective communication techniques to involve patients

Table 2.4 Strategy levels of patient- and family-centred care

Interpersonal level	Clinical level	Structural level
Adopt communication techniques	Ensure shared clinical decisions	Improve access to care
Promote patient narratives	Promote self-care	Improve healthcare physical environment
Build strong partnerships	Improve care transitions	Promote virtual care
Ensure shared decision-making	Support with clinical follow-ups	Promote information technology
Encourage involvement in care		

Source data from Greene SM, Tuzzio L, Cherkin D. A framework for making patient-centered care front and center. Perm J. 2012 Summer;16(3):49–53.

and families in the process of care and earn their trust. In order to 'centralize' care, it is important to understand patient and family preferences, needs, and values. Three routine steps are suggested in order to safeguard patient- and family-centred care in daily practice: (1) building a partnership with the patient, through patient narrative (starting point of the process); (2) strengthening the partnership through shared decision-making; and (3) documenting patient preferences, beliefs, values, and involvement in care and decision-making. Also, regular investigations into patients' and families' experience of care could help find areas of improvement, with the last objective to monitor the quality of care offered.

Clinical level of care

The clinical level of care refers essentially to the care delivered by the professional teams. In order to ensure higher standards of care, providers should adopt clinical decisions according to the best available evidence and, at the same time, ensure active patient and family involvement.[66,67] However, the needs of patients surpass clinical needs and, therefore, they should be empowered to achieve more autonomy. A further element of patient- and family-centred care is the promotion of self-care for individuals with chronic illnesses and their families. In this context, the engagement of patients is viewed as a more active role in the care process. This is an important objective of all healthcare systems, especially in previous recent decades, where the ageing population and the increase in life expectancy have paved the way for the increase in non-communicable diseases. Another aspect of clinical care is to improve care transitions, or the movement of patients across healthcare providers and settings. Pre-discharge interventions should include facilitation of patient engagement, and patient and family education oriented to self-care. Post-discharge interventions should be proactive and encompass facilitation of communication with healthcare providers, additional support (including follow-up phone calls and home visits), and clinical follow-up.

Structural level of care

The structural level of care represents, essentially, the environment where care is delivered. A growing body of literature has been published on the field of the 'healing environments', defined as the healthcare environments that are designed to positively influence the patient's healing process, recovery, and well-being. Recognition of these healing environments represents key progress, as now many structures are still tailored to facilitate clinical activities. For example, doctors' and nurses' stations in hospitals are often distant from patients' beds, and healthcare services are designed such that patients and families are forced to move to services rather than having them wherever they are, with the result of increasing psychological and physical stress. The creation of a healing environment that removes barriers between patients, families, and providers is one of the objectives of the Planet Tree Model. Specifically, the aims of this model, which is being implemented in many institutions around the world, are to (1) demedicalize the individual and family experience, and (2) create more accessible services in the context of care.

Some strategies to improve the healthcare physical environment include, for example, redesigning the waiting areas and the spaces of outpatient services, to ensure that they better meet patient and family needs. Or interventions to improve access to care, including more outreach services in underserved rural and urban areas, minimization of clinic waiting times, and facilitation of appointment-making processes. A structural context should also dedicate proper strategies to information technology, in order to facilitate (1) organization and exchange of patient-related information, which is typically fragmented across and isolated within services and (2) virtual care, a broader term that refers to interactions that do not require patient, family, and providers to be in the same room at the same time. Virtual visits can be one means to ensure continuity of care, and make healthcare systems more patient- and family-centred, as they provide easier access to care and improve effective communication with healthcare providers.[68]

Optimal delivery of patient- and family-centred care cannot prescind from strategies and interventions that are evidence based and multidimensional in nature. Healthcare providers, which are facing increasing pressure to implement patient- and family-centred care into their practice, have to engage in multidisciplinary aspects of care, from building relationships with patients and families, to engaging in organizational leadership strategies. But they are also constantly challenged by the provision of care under conditions of constrained resources, especially in this modern era where the epidemiological transition has determined a tremendous expansion of individuals with chronic illnesses and an increase in costs.

Patient- and family-centred care in cardiovascular conditions

Cardiovascular diseases are recognized as a major health problem worldwide. According to the literature, they represent the leading cause of death (see Chapter 1). For example, in the US, they account for 17% of all health expenditure.[69] However, the burden of cardiovascular diseases comes not only from mortality but also from the consequences of living with the disease. As an example, coronary artery disease (the most common disease of the heart), is a major cause of disability in developed countries, and also a primary contributor to the development of heart failure, which in turn is the principal cause of hospitalizations in older adults.

A patient- and family-centred care approach is increasingly being recognized as an important component of the treatment and management of cardiovascular diseases. Recent developments have heightened the need for further implementation of patient- and family-centred care interventions in cardiovascular nursing and medicine, particularly during the initial periods following an acute cardiac event (e.g. acute coronary syndrome, heart failure, and ventricular arrhythmias). A systematic review found that the highest effectiveness of patient- and family-centred care interventions was reached when delivered to acute patients, for example, those being affected by myocardial infarction. However, there is substantial evidence of positive effects also when patient- and family-centred care is implemented for chronic patients with exacerbations. With regard to this, the experience of Ekman and colleagues (2012) is noteworthy.[70] They implemented a randomized controlled trial by recruiting patients with chronic heart failure hospitalized for worsening of symptoms. The study intervention was based on three patient- and family-centred care goals (initiating, working, and safeguarding the partnership) and provided evidence of a significant reduction in hospital readmissions and maintenance of functional performance.[70]

In addition, a retrospective study suggested that patient- and family-centred care was able to reduce mortality in veteran patients hospitalized for acute myocardial infarction, although the estimation of the 'technical' quality of care was not proven directly, rather by means of measures of adherence to international guidelines. A more recent study by Fors and colleagues (2015) implemented a detailed patient-centred care intervention for patients affected by acute coronary syndrome, to facilitate discharge from hospital and return to everyday life. The intervention comprised a care planning and decision-making process performed collaboratively by patients and healthcare professionals. It included a first step (inpatient stay) concerning listening to patient narratives and reaching a joint agreement on the care plan. A second step was then performed during outpatient care visits, to discuss the health status, and a third final step (the most important one) was instead dedicated to primary care. The benefits of this approach were a reduced length of stay, a minor uncertainty about the disease and treatment, and a significant improvement in quality of life and self-efficacy. One of the fundamental aspects to improve the health of patients affected by cardiovascular diseases is the implementation of practice guidelines. In 2015, the ESC produced five guidelines; one of them was to support the management of patients with ventricular arrythmias and the prevention of sudden cardiac death. This initiative, to which a team of nurses also participated, was important because it emphasized the patient- and family-centred care approach in the emergency context. Two strategies were particularly recommended: the involvement of an interdisciplinary team and the involvement of the families.

But what exactly are the opinions and views of cardiac patients concerning patient- and family-centred care? In a recent qualitative study, 18 cardiac patients hospitalized in coronary care units were interviewed. The study found that the most important perceived themes regarding patient- and family-centred care included the management of their uncertainty, more flexibility of care, more effective and emphatic communication, and the importance of making independent decisions in the care process. The results of this study are important because, to date, little attention has been given to cardiac patients' perceptions towards patient- and family-centred care and, more importantly, they confirm once more that such perceptions match the key principles of a patient- and family-centred care approach.[71]

Patient- and family-centred care as a support to self-care in cardiovascular conditions

Unfortunately, individuals who develop a cardiovascular illness have a higher risk of subsequent cardiovascular events (e.g. stroke and myocardial infarction), so it is important they engage in preventive lifestyle behaviours (physical activity and exercise, diet, smoking cessation, etc.) and perform an adequate level of self-care.[72] Self-care, defined as the decision-making process performed by patients to promote their health and manage their illness, represents a fundamental aspect of patient- and family-centred care because it requires the individuals to become the main actors who are responsible for their care. In the cardiovascular field, self-care has been extensively studied in patients affected by heart failure. Initially, Riegel and colleagues developed the 'situation-specific theory of heart failure self-care', which was then followed by the 'middle range theory of self-care of chronic illness', in order to describe how self-care works in individuals with heart failure and chronic illnesses, respectively. These theories, which are quite similar, identify three components of self-care: (1) self-care maintenance, that is, the actions performed by patients to promote health and keep the chronic illness stable (e.g. physical exercise, diet, medication adherence); (2) self-care monitoring and symptom perception, that is, the process of monitoring signs and symptom of an illness (e.g. keeping a record of body weight); and (3) self-care management, namely the process of decision-making after detecting signs and/or symptoms (e.g. consulting the healthcare providers because of a symptom).

In heart failure studies, researchers have found that self-care can improve a variety of outcomes including quality of life, mortality, healthcare utilization, and symptoms. But there is also evidence of self-care benefits in other populations, such as hypertension, coronary heart disease, and atrial fibrillation, where in general there is a significant improvement in lifestyle modifications, self-monitoring, and medication adherence. Patients also rely on their families, relatives, or friends for the management of their care. These individuals are called informal caregivers and contribute to a variety of self-care tasks including accompanying patients to medical appointments, monitoring health conditions, and communicating with healthcare providers. Similar to self-care, caregiver contributions have also shown a positive impact on patients' outcomes, particularly on medication adherence, health behaviours, psychological health, quality of life and healthcare utilization, and patient clinical events (hospitalizations, access to emergency services, and mortality).

Caregiver contributions to self-care have been defined, in the context of heart failure, as:

> **[T]he process of recommending to (or substituting for) the patient to perform those behaviors that help to (1) maintain stability of heart failure conditions (caregiver contribution to self-care maintenance), (2) facilitate heart failure symptom monitoring and perception (caregiver contribution to symptom monitoring and perception), and (3) respond to the signs and symptoms of an HF exacerbation when they occur.**[73]

Self-care should be considered an important target of patient- and family-centred cardiovascular care, due to the fact that such diseases are complex in nature and often manifest with symptoms that can limit physical, social, and mental abilities, as well as impair quality of life. With advanced cardiovascular conditions, patients may not be able to overcome the difficulties in self-managing their illness, so it is necessary to involve caregivers from the very beginning of the care planning. Therefore, assessing both self-care abilities of patients and the levels of contributions of caregivers to self-care may allow an understanding of the extent of their active participation in the management of the disease. Other indispensable patient- and family-centred care strategies should encompass the implementation of personalized educational interventions focused on (1) closing knowledge gaps, (2) sustaining motivation and self-efficacy, and (3) strengthening specific self-care skills and abilities.

Barriers to implementing quality care

Failures to provide adequate care or 'care left undone' are frequently reported as safety and quality gaps, and have been under intense scrutiny. High-profile incidents of poor care led to increased development of policies, strategies, and research groups focused on fundamental aspects of nursing care.[14] Failures in fundamental or basic care constitute significant risks for patients, often leading to wider patient safety failures as hospital-acquired infections or issues in nutrition and hydration in older people.[14] There has been some debate around whose role it is to deliver this care as it is increasingly delegated to other care staff.[10] It has been suggested that nurses tend to see fundamental care as minor physical tasks often devalued and invisible in a technological era, for which they do not have time, whereas it is highly valued by patients whose experience of healthcare is sensitive to nursing quality.[10] Suboptimal nursing care can lead to patient distress and dissatisfaction as they expect nurses to be well educated and competent but also compassionate and caring.[10]

Another source of quality care failure is a healthcare context that tends not to value these attributes, placing more importance on cost-effectiveness outcomes rewarding 'task and time' nursing rather than personalized care. Missing or incomplete nursing care has been clearly associated with nurse staffing levels and the replacement of registered nurses with less skilled workers.[10] This kind of restructuring initiatives lead to less time spent on direct caregiving, less mentoring of staff nurses, and undermine nurses' clinical leadership; all resulting in higher levels of dissatisfaction and lower meaningful nurse–patient relationships.[16] Excessive administrative tasks, paperwork, and data collection are taking away nurses' time to spend on direct care; for an hour of patient care, 30–60 minutes are needed for subsequent paperwork.[16] This is endorsed by international debate relating failures in nursing care with nurses' inability to provide compassionate care, such as comforting and talking to patients, when workloads intensify.[14]

Nurses report that the most enjoyable feature of nursing is helping patients and their families, but complain that 40% or less of their time is spent on direct patient care. Surveys describing nurses' last shift report high percentages of care left undone; 20–30% of the patients did not receive adequate skin or oral care, 28% of nurses were not able to provide patients with necessary education or family instructions, and up to 40% were not able to comfort or talk with their patients.[74] Studies about burnout, and the reasons nurses want to leave the profession, reveal that nurses are profoundly dissatisfied when they have not been able to provide the personalized care they want to.

Technology has also been blamed for interfering with 'care' in the broad sense of the term, moving away from high-touch care. There is a growing use of robotics for fundamental care provision (i.e. to provide feeding assistance or robot bathtubs in elder care). The challenge to nursing is to humanize the use of technology exerting influence on how it can and should provide fundamental care and not forgetting the importance of personal caring and touch.

Poor conceptual definition and lack of agreement surrounding components of fundamental aspects of nursing care prevents the development of robust evidence, and underlines problems with the delivery of such care. Limited data on the effectiveness of the intervention undermines a refocus on fundamental nursing care: developing a consensus definition of fundamental nursing care will facilitate the development of adequate metrics. Different interpretations have contributed to the lack of clarity of the concept referring, for example, to fundamental needs (i.e. hygiene), aspects of nursing care (i.e. honesty), and outcomes or factors required to address these needs. The lack of consensus of general or common descriptors and the dissimilar inclusion of elements (i.e. low reference to comfort, pain management, privacy, and dignity) have also contributed to misunderstanding.[10] This confusion is also influenced by the diversity of terms used to describe fundamental care, such as essence of care, essentials of care, and basic nursing, as a synonym of compassionate care and the frequent use of 'fundamental care' and 'fundamentals of care' as interchangeable terms. Nurses therefore have a critical role to play in collecting data to demonstrate efficacy of our interventions. Despite progress in nursing practice and research, there is still not enough knowledge of what elements of the fundamentals of nursing care matter to patients and how this agrees or differs with caregivers.[10]

Qualitative studies have examined patients' subjective experience/perception underlying fundamental care.[10] Reports from stroke survivors describe the psychosocial and emotional impact tailored to physical needs (i.e. eating) and how their integration in care, involving them in setting achievable targets, helped them to regain independence and self-esteem. Studies in these patients also highlight that distressing experiences were more evident than positive ones; independently of the clinical outcome, patients retained vivid memories after their acute stroke phase. Biographical disruption, poor narratives of patient–carer relationship, long-stay patients' intensive care unit experiences (including lack of families being present/involved), and other patients' and families' perspectives of inadequacies in nursing care are some challenges nurses must be aware of and constitute areas where more analysis of patients' experience data is needed to provide insight into current practice and how it addresses aspects of care most valued by patients and families.

A third dimension creating barriers to high-quality care exists within the health system or the context. Failures of care are not solely the responsibility of nurses as several conditions can enable or hinder care at different levels.[10] Resources (equipment and human), policy, culture, leadership, feedback, and standardized evaluation have been identified as system enablers.[10] Some authors emphasize that unless changes of core values and attitudes within healthcare systems occur, fundamentals of care will not be improved. Environment and culture are relevant challenges to the provision of patient- and family care, especially in intensive care units such as coronary care units. Literature about the fundamentals of nursing care appears confusing, with authors providing lists of nursing activities, using different definitions of fundamentals and fundamental or compassionate care.[10] Greater visibility of fundamental nursing care is needed to understand how it can contribute to patient experience and outcomes. Nurses have been called to action internationally to produce evidence for clinical practice in the fundamentals of care in a reliable, replicable, and robust manner.

A major identified barrier is uncertainty or ignorance about the qualifications and competence of nursing leaders by other professionals, managers, and even patients. Gaps in role clarification and collaborative leadership, lack of operationalization of team functioning, or conflict resolution adds to this difficulty. Varying levels of authority; misunderstanding of current roles and responsibilities; and different interests, goals, expectations, styles, and experience can interfere with communication and generate conflict. Some critical factors such as systemic determinants, organizational structures, context, and workplace culture may be beyond the control of the team. Tools, procedures, management influences, professional practice regulation, institutional policies, and the physical environment are relevant for the full scope of practice within an interdisciplinary approach.

Health organizations and managers must establish workplace cultures that embed innovation and excellence where staff are respected and valued, with positive practice environments providing development and support to the health team. Local empowerment will create local solutions and a better understanding of workflow in members of the interdisciplinary team. This requires radical shifts in service delivery and philosophy (i.e. flexibility of roles), values, and norms of the system with explicit commitment to innovation and learning (both formal and informal education).[75]

Nurses have been identified as pivotal in team building and in creating a culture of collaboration for safe, high-quality care, especially for cardiovascular patients. Nurse-coordinated care in the interdisciplinary team has proven to be effective, especially in preventive cardiovascular care, but it depends on several factors such as training, knowledge, professional confidence, and evidence-based practice. Newly graduated nurses frequently lack intradisciplinary expertise while postgraduate training of nurses largely determines their role on a cardiovascular team.[20] Programmes led by specialist nurses that include general practice nurses, dietitians, and physical activity specialists have achieved significant results in cardiovascular risk management related to diet, physical activity, and blood pressure.[20] This translates into benefits such as increased follow-up, fewer angina symptoms and hospital admissions, lower mortality, as well as better general health.

Moreover, physicians recognized their lack of knowledge about diet and physical activity regimens in specific medical conditions as well as lack of the competencies for effective lifestyle counselling for cardiovascular patients, whereas experienced clinicians have reported that working within a nurse-led professional collaborative practice model has increased their knowledge, leading to changes in behaviour and practice.[20] Systematic socioeconomics reviews have provided robust evidence of nurse-led inpatient units compared with doctor-led units with better outcomes such as functional status, well-being, readmissions, and mortality. In nurse-led primary care, patient satisfaction also tends to be higher. Key organizations recognize the importance of interdisciplinary working and the role of nursing as an essential component and provider of highly skilled cardiovascular care in the team. This will improve as more nurses are encouraged globally to embrace leading roles in evidence-based practice, advocacy, and collaboration between disciplines.

Conclusion

In this chapter, we have explored the delivery of high-quality cardiovascular care through the adoption of the WHO framework for quality care. High-quality care needs to be safe, effective and evidence based, timely, equitable, efficient, and, most importantly, people-centred. Nurses make up the largest group of healthcare workers, and therefore have a central role in ensuring that care is of high quality across the life course. Nurses need to advocate for safe practice, and to do so we must be able to access and apply the latest evidence. It is essential that nurses are able to critique research and understand the quality of the research on which we base our decisions to provide care. Using the ESC Guidelines and derivative products is one way to ensure that our decisions are based on the best evidence available.

Nurses need to develop cultural competence to address the disproportionate burden of disease among culturally and linguistically diverse groups to ensure that care is equitable. In doing this, we explored the links between efficient care and quality of care indicators. We also discussed PROMs and PREMs as important measures of quality care. These measures help us to remember how important it is to keep the patient and the family at the centre of everything we do.

Finally, this chapter reviewed the barriers to high-quality care, and the way nurses can overcome these by working with health systems to implement practice that enables provision of high-quality care, by investing in educational opportunities for nurses and embedding innovation and excellence in all we do.

References

1. World Health Organization, Organisation for Economic Co-operation and Development, International Bank for Reconstruction and Development/The World Bank. Delivering quality health services: a global imperative for universal health coverage. World Health Organization; 2018. https://apps.who.int/iris/handle/10665/272465.
2. Institute of Medicine. Crossing the Quality Chasm: A New Health System for the 21st Century. Washington, DC: National Academies Press.
3. Strome TL. Developing and using effective indicators. In: Healthcare Analytics for Quality and Performance Improvement. Hoboken, NJ: John Wiley and Sons; 2013:115–27.
4. Butler M, Schultz TJ, Halligan P, Sheridan A, Kinsman L, Rotter T, et al. Hospital nurse-staffing models and patient- and staff-related outcomes. Cochrane Database Syst Rev. 2019;4:CD007019.
5. Registered Nurses Association of Ontario. Position statement: excellence in clinical nursing practice. 2004. https://rnao.ca/policy/position-statements/excellence-clinical-nursing-practice.
6. Coulon L, Mok M, Krause KL, Anderson M. The pursuit of excellence in nursing care: what does it mean? J Adv Nurs. 1996;24(4):817–26.
7. Paans W, Wijkamp I, Wiltens E, Wolfensberger MV. What constitutes an excellent allied health care professional? A multidisciplinary focus group study. J Multidiscip Healthc. 2013;6:347–56.
8. Hickey PA. Excellence by design: the Patricia A. Hickey award for excellence in cardiovascular nursing. World J Pediatr Congenit Heart Surg. 2017;8(6):721–25.
9. Norekvål TM, Deaton C, Scholte op Reimer WJM. The European Council on Cardiovascular Nursing and Allied Professions: toward promoting excellence in cardiovascular care. Prog Cardiovasc Nurs. 2007;22(4):217–20.
10. Kitson A, Conroy T, Kuluski K, Locock L, Lyons R. Reclaiming and Redefining the Fundamentals of Care: Nursing's Response to Meeting Patients' Basic Human Needs. Adelaide: School of Nursing, the University of Adelaide; 2013.
11. Fitzpatrick JJ. Joint Commission on Accreditation of Health Care Organizations White Paper: health care at the crossroads: strategies for addressing the evolving nursing crisis. Policy Pol Nurs Pract. 2003;4(1):71–74.
12. Clarke SP. Nurse staffing in acute care settings: research perspectives and practice implications. Jt Comm J Qual Patient Saf. 2007;33(11 Suppl):30–44.
13. Hughes R. Patient Safety and Quality: An Evidence-Based Handbook for Nurses. Rockville, MD: Agency for Healthcare Research and Quality; 2008.
14. Richards DA, Hilli A, Pentecost C, Goodwin VA, Frost J. Fundamental nursing care: a systematic review of the evidence on the effect of nursing care interventions for nutrition, elimination, mobility and hygiene. J Clin Nurs. 2018;27(11–12):2179–88.
15. Nursing and Midwifery Council. Standards for competence for registered nurses. 2014. https://www.nmc.org.uk/globalassets/sitedocuments/standards/nmc-standards-for-competence-for-registered-nurses.pdf.
16. Draper DA, Felland LE, Liebhaber A, Melichar L. The role of nurses in hospital quality improvement. Res Brief. 2008;3:1–8.
17. Driscoll A, Grant MJ, Carroll D, Dalton S, Deaton C, Jones I, et al. The effect of nurse-to-patient ratios on nurse-sensitive patient outcomes in acute specialist units: a systematic review and meta-analysis. Eur J Cardiovasc Nurs. 2018;17(1):6–22.
18. Aiken LH, Sermeus W, Van den Heede K, Sloane DM, Busse R, McKee M, et al. Patient safety, satisfaction, and quality of hospital care: cross sectional surveys of nurses

and patients in 12 countries in Europe and the United States. BMJ (Clin Res Ed). 2012;344:e1717.
19. Michaels AD, Spinler SA, Leeper B, Ohman EM, Alexander KP, Newby LK, et al. Medication errors in acute cardiovascular and stroke patients: a scientific statement from the American Heart Association. Circulation. 2010;121(14):1664–82.
20. Jennings C, Astin F. A multidisciplinary approach to prevention. Eur J Prev Cardiol. 2017;24(3 Suppl):77–87.
21. Ley SJ. Evidence-based practices for patients with cardiac disease. Prog Cardiovasc Nurs. 2009;24(1):34–35.
22. Ball JE, Griffiths P, Rafferty AM, Lindqvist R, Murrells T, Tishelman C. A cross-sectional study of 'care left undone' on nursing shifts in hospitals. J Adv Nurs. 2016;72(9):2086–97.
23. Parent N, Vissandjée B. Evidence-based cardiovascular nursing practice: why? For whom? Where and how? Can J Cardiovasc Nurs. 2008;18(3):26–30.
24. Jeffs L, Muntlin Athlin A, Needleman J, Jackson D, Kitson A. Building the foundation to generate a fundamental care standardised data set. J Clin Nurs. 2018;27(11–12):2481–88.
25. Granero-Molina J, Fernández-Sola C, Mateo-Aguilar E, Aranda-Torres C, Román-López P, Hernández-Padilla JM. Fundamental care and knowledge interests: implications for nursing science. J Clin Nurs. 2018;27(11–12):2489–95.
26. Jaarsma T, Deaton C, Fitzsimmons D, Fridlund B, Hardig BM, Mahrer-Imhof R, et al. Research in cardiovascular care: a position statement of the Council on Cardiovascular Nursing and Allied Professionals of the European Society of Cardiology. Eur J Cardiovasc Nurs. 2014;13(1):9–21.
27. Jylhä V, Oikarainen A, Perälä M, Holopainen A. Facilitating evidence-based practice in nursing and midwifery in the WHO European Region. World Health Organization; 2017. https://www.euro.who.int/en/health-topics/Health-systems/nursing-and-midwifery/publications/2017/facilitating-evidence-based-practice-in-nursing-and-midwifery-in-the-who-european-region-2017.
28. Russell KL, Holloway TM, Brum M, Caruso V, Chessex C, Grace SL. Cardiac rehabilitation wait times: effect on enrollment. J Cardiopulm Rehabil Prev. 2011;31(6):373–77.
29. Kavanagh P. Nursing & midwifery quality care-metrics (QCM)—the journey. Int J Integr Care. 2017;17(5):A441.
30. Lohr KN. Medicare—Vol. I A strategy for quality assurance; Medicare—Vol. II A strategy for quality assurance—sources and methods. J Healthc Qual. 1990;12:31.
31. Silverio A, Cavallo P, De Rosa R, Galasso G. Big health data and cardiovascular diseases: a challenge for research, an opportunity for clinical care. Front Med (Lausanne). 2019;6:36.
32. McConnell KJ, Lindrooth RC, Wholey DR, Maddox TM, Bloom N. Management practices and the quality of care in cardiac units. JAMA Intern Med. 2013;173(8):684–92.
33. The Health Foundation. The Measurement and Monitoring of Safety. London: Health Foundation; 2013.
34. Small J. Institute for Healthcare Improvement (IHI). Encyclopedia of Health Services Research. Thousand Oaks, CA: SAGE Publications, Inc.
35. Defeo JA, Juran JM. Juran's Quality Handbook: The Complete Guide to Performance Excellence (6th ed). New York: McGraw-Hill Professional; 2010.
36. Ham C, Dixon A, Brooke B. Transforming the Delivery of Health and Social Care. London: King's Fund; 2012.
37. Langley GJ, Moen RD, Nolan KM, Nolan TW, Norman CL, Provost LP. The Improvement Guide: A Practical Approach to Enhancing Organizational Performance. Chichester: John Wiley & Sons; 2009.
38. The Health Foundation. Quality Improvement Made Simple. London: Health Foundation; 2013.
39. Moen RD, Nolan TW, Provost LP. Quality Improvement Through Planned Experimentation. New York: McGraw-Hill; 1999.
40. Scoville R, Little K, Rakover J, Luther K, Mate K. Sustaining Improvement. Institute for Healthcare Improvement White Paper. Cambridge, MA: Institute for Healthcare Improvement; 2016.
41. Provost L, Murray S. The Healthcare Data Guide. San Francisco, CA: Jossey-Bass; 2011.
42. Alderwick H, Charles A, Jones B, Warburton W. Making the Case for Quality Improvement: Lessons for NHS Boards and Leaders. London: King's Fund; 2017.
43. The Health Foundation. Overcoming Challenges to Improving Quality. London: Health Foundation; 2012.
44. Batalden PB, Davidoff F. What is 'quality improvement' and how can it transform healthcare? Qual Saf Health Care. 2007;16(1):2–3.
45. Topol E. The Topol Review: Preparing the Healthcare Workforce to Deliver the Digital Future. An Independent Report on Behalf of the Secretary of State for Health and Social Care. London: Health Education England; 2019.
46. Smith SC, Fonarow GC, Piña IL, Suter R, Morgan L, Taubert K, et al. Improving quality of cardiac care: a global mandate. Rev Esp Cardiol (Engl Ed). 2015;68(11):924–27.
47. de Heer F, Gökalp AL, Kluin J, Takkenberg JJM. Measuring what matters to the patient: health related quality of life after aortic valve and thoracic aortic surgery. Gen Thorac Cardiovasc Surg. 2019;67(1):37–43.
48. Weldring T, Smith SMS. Patient-reported outcomes (PROs) and patient-reported outcome measures (PROMs). Health Serv Insights. 2013;6:61–68.
49. Kingsley C, Patel S. Patient-reported outcome measures and patient-reported experience measures. BJA Educ. 2017;17(4):137–44.

50. Doyle C, Lennox L, Bell D. A systematic review of evidence on the links between patient experience and clinical safety and effectiveness. BMJ Open. 2013;3(1):e001570.
51. Black N, Varaganum M, Hutchings A. Relationship between patient reported experience (PREMs) and patient reported outcomes (PROMs) in elective surgery. BMJ Qual Saf. 2014;23(7):534–42.
52. Bradley SM, Strauss CE, Ho PM. Value in cardiovascular care. Heart. 2017;103(16):1238–43.
53. Nilsson E, Orwelius L, Kristenson M. Patient-reported outcomes in the Swedish National Quality Registers. J Intern Med. 2016;279(2):141–53.
54. McNamara RL, Spatz ES, Kelley TA, Stowell CJ, Beltrame J, Heidenreich P, et al. Standardized outcome measurement for patients with coronary artery disease: consensus from the International Consortium for Health Outcomes Measurement (ICHOM). J Am Heart Assoc. 2015;4(5):e001767.
55. Benstoem C, Moza A, Meybohm P, Stoppe C, Autschbach R, Devane D, Goetzenich A. A core outcome set for adult cardiac surgery trials: a consensus study. PLoS One. 2017;12(11):e0186772.
56. Wiering B, de Boer D, Delnoij D. Patient involvement in the development of patient-reported outcome measures: a scoping review. Health Expect. 2017;20(1):11–23.
57. Kim J, Henderson RA, Pocock SJ, Clayton T, Sculpher MJ, Fox KAA, et al. Health-related quality of life after interventional or conservative strategy in patients with unstable angina or non–ST-segment elevation myocardial infarction: one-year results of the third Randomized Intervention Trial of unstable Angina (RITA-3). J Am Coll Cardiol. 2005;45(2):221–28.
58. Black N. Patient reported outcome measures could help transform healthcare. BMJ. 2013;346:f167.
59. Rawson JV, Moretz J. Patient- and family-centered care: a primer. J Am Coll Radiol. 2016;13(12 Pt B):1544–49.
60. Ringdal M, Chaboyer W, Ulin K, Bucknall T, Oxelmark L. Patient preferences for participation in patient care and safety activities in hospitals. BMC Nurs. 2017;16:69.
61. Wolf DM, Lehman L, Quinlin R, Zullo T, Hoffman L. Effect of patient-centered care on patient satisfaction and quality of care. J Nurs Care Qual. 2008 Oct-Dec;23(4):316–21. doi:10.1097/01.NCQ.0000336672.02725.a5. PMID: 18806645.
62. Counsell SR, Holder CM, Liebenauer LL, Palmer RM, Fortinsky RH, Kresevic DM, Quinn LM, Allen KR, Covinsky KE, Landefeld CS. Effects of a multicomponent intervention on functional outcomes and process of care in hospitalized older patients: a randomized controlled trial of Acute Care for Elders (ACE) in a community hospital. J Am Geriatr Soc. 2000 Dec;48(12):1572–81. doi:10.1111/j.1532-5415.2000.tb03866.x. PMID: 11129745.
63. Casimir YE, Williams MM, Liang MY, Pitakmongkolkul S, Slyer JT. The effectiveness of patient-centered self-care education for adults with heart failure on knowledge, self-care behaviors, quality of life, and readmissions: a systematic review. JBI Database Syst Rev Implement Rep. 2014;12(2):188–262.
64. Nutting PA, Miller WL, Crabtree BF, Jaen CR, Stewart EE, Stange KC. Initial lessons from the first national demonstration project on practice transformation to a patient-centered medical home. Ann Fam Med. 2009;7(3):254–60.
65. Khatib R, Lee GA, Marques-Sule E, Hopstock LA, O'Donnell S, Svavarsdóttir MH, et al. Evaluating the extent of patient-centred care in a selection of ESC guidelines. Eur Heart J Qual Care Clin Outcomes. 2020;6(1):55–61.
66. Ekman I, Swedberg K, Taft C, Lindseth A, Norberg A, Brink E, et al. Person-centered care—ready for prime time. Eur J Cardiovasc Nurs. 2011;10(4):248–51.
67. Siminoff LA. Incorporating patient and family preferences into evidence-based medicine. BMC Med Inform Decis Mak. 2013;13(Suppl 3):S6.
68. Donelan K, Barreto EA, Sossong S, Michael C, Estrada JJ, Cohen AB, et al. Patient and clinician experiences with telehealth for patient follow-up care. Am J Manag Care. 2019;25(1):40–44.
69. Chou AF, Homco JB, Nagykaldi Z, Mold JW, Daniel Duffy F, Crawford S, Stoner JA. Disseminating, implementing, and evaluating patient-centered outcomes to improve cardiovascular care using a stepped-wedge design: healthy hearts for Oklahoma. BMC Health Serv Res. 2018;18(1):404.
70. Ekman I, Wolf A, Olsson LE, Taft C, Dudas K, Schaufelberger M, Swedberg K. Effects of person-centred care in patients with chronic heart failure: the PCC-HF study. Eur Heart J. 2012;33(9):1112–19.
71. Esmaeili M, Cheraghi MA and Salsali M. Cardiac patients' perception of patient-centred care: a qualitative study. Nursing in critical care. 2016;21:97–104.
72. Riegel B, Moser DK, Buck HG, Dickson VV, Dunbar SB, Lee CS, et al. Self-care for the prevention and management of cardiovascular disease and stroke: a scientific statement for healthcare professionals from the American Heart Association. J Am Heart Assoc. 2017;6(9):e006997.
73. Vellone E, Riegel B, Alvaro R. A situation-specific theory of caregiver contributions to heart failure self-care. J Cardiovasc Nurs. 2019;34(2):166–73.
74. Olley R, Edwards I, Avery M, Cooper H. Systematic review of the evidence related to mandated nurse staffing ratios in acute hospitals. Aust Health Rev. 2019;43(3):288–93.
75. Prime Minister's Commission on the Future of Nursing and Midwifery in England. Front Line Care: Report by the Prime Ministers Commission on the Future of Nursing and Midwifery in England. 2010. https://webarchive.nationalarchives.gov.uk/20100331110913/http://cnm.independent.gov.uk/wp-content/uploads/2010/03/front_line_care.pdf.

3 Key considerations for continuing professional development and specialization

LIS NEUBECK, JENNIFER JONES, IZABELLA UCHMANOWICZ, SUE KOOB, CATRIONA JENNINGS, MARÍA TERESA LIRA, SHIRLEY INGRAM, AND DONNA FITZSIMONS

CHAPTER CONTENTS

KEY MESSAGES

- Nurses are on a lifelong learning journey.
- Using the core curriculum enables a framework for learning.
- There is some disparity in description of specialist and advanced practice roles, but all require additional education beyond initial qualification.
- Reflection is an important part of learning.
- Leadership in nursing is critical to ensure high-quality patient care.
- Professional societies and associations provide important support for lifelong learning and development of core skills.

Introduction

In this chapter, we will look at continuing professional development in nursing. Continuing professional development is described internationally by a variety of terms. These include continuing nursing education, life-long learning, and professional skills development (among others). While there is no universally agreed term for continuing professional development, there is a generally accepted understanding of its purpose—to help nurses maintain an updated skill set so that they are able to care for patients safely and competently. Given the current climate of an ageing population and the increasing incidence of non-communicable disease, and in particular cardiovascular disease (CVD), nurses, who are the largest healthcare workforce worldwide, are called upon to continue their efforts in the development of high-quality healthcare services, as discussed in Chapter 2. Nurses do not exist in isolation from other health professionals, in fact they are required to work in an integrated and interdisciplinary way with physicians, allied health professionals, and indeed other disciplines outside the healthcare domain such as social care services. One way that nurses contribute to service development and improvement is to enter into specialization in cardiovascular care and develop advanced practice skills. In order to develop as specialists, nurses need to access appropriate educational programmes to prepare them for these roles. In addition, these programmes provide stepping stones towards advanced practice. Service improvements and innovations are more likely to happen when professionals are able to reflect on their clinical practice and use their experience to make positive improvements. This influences what happens on both an individual and bigger picture level. Nurses can find opportunities for getting involved in research and service development by linking into organizations that support funding for their research and provide mentorship and opportunities for leadership. Implementing research findings in practice is essential to improving care for our patients. Mentorship and leadership provided by nurses for nurses is also an imperative to create a culture for quality in care (see Chapter 2).

Nursing education across the career trajectory

Across the globe, nurse education is moving towards university-based models. The evolution of nursing from hospital-based training to bachelor of nursing and graduate programmes is as a result of increasing knowledge of the effectiveness of nursing care and the ability of nurses to manage complex cardiovascular conditions. Educational programmes for cardiovascular nurses need to ensure that cardiovascular nurses are 'fit to practise', with the necessary knowledge and skills to ensure optimal care.[1] It is well known that skilled nurses reduce morbidity and mortality. In a study reporting discharge data of more than 400,000 patients, a 10% increase in the ratio of bachelor degree-prepared nurses resulted in a 7% decrease in morbidity.[2] Similarly, an Australian review highlighted the association between workforce, qualifications, and quality of care, and found critical thinking and clinical skills increase incrementally, with increased nursing qualifications.[3]

Despite the strong evidence for degree-based education programmes for nurses, there is still disparity in the delivery of education across Europe. Consequently, the Education Committee of the European Society of Cardiology (ESC) Association of Cardiovascular Nursing and Allied Professions (ACNAP) (formerly the Council of Cardiovascular Nursing and Allied Professions) developed the core curriculum for education of cardiovascular nurses.[4] The Education Committee reviewed existing curricula, international publications, and policy documents and developed a core curriculum underpinned by educational theory with eight major themes (➤ Box 3.1).

The core curriculum was designed as a document to inform discussions about the harmonization of the continuing professional development of cardiovascular nurses across health services and educational institutions in Europe. Across each of these themes, nurses move from novice to expert following Benner's model

Box 3.1 Core curriculum major themes

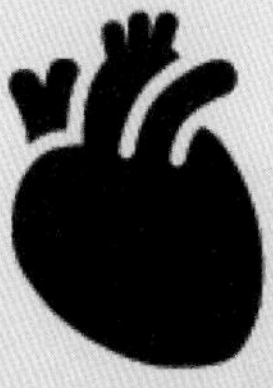

Fundamentals of cardiovascular pathophysiology

- Anatomy, pathophysiology, and clinical manifestations
- Recognizing clinical deterioration
- Atherosclerotic heart disease
- Heart rhythm and conduction
- Structural abnormalities
- Heart muscle disorders

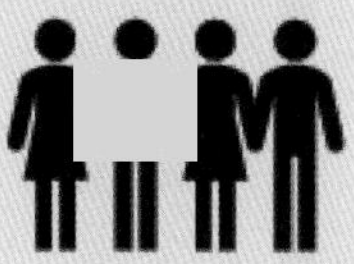

Optimizing cardiovascular health for people and populations

- Global CVD burden
- Coronary risk factos
- Risk assessment
- Behaviour change
- Interventions to aid prevention

Assessment, planning, and managing care

- Cardiovascular assessment
- Diagnostic tests
- Ectrocardiogram skills
- Life support skills
- Pharmacology
- Nursing care plans

Principles and practices of person-and family centred care

- Person-centred care
- Shared decision-making
- Reflective practice
- Tools and approaches

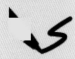

Education and communication

- Education and adult learning
- Communication skills
- Health literacy

Emotional and spiritual well-being

- Emotional resources and self-care
- Prevalence of maladaptation
- Screening tools
- Nursing interventions

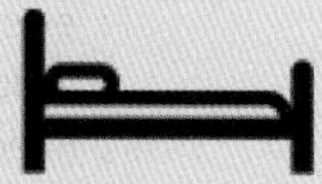

Physical well-being and comfort

- Patient safety
- Symptom management
- Exercise and rehabilitation
- End of life care

Evaluation of the quality of care

- Systems and organizational theory
- Quality care a quality indicators
- Care coordination
- Risk assessment, patient safety, adult, and evaluation
- Role of technology in patient safety

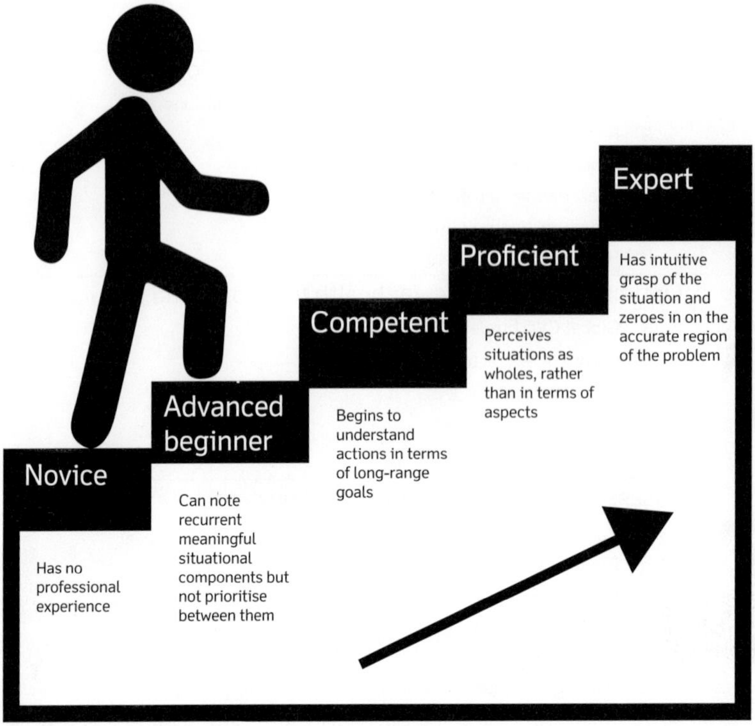

Fig. 3.1 The continuum of nursing experience.
Source data from Benner P, From Novice to Expert: Excellence and Power in Clinical Nursing Practice, Commemorative Edition, 2001.

(2001),[5] recognizing that the process of becoming a skilled cardiovascular nurse occurs on a continuum over time. Accordingly, nurses move through the five levels of proficiency: novice, advanced beginner, competent, proficient, and expert (➤ **Fig. 3.1**).[5] This provides a vision for the future of how nurses can advance from novices to becoming experts and leaders in cardiovascular care.

Global standards in cardiovascular nursing competence are important, as nurses are highly mobile, and are frequently incentivized to move country to meet nursing shortages.[6] Within England alone, over 13.8% of National Health Service staff report a non-British nationality.[7] Some 67,559 staff are nationals of European Union countries and a further 63,818 staff come from Asia. Therefore, mechanisms need to be in place to ensure that internationally trained nurses have acceptable standards of practice underpinned by core curricula and competency-based education, such as the ACNAP core curriculum to ensure standardized levels of practice.[6] Nurses comprise the largest portion of the healthcare workforce, with around 28 million nurses working globally.[8]

With a highly mobile population, it is imperative to understand the significant contribution that nurses make in reducing the global burden of CVD across healthcare services. However, this contribution can be recognized only if cardiovascular nurses are appropriately educated and trained, equipped with the required knowledge and skills, and supported by relevant certifications. Therefore, it is an immediate priority for ACNAP to support the dissemination of the core curriculum to ensure that the comprehensive, explicit standards/guidelines encompassing educational preparation, roles, and competencies for cardiovascular nurses globally are accessible. Lifelong learning is required to ensure the maintenance of competencies, which then helps to assure quality cardiovascular care.

What is specialization and advanced nursing practice?

One of the key challenges is the variety of definitions which surround the concepts of specialization and advanced nursing practice, which are underpinned by research,

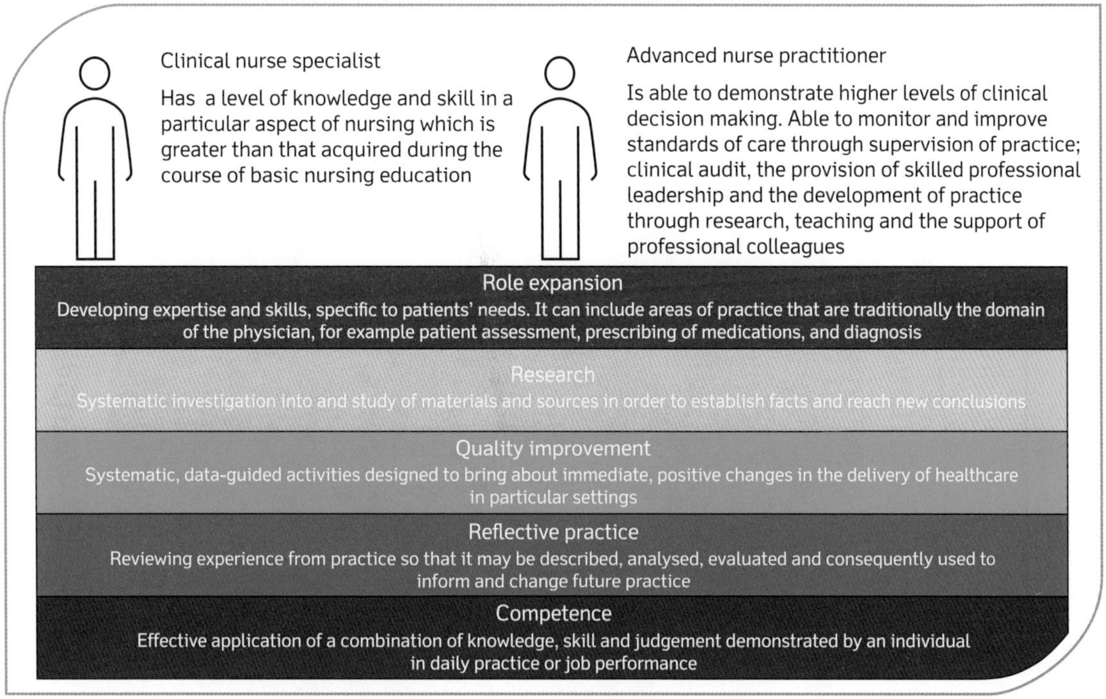

Clinical nurse specialist
Has a level of knowledge and skill in a particular aspect of nursing which is greater than that acquired during the course of basic nursing education
Advanced nurse practitioner
Is able to demonstrate higher levels of clinical decision making. Able to monitor and improve standards of care through supervision of practice; clinical audit, the provision of skilled professional leadership and the development of practice through research, teaching and the support of professional colleagues
Role expansion
Developing expertise and skills, specific to patients' needs. It can include areas of practice that are traditionally the domain of the physician, for example patient assessment, prescribing of medications, and diagnosis
Research
Systematic investigation into and study of materials and sources in order to establish facts and reach new conclusions
Quality improvement
Systematic, data-guided activities designed to bring about immediate, positive changes in the delivery of healthcare in particular settings
Reflective practice
Reviewing experience from practice so that it may be described, analysed, evaluated and consequently used to inform and change future practice
Competence
Effective application of a combination of knowledge, skill and judgement demonstrated by an individual in daily practice or job performance

Fig. 3.2 The foundations of specialization and advanced nursing practice.

continuing professional development, quality improvement, role expansion, and reflective practice (➤ **Fig. 3.2**).

In the absence of an international definition or title for nurses in expanded roles, the definition of 'advanced nursing/nurse practice' is used by the International Council of Nurses (ICN) to describe 'a registered nurse who has acquired expert knowledge, complex decision-making skills and clinical competencies for expanded practice, which is shaped by the country in which s/he is credentialed to practice'.[9] Ryley and Middleton (2016) suggest that advanced practice is a level of practice rather than a specific role.[10] However, a clear and legal title for the advanced practice nurse protects both the public and the practitioner and provides role clarity for all. Internationally, titles are many and varied; however, the terms clinical nurse specialist (CNS) and advanced nurse practitioner (ANP) are used frequently.[9,11] In Ireland, for example, these titles have now shaped the model of graduate to advanced practice,[12] providing a clear framework from graduate nurse to ANP (➤ **Fig. 3.3**).

Cardiovascular advanced nursing practice in Europe

The evidence shows that care provided by ANPs improves patient outcomes, is safe, acceptable, and cost neutral and ANPs now make up a growing percentage of the nursing workforce.[13] The US leads the way with a level of 5.6%, Canada 1.4%, the Netherlands 1.5%, and Ireland has projected growth from 0.2% to 2% of ANPs by 2021.[14] Advanced practice cardiovascular nursing in Europe is already in evidence, especially in the area of heart failure, with the ESC suggesting every hospital that manages patients with heart failure should employ a heart failure specialist nurse.[15] Cardiac rehabilitation recommends the inclusion of a cardiovascular nurse specialist as a team member in Portugal[16] and individual nurses have provided evidence of ANP benefits in cardiology services.[17]

Role expansion—a prerequisite for specialization and advanced practice

Role expansion of the general nurse is common in modern nursing and there is potential for the role expansion of nurses in line with health service needs.[18] Cardiovascular medicine has evolved into many specialities as evidenced by the affiliated groups of the ESC (seven Associations, seven Councils, and 15 Working Groups). With increasing specialization and evolving evidence-based care, patients' needs have become more complex and cardiovascular nursing has had to expand and specialize to provide expert

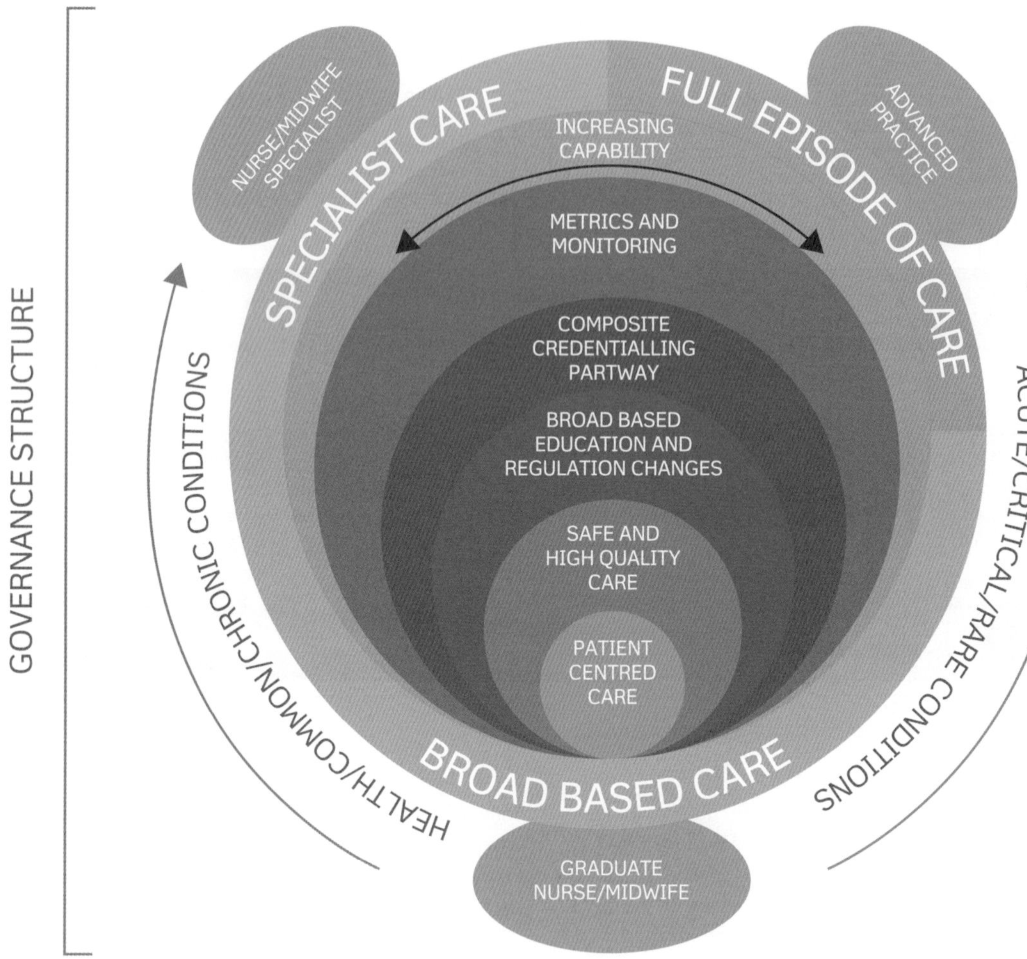

Fig. 3.3 Model of Advanced Practice.

Reproduced by kind permission of The Department of Health, Ireland. A Policy on the Development of Graduate to Advanced Nursing and Midwifery Practice.

care. In response to this, ANP roles have developed in many countries with cardiovascular medicine at the forefront. The American Heart Association suggests that advanced nursing roles within cardiology add to the quality of patient care and are cost-effective.[19] Cardiovascular medicine provides the nurse who wishes to expand their role with a variety of specialist areas in which to practise, as a generalist, specialist, or ANP. Historically, role expansion to 'specialist' nurse has been driven by the individual nurse in collaboration with the cardiologist[20] and while some countries in Europe have developed strategies for role development,[14] individual vision, drive, and determination remain the key drivers of specialist and advanced practice.

The goal of role expansion is to improve the quality of care provided by nurses, through enhanced competencies which expand the nurse's skills, capacity, and ability to deliver expert care.[18] Role expansion in cardiology nursing includes developing expertise and skills specific to patients' needs and can include areas of practice that are traditionally the domain of the physician, for example, patient assessment, prescribing of medications, and diagnosis. Role expansion brings an increase in autonomy[18] and consequently increased professional accountability within each individual professional's scope of practice. For example, Scope of Practice in Ireland is described as 'the range of roles, functions, responsibilities and activities which a registered nurse or registered midwife is educated, competent and has authority to perform'.[21] Internationally, it may define practice limitations within which the nurse may practise legally.[9] An Organisation for Economic Co-operation and Development (OECD) report reviewed the development of ANPs in 12 countries, ten of which were European, and found that ANPs improve access, reduce waiting times, and provide equal quality care to that of physicians with a high level of patient satisfaction.[13]

Education to achieve specialization and advanced practice status

Although a cardiovascular nurse's education may begin in the coronary care unit, cardiac surgical unit, and/or cardiac catheterization laboratory, there are many routes into cardiovascular nurse specialization. Working in acute environments exposes the nurse to a variety of cardiac conditions, interdisciplinary teamwork, and emergency nursing actions, and facilitates the beginning of electrocardiogram interpretation, a specialist skill vital in all aspects of specialist cardiovascular care. However, primary care is an excellent environment to develop holistic skills in cardiovascular risk factors and prevention. There is no right way or wrong way to become a cardiovascular nurse specialist, but continuing professional development is the hallmark of specialization. The ICN suggests the ANP is educated to master's degree level, but this varies by country.[22] In Ireland, for example, the CNS is educated to postgraduate diploma level in the specialist area of practice, while the ANP is educated to a master's level qualification.

As cardiovascular care covers many different conditions, treatments, and interventions, in addition to the core curriculum[4] described earlier, specialist curricula are also required to inform the continuing professional development of cardiovascular nurses and complement the core curriculum. Heart failure, for example, is a global and complex condition in which ANP roles have evolved and grown.[23] The Heart Failure Association of the ESC, in collaboration with ACNAP, has developed a heart failure-specific educational curriculum for nurses.[24] The American College of Cardiology is developing competencies for ANPS that are similar to those for physician training and specific to the care of cardiovascular patients.[19] Similarly, the European Association of Percutaneous Coronary Intervention has developed a certification to assure optimal quality in interventional cardiology by assessing the knowledge and attitudes of nurses and allied professionals. Although national standards for cardiovascular care have not been comprehensively developed, the ESC generates a variety of guidelines that provide nurses with a clinical framework to benchmark clinical practice and be safe in the knowledge that they are providing evidence-based care.

Regulation, barriers, and enablers

Regulation of advanced nursing practice is vital to protect both the patient and the practitioner and ensures safe and competent nursing care from skilled providers. In Europe, the extensive nursing workforce is not all at graduate level,[4] with some countries requiring state licensing instead of professional registration. In a survey of European countries to determine international ANP regulation, it was found that CNS posts existed in nine countries with formal regulation provided in four countries.[11,22] In addition, these surveys revealed that ANP posts existed in nine countries, with formal regulation in Ireland, Norway, the Netherlands, and Spain.

In response to an ageing population, chronic disease, delayed access to care, and extended waiting lists, policies on the development of graduate to advanced nursing (and midwifery) have been developed.[14] The goal of policies are to support nurses to progress from graduate to ANP within 1–2 years, moving from competent to capable, novice to expert. Policy documents will now enable nurses to develop in a structured way. Other enablers to ANP include role clarity, working within a team of ANP, belonging to ANP associations locally and internationally, national policy, graduate education, support of clinical mentors, and being part of a clinical indemnity scheme for legal protection and representation.[14,19] Specific barriers to becoming an ANP have been described by nurses, including lack of role clarity and lack of national policies (➤ Box 3.2).

Clinical experience and core competencies

Clinical experience in a specific area of cardiovascular care often shapes the ANP speciality. The difference between a general registered nurse and an ANP within a speciality is the depth of knowledge and critical thinking skills the ANP brings to the area.[9] The ICN has devised competencies for the general nurse and a framework for the nurse specialist.[25] A CNS will hone their focus of knowledge and experience into a specific speciality such as heart failure. However, an ANP will extend into the 'medical' domain, diagnosing and managing the patient, within a particular speciality. As such, they expand their level of knowledge and competence from that of a specialist nurse.[9]

Box 3.2 Barriers to advanced nursing practice frequently cited by nurses

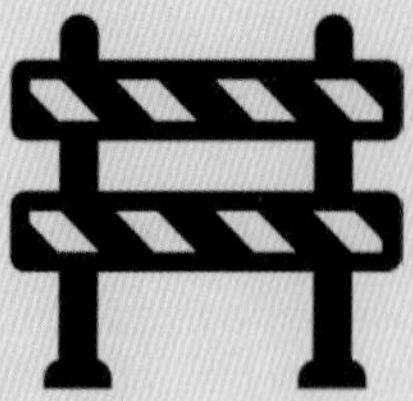

- Lack of role clarity
- Lack of national policies
- Limited financial support
- Large caseloads
- Working alone
- No mentorship
- Lack of regulation
- Undervalued roles
- Limited access to diagnostics
- Opposition of other healthcare providers
- Unwillingness of physicians to delegate or provide clinical supervision
- Lack of insurance support
- Varied role titles leading to lack of identification with roles of others
- Limitations to nurse prescribing

National standards of the duration of clinical experience required to practise as an ANP vary; the US requirement is 4–6 years' experience, and Ireland is now reduced to 2 years from 5 years to achieve ANP level. Specific supervised experiential learning requirements for ANP also vary by country, with the US requiring 750 hours and Ireland 500 hours.[14] European countries also have specific frameworks for advanced practice such as in Wales[10] and in Germany.[9]

The ANP leads a service, thereby taking responsibility and clinical accountability for a specified caseload, which includes diagnosis and management planning. Many ANPs practise autonomously, including completing an episode of care and discharging or referring the patient to another service or clinician. While some practice aspects overlap, including advanced physical assessment and diagnosis, nursing knowledge and experience inform the ANP's autonomous decision-making.[20]

Competence

The ICN suggests that 'competence' is 'the effective application of a combination of knowledge, skill and judgement demonstrated by an individual in daily practice or job performance'.[25] In Ireland, competence is 'the effective and creative demonstration and deployment of advanced knowledge and skill in human situations, based on professional attitudes, emotions, values, and sense of self-efficacy of each ANP, as well as advanced knowledge of procedures'.[14]

Core competencies of the clinical nurse specialist—based on the Irish model (Office of the Nursing and Midwifery Service Director)

The CNS will often work within the multidisciplinary team and closely with medical colleagues to provide specialized assessment, planning, delivery, and evaluation of care utilizing protocol-driven guidelines.[14] In Ireland, the CNS must have at least 1 year of experience in the specialist area of care and provide evidence of experience and education relevant to the area of practice. The CNS role in Ireland centres on five core competencies (➤ Fig. 3.4).

Internationally, it is recognized that heart failure specialist nurses play an essential role within a multidisciplinary heart failure management programme with roles including the provision of education to patients and their families, optimization of disease-modifying medications, and monitoring and early detection of indicators of clinical decompensation.[24]

Core competencies of the advanced nurse practitioner

Registered ANPs work in partnership with other healthcare colleagues and provide holistic assessment, diagnosis, autonomous decision-making regarding treatment, interventions, and discharge from an episode of care as per the core concepts (➤ Fig. 3.5 and ➤ Box 3.3). Despite the described competencies, some role crossover is evident in Europe due to differing role titles.

In the current climate of medical practitioner shortages, it is tempting to perceive the ANP as a replacement for the physician. As the nursing role expands, there is a crossover with roles and skills traditionally undertaken by other healthcare professionals, such as physicians,[9] and this is most apparent in the ANP role where comparison is often made. This can either enhance professional collaboration or divide. Nursing is more than just a set of tasks and a competency-led model of care can ensure that the ANP is bringing the 'core values' of nursing care to her or his advanced practice.[12]

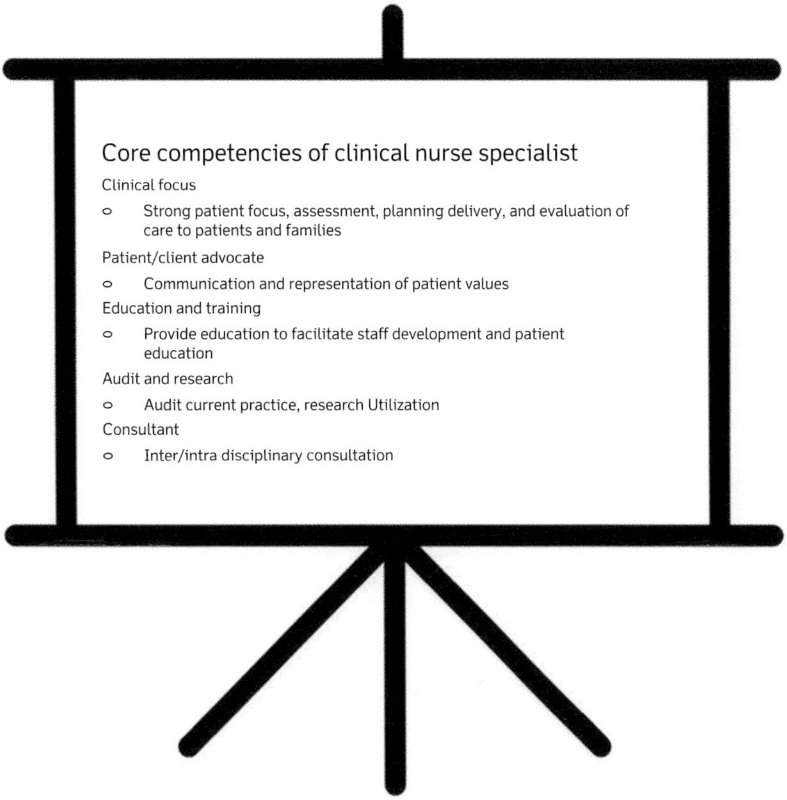

Fig. 3.4 The five core concepts of the CNS role in Ireland.

Prescribing/referral of medications and/or ionizing radiation

Prescribing medications and referring for X-ray are advanced skills traditionally in the physician's remit. With the success of nurse prescribing of medications[26] and radiation,[27] other healthcare professionals are becoming prescribers.[28] Nurse prescribing is beyond the scope of this chapter (see Chapter 12) but is considered an integral component of ANP in several European countries (Ireland, the UK, the Netherlands, and Sweden) with varying restrictions, education, and regulation.

Advanced nursing practice varies greatly throughout Europe. In Ireland, there is now a clearly defined pathway from general, specialist, to ANP. Although direction and regulation may be lacking in many countries, advanced nursing practice roles have traditionally been developed by pioneering, innovative, and driven cardiovascular nurses.[23,29] Using advanced nursing practice networks internationally and nationally can provide nurses with direction and support (➤ Box 3.4) and ESC Guidelines provide evidence-based care pathways for the varied specialities. Schober's (2016) ICN publication provides a wealth of information on advanced nursing practice with excellent sections on role development.[9] ANPs provide safe, patient-focused care and are entrepreneurs and leaders.[30] Cardiology nursing provides many opportunities to achieve this.

Timely and efficient integrated care: the role of teamwork and collaboration

Healthcare models have evolved in response to more complex patient needs and services facing major challenges to operate more efficiently to cope with population changes.[31] An ageing population due to higher life expectancy, exponential increase in chronic and lifestyle-related

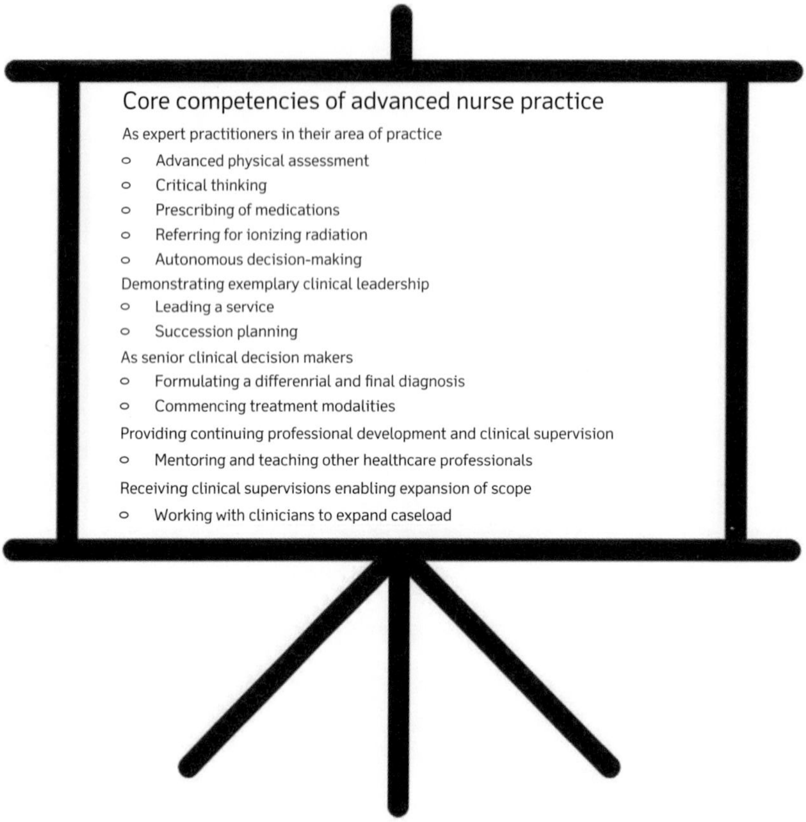
Core competencies of advanced nurse practice
As expert practitioners in their area of practice
Advanced physical assessment
Critical thinking
Prescribing of medications
Referring for ionizing radiation
Autonomous decision-making
Demonstrating exemplary clinical leadership
Leading a service
Succession planning
As senior clinical decision makers
Formulating a differenrial and final diagnosis
Commencing treatment modalities
Providing continuing professional development and clinical supervision
Mentoring and teaching other healthcare professionals
Receiving clinical supervisions enabling expansion of scope
Working with clinicians to expand caseload

Fig. 3.5 Core competencies of advanced nurse practice.

illnesses such as cardiovascular conditions, and chronic mental or physical illnesses/disabilities will continue to present significant challenges that will require skilled care.[32] Due to the complexity of CVD, no single profession is able to provide safe and effective care, or have the knowledge, skills, or resources to meet all of these requirements.[31] Several examples of integrated, collaborative, and comprehensive care models have been proposed which promote teamwork rather than single disciplines working in silos.[31,33]

The term 'collaboration' is widely used, but may be misunderstood because its meaning is dependent on particular settings.[34] We can consider three modes of cross-disciplinary, team-based care as defined in ➤ Table 3.1. These are all proven effective across the spectrum of management of CVD with reduced hospitalizations, length of stay, and mortality.[35]

Several elements (principles, competencies, determinants, drivers, and barriers) of collaborative practice have been described in the literature (➤ Fig. 3.6).[36]

Morley and colleagues highlight key determinants of team collaboration related to structural, psychological, and educational factors[34]:

- Structural determinants (opportunity).
- Psychological determinants (willingness).
- Educational determinants (ability).

They also classify elements in three axes: content, processes, and behaviours of the team, where processes are related to organizational structures.[34] The articulation of these elements helps us to understand, develop, and contextualize a framework for effective interprofessional teamwork. This is also useful for teaching and assessing interprofessional teamwork competencies and identifying strengths, as well as areas needing improvement.[37] Team training has been identified as a critical curricular need, both at undergraduate and postgraduate levels, advocating more shared interprofessional learning to create common teamwork competencies.[37]

Box 3.3 An example of the advanced nurse practitioner role in chest pain assessment in the emergency department

Chest pain is a principal presenting complaint to this tertiary care hospital. Presentations had increased from 5% of all presentations in 2009, to 11% in 2018. In 2009, 48% of all patients presenting with chest pain were admitted to hospital, often remaining on a trolley in the emergency department for several days, while awaiting an inpatient bed/further investigation. This presented a real problem for the hospital with reduced access to emergency bed capacity, growing numbers of patients cared for on trolleys, and increased use of available in-hospital beds. The primary goal of the evaluation of the patient who presents with chest pain is to accurately risk stratify and either identify, or exclude, a diagnosis of acute coronary syndrome.

The ANP assesses the patient with chest pain in the emergency department autonomously. The ANP performs a comprehensive assessment of health history, advanced physical assessment (including auscultation of heart sounds), electrocardiogram interpretation, blood testing and interpretation, chest X-ray referral, and risk stratification. Utilizing ESC Guidelines and clinical acumen, the ANP rules in/out acute coronary syndrome and other serous causes (i.e. pulmonary embolism as a priority) and then assesses for possible stable heart disease and/or a non-cardiac cause for the chest pain. Health promotion is a core component of the care that is provided.

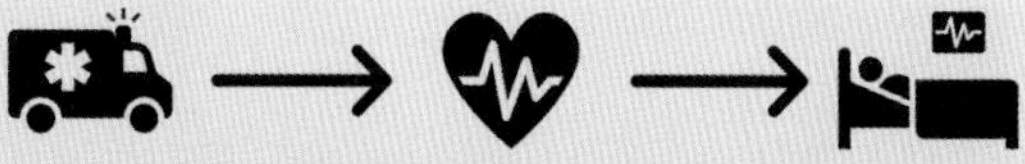

Once acute coronary syndrome/cardiac chest pain is ruled out and the patient categorized as being at low–intermediate risk of a major adverse cardiac event in 30 days, the ANP discharges them to primary care. If there is a potential differential diagnosis of stable angina, the ANP discharges the patient to the joint ANP/CNS-led chest pain clinic for exercise stress testing within 72 hours. The ANP reports on the exercise stress test, refers for invasive testing, prescribes medications if required, and/or discharges the patient who receives a diagnosis while avoiding hospital admission. Although the ANP practises autonomously, and the majority of their patients do not see a physician, they work as part of the interdisciplinary cardiology team as, inevitably, there will be cases outside the ANP's scope of practice.

The cardiology ANP-led chest pain service has delivered remarkable patient benefits in the last 8 years with limited resource investment including the avoidance of almost 600 inpatient admissions per year. Within the first year, acute hospital admissions were reduced by 36%, and waiting on emergency department trolleys by 60%, contributing to significant savings for the hospital.

Reflective practice

An important part of continuing professional development and improvement of the quality of services is reflective practice. The reflective practitioner will find opportunities for improvements in service development because they will always consider how better to conduct care, especially in the event of care practice going particularly well or going wrong. Developing skills for critical evaluation of the application of research and evidence-based guidelines to everyday clinical practice is essential. However, this should be in the context of a critical awareness of the limitations that clinicians and service providers face in their ability to develop and deliver services that adhere to these guidelines.

Critical reflection on the quality of care centres on a number of factors which include the philosophy of care, moral dilemmas in decision-making, clinical decision-making, and audit, research, and evaluation (➤ **Fig. 3.7**).[38]

Reflective practice is an important learning process involving capturing an experience and analysing and evaluating it in order to improve practice. Knowledge does not ensure good practice. Likewise, experience alone does not lead to learning. For example, breaking bad news is a skill that can be taught and theoretically applied but it is the deliberative reflection on this experience that forms the essential integration of knowledge to practise, enabling self-development and better patient care going forward. Reflective practice is also integral to development of the nursing profession and is a central feature in the revalidation process.[39] Consequently, acquisition and implementation of this important skill is essential to nursing practice. The following aims to provide nurses with an understanding of reflective clinical practice and why it matters, together with practical guidance on how to effectively apply reflection into clinical practice.

Reflective clinical practice: what is it and why does it matter?

The concept of reflective practice originated in 1984 from Donald Schon.[39] It is recognized as an essential skill that

Box 3.4 Examples of advanced nursing practice networks in Europe

ICN Nurse Practitioner/Advanced Practice Nursing Network
https://international.aanp.org/Practice/APNRoles#ICNGlobalAPN

The Irish association of Advanced Nurse & Midwife Practitioners
www.iaanmp.com

German Networks Advanced Practice Nursing & Advanced Nursing Practice
www.dnapn.de

Royal College of Nursing
https://www.rcn.org.uk/library/subject-guides/advanced-nursing-practice

NHS Scotland
https://www.nhsggc.org.uk/about-us/professional-support-sites/nurses-midwives/advanced-nurse-practitioners/

Table 3.1 Definitions of cross-disciplinary team-based care

Type of cross-disciplinary team	Definition
Multidisciplinary—'multi-' means 'more than one'	Mixed-discipline practitioners who tend to work in relative isolation with particular unshared goals
Interdisciplinary	Implies not only collaboration but also interaction of professionals from different backgrounds bringing together expertise to achieve common goals through cohesive shared plans, in a more profound level considering the patient and family 'as a key member of the care team'
Transdisciplinary	Also includes non-healthcare partners, and encourages team members to move beyond their discipline integrating expertise to solve problems and generate new knowledge Reported examples of this model include family-initiated escalation of care and palliative cardiovascular care

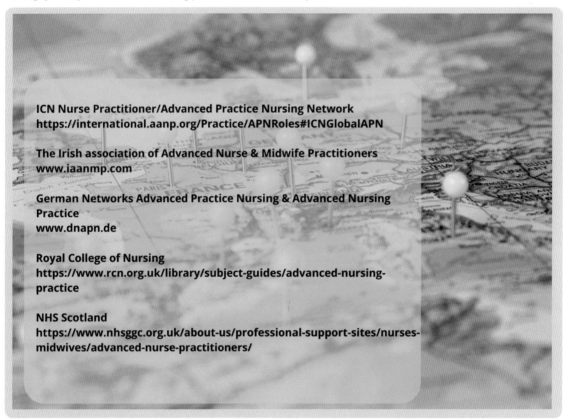

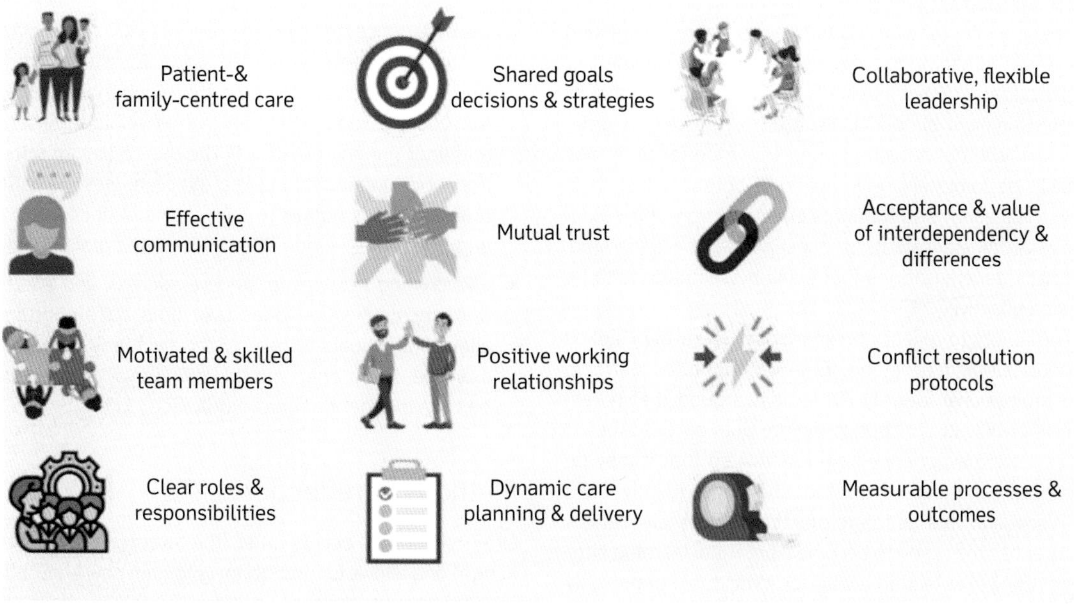

Fig. 3.6 Key elements required for effective interdisciplinary teamwork.

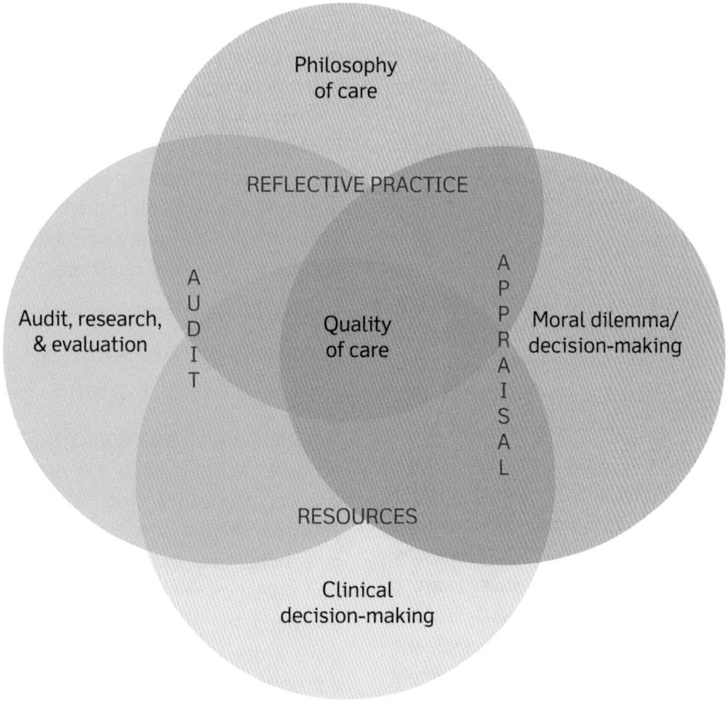

Fig. 3.7 Critical reflection on daily reality.

Reproduced from Esterhuizen P, Freshwater D, Freshwater C, et al. Clinical supervision and reflective practice, Int Textb Reflective Pract Nursing, Chichester Wiley-Blackwell 2008; 119–136 with permission from John Wiley and Sons.

should be applied at every level of nursing practice. In essence, it allows for learning from experiences by 'making sense' of them through a process of *describing, analysing,* and *evaluating*.[40] Gibbs clearly captures this, stating: 'It is not sufficient simply to have an experience in order to learn. Without reflecting upon this experience, it may quickly be forgotten, or its learning potential lost. It is from the feelings and thoughts emerging from this reflection that generalisations or concepts can be generated. And it is generalisations that allow new situations to be tackled effectively.'[41]

The ability to reflect on experiences is strongly linked to deep learning, development of self-regulated learning, and professional identity. While it is argued that reflection is a difficult concept to define, Bulman describes it as 'reviewing experience from practice so that it may be described, analysed, evaluated and consequently used to inform and change future practice'.[42] Every clinical encounter has the scope to become a potential learning situation. Clinical reflection allows for individuals to not only learn from mistakes and poor choices but also to acknowledge when things have gone well.

There are many reasons why reflection in clinical practice is important, including:

- *Development of practice*: reflective clinical practice assists nurses to sort through information, negotiate the confusing or complex situations within their practice, and to examine the context of practice from a variety of perspectives. This enables practitioners to gain a deeper understating of the issues and to identify the best course of action to optimize outcomes in practice. Nurses who take the time to reflect on their daily experiences have been shown to provide enhanced nursing care, have a better understanding of their actions, which in return develops their professional skills.[43] Ultimately this learning both enhances development of nursing practice as well as providing better care to the patients.
- *Continual professional development and revalidation*: reflective clinical practice is also a requirement for many regulated health professions, including nursing. Demonstrating evidence of critical reflection and the ability to identify one's own strengths and weaknesses, together with the development of a needs-driven learning plan that aims to continually enhance competence, is key to demonstrating continual professional development, maintaining registration, and is also a core requirement in nursing revalidation.[2]
- *Coping with emotions*: nurses suffer emotional trauma and reflective practice facilitates coping. The process of reflection has been shown to help nurses to recognize the experience that caused them distress or uneasiness in order to gain a better understanding of their personal response, disperse the emotional load, and think deeply about what they learned about themselves and their nursing practice.[44] The day-to-day emotional impact of nursing can take a toll on nurses. Reflective practice allows nurses to have a safe outlet to discuss and better understand their feelings and practice.
- *Overcoming barriers to achieve success and positive outcomes*: reflection does take time but importantly allows individuals to take a step back and objectively examine situations, and identify ways to overcome barriers in order to improve quality.

Methods of reflection

Often reflection occurs after the event (reflection-on-action) and allows for practitioners to gain new knowledge from experiences through a process of thinking about what happened, analysing the actions that were performed, and identifying what would change the outcome next time. Reflection can also occur prior to and during an event or experience. Reflection-in-action is more advanced and involves practitioners reflecting on practice while it is happening, where gains in understanding enable a situation and outcome to change in real time.

Commonly, reflection is informal with no formalized recording. For example, individuals may think about a particular incident that day or a group or team of individuals may look at a particular situation together and learn from each other. It is useful to structure these informal reflections using three key questions[40]:

1. What went well?
2. What did not go so well?
3. What would you do differently next time?

More formalized reflection, such as producing a written account, provides for a more meaningful reflection and enables deeper learning. There are many different examples of frameworks that can be helpful to structuring reflections.[45] For example, Boud and colleagues highlight that reflection is returning to that whole experience and analysing the situation.[46] Re-evaluating the experience gives a new perspective on that experience, resulting in a possible change of behaviour. This framework also acknowledges that change in practice is dependent on an individual's readiness for application and commitment to action (➤ Fig. 3.8).

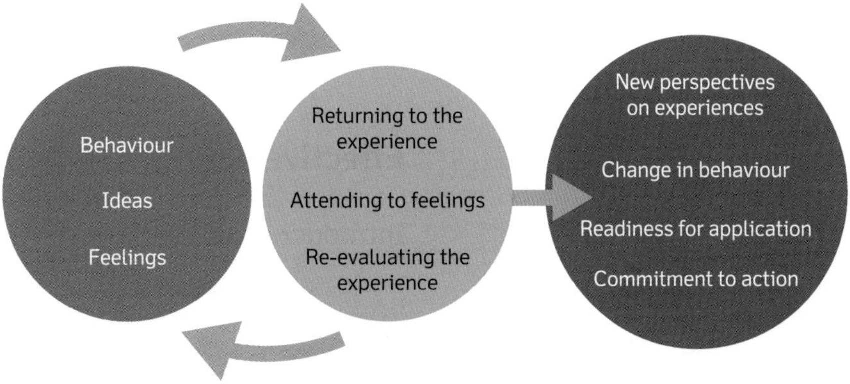

Fig. 3.8 Boud's framework for refection.

Source data from Boud D, Keogh R, Walker D. Reflection: Turning experience into learning. Routledge, 2013.

Gibbs' reflective cycle (➤ Fig. 3.9) builds on Boud's model and acknowledges that personal feelings influence the situation. This framework breaks down reflection into further stages of evaluation and analysis and recognizes there is a clear link between the learning that has happened from the experience and future practice.

Practice application

As highlighted previously, reflective practice is an important process. From students to practising nurses, reflection encourages growth and helps nurses continue to provide the best care to patients. A greater emphasis

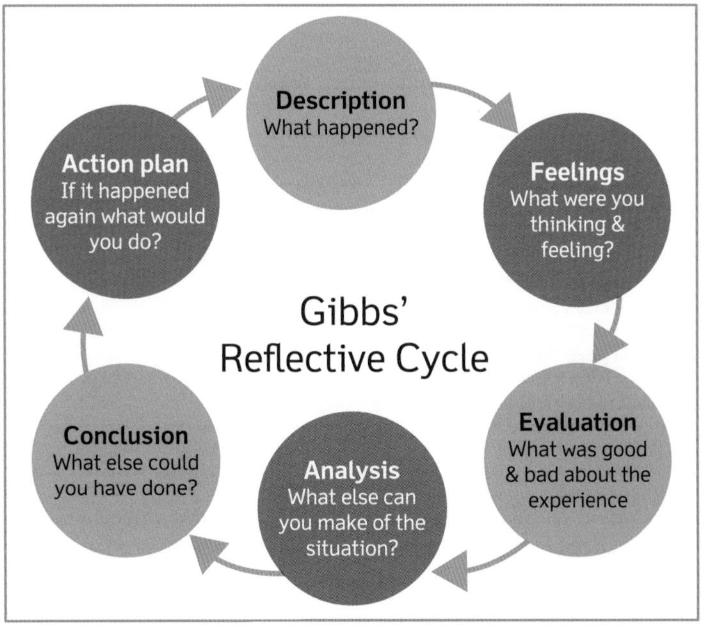

Fig. 3.9 Gibbs' reflective cycle.

Source data from Gibbs G. Learning by doing: A guide to teaching and learning methods. Further Education Unit, Oxford Polytechnic, 1998.

is now being placed on continuous professional practice with many professional bodies requiring the submission of written reflections to be provided as evidence of learning. Gibbs' framework (➤ **Table. 3.2**) provides a useful template to support nurses in this important process.

In summary, clinical reflection is a vital tool in nursing practice. It enables individuals to learn from their experiences and actions, resulting in better understanding, knowledge, and, ultimately, better patient care. Reflective ability is a learned skill of critical thinking and situation analysis that can be developed. Nurses at every level of their career are encouraged to draw on existing frameworks to support this important learning process. Developing a portfolio of reflections and journal keeping are particularly encouraged together with ensuring to seek feedback and to reflect on that feedback. Professional practice requires competency and the ability to think reflectively, with many regulatory bodies now requiring evidence of critical reflection. Consequently, acquisition and implementation of this important skill is essential to nursing practice.

Effective nursing leadership

Introduction

Leadership is an essential feature of any healthcare organization, enabling the delivery of high-quality patient care by balancing issues such as welfare of personnel, general resource management, and cost-efficiency alongside the organizational vision. The mission, attitude, and behaviours of a healthcare organization begin with its leadership, which creates the vision and purpose of the organization.

Table 3.2 Example template for written reflections using Gibbs' cycle.

Description	*What learning did I apply to real-world clinical practice?*
	What exactly did I do and how would I describe it precisely?
Feelings	*How exactly did I feel during this application of my learning?*
Evaluation	*What was I trying to achieve?*
	Why did I choose that particular action?
	What went well?
	What did not go so well?
	What criteria am I using to judge success?
Analysis	*What sense can I make of this in light of my past experience?*
	What factors were influencing me?
	Could I have handled this better in a similar situation?
	How do I now feel about this experience?
	Can I support myself or others better as a consequence?
	Faced with that experience again, what would I do?
Conclusion	*What can be concluded, in a general sense, from these experiences and the analyses I have undertaken?*
	What can be concluded about my own specific ways of working?
Action plan	*What am I going to do differently in this type of situation next time?*
	What steps am I going to take on the basis of what I have learnt?

All nurses are leaders

The notion that leadership is the domain of the more experienced, senior, or powerful nurse is outdated, and recent literature confidently asserts that every nurse is a leader, responsible for the quality of care that they personally provide and that delivered by their team.[47] A devolved, rather than hierarchical, leadership structure encourages opportunities for healthcare improvement and fosters innovation at team and organizational levels. A key component of your role as a cardiovascular nurse is to recognize and respond to opportunities for healthcare improvement, offering every patient the highest standards of care. The ACNAP Be Guideline Smart Initiative (https://www.escardio.org/Sub-specialty-communities/Association-of-Cardiovascular-Nursing-&-Allied-Professions/Education/be-guidelines-smart) has produced a range of resources that educate and empower nurses like you to advocate for the patient and challenge suboptimal care. These types of educational resources enable cardiovascular nurses at all levels to demonstrate their leadership potential and strategies for change. You are encouraged to join ACNAP and learn more on how to unleash your own leadership potential.

What is leadership in nursing and why is it important?

Definitions of leadership are illusive and conflicting. Leadership has been variously defined as the ability to bring individuals to success with the minimum conflict and the maximum cooperation, allowing leaders to be able to make decisions using authority,[48] or 'the process of getting people to do their best to achieve a desired result. It involves developing and communicating a vision for the future, motivating people and gaining their engagement'.[49] These definitions show how the concept varies within the literature and across different settings, so this section aims to provide a more holistic understanding of the leadership concept, with key leadership theories outlined in ➤ Table 3.3.[50]

The debate around whether leaders are born or made largely concludes that because leadership is a social construct, it can be fostered, developed, and modulated for different circumstances.[47] There are also different perspectives on the factors that may influence effective leadership and how these can lead to transformation in service delivery. A key facet is that leadership is relational—and that effective leaders have an impact, by effecting a change in the behaviour of others. The concept of emotional intelligence has been proffered as a key mechanism by which such change is achieved.[47] The Cumulative Index to Nursing and Allied Health Literature (CINAHL) defines emotional intelligence as the intentional and intelligent use of emotions to help guide behaviour and thinking. Nurses are consistently regarded across many different cultures as compassionate and trustworthy, and those emotions have now been recognized as central components of effective healthcare leadership. Research

Table 3.3 Summary of traditional leadership theories

Great man theories	Based on the belief that leaders are born with innate qualities and are destined to become leaders
Trait theories	Leaders possess certain traits that are positive in nature. Fits in well with 'great man theories'
Behaviourist theories	Focuses on what leaders do rather than on their qualities
Situational leadership	Leadership is specific to the situation; leaders will adapt their style according to the specific situation they are in
Contingency theory	This is a refinement of situational leadership. Focuses on identifying situational variables and matching this with a specific leadership style to suit
Transactional theory	Emphasizes the relationship between leaders and followers, focusing on mutual benefits
Transformational theory	Change is the central concept and leadership is about empowering followers to excel in their performance

Source data from Bolden R, Gosling J, Marturano A, et al. A Review of Leadership Theory and Competency Frameworks. Exeter, 2003.

conducted regarding nursing leadership has revealed that a culture of effective leadership within the field of healthcare is associated with improved patient outcomes, higher job satisfaction, and reduced nursing staff turnover rates.[51]

What kinds of leadership work best in nursing?

There are many different styles of leadership available (➤ **Table 3.3**), but to be successful, nurse leaders require high levels of cognitive ability in order to consistently coordinate all elements of the clinical setting and effectively quality assure patient-centred clinical nursing care practices. Within this context, transformational leadership has been regarded favourably in hospital, primary care, and community settings.[52] Transformation refers to a process of interaction between the leader and the other staff, that moves them towards workplace goal achievement. Pullen claims that transformational leadership generates positive change in people and social systems with the ultimate goal of changing followers into leaders.[53] The concept focuses on inspiring the team to carry out their responsibilities to the best of their abilities, whereby the leader creates a 'shared vision' of the future that others buy into.[54] The leader will earn respect from followers by role modelling exemplary behaviour that inspires others to emulate similar traits, transforming the quality of healthcare provision among nursing staff. Innovation based on problem-solving initiatives and transmission of values along with ethical principles are significant in this transformational form of leadership.

While many of these behaviours are irrefutable, more recently the concept of transformational leadership has been challenged because of its hierarchical approach, conflicting evidence that it produces superior outcomes,[55,56] and concern that it is an idealistic concept[57] that puts unrealistic pressure on individuals. Providing the highest standards of patient care is extremely challenging for nurses in the post-coronavirus 2019 (COVID-19) era, with its continually changing and demanding healthcare environment. One of the biggest problems experienced within the sector is enabling staff to influence change and motivate teams towards patient-centred care in such adverse circumstances. With considerable cost-efficiencies required in healthcare to deliver affordable services, the sector is under pressure—staff shortages exist right across the international healthcare workforce, stress levels are high, and burnout is common.[58] All too often, nurses seem pulled between increasing their productivity and delivering safe and effective care and there is clear evidence that such job strain in nurses impacts their own health outcomes.[59] The COVID-19 pandemic has emphasized the interconnectedness of global healthcare and the imperative of collaboration in solving current healthcare challenges. It is in this context that compassionate leadership has emerged as potentially of greater value to nursing and the healthcare professions than process-orientated styles of leadership, given the nature of our work and the goals we aspire to.[60]

Compassionate leadership in healthcare

Compassionate leadership encourages a move away from heroic models of leading, to a more collaborative approach in which all members of the healthcare team are seen and heard. Advocating for patients is a priority and because values and goals are shared within teams, there can be more devolved decision-making at all levels in the organization.[61] ➤ **Table 3.4** outlines the strategies needed to create a compassionate culture within the workplace.[62] It is evident that this is a devolved approach to leadership, but the important point is that it starts at the level

Table 3.4 The essence of effective healthcare leadership

1	Support, trust, and compassion
2	Valuing diversity and fairness
3	Building effective teams
4	Building relationships across boundaries
5	Promoting learning and innovation
6	Promoting others' development and leadership
7	Ensuring effective performance
8	Ensuring necessary resources are available and used well
9	Ensuring direction and alignment
10	Developing positivity, pride, and identity

Source data from West MA, Chowla R. Compassionate leadership for compassionate health care. In: Gilbert P (ed) Compassion: Concepts, research and applications. London: Routledge, pp. 237–257.

of the individual. Each one of us as nurses can make the move to a compassionate culture, starting with ourselves. Edmondson[63] underlines the importance of being authentic—open to change and honest enough to stand over our mistakes. He advocates a 'humble curiosity', where appreciation and gratitude breed a culture of optimism that makes commitment and motivation palpable within yourself and your team.

Identifying new leaders is critical to the future success of nursing. It is important for nursing staff to build effective nursing leadership structures for better clinical care, contributing to patient safety outcomes in everyday nursing practice.

Clinical leadership in nursing

In the nursing literature, the concept of nursing clinical leadership is frequently linked to management and official roles.[64] A clinical leader is described as a nurse directly involved in offering clinical care that continuously improves the quality of patient experience and outcomes by influencing other people.[64] Nursing leadership necessitates instilling in the workplace a culture of professional and modern patient-centred nursing personnel. Kreindler[65] explores the politics of patient-centred care, explaining that leaders should emulate the positive aspects of each group's focus while guiding them towards putting patients first. Effective nursing leadership is important in all forms of work settings within clinical nursing practice, and especially in acute settings where swift decision-making is crucial to save lives. This is the case with clinical leadership in cardiovascular nursing, in which engagement as a nurse in a healthcare environment indisputably fits into that context. The major raison d'être for leadership in nursing is to determine the most suitable goals and objectives for the organization in relation to quality patient care.[48] Therefore, effective leadership is key to establishing successful nursing teams within the clinical environment.

In summary, leadership is an important aspect of any healthcare organization that enables the delivery of high-quality patient care by balancing issues such as welfare of personnel, general resource management, and the organizational vision as a whole. Definitions of leadership have evolved over recent years and it is now regarded as a collaborative and devolved process in which all nurses are recognized as leaders. This section has discussed the concept of leadership, explored key perspectives, and emphasized the importance of nursing leadership in enhancing patient outcomes as well as nurturing teamwork in organizations. It has considered clinical leadership in cardiovascular nursing and underlined the principles of emotional intelligence and compassionate leadership approaches in delivering effective nursing care in today's challenging clinical context. Cardiovascular nurses should be equipped with requisite knowledge, expertise, and support to become leaders in cardiovascular care. Self-reflection is a key component of effective leadership and the ACNAP website has a range of resources for you to learn more and to really grow your leadership potential within cardiovascular nursing.

Getting involved with professional societies, associations, and heart foundations

What professional development opportunities do societies, associations, and foundations provide for nurses working in cardiovascular care?

Developing a profile as a nurse is an important part of continuing professional development. An important route to achieving such a profile includes joining and linking in with professional associations, societies, and heart foundations. These groups can provide several opportunities such as furthering education, funding and mentoring for doctoral, postdoctoral studies, and other research, networking with colleagues beyond the confines of one's institution, and leadership. They can also provide support to patients and caregivers, influence policy, and advocate for both professionals and patients. Many of these groups produce educational materials and programmes, publish and disseminate research in journals, and offer patient and carer support groups.

Most associations serve as a primary source for lifelong learning. They offer a wide range of professional development opportunities including tools and resources to increase knowledge and build professional skills. They offer networking opportunities to access and connect with healthcare professionals facing similar work and patient-related challenges. They are a valuable resource for sharing best practices in cardiovascular care.

As the science around CVD evolves and demands on health professionals' time and attention continue to increase, lifelong learning is critical for providers and patients so that healthcare can be delivered at its highest level. Associations and societies are the cornerstone for the timely dissemination of new and important healthcare information.

It is especially important for nurses to become involved in professional groups. Nurses represent the largest segment of the healthcare workforce, are considered the most trustworthy of all professions (http://www.gallup.com/poll/1654/honesty-ethics-professions.aspx), and they play a critical role in our schools, hospitals, community health centres, long-term care facilities, and home care. These groups also work to ensure that nurses contribute to CVD guideline development committees, health-related boards, panels, and commissions.

The Institute of Medicine (IOM) report,[66] *The Future of Nursing: Leading Change, Advancing Health*, recommended increasing the number of nurse leaders in pivotal decision-making roles on boards and commissions that work to improve the health of everyone in the US. National and international nursing organizations continue to raise awareness that all healthcare-related boards and commissions benefit from having the unique perspective of nurses.

The Preventive Cardiovascular Nurses Association is a leading nursing organization dedicated to the prevention of CVD and stroke. The Preventive Cardiovascular Nurses Association's mission supports the important role of nursing in CVD and stroke prevention internationally by establishing and supporting the Global Cardiovascular Nursing Leadership Forum (GCNLF). The GCNLF explores ways in which nursing and global nursing organizations can support the established cardiovascular risk reduction and stroke reduction goal set by the World Health Organization to reduce deaths from non-communicable diseases by 25% by 2025. Recognizing that nurses and nursing organizations are on the frontlines of patient education, the GCNLF works to engage and mobilize an international community of nursing leaders to promote prevention through research, education, policy, and advocacy. In addition, the GCNLF aims to develop a mechanism for outreach to low- and middle-income countries where organized nursing practice and leadership is not well established or supported for the prevention of and rehabilitation from CVD and stroke.

ACNAP is one of seven associations of the ESC. The mission of ACNAP is to support nurses and allied professionals throughout Europe and more globally to deliver the best possible care to patients with CVD and their families. ACNAP provides a diverse portfolio of activities, including education, research, and mentorship. ACNAP has developed a core curriculum with key themes to support the continuing professional education of nurses working in cardiovascular settings; a portfolio of e-learning, which offers webinars and a clinical case gallery to help nurses and allied professionals learn from real-life, practice-based scenarios; a comprehensive Guidelines Implementation Toolkit, 'Be Guidelines Smart'; and one of the most highly ranked journals in the field, the *European Journal of Cardiovascular Nursing*.

Summary

Globally, nurses and nursing organizations are a central and essential component of research, practice, policy, and advocacy initiatives designed to promote CVD and stroke prevention. Nurses are an important part of the healthcare team in addressing the needs of patients and are uniquely positioned to play a major role in reducing the burden of CVD and stroke. Providing nurses with improved training, networking opportunities, and access to professional and patient education materials will save lives, improve quality of life, and reduce healthcare costs for those at risk for, or already living with, CVD or stroke.

Conclusion

In this chapter, we have examined the role of continuing professional development through the lens of the ESC core curriculum for cardiovascular nursing. Although there are challenges in defining what a CNS and ANP are, advanced nursing practice must be 'grounded in direct care or clinical work'.[67] It is essential that these roles are clearly defined and protected to ensure the safety of the public, and so that all team members have a clear understanding of what the CNS or ANP are able to do. Continuing professional development is essential to increase skills, and is widely endorsed as an essential part of every nurse's role. It is therefore critical that we work together as a team to best deliver patient- and family-centred care. Nurses exist as part of a skilled transdisciplinary team which is fostered by mutual trust, positive working relationships, and clear roles and responsibilities.

To enable high-quality care, continuing professional development requires nurses to become skilled at reflective practice, firstly to be able to critically reflect on our daily reality. Using a model, such as Gibbs' reflective cycle, nurses can form a detailed assessment of their reaction and form an action plan for what we should do if the same situation were to arise again. Skilled reflection is important for nurse leaders, who need to be able to reflect on how a team works together to improve patient- and family-centred care.

Developing new nursing leaders is critical to the future success of nursing. It is important for nursing staff to build effective nursing leadership roles such as team leadership and transformational leadership, among others, for better clinical care and patient safety outcomes every day in nursing practice. Leaders and aspiring leaders are encouraged to engage with professional societies, associations, and heart foundations, as these are important sources of support and continuing professional development.

References

1. World Health Organization. Preparing a Health Care Workforce for the 21st century: The Challenge of Chronic Conditions. Geneva: World Health Organization; 2005.
2. Aiken LH, Sermeus W, Van den Heede K, et al. Patient safety, satisfaction, and quality of hospital care: cross sectional surveys of nurses and patients in 12 countries in Europe and the United States. BMJ. 2012;344:e1717.
3. Driscoll A, Grant MJ, Carroll D, et al. The effect of nurse-to-patient ratios on nurse-sensitive patient outcomes in acute specialist units: a systematic review and meta-analysis. Eur J Cardiovasc Nurs. 2018;17(1):6–22.
4. Astin F, Carroll D, De Geest S, et al. A Core Curriculum for the Continuing Professional Development of Nurses Working in Cardiovascular Settings: developed by the Education Committee of the Council on Cardiovascular Nursing and Allied Professions (CCNAP) on behalf of the European Society of Cardiology. Eur J Cardiovasc Nurs. 2015;14(2 Suppl):S1–S17.
5. Benner P. From Novice to Expert (Commemorative Edition). Upper Saddle River, NJ: Prentice Hall Health; 2001.
6. Parker V, McMillan M. Challenges facing internationalisation of nursing practice, nurse education and nursing workforce in Australia. Contemp Nurse. 2007;24(2):128–36.
7. Baker C. NHS staff from overseas: statistics. House of Commons Library; 2020. https://commonslibrary.parliament.uk/research-briefings/cbp-7783/.
8. World Health Organization. State of the world's nursing 2020. 2020. https://apps.who.int/iris/rest/bitstreams/1274201/retrieve.
9. Schober M. Introduction to Advanced Nursing Practice. Cham: Springer; 2016.
10. Ryley N, Middleton C. Framework for advanced nursing, midwifery and allied health professional practice in Wales: the implementation process. J Nurs Manag. 2015;24(1):E70–76.
11. Carney M. Regulation of advanced nurse practice: its existence and regulatory dimensions from an international perspective. J Nurs Manag. 2015;24(1):105–14.
12. Office of the Chief Nursing Officer. Position paper one; values for nurses and midwives in Ireland, June 2016. Department of Health; 2016. https://www.nmbi.ie/NMBI/media/NMBI/Position-Paper-Values-for-Nurses-and-Midwives-June-2016.pdf.
13. Delamaire ML, Lafortune G. Nurses in Advanced Roles: A Description and Evaluation of Experiences in 12 Developed Countries. OECD Health Working Papers 54. Paris: OECD Publishing; 2010.
14. Department of Health. A policy on the development of graduate to advanced nursing and midwifery practice. 2019. https://health.gov.ie/wp-content/uploads/2019/07/2644-HE-advanced-NursingMidwiferyPracticePolicy-WEB-v2.pdf.
15. McDonagh TA, Blue L, Clark AL, et al. European Society of Cardiology Heart Failure Association Standards for delivering heart failure care. Eur J Heart Fail. 2011;13(3):235–41.
16. Abreu A, Mendes M, Dores H, et al. Mandatory criteria for cardiac rehabilitation programs: 2018 guidelines from the Portuguese Society of Cardiology. Rev Port Cardiol (Engl Ed). 2018;37(5):363–73.
17. Patel K, Brennan C. 63. Assessing the efficacy of a nurse-led cardioversion service on clinical outcomes. Heart. 2015;101(Suppl 4):A34.2–35.
18. Department of Health. Strategic framework for role expansion of nurses and midwives: promoting quality patient care. 2011 (last updated 2020). https://www.gov.ie/en/publication/c23ef1-strategic-framework-for-role-expansion-of-nurses-and-midwives-promot/.
19. Scordo KA, Stanik-Hutt JA, Melander S, Wyman JF, Madgic K. The advanced practice nurse as a member of the cardiovascular team. Adv Pract Nurs. 2016;1:4.
20. Ingram S. Advanced nurse practitioner registration in Ireland: an RANP cardiology's experience. Br J Card Nurs. 2014;9(4):177–85.
21. Nursing and Midwifery Board of Ireland. Scope of nursing and midwifery practice framework. 2015. https://www.nmbi.ie/Standards-Guidance/Scope-of-Practice/.
22. Heale R, Rieck Buckley C. An international perspective of advanced practice nursing regulation. Int Nurs Rev. 2015;62(3):421–29.
23. Ryder M. Is heart failure nursing practice at the level of a clinical nurse specialist or advanced nurse practitioner? The Irish experience. Eur J Cardiovasc Nurs. 2005;4(2):101–105.
24. Riley JP, Astin F, Crespo-Leiro MG, et al. Heart Failure Association of the European Society of Cardiology

heart failure nurse curriculum. Eur J Heart Fail. 2016;18(7):736–43.
25. International Council of Nurses. ICN Framework of Competencies for the Nurse Specialist (ICN Regulation Series). Geneva: International Council of Nurses; 2009.
26. Drennan J, Naughton C, Allen D, et al. National Independent Evaluation of the Nurse and Midwife Prescribing Initiative. Dublin: University College Dublin; 2009.
27. Drennan J, Naughton C, Griffins M, et al. An Evaluation of the HSE Guiding Framework for the Implementation of Nurse Prescribing of Medical Ionising Radiation (X-Ray) in Ireland. Dublin: Health Service Executive; 2014.
28. Royal College of Nursing. Clinical Imaging Requests from Non-Medically Qualified Professionals. London: Royal College of Nursing; 2008.
29. Blue L, McMurray J. How much responsibility should heart failure nurses take? Eur J Heart Fail. 2005;7(3):351–61.
30. Pearson H. Concepts of advanced practice: what does it mean? Br J Nurs. 2011;20(3):184–85.
31. Jennings C, Astin F. A multidisciplinary approach to prevention. Eur J Prev Cardiol. 2017;24(3 Suppl):77–87.
32. Kitson A, Conroy T, Kuluski K, et al. Reclaiming and Redefining the Fundamentals of Care: Nursing's Response to Meeting Patients' Basic Human Needs. Adelaide: School of Nursing, University of Adelaide.
33. Chamberlain-Salaun J, Mills J, Usher K. Terminology used to describe health care teams: an integrative review of the literature. J Multidiscip Healthc. 2013;6:65–74.
34. Morley L, Cashell A. Collaboration in health care. J Med Imaging Radiat Sci. 2017;48(2):207–16.
35. Baptiste D, Li Q, Milesky JL, et al. Advancing cardiovascular care through nursing research, quality improvement, and evidence-based practice. Shanghai Chest. 2019;3:13.
36. World Health Organization, Organisation for Economic Co-operation and Development, International Bank for Reconstruction and Development. Delivering quality health services: a global imperative for universal health coverage. World Health Organization; 2018. https://apps.who.int/iris/handle/10665/272465.
37. Hepp SL, Suter E, Jackson K, et al. Using an interprofessional competency framework to examine collaborative practice. J Interprof Care. 2015;29(2):131–37.
38. Esterhuizen P, Freshwater D. Clinical supervision and reflective practice. In: Freshwater D, Taylor B, Sherwood G (Eds) International Textbook of Reflective Practice in Nursing. Chichester: Wiley-Blackwell; 2008:119–36.
39. Schon DA. The Reflective Practitioner: How Professionals Think in Action. New York: Basic Books; 1984.
40. Ingram P, Murdoch M. How to reflect on your practice. Nursing in Practice; 2019. https//www.nursinginpractice.com/professional/how-to-reflect-on-your-practice/.
41. Gibbs G. Learning by Doing: A Guide to Teaching and Learning Methods. Oxford: Further Education Unit, Oxford Polytechnic; 1998.
42. Mabbott I. Reflective practice in nursing. Nurs Manage. 2012;19:8.
43. Caldwell L, Grobbel CC. The importance of reflective practice in nursing. Int J Caring Sci. 2013;6(3):319–26.
44. Rees KL. The role of reflective practices in enabling final year nursing students to respond to the distressing emotional challenges of nursing work. Nurse Educ Pract. 2013;13(1):48–52.
45. Bolton G. Narrative writing: reflective enquiry into professional practice. Educ Action Res. 2006;14(2):203–18.
46. Boud D, Keogh R, Walker D. Reflection: Turning Experience into Learning. London: Routledge; 2013.
47. Carragher J, Gormley K. Leadership and emotional intelligence in nursing and midwifery education and practice: a discussion paper. J Adv Nurs. 2016;73(1):85–96.
48. Ceylan H. Leadership in nursing. J Nurs Res Pract. 2018;2(2):20–21.
49. Armstrong M. Armstrong's Handbook of Management and Leadership: A Guide to Managing for Results. London: Kogan Page.
50. Bolden R, Gosling J, Marturano A, et al. A Review of Leadership Theory and Competency Frameworks. Exeter: Centre for Leadership Studies, University of Exeter; 2003.
51. Sfantou DF, Laliotis A, Patelarou AE, et al. Importance of leadership style towards quality of care measures in healthcare settings: a systematic review. Healthcare (Basel). 2017;5(4):73.
52. Solman A. Nursing leadership challenges and opportunities. J Nurs Manag. 2017;25(6):405–406.
53. Pullen RL. Leadership in nursing practice. Nurs Made Incred Easy! 2016;14(3):26–31.
54. Martin J, McCormack B, Fitzsimons D, et al. The importance of inspiring a shared vision. IPDJ. 2014;4(2):4.
55. Brewer CS, Kovner CT, Djukic M, et al. Impact of transformational leadership on nurse work outcomes. J Adv Nurs. 2016;72(11):2879–93.
56. Hutchinson M, Jackson D. Transformational leadership in nursing: towards a more critical interpretation. Nurs Inq. 2012;20(1):11–22.
57. Fast O, Rankin J. Rationing nurses: realities, practicalities, and nursing leadership theories. Nurs Inq. 2017;25(2):e12227.

58. Krystal JH, McNeil RL. Responding to the hidden pandemic for healthcare workers: stress. Nat Med. 2020;26(5):639.
59. Vesterlund GK, Keller AC, Heitmann BL. Changes in job strain and subsequent weight gain: a longitudinal study, based on the Danish Nurse Cohort. Public Health Nutr. 2017;21(6):1131–38.
60. Trzeciak S, Mazzarelli A. Compassionomics: The Revolutionary Scientific Evidence that Caring Makes a Difference. Pensacola, FL: Studer Group; 2019.
61. de Zulueta PC. Developing compassionate leadership in health care: an integrative review. J Healthc Leadersh. 2016;8:1–10.
62. West MA, Chowla R. Compassionate leadership for compassionate health care. In: Gilbert P (Ed) Compassion: Concepts, Research and Applications. London: Routledge; 2017:237–57.
63. Edmondson AC. The Fearless Organization: Creating Psychological Safety in the Workplace for Learning, Innovation, and Growth. Hoboken, NJ: John Wiley & Sons; 2018.
64. Al-Dossary RN. Leadership in nursing. In: Alvinius A (Ed) Contemporary Leadership Challenges. InTechOpen; 2017. https://www.intechopen.com/books/contemporary-leadership-challenges/leadership-in-nursing.
65. Kreindler SA. The politics of patient-centred care. Health Expect. 2015;18(5):1139–50.
66. Shalala D, Bolton LB, Bleich MR, et al. Institute of Medicine: The Future of Nursing: Leading Change, Advancing Health. Washington, DC: The National Academic Press; 2011.
67. Lee G, Hendriks J, Deaton C. Advanced nursing practice across Europe: work in progress. Eur J Cardiovasc Nurs. 2020;19(7):561–63.

Section 2: Holistic nursing care: assessment, intervention, and evaluation

4 Anatomy and physiology of the healthy heart

GERALDINE LEE, GABRIELLE MCKEE, ANDREAS PROTOPAPAS, AND IAN D. JONES

CHAPTER CONTENTS

This chapter provides a basic introduction to cardiac anatomy and physiology of the heart and the conduction system along with a description of the electrical and mechanical characteristics of the cardiac cells. The chapter concludes with an overview of the normal parameters of the electrocardiograph that can be used as a framework to structure a process of systematic analysis. This approach can be applied to abnormal electrocardiographs and rhythm strips presented in the chapters outlining the care of patients with cardiac conditions.

KEY MESSAGES

- A normally functioning heart is essential to create a pressure gradient in the blood vessels that will enable blood flow to the organs.
- The coronary circulation is adapted to meet the high metabolic needs of the heart because it has a greater blood flow, an extensive capillary network, and greater oxygen extraction than other organs.
- The heart contains myocardial cells and autorhythmic cells that enable it to conduct electricity and contract, respectively.
- While the heart possesses its own internal automaticity, its activity is influenced by a combination of factors, the most important of which are neural and hormonal.
- Heart rate is ordinarily determined by the pacemaker activity of the sinoatrial node, which has the highest intrinsic firing rate of the automaticity cells.
- The cardiac cycle describes all of the activities of the heart through a single complete heartbeat.
- The 12-lead electrocardiogram is composed of specific components that reflect the action potential—P wave, QRS complex, and T wave.
- A 12-lead electrocardiogram should be reviewed in a logical, comprehensive manner examining each of the leads so that rate, rhythm, axis, and any abnormalities can be detected.

Introduction

To understand how the human heart and circulation works, it is helpful to have an overview of the key anatomical and physiological features. The study of human anatomy and physiology has been described as the study of life. This branch of science asks questions about the structure and internal workings of human beings and how they interact with the world around them. The circulatory system describes the heart, blood vessels, and properties of the blood and how the circulation functions. It is important to understand how the heart and circulation functions in health so that pathological changes, along with clinical sequelae, can be recognized. The Greek physician Galen is credited with being one of the first scientists to hypothesize how the heart and circulation worked. Legend has it that he discovered the pulmonary circulation in 129 AD. Some 30 years later, in his role as chief physician to the gladiators in Pergamum, he was able to observe the beating hearts of wounded gladiators. This marked a major step forward in understanding how the heart and circulation worked.[1]

Despite this, for several centuries scientists thought that blood was circulated through the body by the lungs. In the 1600s, Harvey, an English scientist, was said to be the first to describe how the systemic circulation functioned with the heart propelling the blood through the brain and body. The heart is indeed an amazing organ with unique physiological properties not shared by any other organ in the human body.

Blood vessels and the control of blood flow

Overview of the circulatory system

The circulatory system consists of two major components: the blood vessels and the heart. The heart is the pump that maintains blood flow within the system and the blood vessels function as the transport system. The circulatory system is referred to as a single closed system and the volume within it stays relatively constant. Within this system there are two circulations, utilizing the two synchronous pumps of the right side and the left side of the heart (➤ Fig. 4.1). The circulatory system has multiple functions. These include the transport of gases, nutrients, and wastes, the regulation of blood pressure, acid–base balance, fluid balance, and body temperature. The right side of the heart receives blood from the venous circulation of the body and brain and pumps it to the lungs for oxygenation and carbon dioxide release, while the left side of the heart receives oxygenated blood from the lungs and pumps it to the body and brain.

The system is made up of five types of blood vessels which when combined would cover 100,000 km. The blood vessels can be grouped into three main categories: arteries, capillaries, and veins (➤ Fig. 4.2). Arteries, and their smaller counterparts arterioles, generally carry oxygenated blood away from the heart to the tissues. Veins, and their smaller counterparts venules, generally carry deoxygenated blood from the tissues to the heart. In

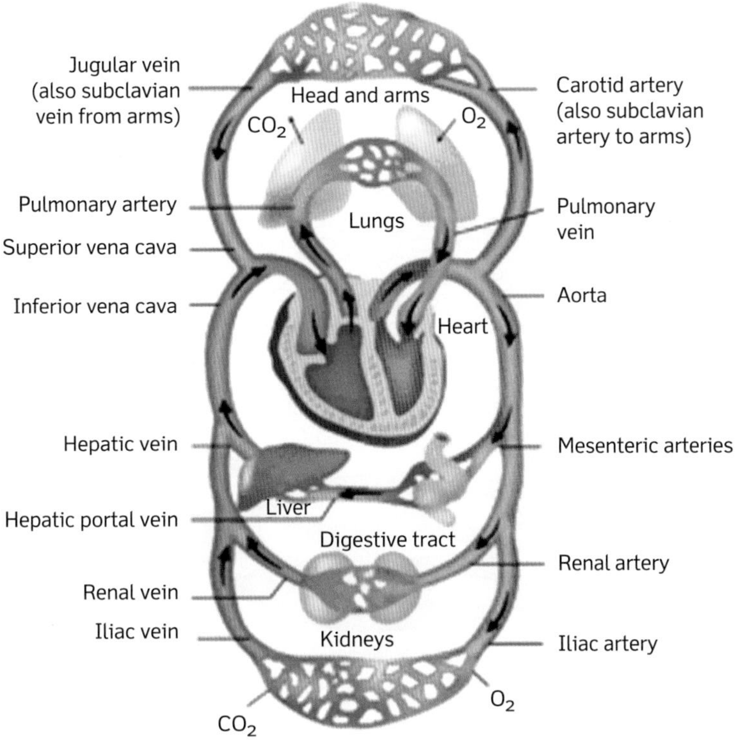

Fig. 4.1 The circulation of blood in the body.

this section, we will describe the structure of blood vessels and then review the functional aspects describing fluid exchange, blood pressures, vasodilatation, and vasoconstriction.

The overall structure of blood vessels

The different types of blood vessels in the human body consist of between one and three layers, reflecting their function (➤ **Fig. 4.2**). The innermost layer is called the tunica intima and is better known as the endothelium. This layer is common to all blood vessels and is in direct contact with the blood that flows through the hollow opening inside the blood vessel called the lumen. It has the same basic structure across all blood vessels—a single layer of squamous epithelium, a basement membrane that acts as a structural support, and an elastic layer on the outside. The next major layer is the muscular layer, or the tunica media, which is made up of both smooth muscle and elastic fibres. The proportion of these layers differs across arteries, arterioles, veins, and venules and this layer is completely absent from capillaries. The outmost layer is the tunica externa, which is made up of elastic and collagen fibres and is absent in capillaries.

The structure and function of arteries

Arteries are blood vessels that usually transport blood away from the heart. They contain all three layers: the tunica intima, tunica media, and tunica externa (➤ **Fig. 4.2**). They differ in diameter at rest from 1 cm to 0.1 mm and differ in the amount of muscle and elastic that is present, particularly in the tunica media. Arteries have the largest tunica media layer of all blood vessels and, depending on the artery, the amount of elastic fibres present differs substantially. The largest arteries of the body, those of the pulmonary trunk and the aorta, tend to have greater proportions of elastic fibres and a wider lumen than other arteries. These characteristics allow these large arteries to act as temporary reservoirs for blood leaving the heart. This helps to regulate the intermittent pumping of blood from the heart to create a more consistent flow and pressure. These large elastic arteries empty into smaller, more muscular arteries which have the capacity to constrict and

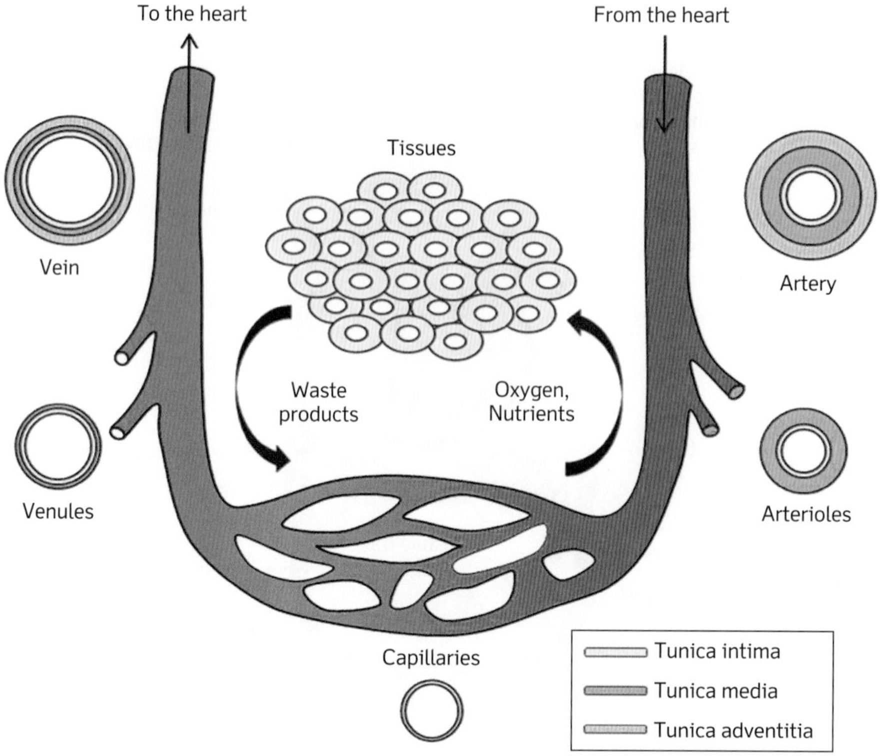

Fig. 4.2 The main blood vessels of the body.

dilate, enabling them to play an important role in regulating the distribution of the blood throughout the body. When blood leaves the heart, it is at its highest pressure; the strong muscular structure of the arteries (the dominant tunica media muscular layer and elastic layer) minimizes the loss of pressure as blood flows through these vessels, compared to other blood vessels (➤ **Fig. 4.3**). This facilitates the maintenance of blood flow in the circulatory system.

From birth, exposure of the endothelium to shear stress and multiple cardiovascular risk factors lead to the accumulation of fatty streaks, seen from the age of 1 year, and eventually plaques beneath the endothelium surface. This accumulation changes the characteristics of the endothelium and tunica media, eventually developing into atherosclerosis[2] (see Chapter 6 for more detail).

The structure and function of the arterioles

Arterioles have a similar structure to arteries and have three layers. However, they are smaller in diameter and their thick walls take up a greater proportion of the overall vessel, leaving a small vessel lumen for blood to flow through (➤ **Fig. 4.2**). The tunica media is predominantly muscle and as the blood vessel gets closer to the capillaries, this layer gets thinner. At the junction with the capillary, there is a sphincter that controls flow into the capillary. These precapillary sphincters are important in the regulation of blood flow to tissues. The endothelium, which lines arteries and arterioles, is surrounded by a thin layer of connective tissue. The cells of the endothelium secrete many substances that are important in blood clotting, vascular permeability, and vasoconstriction and vasodilatation which control blood flow to the tissues.

Control of blood flow

The proportion of blood in the capillary beds is increased by the relaxation of the precapillary sphincters and the smooth muscle of the tunica media. This relaxation causes the vessel lumen to enlarge and consequently decreases the blood pressure in the small arteries and arterioles (➤ **Fig. 4.3**). This relaxation is

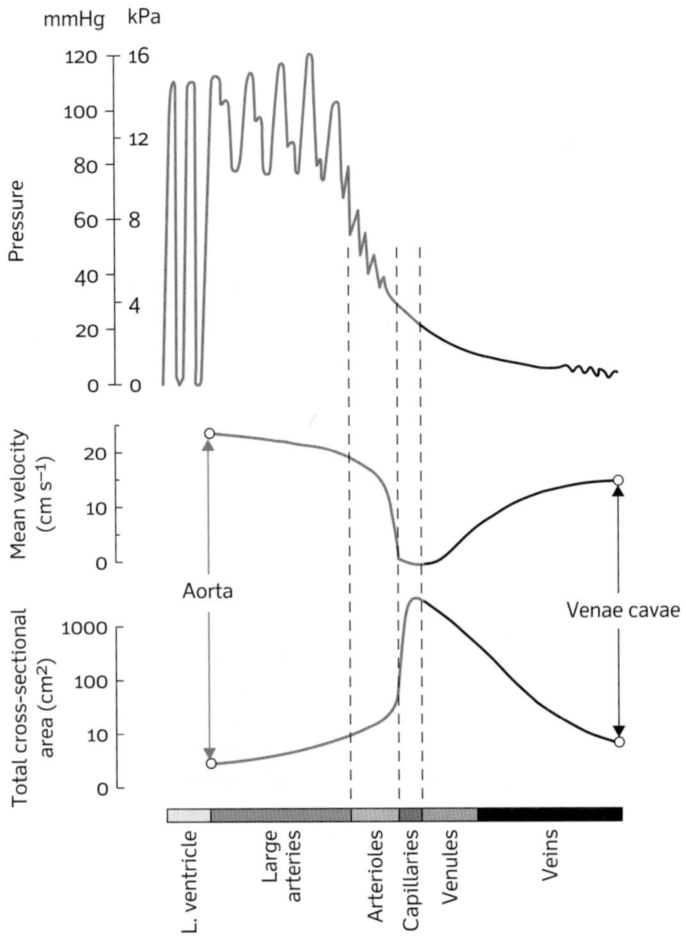

Fig. 4.3 Pressure, blood flow/velocity, and cross-sectional lumen size of blood vessels.

Reproduced from Pocock, G., and Richards, C. Human Physiology, Third Edition, Oxford University Press, Oxford, UK, Copyright © 2006 with permission from Oxford University Press.

termed vasodilatation and can result from sympathetic nervous system activation of blood vessels in some organs, release of local vasodilators, and metabolic vasodilators (➤ Table 4.1). Vasoconstriction is the opposite, with an increase in vessel muscle contraction, resulting in decreased lumen size and increased blood pressure in the vessel. It is caused by hormones, local hormones, and the sympathetic nervous system in some vessels. The coronary circulation of the heart is strongly influenced by the metabolic vasodilators, particularly adenosine, during exercise. In an average individual with healthy arteries, these mechanisms facilitate increased blood supply to the myocardium of the heart to meet the increased aerobic needs of the heart as it moves from normal cardiac muscle contraction and beating at 70 beats per minute (bpm) to increased force of contraction and heart rate required, for example, during exercise.

The structure and function of capillaries

Capillaries differ from all other blood vessels in that they have only one main layer, the endothelium, which is surrounded by a basement membrane (➤ Fig. 4.2). These are very small vessels, ranging from 4 to 10 μm in diameter and up to 1 mm long. Although the smallest of the blood vessels, they make up 80% of the 100,000 km of blood vessels within the body. The capillaries fulfil the main function of the circulatory system by exchanging gases and nutrients between the blood and the tissues. They form capillary beds that are in close contact with almost every

Table 4.1 Vasoconstriction and vasodilatation

Main vasoconstrictors	Main vasodilators
Noradrenaline (adrenaline) via α receptors, i.e. in skin	Adrenaline (noradrenaline) via β_2 receptors, i.e. in coronary vessels and skeletal muscle
Angiotensin II	Local vasoactive chemicals from the endothelium: nitric oxide, histamine, bradykinin, serotonin, prostacyclin
Antidiuretic hormone	Metabolic vasodilators: increased carbon dioxide, hydrogen, and adenosine (a by-product of adenosine triphosphate metabolism) or decreased oxygen
Endothelin (from the endothelium), thromboxane	Atrial natriuretic peptide

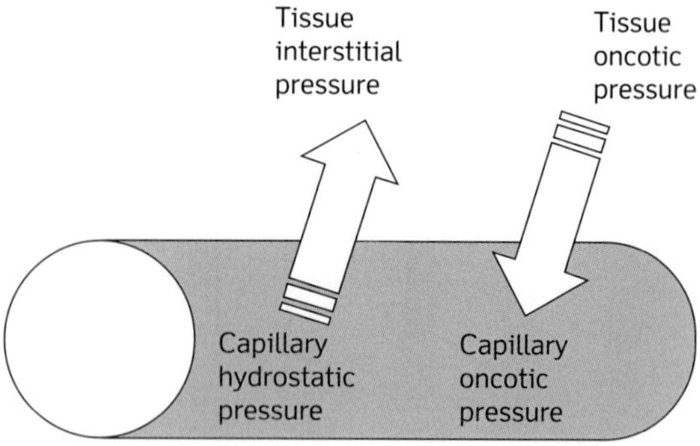

Fig. 4.4 Capillary pressures and capillary fluid exchange. The left portion of the diagram reflects the pressures in the arterial end of the capillary, where the outward force of the capillary hydrostatic pressures is dominant and results in fluid moving from the capillary into the interstitium. The right side reflects the venous end of the capillary where the capillary osmotic/oncotic pressure is dominant and results in fluid being drawn back into the capillary.

cell in the body, which enables them to fulfil this important function. The extensiveness of the capillary bed and the structure of the capillary vary depending on metabolic requirements of the tissues. Tissues that have high oxygen demands, such as muscle, tend to have large capillary networks. While some tissues, such as cartilage, are avascular with no capillary beds, necessitating the exchange of nutrients and gases to move through surrounding tissues.

The structure of the capillary is designed for its function of exchange. The capillary uses two different types of gradient to facilitate exchange: pressure gradients for the movement of fluid and concentration gradients for the diffusion of gases and nutrients. Exchange will occur between the blood in the capillaries and the surrounding interstitium and then with the cells, if a gradient is present. Oxygen will therefore move from the blood, where levels of oxygen are high, to the tissue where the levels are low due to the usage of oxygen during metabolism. The reverse is true of carbon dioxide, which moves from the tissues, where metabolism created high levels, to the blood which has low levels. Fluid exchange due to pressure gradients is rather more complex as two pressures are involved. At the arterial end of the capillary, hydrostatic pressure, due to the blood pressure in the capillary, is high and pushes fluid into the interstitium which has a low hydrostatic pressure. In opposition to this, osmotic/oncotic pressure is at work. This pressure is mainly due to the presence of proteins. In the arterial capillary, the large amount of protein in the blood osmotically attracts fluid and attempts to pull fluid from the tissues. However, at the arterial end of the capillary, the dominant force is the hydrostatic pressure and there is net movement of fluid into the surrounding tissue, approximately 24 L of fluid every day (➤ **Fig. 4.4**). The opposite is true at the venous end of the capillary. Here, the hydrostatic pressure in the capillary is low and the osmotic pressure remains the same, and is higher than the hydrostatic pressure, so fluid is pulled into the venous capillary, about 21 L per day. The excess is returned to the circulatory system by the lymphatic system. However, there are some reasons that will cause fluid to remain in the tissues and surrounding interstitial fluid. The most common of these are increased capillary pressure or capillary permeability, a reduction in lymphatic drainage, or a decrease in plasma proteins.

The structure and function of veins

Blood flows from the capillaries into the venules and then the veins. Veins carry blood back from the tissues to the heart. Veins have a three-layered structure similar to arteries but differ in that the tunica media—the muscle layer—is much thinner (➤ **Fig. 4.2**). This means that the vessel walls are very compliant and act as a reservoir, containing approximately 60% of the system's blood. Veins have a large lumen and the pressure within them is relatively low (➤ Fig. 4.3). Because of the structural weakness of the veins and the low pressure of this system, venous return to the heart is slow and is augmented by valves in the larger veins, which prevent backflow, and pumping due to surrounding skeletal muscle contraction. Contraction of the skeletal muscle exerts pressure on the veins and squeezes blood back to the heart. Venous return is also facilitated by vasoconstriction which can be stimulated by sympathetic nerves. The slowness of flow through the veins can lead to the stasis of blood, particularly behind the valves, which can increase the risk of venous thrombi development.

Overview of cardiac anatomy

Key features

The heart is the core of the cardiovascular system, a hard-working muscular organ that contracts rhythmically and automatically. It plays a major role as a pump that ensures the continuous flow of blood in the body, pumping blood through the circulation by developing a pressure gradient. To do this it functions as two pumps acting synchronously—the right side pumps blood to the pulmonary circulation, and the left side to the systemic circulation. The heart has its own circulation system called the coronary circulation to The sinoatrial node generates electrical impulses that stimulate the cardiac muscle. This causes the contraction of the chambers of the heart which powers blood into the circulation. The combinations of mechanical and electrical events that occur with each beat of the heart is collectively known as the cardiac cycle (see 'Mechanics of the heart'). The human heart is about the size of an adult closed fist and weighs about 250 g and 300 g in the average adult female and male, respectively. The heart is one of the few muscular organs in the body that works every second, every minute, of every day of your lifetime. At on average 70 bpm in the average lifetime, this amounts to approximately 2.5 billion beats.

The heart is normally located in the mediastinum between the lungs. Two-thirds of it lie to the left side of the midline of the chest, and one-third to the right (➤ Box 4.1 and ➤ Fig. 4.5). It has a slightly tilted appearance with the apex, the tip of the left ventricle, resting on the diaphragm. The apex beat is generally auscultated on the midline of the left clavicle in the fifth intercostal space between the fifth and the sixth ribs. The base or top of the heart is much wider and is the location of the entry and exit of the main vessels. It lies mainly under the sternum just below the second rib. The location of the heart may deviate slightly depending on stature. Short individuals tend to have a slightly more horizontal heart orientation and tall individuals a more vertical orientation.

Box 4.1 Did you know?

> In rare cases (1:12,000 adults), a congenital condition means that the heart points to the right side of the heart rather than the left. This condition is called dextrocardia.

The heart is enclosed within a double-walled pericardial sac, also called the pericardium (➤ Fig. 4.5). The outer layer of the pericardium has a fibrous layer that supports and anchors the heart to the diaphragm and surrounding structures and a parietal layer of serous pericardium. The inner layer, the epicardium (mesothelial cells, fat, and connective tissue), covers the outer surface of the heart and is known as the visceral layer of the serous pericardium. The serous layers secrete pericardial fluid. The pericardial fluid accumulates between the pericardium and the epicardium and allows movements of the heart to occur uninhibited and without friction against the surrounding organs.

The heart itself is made up of several more layers. Below the epicardium is the myocardium. It is the thickest layer of the heart which is muscular in structure (cardiomyocytes). The innermost layer of the heart that lines the chambers and valves is called the endocardium (endothelial cells and subendocardial connective tissue).

The heart is made up of four chambers: two atria and two ventricles (➤ Fig. 4.6). The upper chambers of the heart, called atria, have a thin myocardial layer and their main function is the collection of blood that enters the heart from the venous system. The right atrium receives deoxygenated blood from the lower part of the body, via the inferior vena cava, and from the upper part of the body via the superior vena cava. The left atrium receives oxygenated blood from the pulmonary veins.

Two atrioventricular (AV) valves separate the atria from the ventricles; the tricuspid valve on the right side of the heart and the bicuspid, or mitral valve, on the left side of the heart (➤ Fig. 4.6). When the valves in the heart are working effectively, they create a one-way system of blood flow. During most of the cardiac cycle (except when the ventricles contract), the valves are open and their cusps project into the ventricles. The valves are thin, non-muscular, fibrous structures with cusps that are attached by chordae tendineae to papillary muscles in the

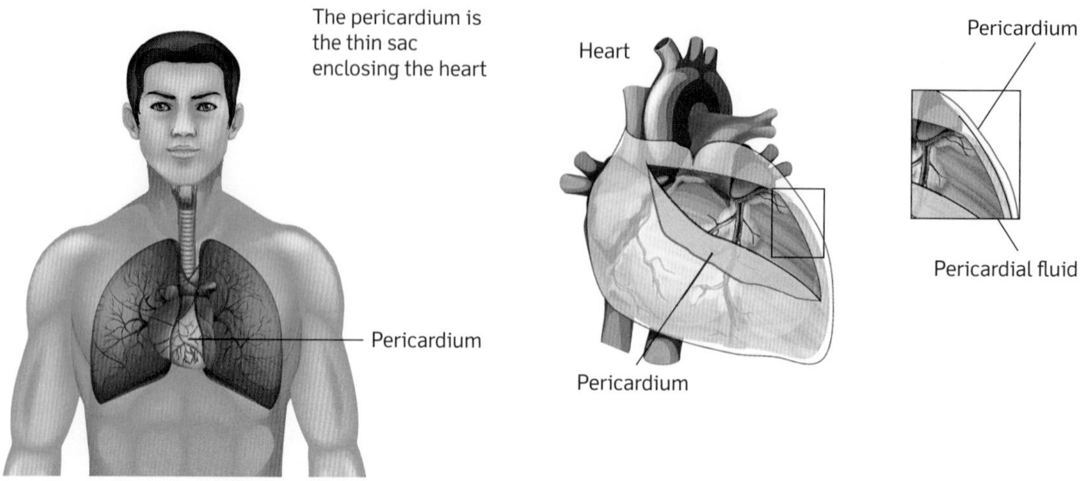

Fig. 4.5 The heart and the pericardium.

walls of the ventricles. When the ventricular muscles of a healthy heart contract, blood attempts to flow from the high-pressure ventricles back to the low-pressure atria. The valves are pushed upwards and overlap on each other to close the valve opening and prevent backward flow. In addition, the papillary muscle contracts which tightens the chordae tendineae. This prevents the cusp moving further backwards into the atria. The mechanism is like opening an umbrella, in that it can only open to a certain degree beyond which it will turn inside out. Valvular thickening and stiffening tend to occur with age (see Chapter 8).

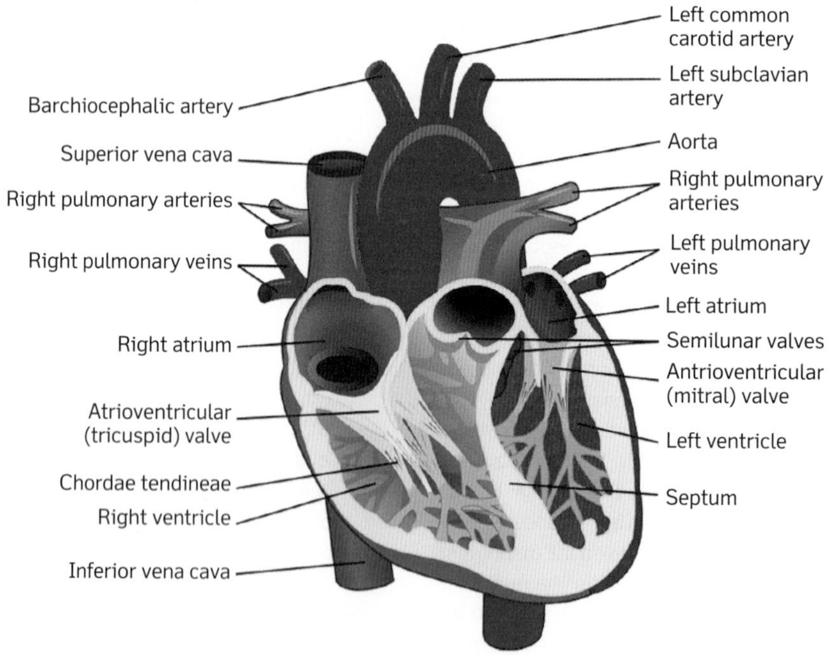

Fig. 4.6 Cross-section of the heart showing the chambers, valves, and major blood vessels.

Box 4.2 Did you know?

Some ultra-endurance athletes have been reported to have left ventricular wall thicknesses that can be up to 19 mm due to the high level of aerobic activity linked to their sport.

The ventricles are the 'pumping chambers' of the heart and have thicker muscle layers compared to the atria which are 'receiving chambers'. The mean thickness of the myocardium in the left ventricle is around 7 mm in women and 9 mm in men (➤ **Box 4.2**). Hypertrophy is the term that describes the excessive enlargement of an organ. This can occur in the heart as a result of pathophysiological changes that occur when the heart has to work harder than normal to maintain its normal output in conditions such as hypertension and heart failure (see Chapter 10). Overwork of the left ventricle can also cause hypertrophy as the heart musculature increases as part of a physiological response to large amounts of aerobic exercise.

The exit vessels from the right and left ventricles are the pulmonary artery and the aorta, respectively (➤ **Fig. 4.6**). They have valves called semilunar valves, which as the name implies, are shaped like a half-moon. They work in the same way as the AV valves and close when blood attempts to flow back into the ventricles. This occurs at the end of ventricular contraction (systole) when the pressure in the ventricles decreases and drops lower than the pressure in the aorta and pulmonary artery.

Coronary circulation

For the heart to fulfil its essential function, it needs an adequate blood supply. This is provided by the coronary circulation (➤ **Fig. 4.7**). The heart tissues receive oxygenated blood from two small blood vessels, the right and left coronary arteries. These are the first vessels to emerge from the root of the aorta. They emerge unseen from behind the right and left cusps of the aortic valve. The coronary arteries progress horizontally thereby encircling the myocardium along the groove between the atria and the ventricles, called the coronary sulcus. The branches of the right and left coronary arteries then radiate down in a crown (corona)-like appearance. The right coronary artery has two main branches. The marginal branch, visible in a frontal view of the heart, moves along the coronary sulcus and supplies blood to the right ventricle and atrium. The descending branch, the posterior interventricular artery, visible in a posterior view of the heart, supplies the right and left ventricle. The left coronary artery has two main branches. The circumflex branch in the coronary sulcus supplies the left atrium and the left ventricle, and the anterior interventricular artery supplies both ventricles. As seen from these descriptions, there is some overlap in the supply from both main arteries, particularly to the ventricles. There is individual variation but, in most people, the right coronary artery is dominant and supplies most of the oxygenated blood to the myocardium.

The coronary arteries supply 250 mL of oxygenated blood per minute to the average-sized heart at rest, a supply

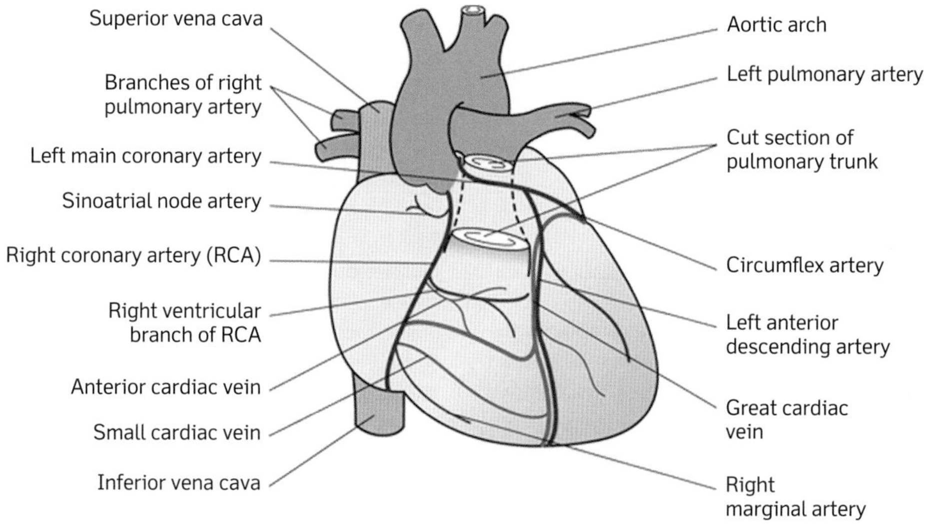

Fig. 4.7 Diagram of the heart showing the coronary circulation.

Box 4.3 Did you know?

A heart rate of over 100 bpm means that the blood flow to the heart muscle is reduced. This is because the coronary arteries fill during diastole (relaxation). A tachycardia leads to a shortened diastole which can cause myocardial ischaemia.

disproportionate to its size compared to other organs in the body. The heart is an essential organ, a hard-working tissue that functions aerobically and is therefore one of the organs whose blood supply is autoregulated. This means that it receives its proportion of blood supply irrespective of small variations in normal blood pressure. The heart also has a more extensive capillary vasculature than other organs, in that nearly every cell is in direct contact with a capillary bed, facilitating fast diffusion of gases and nutrients. In addition, the amount of oxygen extracted from the blood is high, up to 75% compared to the average extraction rate of 25% for most tissues in the body. All of these adaptations help to ensure that the heart maintains its function, a crucial adaptation as without it, circulation would cease.

An important consideration in understanding the mechanics of coronary blood flow is that it is naturally interrupted. During ventricular contraction (systole), blood is ejected through the open aortic valve to the aorta. The cusps of the aortic valve close over the entrance (ostia) to the coronary arteries which reduces blood flow into them at this time (➤ Box 4.3). In addition, the coronary blood vessels that supply blood to the epicardium, myocardium, and endocardium during ventricular contraction (systole) become compressed by the surrounding muscle, particularly in the left side of the heart. This can result in an interrupted coronary blood flow, especially to the endocardial side of the myocardium.

Mechanics of the heart

Contractility

The heart's stroke volume, the volume ejected from the ventricle at each heartbeat, is determined by the preload (stretch of the myocardial fibres, myocytes), the afterload (vascular resistance), the contractility (volume and contractile force), and the synchrony of the ventricles. This is illustrated by the Frank–Starling law that shows the relationship between the ventricular end-diastolic myocardial fibre length and the ventricular performance. According

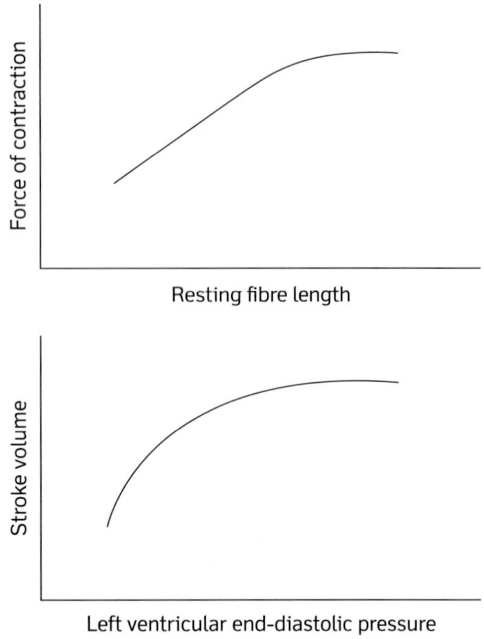

Fig. 4.8 The Frank–Starling law of the heart.

to the Frank–Starling law, an increase in venous return will increase the ventricular end-diastolic pressure and thereby stretch the cardiac myocytes prior to contraction (➤ Fig. 4.8).

The stretch increases the sarcomere length, which results in an increased generation of force. This enables the heart to eject the additional venous return and thereby increase the stroke volume. One can think of it as a slingshot: the harder you pull the rubber band, the more force is accumulated, and the longer the shot will be.

During exercise, the cardiac output, the volume ejected from the heart per minute, increases by three to four times compared to the resting state, but the stroke volume can only increase by 40–60%. Thus, the ability to increase heart rate is of key importance to increase blood flow to meet the metabolic demand from the working muscles during exercise. At low levels of exercise, the increase in heart rate and contractility are mostly a result of a reduction in vagal tone, while at higher levels of exercise, after the anaerobic threshold has been reached, the sympathetic nervous system becomes dominant. This results in the activation of catecholamines, that increase the heart rate and cardiac contractility and thereby the cardiac output. Catecholamines also cause vasoconstriction and increased systemic vascular resistance leading to an elevation in arterial blood pressure.

Cardiac cycle

The cardiac cycle is a term that describes a series of changes in pressure and volume that occur within the chambers of the heart. Pressure changes are caused by valves opening and closing to direct blood flow. The cardiac cycle consists of alternating periods of contraction (systole) and relaxation (diastole). The pressures that occur within each part of the periods vary. This is important as without the pressure differential blood flow through the heart would not occur. During the cardiac cycle, the electrical phenomena precede the mechanical, and the mechanical precede the auscultatory phenomena. The cardiac cycle includes changes that occur almost simultaneously on both sides of the heart. These changes are similar, although pressures on the right side of the heart are normally much lower than those on the left side.[3–6] Therefore, mostly the events on the left side of the heart are described here. In this description, each of the seven different phases of the cardiac cycle will be presented separately and will include associated electrical events, pressure and volume changes, valve activity, and heart sounds. ➤ Fig. 4.9 shows the cardiac cycle.

Phase 1: atrial contraction

The cardiac cycle begins with atrial contraction or systole:

- *Electrical events*: the electrical depolarization of the atria is represented in the ECG by the P wave. Electrical depolarization leads to the mechanical contraction of the atria.[7,8]
- *Pressure and volume changes*: during atrial contraction, the pressure in the atria increases and the blood is directed through the AV valves (mitral and tricuspid) to the ventricles. During this phase, the left ventricle is in relaxation. Before atrial contraction, the ventricle contains a large amount of blood due to passive filling. At rest and with normal heart rate, atrial contractions account for approximately 10% of ventricular filling. Atrial contraction merely assists ventricular filling with blood, but becomes more significant during exercise, especially in young people. This is because passive ventricular filling time is decreased as the heart rate increases. Therefore, ventricular filling is mainly passive and depends upon venous return.[4] The end of this phase is marked by the end of ventricular diastole when the volume in the ventricle reaches its maximum. This volume of blood in the ventricle is called the end-diastolic volume (EDV). The EDV of the left ventricle is approximately 120 mL. The pressure level at the end of left ventricular diastole is called left ventricular end-diastolic pressure, and is approximately 8–12 mmHg.[8]
- *Valve activity*: the AV valves open because the ventricular pressures are lower than atrial pressures.[4]
- *Heart sounds* (fourth heart sound (S4)): an S4 heart sound is rarely a normal finding (unlike a third heart sound (S3)) although it can be heard in older people.[4,9] During this phase, no heart sounds are normally audible with a stethoscope. However, in cases where the compliance of the walls of the right, or left ventricle, are reduced (e.g. left ventricular hypertrophy), an S4 heart sound may be audible. The S4 is produced by vibrations of the ventricular wall that occur as blood rapidly enters the ventricle during atrial systole.

Phase 2: isovolumetric contraction

The atrial contraction is followed by ventricular contraction (systole):

- *Electrical events*: following depolarization of the atria, the electrical potential travels to the AV node through the bundle of His into the ventricles via the Purkinje fibres. The isovolumetric contraction begins during the QRS complex, which represents the depolarization of the ventricles.[6,10]
- *Pressure and volume*: at the beginning of ventricular systole, the pressure in the ventricles increases rapidly but the total volume does not change. For this reason, this phase is also called 'isovolumetric'. In this phase, the pressure in the ventricles becomes higher than in the atria.[5,6]
- *Valve activity*: the increased pressure within the ventricles causes the closure of the AV valves. Also, the aortic valve remains closed because at this stage the pressure in the aorta is greater than the pressure in the left ventricle. The same occurs in the right ventricle. All valves are closed in this phase of the cardiac cycle.[3,4]
- *Heart sounds* (first heart sound (S1)): the closure of the AV valves generates the S1 which sounds like 'lub' during auscultation with a stethoscope.[9]

Phases 3 and 4: rapid and reduced ejection

The ejection phase is divided into two separate phases—rapid and reduced ejection—which differ in the flow velocity:

- *Electrical events*: the initial part of this period is represented on the ECG by the ST segment. During

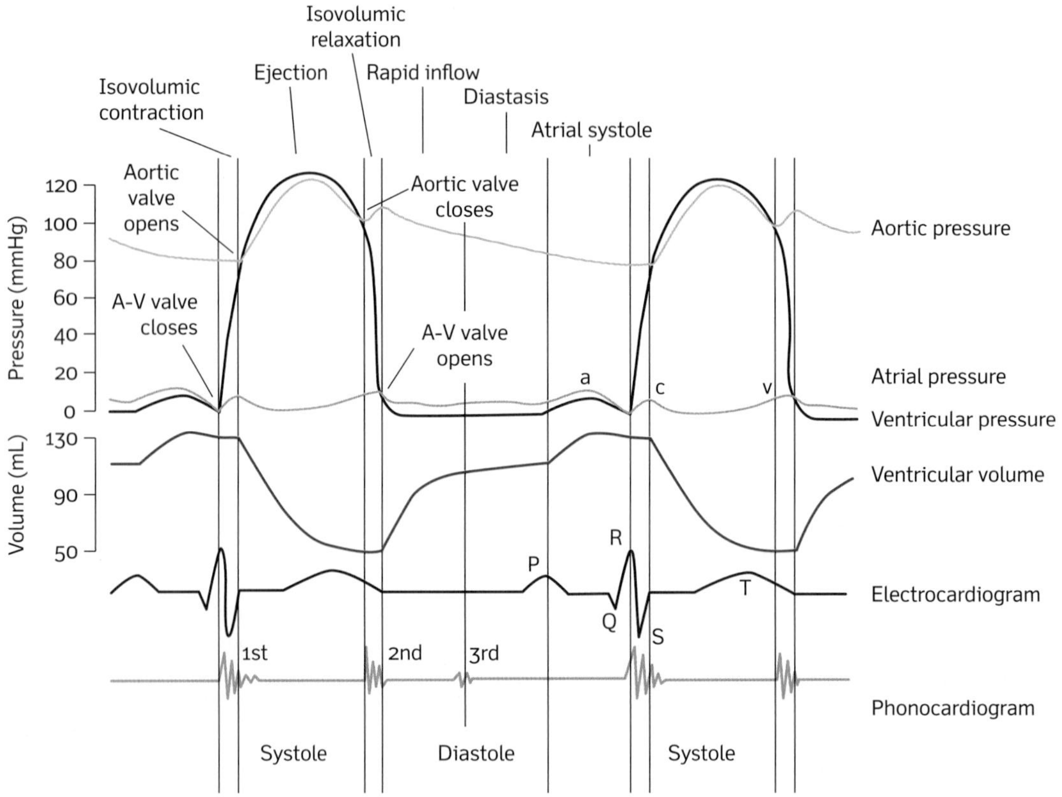

Fig. 4.9 The cardiac cycle.

Daniel Chang MD, Destiny Qx (2011) Wiggers Diagram. Licensed under CC-BY-SA 2.5 via Wikimedia Commons, accessed 24 July 2014, http://commons.wikimedia.org/wiki/File:Wiggers_Diagram.png. This image is licensed under the Creative Commons Attribution– Share Alike 2.5 Generic license. https://creativecommons.org/licenses/by-sa/2.5/.

reduced ejection, part of the repolarization of the ventricles is marked by the T wave on the ECG.[7,11,12]

- *Pressure and volume*: after the end of isovolumetric contraction, the ventricles continue to contract, and the intraventricular pressures increase to a maximum level during these phases. The pressure difference allows blood to be ejected from the left ventricle through the open aortic valve into the aorta at high velocity (rapid ejection). Also, ventricular volume decreases rapidly, and the aortic volume increases. The amount of blood ejected from the left ventricle at each contraction is called the stroke volume. In parallel, the atrial filling begins. Subsequently, ventricular and aortic pressures start decreasing. The end of this phase concludes systole.[3–6]
- *Valve activity*: the aortic valve is forced open because the pressure in the left ventricle is greater (around 80 mmHg) than the pressure in the aorta and remains open as long as ventricular pressure exceeds aortic pressure. During ejection, the AV valves remain closed.[3,8]
- *Heart sounds*: no heart sounds are normally heard. The presence of sounds during systole indicates valve disease (i.e. systolic murmurs).[4,9]

Phase 5: isovolumetric relaxation

- *Electrical events*: the isovolumetric relaxation of ventricles is indicated at the end of the T wave on the ECG.
- *Pressure and volume*: at this point, diastole begins. As the ventricle relaxes, ventricular pressure decreases rapidly and falls below the aortic pressure. During isovolumetric relaxation, the volume in the ventricles remains stable and does not change. For this reason, this phase is also called 'isovolumetric'. The ventricle

does not empty completely during systole and the volume that remains in the left ventricle after ejection is called the end-systolic volume. This is approximately 50 mL of blood. The difference between the EDV and the end-systolic volume (ESV) is called stroke volume (120 − 50 = 70 mL). The division of the stroke volume with the EDV gives us the ejection fraction. The atrial pressure continues to increase as the flow from the pulmonary veins continues.[4–6]

- *Valve activity*: the aortic valve closes because the pressure in the aorta is greater than the pressure in the left ventricle. The pulmonary valve closes shortly after the aortic valve because inspiration delays occlusion. All valves are now closed.[4,9]
- *Heart sounds* (second heart sound (S2)): closure of the aortic and pulmonary valve produces the S2. At the end of inspiration there is a normal split of the S2 due to delayed closure of the pulmonary valve. This sound is heard like 'dub' with a stethoscope.[9]

Phase 6: rapid ventricular filling

- *Electrical events*: no activity, but sometimes a U wave may occur.[10]
- *Pressure and volume*: when the pressure in the left ventricle falls below the pressure in the left atrium, the mitral valve opens, and the ventricle consequently passively and rapidly fills with blood. The volume of the ventricle is increasing rapidly. About 80% of ventricular filling occurs during this phase. However, the pressure in the left ventricle remains low because of relaxation.[3]
- *Valve activity*: the AV valves open because the ventricular pressures are lower than atrial pressures. The aortic and pulmonary valves remain closed.[4]
- *Heart sounds* (S3): during filling, no sounds are heard. Nevertheless, rapid flow of blood from the atria to the ventricles produces the S3, which is normally heard in children. However, the presence of S3 in middle-aged or older adults is indicative of volume overload, such as congestive heart failure.[4,9]

Phase 7: ventricular diastasis or reduced ventricular filling

Ventricular diastasis, or reduced ventricular filling, is the longest phase of the cardiac cycle and involves the final phase of ventricular filling. At a normal resting heart rate, the duration of diastasis is longer than half of the entire cardiac cycle. However, in periods when the heart rate is fast, the duration of the diastole becomes shorter than that of systole. For example, if the heart rate is higher than 200 bpm, the duration of diastole is reduced, and the filling of the ventricles becomes inadequate (reduced EDV). As a result, the stroke volume is reduced, and cardiac output is also reduced. Cardiac output is the product of stroke volume and heart rate: CO = SV × HR. The end of diastasis marks the end of the diastole.[3,4,6]

- *Electrical events*: it represents the beginning of the next P wave.[10]
- *Pressure and volume*: after rapid filling and before the beginning of atrial contraction, the pressure in the atria and ventricles is balanced. Due to the passive filling of the ventricles, the ventricular volume and pressure gradually increases. During this phase, coronary artery blood flow reaches its maximum. The pressure in the aortic and pulmonary valves continues to fall.[4–6]
- *Valve activity*: the AV valves (mitral and tricuspid) remain open and the pulmonary and aortic valves remain closed.[4]
- *Heart sounds*: no heart sounds are normally heard at this time. The presence of sounds during diastole (between S2 and S1) indicate valve disease (i.e. diastolic murmurs).[9]

Auscultation of the heart

Understanding the creation of heart sounds is the basis of effective heart auscultation. Associated with the cardiac cycle, there are four heart sounds. The origin of all sounds is based on the mechanical movement of the heart valves. In summary, S1 is generated by closure of the AV valves during systole, and S2 is generated by closure of aortic and pulmonary valves during diastole. With a stethoscope, these sounds are heard like 'lub–dub'. S3 is associated with rapid ventricular filling and S4 results from the movement of blood during atrial contraction. S3 is heard like 'lub–dub–*dum*' and S4 like '*da*–lub–dub'. Blood turbulence during systole is also known as systolic murmur and during diastole as diastolic murmur.[3,9]

Blood pressure

During ejection, the ventricular contraction produces the pressure necessary for the circulation of blood in the network of blood vessels. Blood pressure readings are important for assessing the haemodynamic status of patients.

Systolic blood pressure (SBP) is the highest pressure that occurs during a cardiac cycle (ventricular contraction). It is the pressure in the artery after blood is pumped out of the left ventricle during contraction. Diastolic blood pressure (DBP) is the lowest pressure measured during the cardiac cycle (ventricular filling). It is the pressure in the arteries during the relaxation of the ventricles when no blood is ejected from the left ventricle.[6,9,13]

Pulse pressure

The different between SBP and DBP is referred to as pulse pressure. For example, if the SBP is 120 mmHg and the DBP is 80 mmHg, the pulse pressure will be 40 mmHg. Narrow pulse pressure may be due to a decrease of stroke volume as it occurs after haemorrhage. Pulse pressure can be used as an indicator of stroke volume.[13] On the other hand, a wide pulse pressure (>80 mmHg) is a sign of moderate to severe aortic regurgitation.[14]

Mean arterial pressure

➤ **Fig. 4.10** shows systolic, diastolic, and mean arterial wave pressures. The mean arterial pressure (MAP) is defined as the average of the arterial pressure in the arterial system during a complete cardiac cycle. It is actually an important indicator of the perfusion level of vital organs and is calculated by the following equation[10,15]:

$$MAP = DBP + (1/3 \times \text{pulse pressure})$$

or

$$MAP = (SBP + (2 \times DBP))/3$$

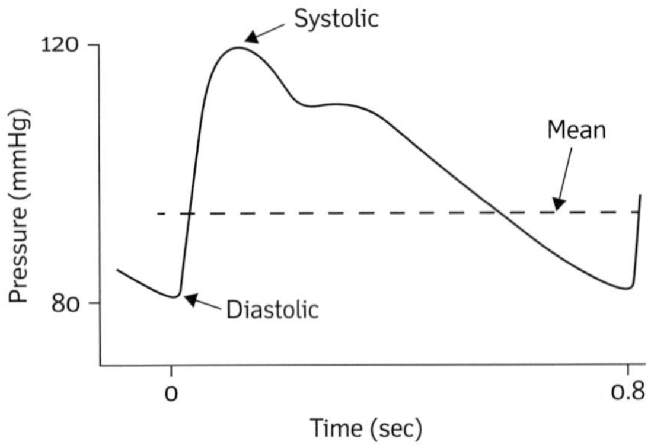

Fig. 4.10 Systolic, diastolic, and mean arterial wave pressures.

Arterial pulse

Each contraction of the left ventricle generates a pressure wave by the ejection of blood into the circulation. This wave is palpated in the arteries as a pulse. Each pulse in the arteries coincides with a cardiac cycle.[9]

Ejection fraction

Ejection fraction is the most commonly used clinical index to evaluate ventricular function. Normally, the ejection fraction is approximately between 55% and 75% and is assessed using echocardiography[4,7,13,16]:

$$EF = \frac{LVEDV - LVESV}{LVEDV} \times 100$$

Where EF, ejection fraction, LVEDV = left ventricular end-diastolic volume, and LVESV = left ventricular end- systolic volume.

Electrical properties of the heart

Myocytes and the cardiac syncytium

Each heartbeat relies on the generation of an electrical impulse. In the normal heart, this impulse stimulates the cardiac muscle cell, or myocyte, to shorten in length and, in turn, stimulates the adjacent myocyte to do the same. This pattern of electrical activity followed by myocyte contraction enables the chambers of the heart to contract in a sequence that allows blood to be moved around and out of the heart accordingly.

In order to achieve this goal, the heart relies on two major cells types:

- Myocardial cells with primary responsibility for contraction (99%) (ventricular and atrial).
- Autorhythmic cells with responsibility for the generation of electrical impulse (1%).

These cells are morphologically, molecularly, and functionally distinct.[17]

Ventricular cardiomyocyte

A typical ventricular myocyte contains a central nucleus (possibly two) and around 150 myofibrils aligned along the cell's axis connecting end to end with neighbouring fibres through intercalated discs.[18] These discs contain desmosomes, strong cable-like filaments that bind myocytes together, and gap junctions that allow ions to travel from one fibre to another. These cell-to-cell junctions form strong mechanical linkages but also enable the transmission of electrical activity from one myocyte to another. Within each of these myocytes a series of subunits of sarcomeres are responsible for cardiac contractility.

Atrial cardiomyocyte

Atrial myocytes are much smaller than ventricular myocytes and have different electrophysiological and contractile properties. Atrial myocytes possess lower and shorter action potentials than ventricular myocytes,[17] enabling the atria to distribute electrical impulses at a higher rate compared to the ventricles. In addition, due to the difference in the presence of myosin, atrial myocytes are known to be able to shorten at a much quicker speed than ventricular myocytes. Myosin is a fibrous protein which, together with actin, plays a key role in muscle contraction.

Sarcomeres

A sarcomere is the most basic unit that makes up striated muscle. Each sarcomere is approximately 2–2.2 μm long in its resting state and contains two chief proteins, actin and myosin. Actin is a thin filament connected to the sarcomere's membrane (Z line), whereas the thicker myosin lies at the centre of the sarcomere with the heads of the myosin molecules producing potential bridges between the myosin and actin filaments.[19] At rest, these bridges are redundant. However, when the cell is stimulated, calcium enters the cell. These additional calcium ions connect with intracellular troponin causing a chain reaction that binds the myosin bridges to the actin filament.[20] However, the angle of connection creates instability and the link is short lived as the actin filament disengages and connects to the next myosin site along the chain. This movement shortens the sarcomere and results in contraction (➤ Fig. 4.11). Contraction ceases when the calcium ions exit the cell with the actin filaments sliding back to their original position, lengthening the sarcomere once again.[21] The energy that enables the movement of these actin filaments along the myosin cross-bridges is provided by adenosine triphosphate, which is produced by the myocyte's many mitochondria. The number of linked bridges and, therefore, the force of contraction is related to the concentration of free calcium ions.[19]

➤ Fig. 4.11 illustrates how the sarcomere is composed of different sections between two Z lines. The A band at the centre remains constant whereas, during contraction, the I bands shorten as the thin filaments in the I band slide between the thick filaments of the A band.

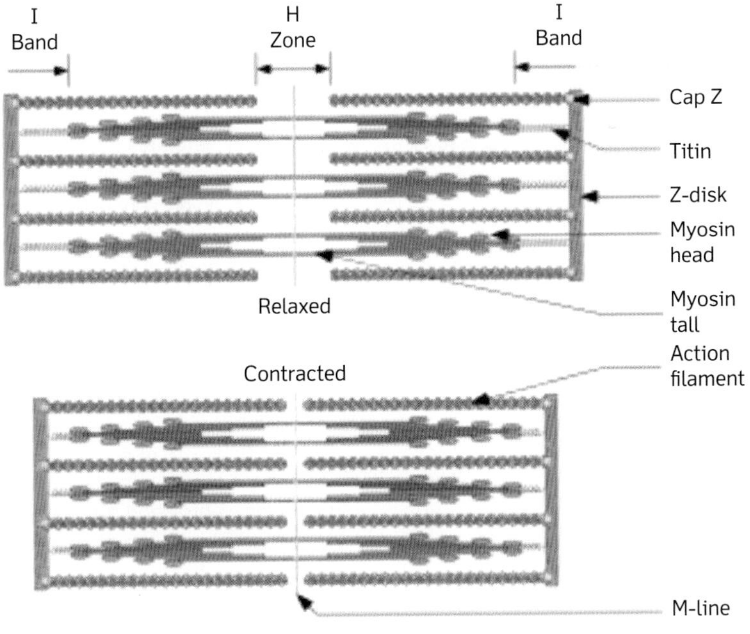

Fig. 4.11 Diagram of a sarcomere during relaxation and contraction.

Autorhythmic cells

The heart is a unique muscle in that it is capable of producing its own electrical impulses and can do so without external influence from the autonomic nervous system. While most cardiac cells are capable of initiating and transmitting electrical impulses, naturally modified autorhythmic cells generate and transmit impulses through a specialized conduction system at a higher rate than other cells within the heart. Autorhythmic cells, unlike myocytes, do not possess a resting action potential, moving constantly between −60 mV prior to depolarization to +20 mV post depolarization and back to −60 mV following repolarization in a three-phase process.[7] These phases are associated with changes in cell permeability altering the rate of, mainly, sodium, potassium, and calcium across the cell membrane.[22] The autorhythmic cell's negative membrane potential (−60 mV) is due to a slow outflow of intracellular potassium, lost through gated ion channels in the cell membrane.[19]

The coordinated way in which the action potential travels through the heart, combined with the mechanical contraction that occurs because of electrical stimulation, enables the heart to pump blood around the body in a synchronized and measured way and by doing so meet the metabolic needs of the body's organs.

Control/regulation of the heart rate and intrinsic heart rate

Heart rate is ordinarily determined by the pacemaker activity of the sinoatrial (SA) node, which has the highest intrinsic firing rate of the automaticity cells (➤ Table 4.2). It is located in the posterior wall of the right atrium. The AV node has the second highest intrinsic firing rate while the Purkinje fibres in the ventricles, which also have automaticity, fire at a very slow rate. Though, as the action potential production in the SA node is faster, before the AV node or Purkinje fibres reach the threshold for an action potential, they are depolarized by the oncoming impulse from the SA node, called an overdrive suppression. There are also ectopic pacemaker cells present in all four cardiac chambers of the heart that can initiate a heartbeat. These ectopic pacemakers can become dominant if the main pacemakers are depressed, their own rhythm is enhanced, or if all conduction pathways are blocked.

Table 4.2 Intrinsic rate of the cardiac pacemakers

Pacemaker	Firing rate (bpm) at rest
SA node	60–100
AV node	40–60
Purkinje fibre	20–40
Atrial ectopic foci	60–80
Junctional ectopic foci	40–60
Ventricular ectopic foci	20–40

Cardiac conduction

The cardiac conduction system enables heart muscle to contract (➤ Fig. 4.12). The electrical signal from the SA node moves through the atria and stimulates them to contract. In the AV node, the conduction of the action potential from the atria to the ventricles is slowed down to allow the ventricles to fill with blood before the contraction. The electrical activity then spreads across the ventricles through the His–Purkinje network, which is the fastest conduction pathway within the heart. The network starts with a bundle of fibres called the bundle of His and that separates into two bundles, the right and left bundle branches located in the septum, and ends in the Purkinje fibres in the apex of the heart, causing the ventricular contraction. The His bundle is placed on the right side of the interventricular septum and the right bundle branch is a direct continuation of the His bundle down the right side of the septum, while the left bundle branch, that is considerably thicker, arises almost perpendicular from the His bundle and perforates the intraventricular septum.

The bundles divide into the Purkinje fibres, a complex network of rapidly conducting fibres that branch over the subendocardial surfaces of both ventricles. The Purkinje cells have a greater conduction velocity of the cardiac impulse than any other tissue in the heart, which allows for a rapid activation of the entire endothelium surface of the ventricles.

The Purkinje fibres have a prolonged refractory period compared to the rest of the conduction system. This refractory period is rate dependent and a low heart rate will have a longer refractory period protecting the ventricles from contracting if a premature atrial depolarization is conducted over the AV node. The AV node refractory period, in contrast, increases at high firing rates, and will protect the ventricle from excitation at excessive atrial frequencies.

Control of the heart rate—neurohormonal/homeostatic systems

While the heart possesses its own internal automaticity, its activity is influenced by a combination of factors, the most important of which are neural and hormonal.

The autonomic nervous system

The SA node

As stated previously, the autonomic nervous system affects, but does not control, the speed of action potential production in the pacemaker cells. Through the release of noradrenaline (norepinephrine), sympathetic nervous system activity will result in an increased heart rate (positive chronotropy), by decreasing the time it takes to produce an action potential in the SA node and increased excitability. The release of acetylcholine will activate the parasympathetic nervous system and reduce the heart rate (negative chronotropy), by increasing the time it takes to produce an action potential in the SA node.

The AV node

The conduction through the AV node may be affected by the release of acetylcholine from the vagus nerve (parasympathetic activation). Moderate vagal activity will generally only prolong the AV conduction time, while intense vagal activity could prevent impulses from passing through the AV node to the ventricles completely. The cardiac sympathetic nerves, on the other hand, enable AV conduction by decreasing AV conduction time and enhance the rhythmicity (depolarization and repolarization) of the latent pacemakers in the AV junction.

Intrinsic heart rate

The intrinsic heart rate is the rate of the SA node after a complete blockade of the autonomic nervous system, on average at 100 bpm. In a healthy heart, the SA node is under constant influence of the autonomic nervous system where the parasympathetic nervous system dominates and regulates the resting heart rate to 60–80 bpm. Generally, an increased heart rate is caused by a decline of parasympathetic activity and a rise in sympathetic activity. A decreased heart rate is accomplished by the opposite, a rise of parasympathetic activity and a decline in sympathetic activity. Other factors such as hormones, baroreceptor activation by a sudden change in blood pressure, cerebral centres in the thalamus or hypothalamus, and respiration might also affect the heart rate and rhythm.

The action potential

The action potential in the heart is a change in voltage across the cell membrane of specialized cardiac cells and plays an important role in coordinating the contraction of the heart. When at rest, the cardiac cell has a negative membrane potential, meaning that the inside of the membrane is more negative than the outside; it is polarized. The reason for this is the concentration of sodium ions (Na^+) and potassium ions (K^+) over the cell membrane. The ions outside the cell are mainly Na^+, while inside the cell K^+ ions are at a higher concentration. This distribution of ions is maintained by an active transport mechanism, the sodium–potassium pump.

The negative potential over the membrane is lowered until it reaches a critical threshold that will start an action potential that changes the cell membrane's permeability for ions. This change in voltage over the cell membrane can be divided into two main phases, the depolarization and the repolarization (rhythmicity) phases. During depolarization, sodium channels open that allow positively charged ions, Na^+, to enter the cell and to make the potential over the cell membrane positive (➤ **Fig. 4.13**). In the ventricular cells, the depolarization opens the voltage-gated calcium channels and releases Ca^{2+} from the T-tubules, the plateau phase. This influx of Ca^{2+} initiates the contraction of the ventricular cell and causes additional Ca^{2+} release from the sarcoplasmic reticulum of the cardiac cell. This is followed by an inactive period known as the refractory period. This period includes the absolute refractory period when Na^+ cannot pass through and thus no action potential can be produced; and the relative refractory period when the cell starts to recover and the membrane potential becomes more negative again and where a stronger-than-usual stimulus would be required to produce an action potential. When the repolarization phase starts, the potassium channels open and allow K^+ to leave the cell, making the membrane potential return to negative and the cell returns to its resting state (➤ **Fig. 4.13**).

Fast- and slow-response action potentials

Two main types of action potentials can be found in the heart. The cells that generate these differ physiologically,

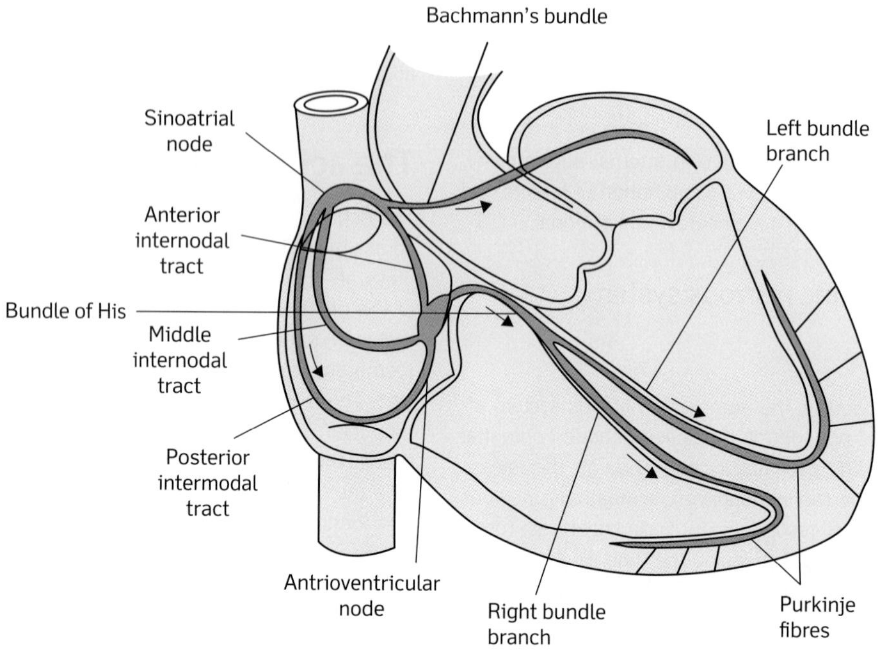

Fig. 4.12 The cardiac conduction system.

both in the type of ion channel expression and in the activation mechanisms. These differences result in the different configurations of the action potential waveform within the heart. The fast-response action potentials occur in atrial and ventricular myocardial fibres and in the Purkinje fibres. The main function of the fast-response action potential is as a conductor that leads the travelling action potential, the cardiac impulse, which results in cardiac contraction. Slow-response action potentials occur in the SA node and the AV node. Cells that have the capacity for automatic action potential generation are important for initiating the contraction of the heart and are called pacemaker cells.

Fast-response action potentials have a very fast upstroke produced by the activation of fast sodium channels, a plateau where efflux of K^+ is balanced electrically by the influx of Ca^{2+} and the repolarization where K^+ leaves the cell (➤ **Fig. 4.13**). Slow-response action potentials, in contrast, have a resting membrane potential that is less negative, the upstroke more gradual, and the plateau less prolonged. All cardiac muscle cells are linked together by gap junctions that make it possible for the action potential to pass from one cell to another, causing the heart to contract.

Action potential and electrocardiogram

The SA node's pacemaker cells provide the signal that synchronizes the heart. The signal from the SA node spreads to, and through, the AV node, normally the only conduction pathway between the atria and the ventricles. The action potentials from the AV node then move through the bundle of His, the right and left bundle branches, and onward to the Purkinje fibres in the ventricle (➤ **Fig. 4.13**). This action potential activity, an electrical signal, will cause the contraction of the heart muscle which can be recorded on the chest surface as an ECG. The components of the ECG represent the depolarization and repolarization of the action potential in the atria and ventricles.

Recording an electrocardiograph

The accurate recording of an ECG is an essential skill. Before recording, the ECG machine should be calibrated so that a 10 mm deflection is produced by 1 mV. Moreover, the paper speed has to be 25 mm/second. Otherwise, any changes on these (paper speed and calibration) must be taken into account before proceeding

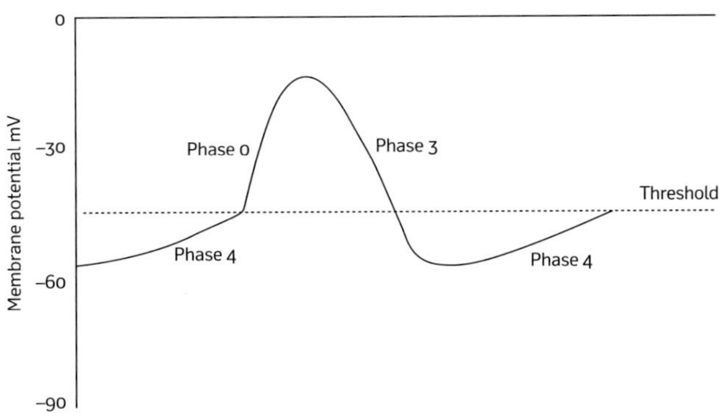

Pacemaker action potential

Phase 0	The membrane potential gradually and spontaneously increases (baseline drift) until a threshold potential is reached at which point 'slow L-type Ca^{2+} channels' open, the resultant influx of Ca^{2+} causing depolarization
Phase 3*	Ca^{2+} channels close; K^+ channels open. K^+ exits the cell down the electrochemical gradient (K^+ is a predominantly intracellular ion) and the cell rapidly repolarizes
Phase 4	Slow leak of cations into the cell via Na^+ leak, T-type Ca^{2+} channels, and Na^+/Ca^{2+} pump leads to gradual drift of the baseline potential until threshold potential is again reached. The gradient of this drift (and hence the frequency of depolarization) is increased by sympathetic stimulation (which opens Ca^{2+} channels) and decreased by parasympathetic stimulation (which opens K^+ channels)

Fig. 4.13 Action potential/depolarization/repolarization.

Reproduced from Gillon, S., Wright, C., Knott, C., McPhail, M., & Camporota, L, Revision Notes in Intensive Care Medicine. Oxford University Press, Oxford, UK: 2016 with permission from Oxford University Press.

with the interpretation of the ECG. The 12-lead ECG is recorded after electrodes are placed at the four limbs and on the surface of the chest. The leads can be divided into two groups: the limb leads that record electrical activity in the frontal plane and the precordial leads that record electrical activity in the horizontal plan.[2–4,6,11]

Limb lead positions

The limb leads consist of three bipolar and three unipolar leads that are applied to right arm, left arm, and left leg. The electrode that is applied on the right leg is used as a ground (neutral electrode).

The three bipolar limb leads (I, II, III)

These leads are called bipolar because they record the potential difference between two points of the body:

- Lead I: the potential difference between right arm and left arm; I = RA–LA.
- Lead II: the potential difference between left leg and right arm; II = LL–RA.

- Lead III: the potential difference between left leg and left arm; III = LL–LA.

The Einthoven triangle

The three bipolar limb leads create the Einthoven triangle (➤ Fig. 4.14). When the lines of the triangle are moved inwards, they form the triaxial lead system.[4,6,11]

According to Einthoven's equation, if we add leads I and II, we have the potential of lead III:

$$\text{Lead I} + \text{lead II} = \text{lead III}$$

This equation helps us to detect if the limb leads are positioned incorrectly. For example, normally, the sum of the R wave in leads I and II must be equal to the sum of the R wave in lead III.

The three augmented vector leads (aVR, aVL, aVF)

These leads are unipolar. They measure the potential difference between a limb lead and a central point:

- aVR: it 'sees' the heart from the right shoulder.
- aVL: it 'sees' the heart from the left shoulder.
- aVF: it 'sees' the heart from the foot.

The hexaxial reference system

As the triangle of Einthoven was used to orient the three bipolar limb leads in space, we can add the other three unipolar leads and form the hexaxial reference system. The centre of the hexaxial system is the heart and in particular

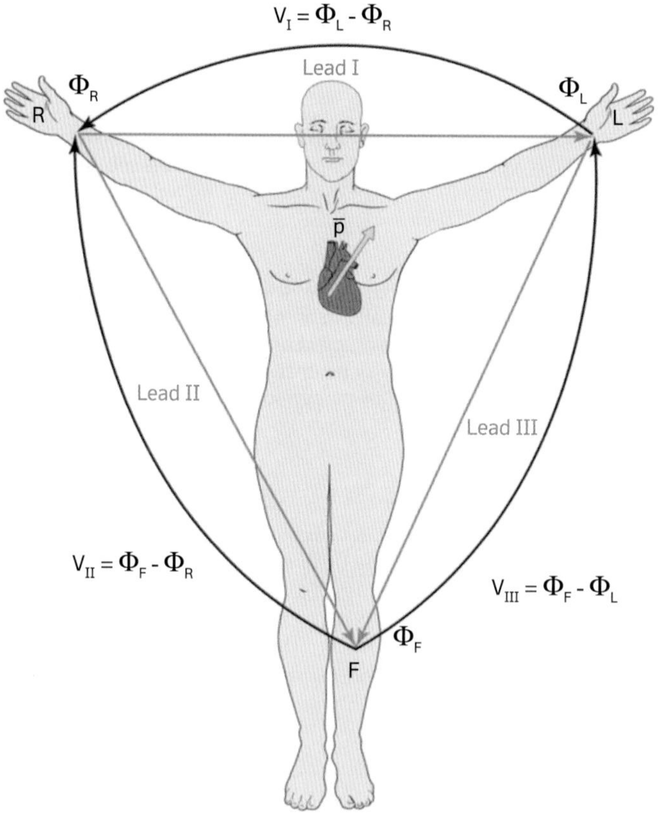

Fig. 4.14 The Einthoven's triangle. V_I = the voltage of lead I, V_{II} = the voltage of lead II, V_{III} = the voltage of lead III. Φ_R = potential at the right arm, Φ_L = potential at the left arm, Φ_F = potential at the left foot.

Reproduced from McGee KP, Martinez MW. ECG Gating and Associated Artifacts. In: McGee K, Martinez M, Williamson E, editors. Mayo Clinic Guide to Cardiac Magnetic Resonance Imaging. 2 ed. Oxford University Press; Oxford, UK 2015 with permission from Oxford University Press.

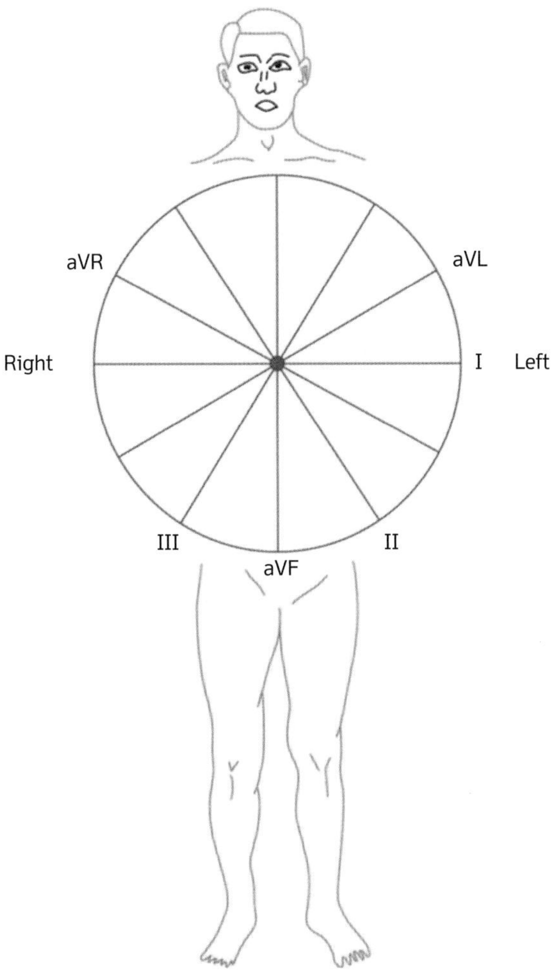

Fig. 4.15 The six limb leads arranged onto the frontal plane.

the interventricular septum. The six limb leads (bipolar and unipolar) are placed at the periphery of the circle (➤ **Fig. 4.15**) and view the centre from different degrees, separating the frontal plane into 12 parts by 30° (➤ **Fig. 4.16**).[4,6,11]

All limb leads are oriented in the frontal plane:

- Lead I: the positive pole is designated as 0° and the negative pole as +/–180°.
- Lead II: the positive pole is designated as +60° and the negative pole as –120°.
- Lead III: the positive pole is designated as +120° and the negative pole as –60°.
- Lead aVR: the positive pole is designated as –150° and the negative pole as +30°.
- Lead aVL: the positive pole is designated as –30° and the negative pole as +150°.
- Lead aVF: the positive pole is designated as +90° and the negative pole as –90°.

Precordial lead positions

There are six precordial leads. The positioning of these leads on the surface of the chest can be seen in ➤ **Fig. 4.17**:

- V1, in the fourth intercostal space just to the right of the sternum.
- V2, in the fourth intercostal space just to the left of the sternum.
- V3, in the middle between V2 and V4.
- V4, in the fifth intercostal space in the midclavicular line.
- V5, in the fifth intercostal space, left anterior axillary line.
- V6, in the fifth intercostal space, left midaxillary line.

Axis determination

While the ventricles are stimulated, electrical axes are created and spread in different directions from one instant to the next. The vector of these forces resulting from the union of several forces applied at the same point is called the mean electrical axis (MEA). In particular, the MEA of the heart is the mean direction of depolarization of the ventricular myocardium in the frontal plane. As previously mentioned, all limb leads are placed in a circle surrounding the heart (hexaxial reference system) and every lead has a positive and a negative pole. Normally, in adults the MEA is between –30 ° and +90° (➤ **Fig. 4.18**). Depending on the MEA level, the mean axis may deviate to the left or to the right (➤ **Box 4.4**).[11,23]

Clinical significance

Left axis deviation

- Left ventricular hypertrophy.
- Left bundle branch block.
- Left anterior hemiblock.
- Inferior myocardial infarction.
- Normal in pregnancy ascites.

Right axis deviation

- Right ventricular hypertrophy.
- Left posterior hemiblock.
- Anterolateral myocardial infarction.
- Right bundle branch block.
- Pulmonary embolism.
- Dextrocardia.

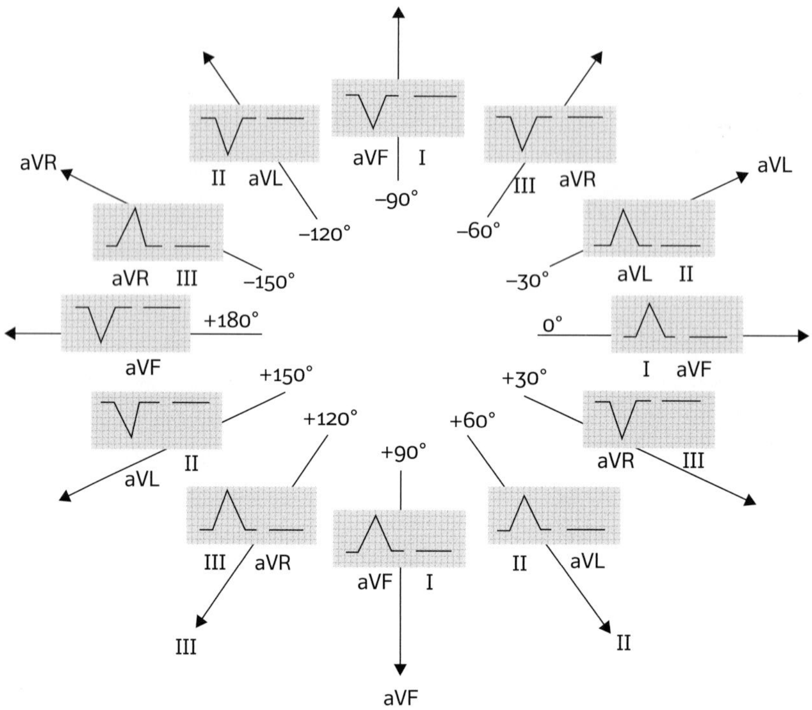

Fig. 4.16 The hexaxial reference system.

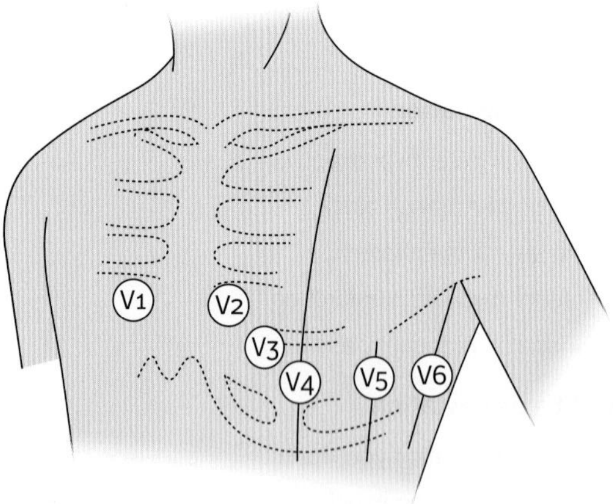

Fig. 4.17 Positions of the precordial leads.

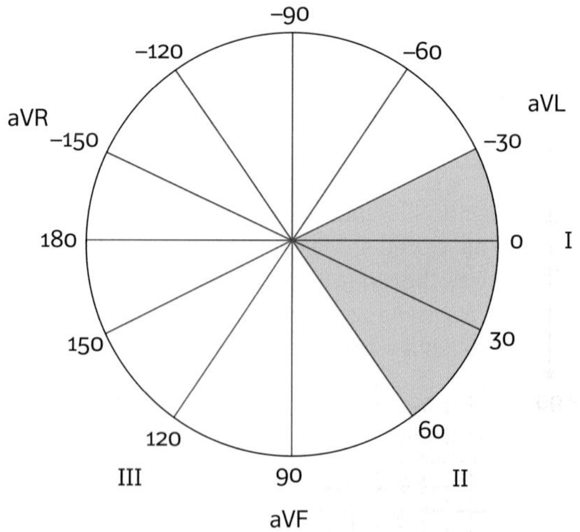

Fig. 4.18 The hexaxial reference system and the normal range for the QRS axis.

Box 4.4 Normal and abnormal ranges of the QRS axis

- Normal (0° to +90°).
- Left axis (−30° to −90°).
- Right axis (+100° to +180°).
- Extreme right axis (+180° to −90°).

How do you calculate the mean axis of the QRS?

There are different ways to calculate the MEA. The most accurate calculation of the axis is to transfer the net deflection of the QRS complex to the hexaxial reference system (➤ Fig. 4.19 and ➤ Fig. 4.20). However, this method is difficult in clinical practice.[6]

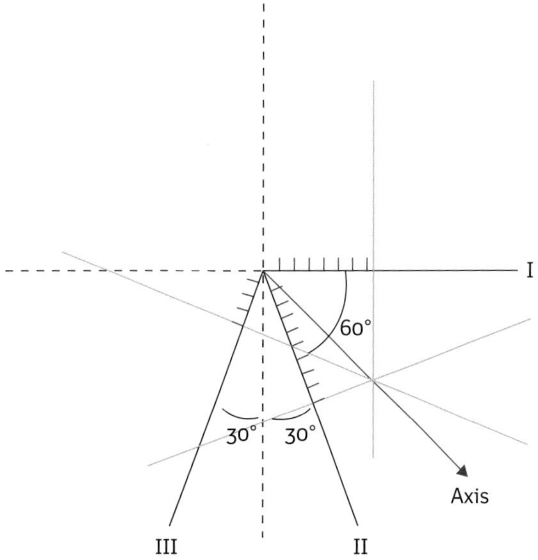

Fig. 4.20 Classical method of axis determination. Calculating the net deflection from three limb leads.

Quick look at the mean axis—an easy approach

Determining the axis from leads I and aVF

In clinical practice, in order to do a more timely assessment of axis deviation, we can consider the normal axis to be between 0° and +90° instead of −30° and +90°. If we divide the hexaxial system into four equal parts, we can examine only leads I and aVF. If we have both positive waves, then the axis is normal. If we have a positive wave in lead I and a negative wave in lead aVF, then the axis is deviated to the left. On the contrary, if we have a negative wave in lead I and a positive wave in lead aVF, then the axis is deviated to the right. Finally, if we have both negative waves in lead I and aVF, the axis is indeterminable (➤ Table 4.3).[23]

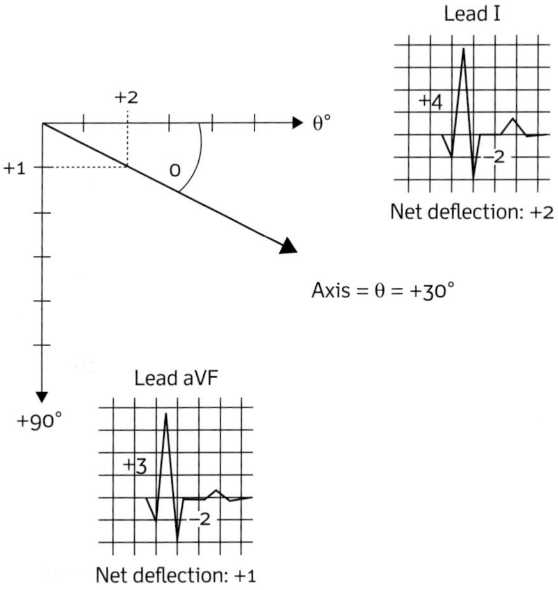

Fig. 4.19 Classical method of axis determination. Calculating the net deflection from two limb leads.

Determining the axis from leads I, II, and aVF

Because the normal axis is between −30° and +90°, the above-described method may miss detection if the axis is

Table 4.3 Calculation of the QRS axis analysing the vector of forces of leads I and aVF

Axis	Lead I	Lead aVF
Normal (0° to +90°)	Positive	Positive
Left axis (−30° to −90°)	Positive	Negative
Right axis (+100° to +180°)	Negative	Positive
Extreme right axis (+180° to −90°)	Negative	Negative

Table 4.4 Calculation of the QRS axis analysing the vector of forces of leads I, aVF, and II

Axis	Lead I	Lead aVF	Lead II
Normal axis (+90° to −30°)	Positive	Positive	Positive
	Positive	Negative	Positive
Left axis (−30° to −90°)	Positive	Negative	Negative
Right axis (+100° to +180°)	Negative	Positive	Negative

between 0° and −30°. In this case, the method summarized in ➤ Table 4.4 may be used by examining leads I, II, and aVF.[23]

ECG analysis and individual parameters of an ECG

ECG components in relation to the action potential

The 12-lead ECG is now part of standard clinical practice and has an important role in aiding diagnosis, monitoring, and screening in cardiovascular disease. The ECG can be broken down into several components and each of these components can potentially detect changes to the cardiac action potential and the electrical conduction through the heart. Being able to read and interpret the 12-lead ECG is an important part of a cardiovascular nurse's role as part of their assessment of the patient. This section will outline each component of the ECG and how it is measured. The 12-lead ECG can be broken down into the following components: P wave, PR interval, Q wave, QRS complex, ST segment, T wave, and QT interval, shown in ➤ Fig. 4.21.

The P wave represents left and right atrial depolarization and precedes the QRS complex. The PR interval is measured from the start of the P wave to the start of the QRS complex. The Q wave is the initial negative (downwards) deflection from the baseline after the P wave. The QRS complex is a measurement of the time taken from onset to completion of ventricular depolarization. After the impulse travels through the septum, the impulse then activates the subendocardial walls and spreads from the endocardium and epicardium through the ventricles. On the ECG, the ventricular activation is seen as a positive tall spike in lead I and known as the QRS complex. The width reflects the time delay from arrival of the depolarization wavefront in the ventricle to total depolarization of both ventricles and as the one of the main properties of the heart is cardiac syncytium, there should be no time delay in depolarization through the ventricles.[24] With the limb leads, the orientation of the

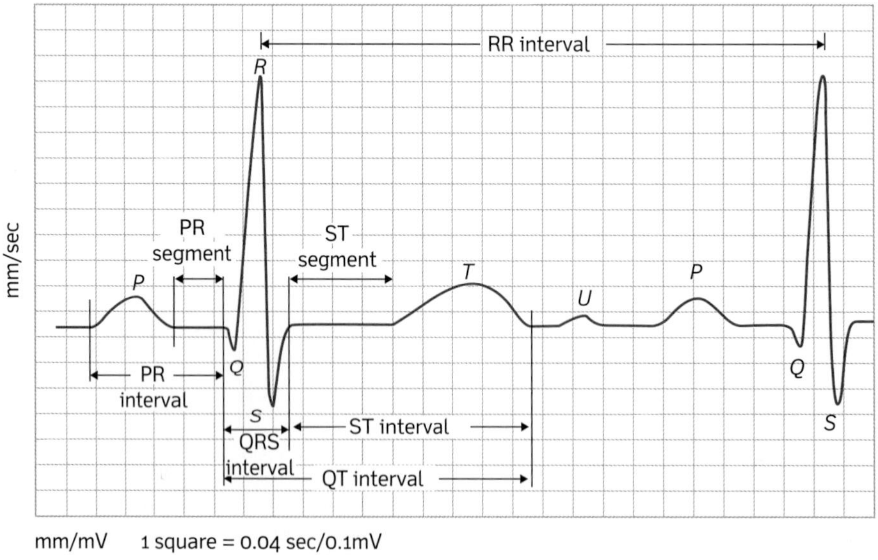

Fig. 4.21 Features of a normal ECG.

QRS complex depends on the direction of the current flow and if the direction is towards a positive electrode, a positive deflection is recorded. An isoelectric trace is recorded when current flow is perpendicular to the lead axis (hence the term isoelectric line). The QT interval is the ventricular repolarization time and is measured from the beginning of the ventricular complex to the end of the T wave (usually best seen in lead II).[25] The R wave is any positive (upwards) deflection of the QRS complex. The ST segment is the early stage of ventricular depolarization and is the interval between the end of the QRS complex (J point) and the onset of the T wave. The T wave represents ventricular depolarization and is the first deflection from the baseline occurring after the QRS complex.[24] The U wave follows the T wave and is usually upright except in aVR.

Using a systematic approach to analysis

For the cardiovascular nurse analysing a 12-lead ECG, there needs to be a systematic approach in which each element of the ECG is examined individually and then an interpretation made based on the analysis. Usually, the specific parameters measured include the following:

- Heart rate (bpm).
- Axis (normal, left, right, extreme, indeterminate).
- Conduction (rhythm and regular or irregular).
- P waves (duration, amplitude, morphology).
- Intervals: PR interval, QT/QTc intervals.
- QRS (duration, amplitude, morphology—in particular amplitude of R waves).
- ST segments (amplitude, morphology—in particular ST elevation or depression).
- T waves (amplitude, morphology).

Using this framework as the basis of your systematic approach will ensure that each component has been examined and analysed and a final interpretation made. ECG interpretation is just one part of the assessment of a patient and is part of the overall assessment which includes patient history and results from blood and enzyme tests (e.g. troponins). Moreover, the presence of disease, race, sex, and prescribed medications can also affect ECG parameters as well as the body size and age of the patient. Nurses need to be familiar with the normal values of these individual ECG components (namely, duration, height, polarity, axis, and shape) for the P wave, PR interval, QRS complex, ST segment, and T waves. The normal characteristics of these components are described in detail in ➤ Table 4.5.

Some characteristics can vary with age (such as the QRS complex and ST segment, for example) and ethnicity (the height of R waves, for example). Therefore, when recording an ECG, the age, sex, and ethnicity of the person needs to be noted so that accurate interpretation can be undertaken.

Reference ranges for the ECG parameters

➤ Table 4.6 shows the normal and abnormal parameters of ECG components which will be described individually.

Heart rate

The heart rate can be calculated using the ECG paper with the time calibration line. It can be calculated by counting the number of large squares between one QRS complex and the next and dividing 300 by this number to obtain the heart rate. If the interval between two beats is 1 second, the heart rate is then 60 bpm. The normal heart rate in an adult with no underlying disease is approximately 70 bpm, but in individuals who are extremely fit with no underlying heart disease, their resting heart rate may be closer to 40 or 50 bpm. A heart rate greater than 100 bpm is a sinus tachycardia and a heart rate less than 60 bpm is sinus bradycardia. Respiration can affect the heart rate during inspiration; this is known as inspiratory sinus arrhythmia and is a normal physiological variant. Along with the heart rate, the axis and conduction must be analysed to determine whether the rhythm is regular or irregular.

Axis

The cardiac axis refers to the general direction in which the depolarization of the heart takes place. The normal range of the QRS axis is −30° and +105° although values can be affected by age, sex, and body morphology. The cardiac axis is usually determined at a glance from leads I, II, and III. If these leads are positive, the axis is normal. Right axis deviation is from +120° to +180° and is associated with tall, thin adults. Left axis deviation is from −30° to −90°. Indeterminate axes (often called 'no man's land' axis) can be observed with downward deflections of leads I and II. An abnormal axis is usually seen with conduction abnormalities, in particular left and right bundle branch block. This conduction abnormality is associated

Table 4.5 Normal characteristics of an ECG in terms of duration, amplitude, polarity, axis, and shape

ECG component	Duration	Amplitude	Polarity	Axis	Shape
P wave	0.08–0. 11 seconds	≤0.25 mV In V1: 0.15 mV Negative deflection <−0.1 mV	+ve: I, II, aVF, V2–V6 −ve: aVR Biphasic: V1 Upright, diphasic, flat, or inverted: III, aVL, V1–V3 Variable: V3	+60° Range 0–75° in frontal plane	Usually smooth
QRS complex	0.05–0.10 seconds Normal Q wave: <0.04 seconds	Varies with age ≥6 mm in V1, V6 ≥8 mm in V2, V5 ≥10 mm in V3, V4 Upper limit of normal is 25–30 mm Rarely >1 mm in V4–V6	+ve to equiphasic: I, II, V3–V6 +ve/−ve/equiphasic: aVF, aVL −ve: aVR Narrow Q or 1–2 mm in I, aVl, V6 Terminal forces: S in V1 and R in V6	−30° to +120° in frontal plane	+ve components: R or r wave −ve component: Q or q or S or s
ST segment		Up to 1 mm is normal >40 years: V2, V3 2 mm	+ve: I, II, V3–V6 −ve: aVR +ve: aVL, aVF but −ve if QRS is <6 mm Varies in III, V1, V2		Rounded and symmetrical
T wave		<5 mm in limb leads and <10 mm in precordial leads Limb leads: <6 mm, tallest in lead II and not less than 0.5 mm in lead I and II Precordial: tallest in V2 and V3, taller in men (6 mm), women 3–4 mm	+ve: I, II, V3–V6 −ve: aVR +ve: aVL, aVF but −ve if QRS is <6 mm Varies in III, V1, V2		Rounded and symmetrical

with underlying cardiovascular disease, especially heart failure.[26–28])

P waves

The P wave represents left and right atrial depolarization. The duration of the P wave is usually 0.08–0.11 seconds and the amplitude is usually between 0.1 mV and 0.3 mV. On average, the voltage is less than 0.25 mV but can have a negative amplitude of −0.1 mV. The P wave is usually positive in leads I, II, aVF, and V2–V6 and negative in aVR and biphasic in V1. It can be either positive or negative in lead V3 and can be flat or inverted in aVL and V1–V3. It can also have a biphasic appearance in V1 (i.e. it has a positive and negative component). The normal P wave axis is 60° and its shape is usually smooth.[29] The P wave is not always present and sometimes not visible in some leads.

A P wave that has increased width and has a notch is associated with left atrial abnormality or right atrial hypertrophy.[30] Left atrial enlargement is observed with a biphasic P wave and a negative component excessively wide P wave in lead II or V1 and a peaked P wave

Table 4.6 Normal and abnormal parameters of ECG components

ECG components	Normal parameters	Abnormal parameters	Causes of abnormal parameters
P wave	Upright in most leads	Inverted Notched or tall	Junctional rhythm Atrial rhythm, atrial hypertrophy
PR interval	Duration 0.12–0.20 seconds	Duration: shorter or longer than normal	Junctional rhythm, Wolff–Parkinson–White syndrome
Q wave	Amplitude <25% of R wave amplitude	Duration 0.04 seconds or longer Amplitude at least 25% of R wave amplitude	Myocardial infarction
QRS complex	Upright, inverted, or biphasic Amplitude:1 mm or more	Duration >0.11 seconds or more	Bundle branch block, ventricular ectopic
QT interval	Duration less than ½ of width of the RR interval	Duration at least ½ RR interval	Long QT syndrome, cardiac drugs, hypothermia, subarachnoid haemorrhage Short QT interval—hypercalcaemia
ST segment	In line with PR or TP segment (baseline) Shortens with increased heart rate	Duration of 0.5 mm or more from baseline	Cardiac ischaemia or infarction, early repolarization, ventricular hypertrophy, digoxin toxicity, pericarditis, subarachnoid haemorrhage
T wave	Upright, asymmetrical. Duration 0.10–0.25 seconds	Peaked, inverted, biphasic, notched, flat, or wide waveforms	Cardiac ischaemia or infarction, subarachnoid haemorrhage, left-sided tension pneumothorax, left bundle branch block, hypokalaemia
U wave	Upright with amplitude <2 mm	Peaked or inverted Amplitude >2 mm	Hypokalaemia, cardiomyopathy, ventricular hypertrophy, diabetes, digoxin, quinidine

associated with right atrial overload and is usually taller in lead I than lead III. An absence of P waves can indicate atrial fibrillation, SA block, atrial standstill, and junctional rhythm with hidden P waves. Inverted P waves in leads II, III, and aVF suggest ectopic atrial beats from low in the atria, retrograde activation from junctional beats, or an AV reentry mechanism.

Intervals

PR interval

The PR interval is the time between the beginning of the P wave and the beginning of the QRS complex and represents the beginning of atrial excitation and the beginning of ventricular depolarization. The normal PR interval is 0.16 seconds and is usually between 0.12 and 0.20 seconds. A shortened PR interval of less than 0.12 seconds is associated with an electrical impulse coming through the AV junction, or one originating from close to the AV node. An example is Wolff–Parkinson–White syndrome where delta waves are seen as a slurring of the upstroke of the QRS complex. A prolonged PR interval is categorized as greater than 0.22 seconds and associated with heart block (see Chapters 6 and 7).[31]

QT/QTc interval

The contraction of the ventricle is marked by the beginning of the Q wave to the end of the T wave. This is known as the QT interval with a duration of less than 0.45 seconds. It represents the interval from onset of ventricular depolarization to ventricular repolarization and varies with the heart rate. The more rapid the heart rate, the faster ventricular depolarization occurs and the smaller the QT interval. A prolonged QT interval is a known side effect of pharmacological agents such as tricyclic antidepressants and can be fatal.[32] To correct for the variation in heart rate, a formula to calculate the QTc interval is used. Bazett's formula is:

$$QTc = \frac{QT\ (\text{seconds})}{\sqrt{R\ \text{to}\ R\ \text{interval}\ (\text{seconds})}}$$

QRS complex

The QRS complex is a measurement of the time taken from onset to completion of ventricular depolarization. The amplitude of the QRS complex can vary with age and ethnicity. The normal duration of the QRS complex is 0.05–0.10 seconds and the normal Q wave is less than 0.4 seconds. The polarity of the QRS complex can be positive to equiphasic in leads I, II, and V3–V6. In leads aVF and aVL, the polarity can be positive, negative, or equiphasic. The axis is usually from −30° to +120° and the shape is usually upright. The Q wave is the first deflection of the complex and is usually downward. The R wave is any upward deflection and it may be preceded by the Q wave or it may be the first deflection. The S wave is the downward deflection that occurs after the R wave. Leads V1–V6 are known as the precordial leads and reflect the thick-walled left ventricle and the R wave becomes taller as the positive current gets closer and closer to the ventricle. The V leads are seen as a good indicator of underlying cardiovascular disease.[33–35] The size of the R wave is measured in V5 and V6 and should be less than 25 mm in older people and less than 30 mm in younger, thin people. The S wave is deepest in V1 and decreases across the rest of the precordial leads (V2–V5) and it should be less than 25 mm deep when measured from the isoelectric line.

There is a lack of consensus regarding the usual QRS complex duration which according to some should be no greater than 0.05–0.10 seconds (50–100 milliseconds) although others state 0.08–0.12 seconds.[24] In bundle branch block, the duration is 0.12 seconds (120 milliseconds) or more, in ventricular hypertrophy it is 0.10–0.11 seconds (100–110 milliseconds). Lead II is a poor lead for showing QRS onset as it is delayed and therefore V1 and V2 are better for measuring QRS duration. The QRS voltage also varies according to age, ethnicity, and in those with thin chest walls.

ST segment

The ST segment is usually 1 mm and in those over 40 years of age the V2 and V3 amplitude can be up to 2 mm. The polarity varies and it is positive in leads I, II, and V3–V6 and negative in aVR. The shape should be rounded and symmetrical. In those of African ethnicity, the ST segment can appear elevated without underlying heart disease and this is why recording ethnicity is important as part of the cardiac assessment.[36] Any ST elevation above 2 mm is associated with myocardial infarction and ST depression is associated with myocardial ischaemia.[37] The greater the ST elevation or depression, the greater the degree of coronary heart disease. However, in patients with known bundle branch block, ST segments cannot be interpreted due to the widening of the QRS complex. Widespread ST-segment elevation can sometimes be seen, and it is associated with pericardial inflammation and usually an echocardiogram is urgently required to confirm the diagnosis.

T waves

The T wave amplitude is less than 5 mm in limb leads and less than 10 mm in precordial leads. Sex differences are seen in the amplitude and polarity of the T wave, but it is usually positive in leads I, II, and V3–V6. The greatest amplitude is in lead II where up to 6 mm is normal. In the precordial leads, the T wave in V3 is usually the tallest and can be up to 12 mm in height. The shape of the T wave is usually rounded and symmetrical. Isolated T-wave inversion is a normal finding that is sometimes seen on a 12-lead ECG. It is not clinically significant unless associated with symptoms or in a patient with known coronary heart disease with progressive, deep, symmetrical T-wave inversion where it is associated with ischaemia.[37] Tall or peaked T waves can also be observed.[38] Abnormal T waves are associated with many clinical pathologies.

U wave abnormalities

The U wave is not always visible on the ECG but if it is present, the U wave should be the same polarity as the proceeding T wave. An abnormal U wave is usually the opposite polarity to the proceeding complex. As can be seen, each ECG component has normal values for amplitude, duration, polarity, and shape and abnormalities have been outlined for all these components. Therefore, examining and analysing each component is important as any abnormality suggests a potential underlying pathology.

Conclusion

This chapter has provided an overview of the structure and function of the heart and circulatory system focusing upon the mechanical and electrical properties. An understanding of these concepts forms the basis of recognizing the signs and symptoms indicative of changes in clinical condition as well as providing important diagnostic information.

References

1. Marieb EN. Holyoke Community College. Human Anatomy and Physiology (10th ed). London: Pearson Education; 2016.
2. Krams R, Bäck M (Eds). The ESC Textbook of Vascular Biology. Oxford: Oxford University Press; 2017.
3. Hamrell BB. Cardiovascular Physiology. Boca Raton, FL: CRC Press; 2018.
4. Klabunde R. Cardiovascular Physiology Concepts. Philadelphia, PA: Lippincott Williams & Wilkins; 2011.
5. Sherwood L. Fundamentals of Human Physiology. Boston, MA: Cengage Learning; 2011.
6. Woods S, Froelicher E, Motzer S, Bridges E. Cardiac Nursing (6th ed). Philadelphia, PA: Lippincott Williams & Wilkins; 2010.
7. Herring N, Paterson DJ. Levick's Introduction to Cardiovascular Physiology. Boca Raton, FL: CRC Press; 2018.
8. Kucia A, Quinn T. Acute Cardiac Care: A Practical Guide for Nurses. Chichester: John Wiley & Sons; 2013.
9. Innes JA, Dover AR, Fairhurst K (Eds). Macleod's Clinical Examination (14th ed). Philadelphia, PA: Elsevier; 2018.
10. Harrison M. Cardiovascular Physiology. Oxford: Oxford University Press; 2017.
11. Goldberger AL, Goldberger ZD, Shvilkin A. Clinical Electrocardiography: A Simplified Approach. Philadelphia, PA: Elsevier Health Sciences; 2017.
12. Rhoades RA, Bell DR. Medical Physiology: Principles for Clinical Medicine (5th ed). Philadelphia, PA: Wolters Klower; 2018.
13. Johnson LR. Essential Medical Physiology. Philadelphia, PA: Elsevier; 2003.
14. Camm AJ, Lüscher TF, Maurer G, Serruys P. ESC CardioMed (3rd ed). Oxford: Oxford University Press; 2018. https://oxfordmedicine.com/view/10.1093/med/9780198784906.001.0001/med-9780198784906.
15. Yealy DM, Callaway C. Emergency Department Critical Care. Oxford: Oxford University Press; 2013.
16. Preston RR, Wilson TE. Lippincott® Illustrated Reviews: Physiology. Philadelphia, PA: Lippincott Williams & Wilkins; 2018.
17. Ng SY, Wong CK, Tsang SY. Differential gene expressions in atrial and ventricular myocytes: insights into the road of applying embryonic stem cell-derived cardiomyocytes for future therapies. Am J Physiol Cell Physiol. 2010;299(6):C1234–C49.
18. Tortora GJ, Derrickson BH. Principles of Anatomy and Physiology. Hoboken, NJ: John Wiley & Sons; 2018.
19. Levick JR. An Introduction to Cardiovascular Physiology. London: Butterworth-Heinneman; 1991.
20. Morton P, Fontaine D. Critical Care Nursing: A Holistic Approach (10th ed). Philadelphia, PA: Lippincott Williams; 2018.
21. Sommer RJ. Cardiac physiology and pharmacology. In: McQueen CA (Ed), Comprehensive Toxicology: Philadelphia, PA: Elsevier; 2010:51–67.
22. Pappano AJ, Wier WG. Cardiovascular Physiology (11th ed). Philadelphia, PA: Elsevier Health Sciences; 2018.
23. Sampson M. Understanding the ECG. Part 6: QRS axis. Br J Card Nurs. 2016;11(4):180–88.
24. Guy D. Pocket Guide to ECGs (2nd ed). Sydney: McGraw Hill; 2005.
25. Conover MB. Understanding Electrocardiography (8th ed). Sydney: Mosby; 2003.
26. Zannad F, Huvelle E, Dickstein K, van Veldhuisen DJ, Stellbrink C, Kober L, et al. Left bundle branch block as a risk factor for progression to heart failure. Eur J Heart Fail. 2007;9(1):7–14.
27. Tabrizi F, Englund A, Rosenqvist M, Wallentin L, Stenestrand U. Influence of left bundle branch block on long-term mortality in a population with heart failure. Eur Heart J. 2007;28(20):2449–55.
28. Imanishi R, Seto S, Ichimaru S, Nakashima E, Yano K, Akahoshi M. Prognostic significance of incident complete left bundle branch block observed over a 40-year period. Am J Cardiol. 2006;98(5):644–48.
29. Scott CC, Leier CV, Kilman JW, Vasko JS, Unverferth DV. The effect of left atrial histology and dimension on P wave morphology. J Electrocardiol. 1983;16(4):363–66.
30. Thomas P, Dejong D. The P wave in the electrocardiogram in the diagnosis of heart disease. Br Heart J. 1954;16(3):241–54.
31. Cheng S, Keyes MJ, Larson MG, McCabe EL, Newton-Cheh C, Levy D, et al. Long-term outcomes in individuals with prolonged PR interval or first-degree atrioventricular block. JAMA. 2009;301(24):2571–77.
32. Oikarinen L, Nieminen MS, Viitasalo M, Toivonen L, Jern S, Dahlof B, et al. QRS duration and QT interval predict mortality in hypertensive patients with left ventricular hypertrophy: the Losartan Intervention for Endpoint Reduction in Hypertension Study. Hypertension. 2004;43(5):1029–34.

33. Wang NC, Maggioni AP, Konstam MA, Zannad F, Krasa HB, Burnett JC Jr, et al. Clinical implications of QRS duration in patients hospitalized with worsening heart failure and reduced left ventricular ejection fraction. JAMA. 2008;299(22):2656–66.
34. Murkofsky RL, Dangas G, Diamond JA, Mehta D, Schaffer A, Ambrose JA. A prolonged QRS duration on surface electrocardiogram is a specific indicator of left ventricular dysfunction. J Am Coll Cardiol. 1998;32(2):476–82.
35. Desai AD, Yaw TS, Yamazaki T, Kaykha A, Chun S, Froelicher VF. Prognostic significance of quantitative QRS duration. Am J Med. 2006;119(7):600–606.
36. Sliwa K, Lee GA, Carrington MJ, Obel P, Okreglicki A, Stewart S. Redefining the ECG in urban South Africans: electrocardiographic findings in heart disease-free Africans. Int J Cardiol. 2013;167(5):2204–209.
37. Larsen CT, Dahlin J, Blackburn H, Scharling H, Appleyard M, Sigurd B, et al. Prevalence and prognosis of electrocardiographic left ventricular hypertrophy, ST segment depression and negative T-wave; the Copenhagen City Heart Study. Eur Heart J. 2002;23(4):315–24.
38. Watanabe Y, Toda H, Nishimura M. Clinical electrocardiographic studies of bifid T waves. Br Heart J. 1984;52(2):207–14.

5 Nursing assessment and care planning in the context of cardiovascular care

EKATERINI LAMBRINOU, DIANE L. CARROLL, HOWARD T. BLANCHARD, ELENI KLETSIOU, FELICITY ASTIN, ALISON WOOLLEY, JO TILLMAN, RICARDO LEAL, AND ROSIE CERVERA-JACKSON

CHAPTER CONTENTS

In this chapter, nursing assessment strategies are explored as they apply to different stages of the care pathway. It starts with the initial assessment, which occurs at the first meeting between nurse and patient. This assessment allows the nurse to determine the adequacy of ventilation and perfusion to ensure early prioritization of care needs, especially regarding life-threatening situations. Commonly used algorithms are shown to facilitate this assessment. Next, a physical examination of each of the body systems is described highlighting, in particular, assessment of the cardiovascular system. Importantly, track and trigger systems to identify deterioration and the need to escalate care in emergency and acute situations are covered. In addition, classic elements of a comprehensive nursing assessment are outlined which aim to determine the baseline physical and emotional status of the patient and family using Gordon's functional health patterns framework. Special assessment considerations for specific cardiovascular conditions are discussed in more detail in other chapters, such as coronary heart disease (Chapter 6), cardiac arrhythmias (Chapter 7), valvular disease (Chapter 8), inherited cardiac diseases (Chapter 9), heart failure (Chapter 10), and prevention and rehabilitation (Chapter 11).

KEY MESSAGES

- Nursing assessment addresses the promotion of health, prevention of illness, and the nursing care of ill people.
- Nursing assessment identifies the immediate and future responses to potential and actual health problems of the cardiovascular patient.
- Care planning aims to address/resolve problems with collaborative goals identified by the cardiovascular patient.
- A physical examination, including a cardiovascular examination, is an essential part of comprehensive nursing assessment providing a wealth of information about the patient.
- The early detection of clinical deterioration is a key component in the care quality and safety agenda.
- The initial assessment in an acute care setting reviews the reason for seeking care and determines adequate ventilation and perfusion to identify the need for early intervention.
- Recognition of deterioration using appropriate track and trigger tools outlined in hospital policies allows nurses to identify the need for escalation of care.
- Timely management of deterioration of patients in emergency situations is facilitated by effective communication with specialist teams with intensive care skills.
- A comprehensive nursing assessment using a holistic patient-centred approach is completed after the initial assessment to gather further data for care planning.
- Using the format of the eleven functional health patterns for assessment, physical examination findings, and a review of diagnostic tests, nurses use their clinical knowledge and reasoning to make judgements that identify problems that are responsive to nursing care.
- With the cardiovascular patient and their family, the nurse confirms the problems, defines the goal to be reached, and uses nursing intervention to reach the patient's goal.

Introduction

Health assessment refers to a systematic method of collecting and analysing data for the purpose of planning patient-centred care. Comprehensive assessment is very important in order to determine an accurate diagnosis and recognize all of the person's needs. Through describing a person's condition and having a holistic approach to identifying their needs, an effective and timely healthcare plan is developed and implemented (see Chapter 11 and Chapter 14).

It is important to point out how a conventional medical assessment differs from a nursing assessment, especially when the role of a nurse is taken into consideration. Virginia Henderson eloquently defined this role several decades ago: 'The unique function of the nurse is to assist the individual, sick or well, in the performance of those activities contributing to health or its recovery (or to peaceful death) that he would perform unaided if he had the necessary strength, will or knowledge.' Medical assessment conventionally collects disease-focused patient information. While this format addresses collaborative care, it does not address the promotion of health, prevention of illness, and the nursing care of ill people. Nursing encompasses autonomous and collaborative care of individuals of all ages, families, groups, and communities, sick or well, and in all settings.[1] Nurses need and collect information that identifies the immediate and future responses to actual or potential health problems of the cardiovascular patient and their family. This information serves as a basis for determining patients' problems that are amenable to nursing care. Therefore, a nursing diagnosis is a clinical judgement concerning a human response to health conditions/life processes, or vulnerability for that response, by an individual, family, group, or community.

Circumstances contributing to the context of care include the setting or environment; the physical, psychological, or socioeconomic circumstances involving patients; and the expertise of the nurse. Because of these

Box 5.1 Types of health assessment

Comprehensive assessment

Involves a detailed history and physical examination performed at the onset of care in a primary care setting or on admission to a hospital or long-term care facility. The comprehensive assessment encompasses health problems experienced by the patient; health promotion, disease prevention, and assessment for problems associated with known risk factors; or assessment for age- and sex-specific health problems (e.g. increased cardiovascular risk for women after menopause; see Chapter 14).

Problem-based/focused assessment

The problem-based or problem-focused assessment involves a history and examination that are limited to a specific problem or complaint (e.g. peripheral/lower extremities oedema; see Chapter 10). This type of assessment is most commonly used in a walk-in clinic or emergency department, but it may also be applied in other outpatient settings (e.g. heart failure clinics). Although the focus of data collection is on a specific problem (e.g. heart failure), the potential impact of the patient's underlying health status also must be considered (in order to find the cause of deterioration).

Episodic/follow-up assessment

This type of assessment is usually done when a patient is following up with a healthcare provider (e.g. heart failure nurse) for a previously identified problem. For example, a patient with heart failure treated by the multidisciplinary team for peripheral oedema might be asked to return for a follow-up visit after completing a prescription of diuretics. An individual treated for an ongoing condition such as heart failure, is asked to make regular visits to the clinic for episodic assessment.

Shift assessment

When individuals are hospitalized, nurses conduct assessments each shift. The purpose of the shift assessment is to identify changes to a patient's condition from the baseline; thus, the focus of the assessment is largely based on the condition or problem the patient is experiencing and the patient's response to the therapeutic plan.

Screening assessment/examination

A short examination focused on disease detection. A screening examination may be performed in a healthcare provider's office (as part of a comprehensive examination) or at a health fair (e.g. European Society of Cardiology congress, heart failure awareness days activities). Examples include blood pressure screening, glucose screening and cholesterol screening.

variables, different types of assessments are performed (e.g. a comprehensive health assessment, a problem-based or focused health assessment, an episodic assessment (e.g. for heart failure, see Chapter 10), a shift assessment, and a screening assessment) (➤ Box 5.1). In some settings, such as a hospital or a community-based primary care setting, a comprehensive history is collected and an examination is performed (see Chapter 11). In an urgent care or emergency department setting (e.g. in an acute coronary syndrome or deteriorated heart failure episode), a problem-based or focused assessment is indicated, although additional subjective and objective data that may have a direct or indirect impact on the management of the patient are collected. In addition, if it is determined that the patient is at risk or in need of further evaluation (e.g. angiography), the patient is referred to the appropriate department (coronary unit/catheterization laboratory) so a comprehensive assessment can be completed.

Components of health assessment include conducting a health history, performing a physical examination, reviewing other data from the health record (as available), and documenting the findings. These steps lead to data analysis and interpretation (discussed later in this chapter) so that a patient-centred plan of care can be developed and implemented. The amount of information collected by the nurse during a health history and the extent of the physical examination depend on the setting, the situation, the patient's needs, and the nurse's experience. The nurse incorporates the patient's knowledge, motivation, support systems, coping ability, and preferences to develop a plan of care that will help the patient maximize his or her potential (➤ Fig. 5.1).[2] Health assessment data are documented so the health status at the time of the healthcare encounter is recorded and the information is available to the rest of the multidisciplinary team involved in the patient's care.

The nursing assessment is the beginning of information collection, and subsequently, nurses continue to collect information at every interaction. The nurse's level of clinical knowledge influences the skilfulness of information

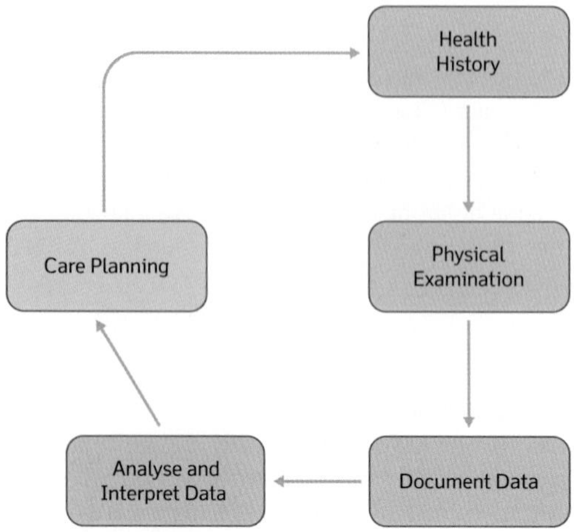

Fig. 5.1 The development of the care plan based on the assessment and data interpretation.

collection and allows for sensitivity to certain cues from the cardiovascular patient. Nurses have the knowledge to make a judgement about the information that permits explanation and prediction. In clinical practice, nurses use their clinical knowledge and reasoning and start to piece information together in a meaningful way. Then, they put a name to the problem, need, or category (nursing diagnosis) on which the nursing care plan will be based.

Health history

The nurse collects *health data* from the patient and compares these with the ideal state of health, taking into account the patient's age, sex/gender, culture, ethnicity, and physical, psychological, and socioeconomic status. Data about the patient's strengths, weaknesses, health problems, and deficits are identified (see Chapter 11 and Chapter 14).

An accurate recording of *medications* including supplements, over-the-counter medications, and herbal remedies and should be recorded and reconciled using electronic data confirmation, if available, from local pharmacies. The list should include names, last dose, and any allergies. Information about the medication and allergies can be taken from the patient and the significant others or caregivers. Also, adherence with medication should be taken into consideration with the appropriate questions asked (see Chapter 12 and Chapter 14) as well as the patient's beliefs and attitudes about their medication therapy. Assessment of level of knowledge of the current medication and its side effects or actions is needed for the upcoming educational planning of the patient with cardiovascular disease (see Chapter 13).

Questions on *allergies* should include all possible allergic agents such as medications, foods, and the environment, as well as the nature of the reaction and its seriousness. Intolerance of medications should also be recorded. Based on the institutional and local policy, allergy history must be documented and be clearly visible to all healthcare team members. Family members should also be made aware of allergic reactions.[3]

Initial assessment

The focus of the initial assessment varies according to the setting and clinical presentation. The initial assessment of all patients presenting to nurses, irrespective of the cardiovascular setting, aims to determine whether the person/patient is haemodynamically stable, adequacy of ventilation and perfusion to assess the need for early intervention for life-threatening situations, whether the person is suffering from an acute cardiac event that would benefit from time-dependent therapy, and the need for symptom management (e.g. see Chapter 6). Therefore, the initial assessment is a key com11ponent of healthcare planning as it helps nurses and other healthcare professionals to prioritize problems and plan timely nursing interventions, especially when urgent action to maintain or to restore adequate ventilation and perfusion is required (➤ Table 5.1).

Starting with the first contact with the patient, initial clinical assessment or the general survey may include stature, overall health status, body habitus, personal hygiene, grooming, skin condition such as signs of breakdown or chronic wounds, breath and body odour, overall mood, and psychological state (see Chapter 11). At the same time, initial vital sign measurements (i.e. temperature, respiratory rate, heart rate, blood pressure with appropriate sized cuff, pulse oximetry reading, and note if on room air or oxygen), and accurately measured weight in kilograms with well-maintained scales and height measurement, so that body mass index (BMI) can be calculated for medication dosing and nutritional intake, should all take place along with the history-taking questions.[4]

Life-threatening conditions must be recognized early, therefore the initial assessment should be structured and detailed, but time-framed, as history taking and patient assessment must not delay interventions or definitive care. Following the algorithms for the assessment,

Table 5.1 Care plan

Plan of care with goals, defining characteristics, and nursing interventions	
Nursing problem	Risk-prone health behaviour—smoking[6]
Goal	Assist patient to quit smoking to reduce a modifiable risk factor
Defining characteristic	Current smoker
Nursing interventions[7]	(See Chapter 11 for more information on how to assist patients with smoking cessation strategies) Advise on quitting smoking Assess motivation and readiness to quit smoking Negotiate strategy to quit smoking Provide smoking cessation assistance Arrange follow-up Identify a support mechanism
Nursing problem	Knowledge deficit related to new diagnosis of exertional angina[6]
Goal	Patient will demonstrate an understanding of this condition, its causes, and appropriate relief measures for chest discomfort
Defining characteristic	New diagnosis of exertional angina
Nursing interventions[7]	Assess knowledge of causes of angina, treatment, and risk factors Identify triggers for angina that can be managed Minimize the symptoms of gastro-oesophageal reflux disease to reduce gastrointestinal symptom burden and assist patient to know difference between gastrointestinal and cardiac discomfort Develop an individualized educational plan: 1. On the proper use of nitroglycerine for chest discomfort 2. How and when to seek emergency medical services Teach use and side effects of other medications for long-term management Address need to reduce modifiable risk factors
Nursing problem	Stress overload related to change in health status and work demands[6]
Goal	Reduce stress from new diagnosis and stressors in the work place
Defining characteristic	Nervousness, alteration in attention
Nursing interventions[7]	Identify stressors both at home and in work environment Recognize family members and colleagues that can provide emotional support and coping strategies to reduce stress Use relaxation therapies such as mindfulness meditation, relaxation response Allied health professional counselling

the assessment should be brief and the need for further assessment and life-supporting intervention should always be considered. An example of such an algorithm is 'SAMPLE' (➤ **Box 5.2**). It provides a simple process to organize this initial assessment and ensure that emergency situations can be assessed in the most optimal way.[5]

Adopting a holistic nursing, patient-centred and not solely a biomedical perspective, is outlined in the Core Curriculum for the Continuing Professional Development of Nurses Working in Cardiovascular Settings.[8] The functional health pattern framework[9] (➤ **Fig. 5.2**) provides a systematic approach to identifying potential or actual

Box 5.2 The SAMPLE algorithm for the assessment of medical emergency situations

S—signs and symptoms.
A—allergies.
M—medications.
P—past medical history.
L—last meal or oral intake.
E—events before the acute situation.

Source data from World Health Organization. The ABCDE and SAMPLE History Approach, World Health Organization 2018.

problems that nurses can consider as part of comprehensive assessment.

This framework has two principal domains, the first being physical well-being and comfort and the second, emotional and spiritual well-being. More detail on what should be assessed for each domain can be seen in ➤ Table 5.2.[10–21] ➤ Table 5.3 provides some examples of questions that can be asked to assess the health perception and management pattern.[9,11,22] It may not be necessary to ask all of the proposed questions. The nurse's clinical knowledge and reasoning will help them to make judgements on which questions to prioritize. See also ➤ Box 5.3[23] for some selected validated cognitive screening tools.

Chief complaint

The first step in the evaluation of a new patient is to record the chief complaint and history. Nurses taking a history and assessing patients should make sure that, when addressing a patient, they use appropriate language relevant to the level of health literacy and use a certified and experienced translator where they are unable to communicate with the patient in their mother tongue. From the very first moment, culturally competent care and respect for privacy should be ensured and maintained throughout the healthcare continuum (see Chapter 14).

There are many algorithms that nurses can use to assess the main complaint. Use of the mnemonics P-Q-R-S-T-A and oPQRSTa (➤ Box 5.4) is considered to be an effective and a reliable approach to the assessment of symptoms and especially chest pain of any origin.[24] They are very useful in assessing other symptoms such as dyspnoea or shortness of breath and also provide a

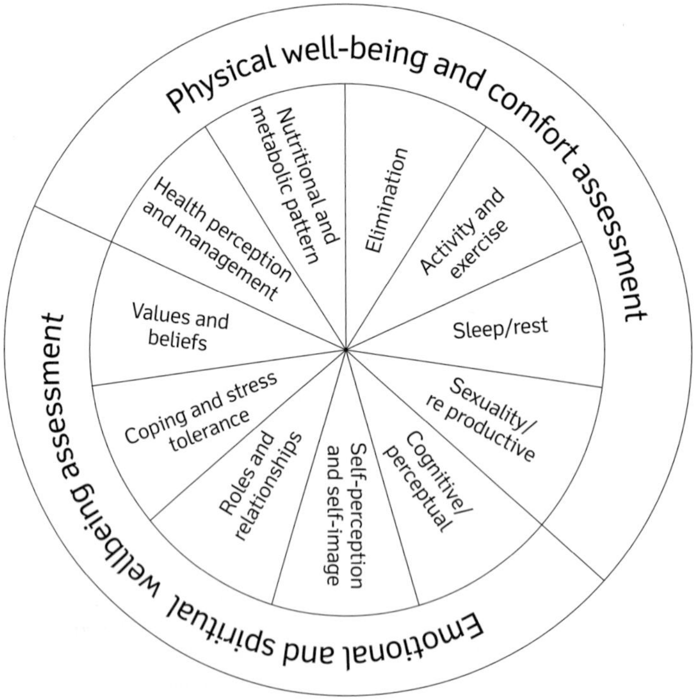

Fig. 5.2 Gordon's eleven functional health patterns.

Table 5.2 Assessment of the eleven functional health patterns

Physical well-being and comfort assessment	Emotional and spiritual well-being assessment
Health perception and management	*Cognitive/perceptual*
1. General perceptions of health, general health management, and disease prevention strategies that may identify a dysfunctional pattern 2. Routines to maintain health, how signs and symptoms are treated, and reasons for seeking healthcare 3. Current and past health practices and future motivation regarding health promotion, e.g. current and past smoking history and attempts at smoking cessation. Smoking is a key cardiovascular risk that nurses can address (see Chapter 11 for more detail on how nurses can address this risk factor) 4. Use and abuse of drugs (e.g. sedatives, amphetamines, opioids, ecstasy, cocaine, heroin, z drugs, and cannabis) 5. Current and past health status 6. Current and past family history of cardiovascular heart disease as an indicator to identify the risk of developing cardiovascular disease 7. Employment and work conditions 8. Social isolation/exclusion 9. Early childhood development 10. Housing 11. Access to healthcare and public health programmes[10]	1. Ability to use cognitive skills (perception, comprehension of ideas, perception, thinking, reasoning, and remembering, capacity for judgement) 2. Ability to use language skills, perception, memory, symbolic and imagery operations, problem-solving and decision-making[9,11] 3. Impaired cognitive functioning as a risk factor for cardiovascular conditions—effect on healthy patterns and behaviours, ability to understand and follow healthcare advice, and influence on medication adherence[12] 4. Need for more in-depth assessment and evaluation with validated specific cognitive screening tools[13] (Box 5.3) 5. Educational level
Nutritional and metabolic pattern (see Chapter 11 Prevention and rehabilitation for more detail on how to conduct a dietary assessment and features of a healthy diet)	*Self-perception and self-image*
1. Food and fluid intake taking into account age, sex, body size, and composition 2. Evaluation of nutrient intake in relation to actual or potential health problems 3. Assessment of food and fluid intake using recall or record 4. Height and weight to calculate BMI—weight in kilograms divided by height in metres squared 5. Cultural food choices, who prepares meals in the home 6. Number of meals eaten outside the home 7. Access to healthy food 8. Financial burden of food 9. Food allergies including response to the allergenic food 10. Use of and abuse of alcohol (CAGE questionnaire available in multiple languages)[14]	1. Evidence of low self-esteem, poor self-image (e.g. body image) 2. General appearance, non-verbal communication (such as body language, posture and movement, eye contact), voice and speech patterns 3. Identify mood disorders, negative feelings or anxiety for the present or future, depression that led to delayed medical advice seeking, or low self-esteem and value of living 4. Where appropriate, use of screening tools for anxiety, depression, or bipolar disorders (relevant to age, cultural level, health literacy, special condition, and educational level)
Elimination (bowels, bladder, and skin)	*Roles and relationships*[15]
1. Regularity and control of elimination patterns (bowels, bladder, and skin) 2. Usual urinary pattern (frequency of urination during the day, difficulty, leaking, pain, waking at night to empty the bladder)	1. Defined roles as identified by patient—importance of these roles in relation to their health situation and the perceived health habits 2. Occupation type and work conditions (working hours, absence leaves, working accident, work stress, level of income, responsibilities, social interactions, occupational satisfaction)

Table 5.2 Continued

3. Usual pattern of bowel elimination (frequency, time of the day, consistency, use of laxatives, changes in bowel pattern, interventions to maintain normal bowel pattern) 4. Maintenance of an intact skin surface—daily hygiene practices, influencing factors, skin problems in the past (see 'Physical examination of the cardiovascular patient' section for more detail) 5. Use of diuretics (hypertension and heart failure)—decrease of fluid adsorption causing constipation 6. Use of cardiovascular medications that increase sun sensitivity 7. Use of anticoagulant and antiplatelet agents—increased bleeding risk (bowels, bladder, skin even with minor injuries) 8. Peripheral oedema for heart failure patients	3. Family roles—who is considered as significant other, family responsibilities, family presence in care planning, function of social support system 4. Impact of age, sex/gender, culture, religious beliefs, and legal issues 5. Family-level problem-solving techniques needed to deal with important health issues, such as health promotion and prevention 6. Burden and strain of caregiving—impact on quality of life, symptoms severity, mortality, and morbidity
Activity and exercise (see Chapter 11 for more detail on how to conduct a physical activity assessment and an outline of benefits of physical activity and exercise on cardiovascular health)	*Coping and stress tolerance*[16]
1. Observation of mobility, posture, and general appearance 2. Usual pattern of a carrying out activities of daily living—ability to use energy, how they feel after engaging in these activities, and how they determine how much activity they can perform 3. Subjective description of exercise and leisure time activities—problems perceived by the patient and family and their actions to relieve these problems 4. Type and amount of exercise performed, attitude, knowledge, and motivation to exercise 5. Leisure time activity includes recreational activity and the amount of time spent on these activities. Changes in these activities and asking about impact on mental health 6. Regular participation in physical activity reduces all-cause and cardiovascular mortality over a wide age range in both males and females.[17] For those patients with risk factors, such as hypertension, lipid disorders, increased body weight, and diabetes, physical activity has a positive effect on reducing these risk factors	1. Perceived levels of stress and potential stressors 2. Previous experiences 3. Coping strategies used to adapt to stressful situations—success and feasibility for use of these strategies in a situation of new or escalating cardiovascular disease
Sleep and rest	*Values and beliefs*
1. Sufficiency and quality of sleep. Length of sleep at night, feeling rested when getting up, napping, difficulty falling asleep, use of sleep medications 2. Influencing factors—age, cultural norms, daily activity, diet, environment, perceived stress level, medications, and illness 3. 24-hour recall of quantity and quality, perception of their sleep experience 4. Appearance of being rested, energy level 5. Influence of medications, and comorbid illnesses, e.g. timing of taking diuretics, beta-blockers 6. Use of stimulants such as caffeine, nicotine, and alcohol can influence sleep patterns	1. Awareness of the personal nature of spirituality 2. Assess spiritual beliefs and appropriate source of support (e.g. chaplaincy, patient's faith community, other professionals and specialized supportive care)[17] 3. Assess spiritual distress[18] and needs[19]

Table 5.2 Continued

Sexuality and reproductive
1. Sexual identity and self-identity, gender identity (sex at birth), gender role behaviour (behaviour exhibited as male or female), and sexual orientation or preference[20] 2. Past and current sexual history and reproductive patterns 3. As appropriate, assess sexual relationships, birth control methods, presence of children, impact of sexual self-identity on health, menstrual cycle experience, and menopause 4. Marginalization (lesbian, bisexual, gay, 'trans', queer (LBGTQ) community) 5. Healthcare access—negative and poorly understood healthcare needs[20] 6. Discrepancies between expression of sexuality attained compared to what is desired 7. Sexual minority women (lesbians, bisexual) display higher rates of modifiable risk factors (smoking and elevated BMI)[21] 8. Sexual minority men (gay, bisexual) display higher rates of smoking 9. Reproductive patterns—cultural and religious norms 10. Unintended pregnancy—provision of contraceptive options if requested 11. Anxiety relating to effect of cardiovascular illness on sexuality and sexual functioning 12. Impact of cardiovascular medication on sexual function 13. Advice for post-myocardial infarction patient on gradual resumption of sexual activity and reduction of alcohol and stressors. Finding a comfortable position to enhance return to sexual activity

methodology to facilitate efficient communication to other healthcare providers. The triage of chest pain patients in the emergency department is based on careful history-taking, physical examination, recording and interpretation of a 12-lead electrocardiogram (ECG) within 10 minutes of arrival, and measurement of cardiac biomarkers.[25] Chapter 6 provides an example of how the initial assessment works for the example of a patient presenting with angina and suspected coronary heart disease.

Assessment of the pain

To assess the intensity of pain, scales such as a numeric rating scale (NRS), a visual analogue scale, a faces pain scale, or the Wong–Baker Faces Pain Rating Scale can be used. The numeric scale 0–10 is still considered to be the gold standard for assessing pain severity. Selection of the appropriate pain assessment tool should be based on the characteristics of the group of patients, their backgrounds, and their communication skills.[26] Examples of an NRS and the Wong–Baker Faces Pain Rating Scale can be seen in ➤ Fig. 5.3 and ➤ Fig. 5.4.

Recognizing emergency situations

The 'ABCDE' (A–E) approach provides a way of systematically assessing vital systems including airway, breathing, circulation, disability, and exposure. The aim of this

Table 5.3 Health perception and management pattern questions

Potential questions for the pattern of health perception and management	1. What made you decide to seek healthcare today? 2. How do you manage signs and symptoms before seeking healthcare? 3. Do you have home remedies that you use for signs and symptoms? 4. How would you define health? 5. What do you routinely do to maintain your health? 6. Do you believe that health is a priority in your life? 7. What makes you feel less healthy? 8. Do you feel it is important to be included in decision-making about your healthcare? 9. Do you trust healthcare professional when it comes to managing your care?
Current health status	1. How would you describe your health status? 2. Compared to a year ago, how would you rate your health? 3. Do you smoke tobacco? If yes, have you tried to quit? 4. Do you use non-prescribed drugs such as opioids, marijuana, cocaine? 5. Do you take any medications prescribe by a healthcare provider? 6. Do you use non-prescription, herbal supplements, or vitamins?
Past health history	1. Birth and childhood illnesses and immunizations 2. Previous illnesses and hospitalizations 3. Accidents or injuries 4. Allergies and reactions
Family history	1. Maternal and paternal family health history 2. Does your race or ethnic affect your health? 3. Do you have a family history of any genetic disorders? 4. How do you obtain and use resources in your community to maintain family health? 5. How does your cultural background influence your health practices?
Environmental history	1. Are you affected by climate? 2. Do seasonal changes affect your health? 3. Do you think air, water, soil, or noise pollution affects your health? 4. What preventive health measure do you and your family follow to counteract the adverse effects of pollution in your environment? 5. Do you feel safe in your home, neighbourhood, and workplace? 6. Do you have and are you able to afford healthy food? 7. Do you have access to affordable healthcare?

Box 5.3 Selected validated cognitive screening tools

Folstein test/Mini-Mental State Examination (MMSE)—also available as a standard version (MMSE-2:SV).[23]

1. Assesses basic cognitive dimensions using simple tasks such as registration and recall, ability to repeat and retain three unrelated words, and then recall after a short intervention task.
2. Assesses orientation to time and place, attention and calculation, naming specific body parts or items, repetition of a sentence with words not often said together, comprehension of a three-stage verbal command, reading and following instructions, writing a sentence, and ability to draw copying intersecting pentagons.
3. Takes 15 minutes to administer.
4. Includes assessment of attention, orientation, registration, recall/short-term memory, language, and visuospatial construction.
5. MMSE-2:SV available in various languages.

Box 5.4 oPQRSTa mnemonic to assess the origin of chest pain and other acute symptoms

1. O—onset: can help to narrow the differential diagnosis. What was the onset? Sudden? Severe at onset? Abrupt? Starts gradually and worsen with exertion? Occurs only when activity creates an oxygen demand? Discomfort begins at lower levels of exercise or at rest?
2. P—what provokes symptoms? What improves or exacerbates the condition? What were you doing when it started? Does position or activity make it worse?
3. Q—quality and quantity of symptoms: is it dull, sharp, constant, intermittent, throbbing, pulsating, aching, tearing, or stabbing?
4. R—radiation or region of symptoms: does the pain travel, or is it only in one location? Has it always been in the same area, or did it start somewhere else?
5. S—severity of symptoms or rating on a pain scale. Does it affect activities of daily living such as walking, sitting, eating, or sleeping?
6. T—time or how long have they had the symptoms. Is it worse after eating, changes in weather, or time of day?
7. A—associated symptoms: what other symptoms do you have besides the chief complaint? How are they connected to the main symptom?

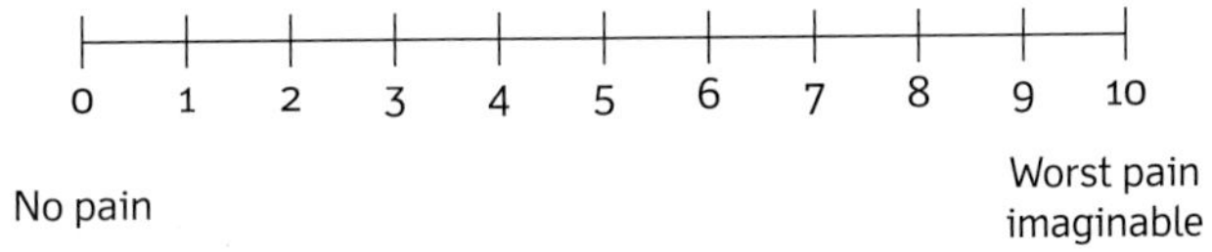

Fig. 5.3 An 11-point NRS (NRS-11).

Reproduced from Basic principles of acute pain. In Brook, P., Connell, J., & Pickering, T. (Eds.), Oxford Handbook of Pain Management. Oxford, UK: Oxford University Press 2011, with permission from Oxford University Press.

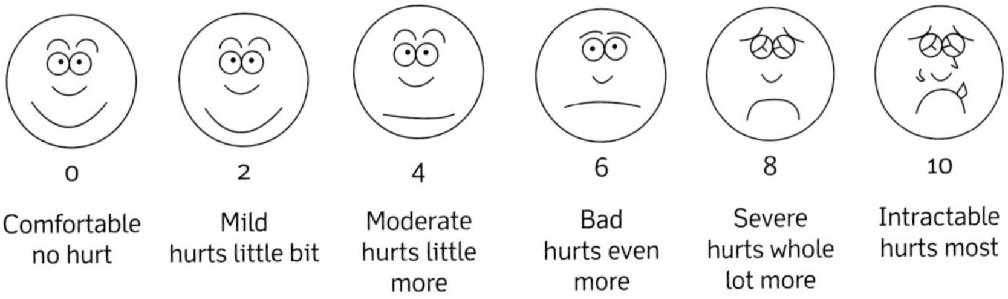

Fig. 5.4 Wong–Baker Faces Pain Rating Scale.

Reproduced from Basic principles of acute pain. In Brook, P., Connell, J., & Pickering, T. (Eds.), Oxford Handbook of Pain Management. Oxford, UK: Oxford University Press 2011, with permission from Oxford University Press.

structured and systematic assessment is to identify and prioritize the patient's most life-threatening problems first. Here also, an algorithm may be useful in establishing common situational awareness among all treatment providers.[27] ➤ Table 5.4 shows the necessary nursing skills to administer this approach.

Physical examination of the cardiovascular patient

A physical examination by a nurse is an essential part of comprehensive nursing assessment providing a wealth of information about the patient. Nurses should

Table 5.4 Assessing vital systems using the ABCD approach

What	Objective	How	Action
A: airway	To establish the patency of the airway and assess the risk of deterioration in the patient's ability to protect their airway	1. Attempt to elicit a vocal response 2. Listen for breath sounds from mouth and nose 3. Check for airway obstruction and possible causes (fluid, foreign body, swelling, altered mental state, ability to swallow saliva, abnormal sounds, chest wall movements)	4. If obstructed, attempt to open airway—head tilt and chin-lift manoeuvre[5,27,28] (➤ Fig. 5.5)
B: breathing	To check presence of breathing and that it has a normal pattern	5. Look, listen, and feel for breathing 6. Check frequency and depth 7. Check number of beats per minute (normal range 12–20 beats per minute (bpm)) 8. Check efficiency (pulse oximetry 97–100%) and arterial blood gases (ABGs) 9. Check for signs of respiratory distress or use of accessory muscles, and adventitious breath sounds, such as crackles or wheezes[29]	10. Administer O_2 if saturation is <94% to increase saturation to between 94% and 99% 11. If history of chronic obstructive pulmonary disease, administer O_2 if saturation is below 90% on room air 12. If patient is short of breath, administer O_2 whatever the saturation level 13. Check for history of breathing problems (dyspnoea on exertion, tachypnoea, orthopnoea, paroxysmal nocturnal dyspnoea), cough (productive or not), and smoking history 14. Use dyspnoea scale to determine symptom severity (e.g. modified Medical Research Council activity-based dyspnoea scale, see ➤ Box 5.5)[30]
C: circulation	To assess function of the cardiac pump	15. Check appearance and skin colour 16. Palpate the pulse (normal range 60–100 bpm) 17. Check capillary refill time—normal <2 seconds 18. Check for signs of poor perfusion (cool, moist extremities, diaphoresis, low blood pressure, tachycardia, absent peripheral pulses)	

Table 5.4 Continued

What	Objective	How	Action
		19. Inspect for pallor, cyanosis, mottling, cool, clammy skin 20. Identify systemic vasoconstriction (decreased skin perfusion, diminished pulses) 21. Check for associated respiratory distress 22. Lethargy, confusion, disorientation, anxiety, and depression may indicate associated reduced cerebral perfusion[3,28]	
D: disability	To assess level of consciousness	23. Use tools to assess level of consciousness i. AVPU (Box 5.6) ii. Glasgow Coma Scale (Box 5.7) 24. Monitor and document neurological status frequently for first 48 hours and compare with baseline 25. Blood glucose (glucose for hypoglycaemia) 26. Be aware of the close relationship between cerebral function and cardiac output and influence of electrolyte and acid–base variations, hypoxia, and systemic emboli 27. Anxiety and restlessness are common signs of hypoxia 28. Confusion and somnolence with worsening ABGs are a sign of cerebral dysfunction due to hypoxaemia 29. In patients with low cerebral perfusion or signs of stroke: i. Observe for right and left limb movements separately ii. Evaluate size, shape, equality, and light reactivity in pupils iii. Observe position and movement of eyes—note whether in mid position or deviated to side or downwards iv. Observe oculocephalic reflex (doll's eyes) (➤ Fig. 5.6) v. Observe for presence or absence of reflexes (blink, cough, gag, and Babinski) (➤ Fig. 5.7)	
E: exposure	To inspect entire body	30. Check for signs of trauma, bleeding, hidden injuries, skin reactions (rash), bites, other lesions, needle marks 31. Remove clothing while respecting dignity[5,27,28]	

Box 5.5 Modified Medical Research Council dyspnoea scale

Grade	Degree of breathlessness scale
0	No breathlessness, except with strenuous exercise
1	Breathlessness when hurrying on the level or walking up a slight hill
2	Walks slower than contemporaries on level ground because of breathlessness or has to stop for breath when walking at own pace
3	Stops for breath after walking about 100 m or after a few minutes on level ground
4	Too breathless to leave the house, or breathless when dressing or undressing

Reproduced from Santos M, Kitzman DW, Matsushita K, Loehr L, Sueta CA, Shah AM. Prognostic Importance of Dyspnea for Cardiovascular Outcomes and Mortality in Persons without Prevalent Cardiopulmonary Disease: The Atherosclerosis Risk in Communities Study. PLoS One. 2016 Oct 25;11(10):e0165111. doi: 10.1371/journal.pone.0165111 with permission from PLOS ONE (https://creativecommons.org/licenses/by/4.0/).

➤ be aware of what is normal, the ranges of normal, and the 'normal' for various disease states as well as the influence of medications. Relevant guidelines of the European Society of Cardiology refer to normal ranges and clinical recommendations for the management of abnormal values (see Chapter 11 and https://www.escardio.org/Guidelines). Also to be taken into account is the impact of patient comorbidities, the outcome of treatments, and medical/surgical interventions. For example, the results of the cardiovascular examination will have specific variations for patients who have a cardiac surgical history, or someone who has had a heart transplant. This review serves only as a baseline for the nurse to reflect on the variability of normal versus pathology for the cardiovascular patient. What to expect of a physical examination in the context of specific cardiac conditions will be covered in later disease-specific chapters.

The physical examination begins with the nurse observing the patient.[31] How easily is the patient roused (Glasgow Coma Scale)? Are they alert when you enter, and do they respond to their name? Do they have appropriate colouring and symmetrical facial responses and features? Can they hear and comprehend a question, formulate an answer, and articulate an appropriate response? A rapid head-to-toe check can be conducted to rule out life-threatening pathology (➤ Box 5.6 and Figs. 5.5–5.7). Bulging neck veins, crushing chest pain with diaphoresis, unilateral absence of lung sounds, tracheal deviation, tearing back pain, or shortness of breath with cyanosis are just some examples of abnormal findings which could be identified when a patient is in distress. Following this, a physical examination should systematically cover each of the body systems.

Box 5.6 AVPU acronym to assess level of consciousness

Alert.
Voice responsive.
Pain responsive.
Unresponsive.

Box 5.7 Glasgow Coma Scale

Glasgow Coma Scale

Response	Scale	Score (points)
Eye Opening Response	Eyes open spontaneously	4
	Eyes open to verbal command, speech, or shout	3
	Eyes open to pain (not applied to face)	2
	No eye opening	1
Verbal Response	Oriented	5
	Confused conversation, but able to answer questions	4
	Inappropriate responses, words discernible	3
	Incomprehensible sounds or speech	2
	No verbal response	1
Motor Response	Obeys commands for movement	6
	Purposeful movement to painful stimulus	5
	Withdraws from pain	4
	Abnormal (spastic) flexion to pain	3
	Extension to pain	2
	No motor response	1

Minor brain injury: 13-15 points, moderate brain injury: 9-12 points, severe brain injury: 3-8 points

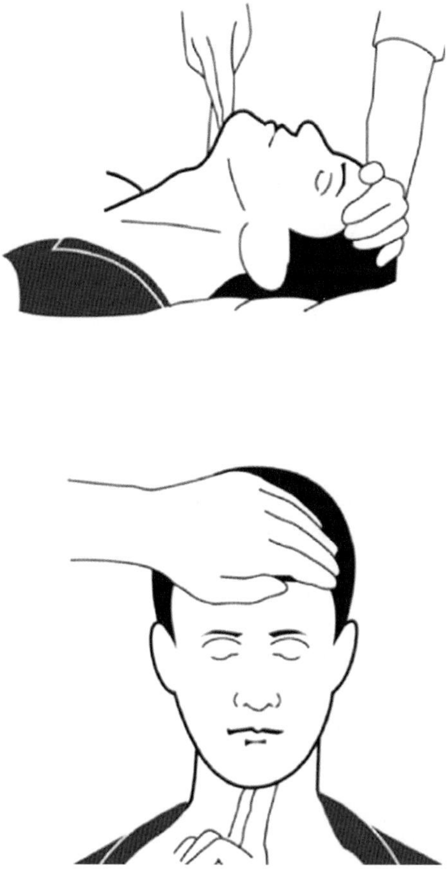

Feature	Response	Score
Best eye response	Open spontaneously	4
	Open to verbal command	3
	Open to pain	2
	No eye opening	1
Best verbal response	Orientated	5
	Confused	4
	Inappropriate words	3
	Incomprehensible sounds	2
	No verbal response	1
Best motor response	Obeys commands	6
	localising pain	5
	Withdrawal from pain	4
	Felxion to pain	3
	Extension to pain	2
	No motor response	1

Fig. 5.5 Head tilt and chin lift manoeuvre to open airway.

Reproduced from Thim T, Krarup NH, Grove EL, Rohde CV, Løfgren B. Initial assessment and treatment with the Airway, Breathing, Circulation, Disability, Exposure (ABCDE) approach. Int J Gen Med. 2012;5:117–21. doi: 10.2147/IJGM.S28478 with permission from Dove Medical Press.

Cardiovascular system

This body system includes the heart, blood, and blood vessels. ➤ Table 5.5 shows the components of this assessment. Specific tests are necessary in different cardiovascular conditions and these are referred to in the relevant chapters (prevention and rehabilitation (Chapter 11), coronary heart disease (Chapter 6), cardiac arrhythmias (Chapter 7), valvular disease (Chapter 8), inherited cardiac diseases (Chapter 9), and heart failure (Chapter 10)). The patient should be positioned so they are relaxed, and have not recently exerted themselves, for example, by just having changed into a gown or walked a short distance.

A complete set of *vital signs*—blood pressure, heart rate, temperature, respiratory rate, oxygen saturation, and peripheral pulses—is the foundation of the physical examination (➤ Table 5.5). Much information can be obtained while manually palpating arterial pulse points (➤ Fig. 5.8). Palpation of a radial pulse provides an estimation of the blood pressure, fullness and characteristics of the blood volume and flow, as well as skin temperature. Palpation of the dorsalis pedis and posterior tibial pulses are a crude indication of lower extremity flow, while concurrently assessing for peripheral oedema.

The regularity as well as speed of the *heart rate* should be documented and the manner it was obtained, that is, through palpating the radial pulse, or auscultating the pulse over the aortic valve at the right second intercostal space, or monitoring the ECG rate. Unless there is an overriding contraindication, bilateral blood pressures should be measured and the values, sidedness, and the method used to obtain, such as manual or automatic device, and size of cuff used, documented in the patient record.[32] Orthostatic hypotension assessment may be indicated in some populations (e.g. older patients). Blood pressure and pulse are recorded at 1 and 3 minutes after standing. Systolic blood pressure decreases of 20 mmHg or greater, or diastolic blood pressure decreases of 10 mmHg or greater, in the first 3 minutes of standing should be reported to a treating clinician as a part of the collaborative assessment as well as for suspected hypertension.[32]

Body temperature is recorded, including the temperature source. Temporal artery, oral, axillary, or pulmonary artery central temperatures are all informative, but trending of temperatures from the same source is required. Vital signs are monitored over time, as multiple data points will be compared when working towards a diagnosis.

Advanced practice nurses or those with special training should auscultate the *heart sounds* (➤ Fig. 5.9) (see also Chapter 4 and Chapter 15). This assessment may reveal pathologies discussed elsewhere in this book (e.g. Chapter 8).

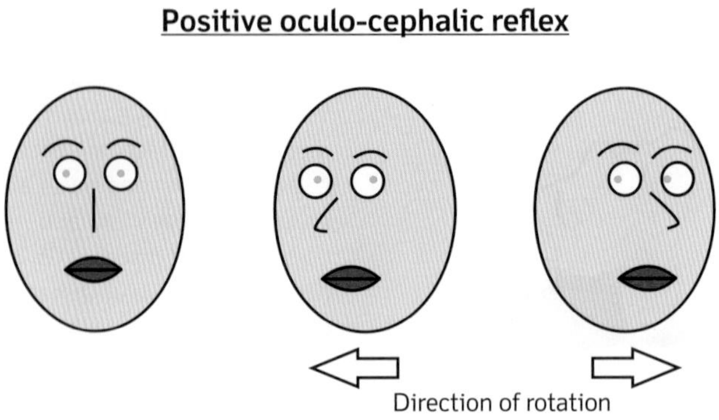

Fig. 5.6 Checking the oculocephalic reflex (doll's eyes).

Electrocardiogram

The 12-lead ECG is included in the routine assessment of the cardiovascular patient. The ECG is sensitive to changes in electrolytes, medication effects, as well as coronary perfusion. It is a low-risk, non-invasive assessment, completed at the bedside without a need to transport the patient, and the results can be reviewed remotely by an appropriate healthcare provider. An ECG is expected to be obtained during a physical examination, prior to

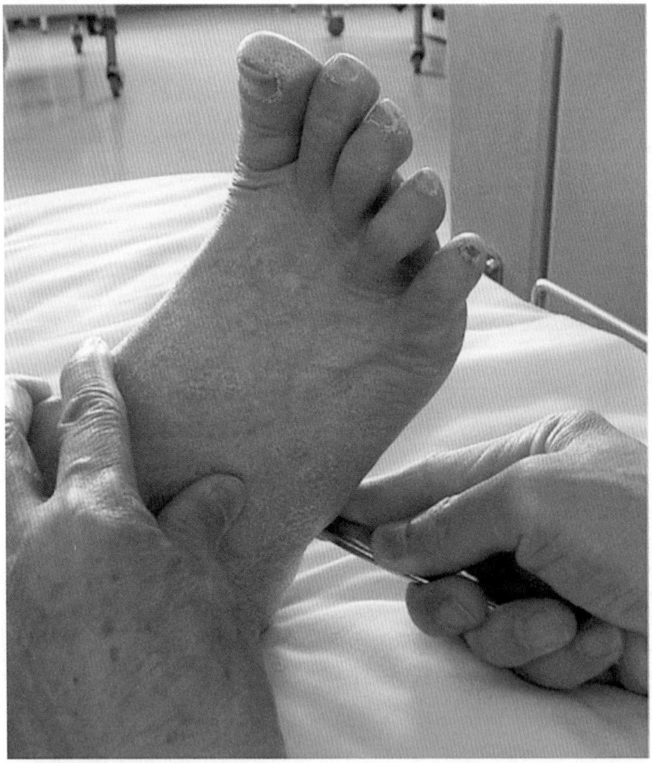

Fig. 5.7 Checking the Babinski reflex.

Reproduced from Shibasaki, H., & Hallett, M., Tendon Reflexes and Pathological Reflexes. In The Neurologic Examination: Scientific Basis for Clinical Diagnosis. Oxford, UK: Oxford University Press 2016 with permission from Oxford University Press.

Table 5.5 Cardiovascular system assessment

Components of assessment		Units of measurement
Vital signs	Bilateral blood pressure	mmHg
	Regularity of heart rate	Beats per minute (bpm)
	Temperature	°C
	Respirations	Per minute
	O_2 saturation	%
Presence of peripheral pulses	Temporal	
	Facial	
	Carotid	
	Brachial	
	Radial	
	Femoral	
	Popliteal	
	Posterior tibial	
	Dorsalis pedis	
Peripheral oedema	Accumulation of fluid in peripheral vascular system (particularly lower limbs)	
12-lead ECG	Representation of the heart's electrical activity	
Biomarkers		
Myocardial ischaemia (see Chapter 6)	Cardiac troponin T, cardiac troponin I, and the high-sensitivity cardiac troponins[33]	
Heart failure (see Chapter 10)	B-type natriuretic peptide (BNP) and N-terminal pro-BNP (NT-proBNP)[33]	
Inflammation marker	High-sensitivity C-reactive protein[17]	
Imaging	Chest X-ray	
	Radionuclide imaging	
	Computed tomography coronary angiography	
	Echocardiography	
Non-invasive	Exercise treadmill test	
	Pharmacological stress test	
Invasive	Coronary angiography	

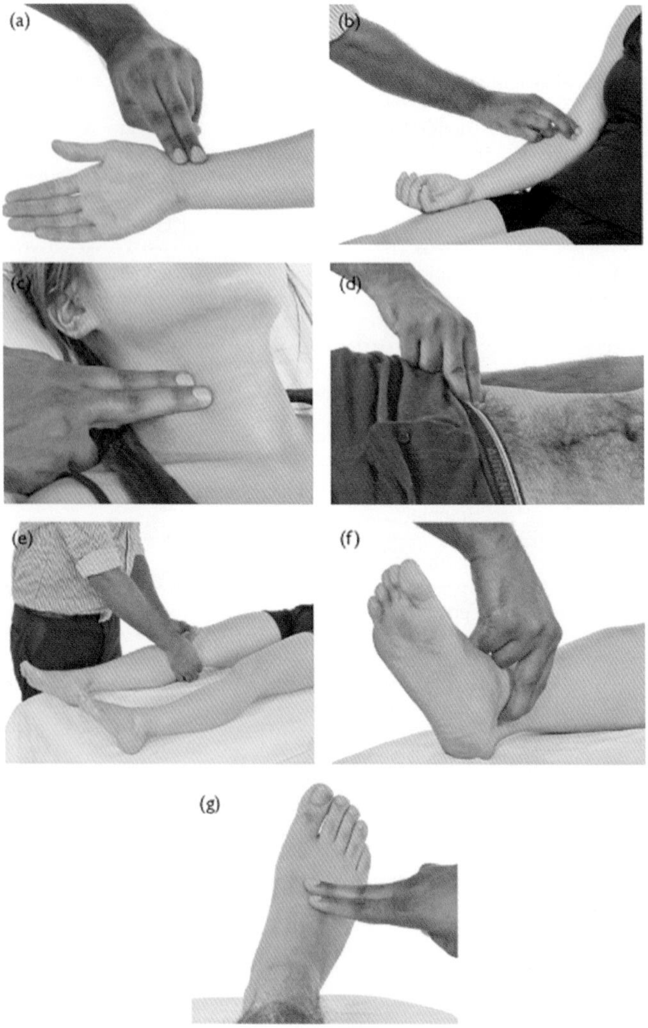

Fig. 5.8 Arterial pulse points.

Reproduced from Thomas, J., & Monaghan, T. The cardiovascular system. In Oxford Handbook of Clinical Examination and Practical Skills. Oxford, UK: Oxford University Press 2014, with permission from Oxford University Press.

procedures or surgery, upon admission to hospital, after a procedure or surgery, with changes in symptoms, or observed change in cardiac rhythm.[33] Initial or serial ECGs may be indicative of life-threatening cardiac pathology in need of immediate intervention and escalation of care (e.g. in acute coronary syndromes; see Chapter 6).[34]

The standard 12-lead ECG records the deflections from the isoelectric line in 12 electrical views using electrodes placed on the four limbs (right arm, left arm, right leg, left leg) and at anatomic locations on the chest (V1 through V6) (➤ **Fig. 5.10**). The six chest electrodes are placed from the patient's right to left: V1 and V2 are parasternal at the fourth intercostal space, V3 is between V2 and V4, V4 is over the fifth intercostal space at the midclavicular line, V5 is at the same level as V4 at the anterior axillary line, and V6 is at the same level as V4 and V5 but at the midaxillary line. Monitoring of the chest electrodes provides information regarding the electrical activity deep to their location. There are variations in lead placement based on local definitions and type of monitoring system so local customs should be followed.

There are two variations of the standard 12-lead ECG which may be obtained to assess electrical activity of the posterior view, or right-sided view. Leads labelled V7 through V9 can be obtained by placing electrodes along the same line as V4, V5, and V6 (➤ **Fig. 5.11**). Lead V7 will be located at the posterior axillary line, V9 will be paraspinal, and V8 will be midway between them, near the

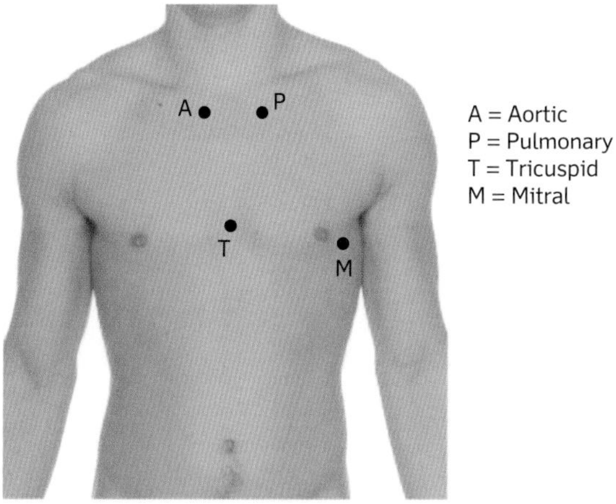

Fig. 5.9 Heart sounds auscultation.

Reproduced from Thomas, J., & Monaghan, T. The cardiovascular system. In Oxford Handbook of Clinical Examination and Practical Skills. Oxford, UK: Oxford University Press 2014, with permission from Oxford University Press.

border of the scapula. Right-sided leads in comparable positions to their placement on the left chest, though they will be labelled V3R, and V4R, will assist in the detection of right ventricular involvement.[34]

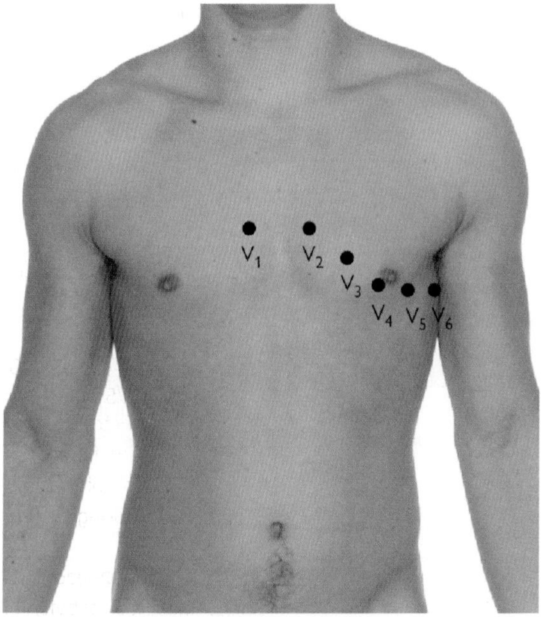

Fig. 5.10 ECG lead placement.

Reproduced from Thomas, J., & Monaghan, T. The cardiovascular system. In Oxford Handbook of Clinical Examination and Practical Skills. Oxford, UK: Oxford University Press 2014, with permission from Oxford University Press.

Detection of ECG changes may be facilitated by comparing the most recently obtained ECG to an ECG measured while a patient is asymptomatic, or symptomatic with chest pain, or with shortness of breath, or other cardiac complaints. ➤ **Fig. 5.12** shows an ECG recording of a normally functioning heart (see also Chapter 4).

Biomarkers

Nurses should review and add appropriate biomarker results to their assessment notes. ➤ **Table 5.5** shows commonly used biomarkers in cardiovascular disease. Biomarker results can vary between laboratories (either differences in units or actual results). Two key aspects to take into account regarding biomarkers are the timing of the sample and trends seen in results in patients from one sample to the next. Biomarker results should be used in conjunction with other cardiac investigations, such as ECG recordings, to facilitate the diagnosis of cardiac injury or type of myocardial infarction.[17,33,34] Cardiovascular nurses should be familiar with their institution's use of biomarkers for such conditions as myocardial ischaemia (see Chapter 6), heart failure (see Chapter 10), and inflammation (see Chapter 6 and Chapter 10).

Imaging

Imaging of the cardiovascular system can be completed with a number of modalities which are outlined in this section and in ➤ **Table 5.5**. Decision-making for undertaking cardiac imaging depends on the assessment of signs and symptoms, laboratory biomarkers, and ECG. When warranted, appropriate healthcare providers will add non-invasive testing, and invasive testing for definitive diagnoses.[35]

Chest X-ray is a basic imaging modality which can provide assessment information for the cardiovascular patient and will likely be included in any interaction.[35] The chest radiograph, along with auscultation of breath sounds, can provide diagnostic information such as the presence and extent of a plural effusion or pneumothorax. Echocardiography is performed to assess cardiac function, structures, and circulatory flow (see Chapters 6, 8, 9, and 10).[35] It is better than ECG in identifying some cardiac abnormalities, such as left ventricular hypertrophy (e.g. in heart failure), but does not improve risk stratification.[14,32] In examination of patients with hypertension, it may include evaluation of left ventricular function (see Chapter 10).[32]

Non-invasive testing includes exercise testing and pharmacological stress and radionuclide imaging directly assesses myocardial viability These tests can aid in assessing the condition of the myocardium under resting and stressed conditions.[33–35]

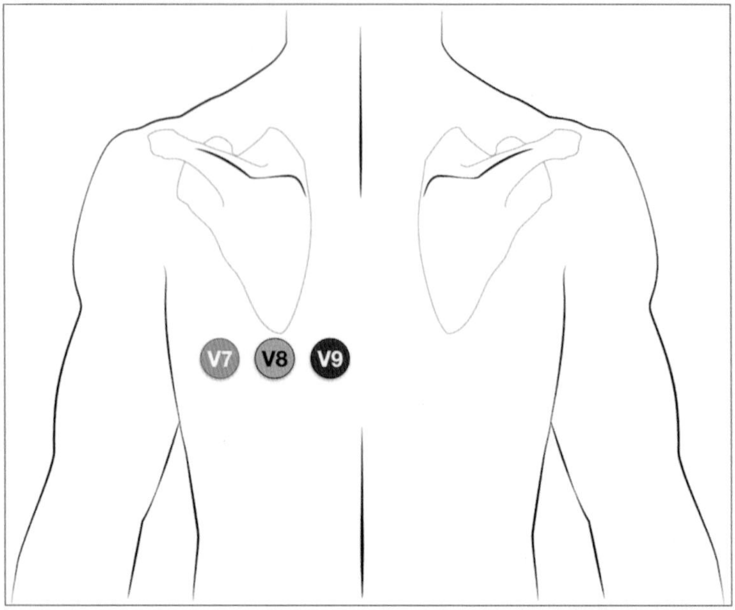

Fig. 5.11 Placement of leads V7–V9.

Invasive tests are used for a more comprehensive assessment. Computed tomography coronary angiography may be used when assessment indicates the possibility of pulmonary embolism or aortic dissection.[17,34,35] Invasive coronary angiography is used for assessment, confirmation, and treatment of coronary artery disease (see Chapter 6).[33,36]

Assessment of other body systems

A physical examination of the cardiovascular patient will also include an assessment of other body systems as outlined in the following sections.

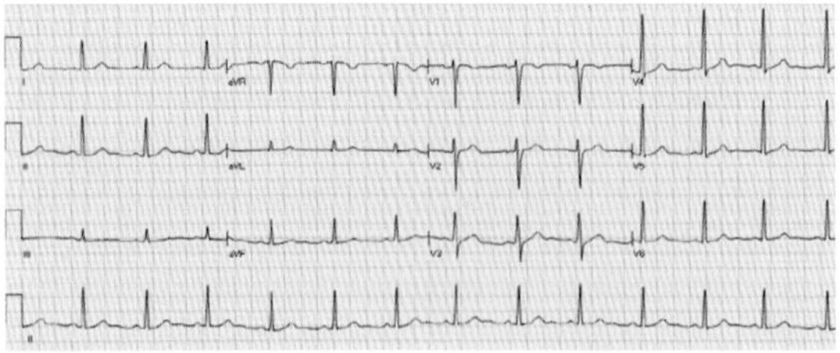

Fig. 5.12 Normal ECG.

Reproduced from Kayani, W. T., Huang, H. D., Bandeali, S., Virani, S. S., Wilson, J. M., & Birnbaum, Y. (2012). ST elevation: telling pathology from the benign patterns. Global journal of health science, 4(3), 51–63. https://doi.org/10.5539/gjhs.v4n3p51. Attribution 3.0 Unported (CC BY 3.0).

Respiratory system

Respiratory function can profoundly impact a patient's performance of routine activities.[37] The assessment of respiratory status can begin at the interview with any known respiratory history or symptoms indicative of pathology, such as shortness of breath, dyspnoea on exertion, cough or sputum production, or the need to be elevated on pillows for sleep. The overall patient history may influence interpretation of thoracic findings. Examination may reveal findings of signs and symptoms of conditions which will need prompt referral to a clinical provider. For example, an examination with sudden onset of shortness of breath after subclavian access may lead to differential diagnosis of tension pneumothorax, or a patient with a splinted leg, who is at risk for deep vein thrombosis, may lead to differential diagnosis of pulmonary embolism. Respiratory rate is challenging to count if regular, and even more so if irregular. In case of irregular breathing, a full minute is needed to quantify. Besides rate and regularity, depth of respiration should be noted. Does the patient appear comfortable or in distress? Are the depths of the respirations constant, slow, and shallow, or deep (Kussmaul—rapid and deep), or are they fluctuating in their depth (Cheyne–Stokes)? Is the patient using accessory muscles, or are they positioning themselves to assist in their breathing? Additionally, is the length of inhalation roughly equal to the length of exhalation?[33]

Assessment of oxygen saturation as measured by pulse oximetry, if available, should be documented, along with a notation of any oxygen therapy in use. How oxygen therapy is being delivered should be documented, litres/minute or fraction of inspired oxygen if the patient is using ambient air. Difficulty in obtaining pulse oxygen saturation or concern for abnormal saturations may be an indication to obtain an arterial blood gas sample to confirm oxygen, carbon dioxide, and pH levels as normal or indicative of a metabolic or respiratory pathology.[37]

Physical assessment of the respiratory system begins with observing attributes of the anterior and posterior chest, such as shape or obvious surgical scars. Normal chest/lung expansion can be assessed by resting both hands on the chest at the lower level of the lung fields and asking the patient to take a deep breath.[37] Palpation of the chest is completed to assess for crepitus, tenderness, and fremitus over lung fields. The posterior lung fields should be percussed to determine if normal, hyper-resonant, or dull, and the patient should be asked to take full breaths through the mouth while auscultating breath sounds. Percussion and auscultation are repeated on the anterior chest.[31,37] It should be noted if the trachea is in its normal midline position.

Neurological system

A more wide-ranging neurological check can be woven into the overall cardiovascular patient assessment, although this is not a substitute for a focused neurological assessment of cranial nerve function, fine motor skills, or subtle differences in limb strength. In speaking with the patient, skilful use of questioning can elicit the orientation level of the patient. Do they know where they are, what they are there for, what the day/date is, or if a special holiday is approaching? Do they have an ease of recall, such as what you talked about when you called them at home, from the shift you shared the day before, or earlier in the examination you are performing?

This level of neurological examination should be routinely performed with a level of sensitivity to detect changes in mentation from such things as delirium caused by extended hospital stay, or the amnestic effects of medications, which may impact the ability of the patient to recall physical limitations or discharge instructions. Has the patient been falling, or losing consciousness? Safety questions can also provide insight into neurological status and provide evidence for possible cognitive impairment and the need for further investigation.[33]

Renal system

The nurse must be aware of several factors in cardiovascular care which interact with renal function. The renal system is dependent upon circulation; therefore, cardiovascular factors directly impact renal function. Renal disease may have detrimental effects on cardiac function and can influence the interpretation of cardiovascular biomarkers.[34] The level of hydration, the amount of fluid intake and output, daily weights, laboratory values for creatinine clearance, blood urea nitrogen, and protein and potassium levels are all reflective of renal function. These parameters impact the clearance of medications and may dictate the need for pre-hydration before a patient has invasive cardiac testing.

For the cardiovascular patient, many invasive cardiac tests involve contrast agents which are cleared through the renal system. Pre-hydration is protective of renal function and may be ordered, particularly for patients who have renal insufficiency or only have one functioning kidney.[33] Patients may require rehydration after withholding anything by mouth, without placing the patient into fluid overload or heart failure.

Physical assessment of the right kidney is possible by palpating the right flank during inspiration. The left kidney is more cephalad and normally is less likely to be felt. Percussion with a closed fist over each kidney is normally felt by the patient without causing intense pain. Sharp pain may be indicative of pathology.[31]

Gastrointestinal system

There is much focus on diets which decrease cardiovascular risk and, in combination with exercise, help in weight control[35] (see also Chapter 11). Measurement of waste circumference is indicative of distribution of weight. Cardiovascular patients need a functioning gastrointestinal system for ingestion of nutrition, absorption of oral medications, and health-related quality of life.

The inpatient diet needs to be monitored. One extreme is the duration of time a patient may be asked to tolerate nil by mouth. Some patients may enter hospital with little reserve and are then held without food prior to an invasive test, or multiple tests over days.

For the cardiovascular patient, gastrointestinal history could be important for knowing about a medical history of oesophageal reflux, whose symptoms could mimic the pain of a myocardial infarction or ischaemia. Nausea and vomiting may cause gastrointestinal distress from medication on an empty stomach but could also be an early indication of a vasovagal response, or an inferior myocardial infarction.

Endocrine, haematological, and immune systems

The presence of diabetes mellitus has been identified as a significant predictor of cardiovascular disease. Due to change in routines, stress, and illness, diabetic patients can be predicted to require increased glucose monitoring and variable dosing of medications for glycaemic control. Nurses participate in the assessment of diabetic patients for level of glycaemic control by recording laboratory values of glycosylated haemoglobin and point-of-care glucose monitoring.[33,35]

Haematological values should be monitored for anticoagulation status, bleeding disorders such as haemophilia, or clotting disorders such as factor V Leiden. Nurses can also assess for recent changes in condition which may not be included in the history but may be significant in the cardiovascular patient. Does questioning elicit reports of unusual bleeding such as oral, nasal, or rectal? Haemoglobin can be checked to rule out anaemia.[35] A significant number of patients with acute coronary syndromes have been shown to be anaemic, which can impact health outcomes.[38]

Immune suppression is induced by combinations of medications after heart transplant to avoid rejection of the transplanted heart. The results of tests for drug levels should be followed to evaluate success in maintaining suppression. Immunosuppressed patients will be assessed for any indication of untoward effects, such as an infection. Immune status can include a history of vaccinations, including current influenza, or pneumonia.[35] Autoimmune disease, such as rheumatoid arthritis, increases risk of cardiovascular disease.[17]

The relationship between thyroid function and cardiovascular disease remains a topic of study. Cardiovascular risk factors as diverse as dyslipidaemia, thrombosis risk, and systemic vascular resistance have been linked to thyroid hormones. It has been concluded that even slight alteration in thyroid function can impact cardiovascular systems functioning.[39] The thyroid is wrapped around the trachea and can be assessed by gently palpating the anterior neck.[31]

Integumentary system

The skin examination is done by exposing an area in bright light to identify deviation from normal for the patient. Visualization of skin is required to assess for discoloration, touching the extremities for assessment of skin temperature, looking for oedema of the feet, legs, and hands, and thinning of skin. The assessment of a patient's skin is also completed to record skin lesions, signs of infection, or skin breakdown.

The cardiovascular patient may have poor circulation due to reduced cardiac output putting them at risk for skin injury during bedrest or procedural inactivity. Medications which increase blood pressure centrally can negatively impact microcirculation, and the application of devices designed to maintain haemostasis at access sites can also put the cardiovascular patient at risk for skin pressure injury. Affected skin areas over possible procedural access sites can also alter a treatment plan.

Care of the deteriorating cardiovascular patient

Emergencies

Cardiovascular emergencies are either sudden events (e.g. acute coronary syndromes) or are preceded by a noticeable deterioration in the patient's condition (e.g. heart failure). They account for approximately 10% of all emergency department visits.[40] Care of the deteriorating patient is a vital skill for all healthcare professionals. Failure to rescue leads to severe harm or death.[36,40,41] The early recognition, assessment, and management of the deteriorating patient is required to prevent cardiogenic shock (CS), may prevent critical care admission, reduce length of stay, reduce costs, and improve survival rates.[41–43] The statistics for survival following in-hospital cardiac arrest are poor, with only 20% of this group returning home.[43,44] Prevention of in-hospital cardiac arrest includes interdisciplinary team education, monitoring of patients, recognition of patient deterioration, and a system to call for help and an effective response.[43,44]

The following sections discuss the main points of recognition, assessment, and management with specific reference to the cardiovascular patient.

Recognition

The earlier deterioration is detected and acted upon, the better the outcome for the patient.[36,43,45] The process of early recognition includes appropriate and timely monitoring of observations and can include cardiac monitoring.[41,45] The biggest challenge health professionals face in the emergency department is to identify rapidly and accurately the small group of patients who require hospitalization for acute management and the larger group with more benign conditions who can be safely discharged from the emergency department.[25,45] All patients should have their heart rate, respiratory rate, blood pressure, level of consciousness, oxygen saturation, and temperature recorded, and in some cases, this should also include fluid balance and specific limb observations for patients at risk of ischaemic limb. The first priority is to identify the patients who need urgent transfer to the catheterization laboratory (see Chapter 6). In case of a haemodynamically unstable patient, initial haemodynamic stabilization (e.g. CS management, drugs, intubation, and mechanical ventilation) may be necessary before the invasive procedure.[25,40] It may be appropriate for patients to have continued monitoring of heart rate, blood pressure, oxygen saturation, respiratory rate, and level of consciousness. This may require change of position on the ward, or movement to a higher level of care to ensure patients have the appropriate level of vigilance.[41] If the patient has a respiratory or cardiac arrest, advanced life support should be commenced and this algorithm used to continue care and treatment.[46,47] The use of track and trigger scores have been identified as useful tools to highlight the deteriorating patient and escalate care appropriately. Healthcare systems in Europe use scoring systems, such as a medical early warning system, to highlight patients who are at risk of deterioration and who may need assessment or intervention by a critical care outreach team. Most tools use a cumulative score comprising heart rate, respiratory rate, systolic blood pressure, level of consciousness, oxygen saturation, and temperature to incorporate into a score which grades the patient's condition.[48] The National Early Warning System 2 (NEWS2) is an example of such a scoring tool and is recommended to be used throughout hospital settings (➤ **Table 5.6**).

Assessment

Patients can be assessed in multiple ways; however, the universal ABCDE approach is well recognized in emergency situations. It ensures all life-threatening reversible causes are identified and prioritized systematically (see 'Recognizing emergency situations').[43,47] The necessary skills for administering this approach are outlined in ➤ **Table 5.4**. There are multiple causes for patient deterioration. ➤ **Table 5.7** shows the main cardiovascular causes or considerations when assessing in a deteriorated patient.

Management

The management of the deteriorating patient requires appropriate and timely escalation and treatment or management plan.[25,36,45,51] Each hospital and department will have its own escalation policy.

Table 5.6 The NEWS2 scoring system and b. trigger score

Physiological parameter	3	2	1	Score 0	1	2	3
Respiration rate (per minute)	≤8		9-11	12–20		21–24	≥25
SpO2 scale 1 (%)	≤91	92-93	94-95	≥96			
SpO2 scale 2 (%)	≤83	84–85	86–87	88–92 ≥93 on air	93–94 on oxygen	95–96 on oxygen	≥97 on oxygen
Air or oxygen?		Oxygen		Air			
Systolic blood pressure (mmHg)	≤90	91–100	101–110	111–219			≥220
Pulse (per minute)	≤40		41–50	51–90	91–110	111–130	≥131
Consciousness				Alert			CVPU
Temperature (°C)	≤35.0		35.1–36.0	36.1–38.0	38.1–39.0	≥39.1	

New score	Clinical risk	Response
Aggregate score 0–4	Low	Ward-based response
Red score score of 3 in any individual parameter	Low–medium	Urgent ward-based response*
Aggregate score 5–6	Medium	Key threshold for urgent response*
Aggregate score 7 or more	High	Urgent or emergency response**

*Response by a clinician or team with competence in the assessment and treatment of acutely ill patients and in recognising when the escalation of care to a critical care team is appropriate.
**The response team must also include staff with critical care skills, including airway management.

Table 5.7 Cardiovascular causes and considerations in a deteriorating patient

Assessment	Signs and symptoms	Cardiovascular-related causes and considerations
Airway—obstruction	Snoring Gurgling Altered voice Grunting Coughing wheezing Cyanosis Difficulty breathing Desaturation	Obstruction due to collapse or loss of consciousness (often caused by the tongue or debris such as vomit obstructing the airway)—consider possible causes such as poor cardiac output, arrhythmia, patients with heart and vascular disease are at higher risk of stroke or myocardial infarction. Don't forget hypoglycaemia as a large percentage of diabetics have cardiovascular disease
	As above Swollen face, lips, tongue Rash Swollen peripheries	Obstruction secondary to airway swelling due to anaphylaxis (histamine-induced angioedema), often patients are commenced on new medications during hospital admissions including antibiotics Urticaria and itching is associated with histamine-induced angioedema (anaphylaxis), has a rapid onset, and will develop into hypotension and shock Angiotensin-converting enzyme inhibitors can also induce angioedema (bradykinin mediated), and less likely angiotensin receptor blockers, antibiotics, and non-steroidal anti-inflammatory drugs .[49,50] Bradykinin-induced angioedema is likely to have a slower presentation and will develop into abdominal, peripheral, and genitourinary swelling. It is important to remember that in both cases the airway may continue to obstruct and requires early airway management. This is an emergency situation and requires a cardiac arrest call to ensure the support of an anaesthetist to manage a difficult airway
Breathing	Tachypnoea/bradypnoea Cyanosis Peripheral oedema Desaturation Pink frothy sputum	Pulmonary oedema or pleural effusion—multiple cardiac cause including heart failure (valvular disease, left or right ventricular dysfunction) or following cardiac surgery
	As above with associated chest pain	Shortness of breath could be a symptom of acute coronary syndrome or myocardial infarction or arrythmia
	As above Associated chest pain Unilateral swollen leg/arm	Pulmonary embolus, admission to hospital is a risk factor for deep vein thrombosis/pulmonary embolism
	As above	Respiratory disease is closely linked with multiple cardiac diagnosis, sometimes undiagnosed such as chronic obstructive pulmonary disease, which could be exacerbated by medications or chest infection
	Unilateral chest movement with reduced air entry Crepitus Surgical emphysema	There are multiple iatrogenic causes of pneumothorax such as central line insertion, following surgery, pacemaker insertion, and tension pneumothorax
	Hyperventilation	Don't forget anxiety as a cause or could exacerbate underlying conditions

Table 5.7 Continued

Assessment	Signs and symptoms	Cardiovascular-related causes and considerations
Cardiovascular	Associated chest pain and shortness of breath Nausea and vomiting Collapse/syncope Cool peripheries Tachycardia Bradycardia	There are multiple causes of cardiovascular collapse, some which have been highlighted above including arrhythmia, poor cardiac output, myocardial infarction, and sepsis (infective endocarditis). Cardiac tamponade which could have been iatrogenically caused
	Normal pulse Hypotension Drug history	Patients on beta-blockers may present with a normal pulse, and therefore may not score on track and trigger scores
	Drug history	Do not forget these patients may be on multiple antihypertensive medications which could cause hypotension
	Incision/box often right upper chest, but sometimes left and abdominal. Past medical history	Arrythmia: don't be fooled by a pacemaker, there could be mechanical failure of pacemaker/implantable cardioverter defibrillator which causes arrythmia *Electrolyte imbalance can cause arrythmia—such as hypo/ hyperkalaemia—consider for those on diuretics*
		Peripheral arterial disease could be the rationale behind a unilateral poor circulation, therefore it is important to assess all peripheries
		Don't forget haemorrhage as a cause, patients post procedure or surgery are at higher risk especially if they are on antiplatelets or anticoagulation or both
Disability	Reduced level of consciousness	As discussed in 'Airway'—collapse could be caused by multiple cardiac causes
		Toxins, medications, and illicit drugs can cause reduced level of consciousness
		Cardiac patients are at higher risk of ischaemic or haemorrhagic stroke if on anticoagulation
		Don't forget hypo- or hyperglycaemia
		Inpatients are at higher risk of hypo- and hyperdelirium

It is very important to become familiar with your local escalation policy, including the track and trigger graded response, how to make an emergency call, and how to make cardiac arrest calls. Some hospitals will have a team of healthcare providers with intensive care skills and equipment who will target the deteriorating patient in non-critical care settings. There are multiple names for these including 'patient at risk team', 'rapid response team', 'medical emergency team', or 'outreach team'. It is essential to establish if there is one in your hospital and how to activate this service.[41,43] There are several factors which could influence activation of these teams.[52]

Effective communication in emergency situations improves collaboration, efficiency, and shared situational awareness.[40,53] A tool can be used to communicate effectively with the multidisciplinary team during an emergency situation such as 'SBAR'.[54] The SBAR tool recommends splitting a scenario into the following categories:

1 Situation (patient's current state).
2. Background (clinical context).
3. Assessment (what have you found).
4. Recommendations (treatment suggestions).

This ensures shared information is relevant and pointed. It ensures that a concise rationale and action plan is supplied for the required treatment. There are other tools that you may find useful to hone your communication skills such as interprofessional simulation training.[55]

The management plan for these patients requires treatment of underlying causes, which may not be apparent without further tests or investigations. The management plan should include the simple bedside tests: blood tests including full blood count, renal and liver function, coagulation, and venous blood gas or arterial blood gas; ECG; chest radiograph; and echocardiogram. These patients may require further investigations such as computed tomography scans or coronary angiogram, or they may require transfer to a different area of care, ensuring patient safety on transfer.[25,36,45,51]

This section has dealt with the physical signs and symptoms, and emergency management. It is also important to support the patient and their family. They are likely to be scared and anxious; giving them information and psychological support is a vital part of your role as a nurse. Effective communication with the patient and family will decrease their anxiety and aid understanding of the current situation.

It is also important to consider that in some cases treatment will not be effective and this may lead to end of life care and palliation. In an acute deterioration, this is a difficult situation for patients and families to comprehend, especially if the patient appeared well prior to this. Ensuring effective communication, care, and consideration is paramount to their management. Most settings have a palliative care team who can support the patient, family, and clinicians to ensure a holistic care plan.

Conclusion

Emergency patient care requires quick and accurate decision-making to distinguish high-acuity patients. The priority for the interdisciplinary team is to recognize and stabilize patients with emergent cardiovascular conditions that include, but are not limited to, myocardial ischaemia/infarction and potentially life-threatening arrhythmias. Cardiac monitoring is one of the most commonly used diagnostic practices in such cases, and emergency nurses are poised to use valuable information revealed in ECG waveforms for early triage and risk stratification.

The patient at risk or in acute cardiogenic shock

Cardiogenic shock—definition

CS is a clinical syndrome characterized by the inability of the heart to deliver an adequate amount of blood to the tissues to meet resting metabolic demands, because of impairment to its pumping function.[56] Heart failure of any aetiology can lead to acute CS, but it is estimated that up to 70% of cases result from acute myocardial infarction[57] and 5–10% of patients with acute myocardial infarction develop CS.[58,59] It is a life-threatening condition, with an in-hospital mortality rate between 30% and 60%, and it requires urgent evaluation in a hospital setting.[51,60]

Cardiogenic shock—diagnosis

CS is diagnosed by clinical assessment and most commonly presents as hypotension (systolic blood pressure <90 mmHg) despite adequate circulating volume with signs of hypoperfusion.[60] However, occasionally CS presents as peripheral hypoperfusion with well-maintained systolic blood pressure (non-hypotensive CS) due to compensatory vasoconstriction.[61] Clinical signs of hypoperfusion are associated with a greater risk of in-hospital mortality regardless of blood pressure. Therefore, it is important to assess for hypoperfusion (➤ Table 5.8). While reduced cardiac index and elevated pulmonary capillary wedge pressure typically reflect CS, these parameters are not required for diagnosis.[51]

Table 5.8 Signs, symptoms, and biochemical indicators of hypoperfusion

Clinical signs and symptoms of hypoperfusion	Biochemical indicators of hypoperfusion
Cold and/or clammy extremities	Elevated serum lactate
Oliguria	Elevated serum creatinine
Mental confusion	Metabolic acidosis
Dizziness	
Narrow pulse pressure	

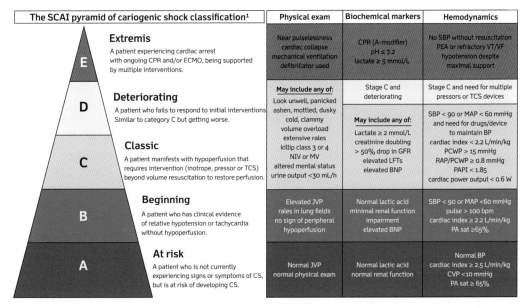

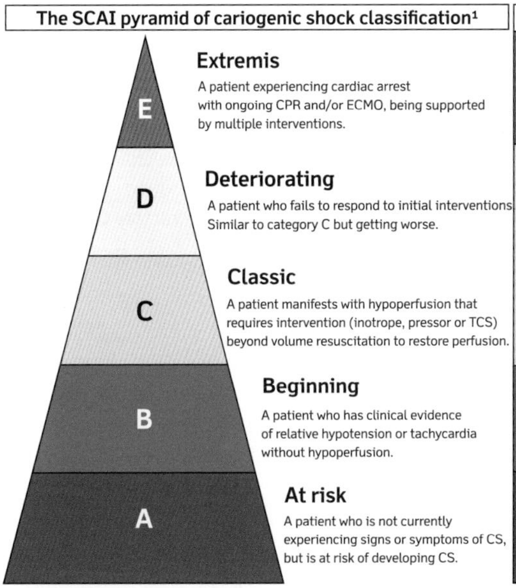

The SCAI pyramid of cariogenic shock classification¹
E
Extremis
A patient experiencing cardiac arrest with ongoing CPR and/or ECMO, being supported by multiple interventions.
D
Deteriorating
A patient who fails to respond to initial interventions. Similar to category C but getting worse.
C
Classic
A patient manifests with hypoperfusion that requires intervention (inotrope, pressor or TCS) beyond volume resuscitation to restore perfusion.
B
Beginning
A patient who has clinical evidence of relative hypotension or tachycardia without hypoperfusion.
A
At risk
A patient who is not currently experiencing signs or symptoms of CS, but is at risk of developing CS.

<table>
<tr><th>Stage</th><th>Physical exam</th><th>Biochemical markers</th><th>Hemodynamics</th></tr>
<tr><td>E</td><td>Near pulselessness
cardiac collapse
mechanical ventilation
defibrillator used</td><td>CPR (A-modifier)
pH ≤ 7.2
lactate ≥ 5 mmol/L</td><td>No SBP without resuscitation
PEA or refractory VT/VF
hypotension despite maximal support</td></tr>
<tr><td>D</td><td rowspan="2">May include any of:
Look unwell, panicked
ashen, mottled, dusky
cold, clammy
volume overload
extensive rales
killip class 3 or 4
NIV or MV
altered mental status
urine output <30 mL/h</td><td>Stage C and deteriorating</td><td>Stage C and need for multiple pressors or TCS devices</td></tr>
<tr><td>C</td><td>May include any of:
Lactate ≥ 2 mmol/L
creatinine doubling
> 50% drop in GFR
elevated LFTs
elevated BNP</td><td>SBP < 90 or MAP < 60 mmHg and need for drugs/device to maintain BP
cardiac index < 2.2 L/min/kg
PCWP > 15 mmHg
RAP/PCWP ≥ 0.8 mmHg
PAPI < 1.85
cardiac power output < 0.6 W</td></tr>
<tr><td>B</td><td>Elevated JVP
rales in lung fields
no sign of peripheral hypoperfusion</td><td>Normal lactic acid
minimal renal function impairment
elevated BNP</td><td>SBP < 90 or MAP <60 mmHg
pulse > 100 bpm
cardiac index ≥ 2.2 L/min/kg
PA sat ≥65%</td></tr>
<tr><td>A</td><td>Normal JVP
normal physical exam</td><td>Normal lactic acid
normal renal function</td><td>Normal BP
cardiac index ≥ 2.5 L/min/kg
CVP <10 mmHg
PA sat ≥ 65%</td></tr>
</table>

Fig. 5.13 SCAI classification for cardiogenic shock.

Reproduced from Baran DA, Grines CL, Bailey S, etal. SCAI clinical expert consensus statement on the classification of cardiogenic shock: This document was endorsed by the American College of Cardiology (ACC), the American Heart Association (AHA), the Society of Critical Care Medicine (SCCM), and the Society of Thoracic Surgeons (STS) in April 2019. Catheter Cardiovasc Interv. 2019 Jul 1;94(1):29–37. doi: 10.1002/ccd.28329 with permission from John Wiley and Sons.

Cardiogenic shock—classification

The Society for Cardiovascular Angiography and Interventions (SCAI) classification describes five stages of CS, from 'At risk' to 'Extremis' (➤ **Fig. 5.13**).[62]

The classification system incorporates the variability of CS presentation and aetiology, allows for reassessment and reclassification at the bedside, and correlated well with mortality risk when validated in a large cohort study.[63]

Cardiogenic shock—management

Initial assessment

1. Full physical assessment for signs of hypoperfusion.
2. Monitoring of vital signs including continuous arterial blood pressure, pulse pressure, heart rate, ECG, and peripheral oxygen saturation.
3. Insertion of arterial and central venous catheters to allow for invasive monitoring of arterial and central venous pressure; serial measurement of arterial blood gas, central venous oxygen saturation, serum pH, lactate, and electrolytes; and safe administration of vasoactive medication.
4. 12-lead ECG.
5. Echocardiography.
6. Chest X-ray.
7. Laboratory testing of full blood count, coagulation, serum electrolytes, serum creatinine, liver function tests, and troponin.
8. Pulmonary artery catheter insertion is not recommended for all patients with CS but should be used for patients who remain hypoperfused and hypotensive despite intervention (SCAI stage D), patients with advanced right heart failure, and patients with mixed shock.[51] A pulmonary artery catheter allows for measurement of cardiac index and pulmonary capillary wedge pressure.
9. In the context of an acute coronary syndrome, coronary angiography is recommended within 2 hours from admission to hospital.[60]

Initial management

Initial management of patients with CS consists of fluid challenge followed by inotropes and vasopressors if required to increase cardiac output and blood pressure, and therefore improve organ perfusion (➤ **Table 5.9**).

Table 5.9 Initial management of patients with cardiogenic shock

Pre-hospital	Focus on stabilizing the circulation and oxygenation Identify and treat the underlying precipitating factor
Hospital—tertiary care centre with the capacity for 24/7 cardiac catheterization, intensive care facilities, and availability of short- and long-term MCS	Restore organ perfusion with medical or mechanical therapies Perform revascularization or surgery if required Plan long-term support or palliation if refractory CS

Fluid management

Fluid administration is used to increase stroke volume. If there are no signs of fluid overload, consider the administration of 250 mL of fluid over 15–30 minutes; measure effects on invasive and/or non-invasive cardiac output measures.

Inotropes/vasopressors

After fluid challenge, inotropes and/or vasopressors should be used to increase heart rate, contractility, and/or afterload and therefore improve cardiac output and/or blood pressure. Usually administered as continuous intravenous infusions, these medications can increase myocardial oxygen consumption and raise the risk of arrhythmias. Use is guided by continuous monitoring of haemodynamics and perfusion. Noradrenaline (norepinephrine) should be used as a first-line vasopressor, in preference to adrenaline (epinephrine), to improve perfusion pressure, measured by mean arterial pressure greater than 60 mmHg.[51] If positive inotropes are required, dobutamine is used commonly, while levosimendan may be beneficial for patients with ongoing beta-blockade and to reduce pulmonary vascular resistance in cases of right ventricular failure or pulmonary hypertension. In non-ischaemic patients, milrinone can be considered, in combination with vasopressin if required to maintain blood pressure.[60] Escalating and combination inotrope and vasopressor therapy points to refractory CS and consideration for alternative treatment such as mechanical circulatory support (MCS).[59]

Respiratory support

Respiratory support may be required to correct hypoxaemia and hypercapnia, manage pulmonary congestion, and reduce myocardial oxygen demand by facilitating deep sedation and suppressing spontaneous respiratory effort. Almost all patients will require oxygen therapy, while 60–80% of patients require invasive mechanical ventilation.[51]

Renal support

Acute kidney injury occurs in one-third of patients with CS. The requirement for renal replacement therapy to manage acute kidney injury is associated with worse prognosis.[51] Continuous renal replacement therapy modalities are recommended over intermittent haemodialysis.

Cardiogenic shock—mechanical circulatory support

Patients with refractory CS (SCAI stages D and E) might require MCS, a group of device-based therapies which increase systemic blood flow and maintain organ perfusion while avoiding cardiotoxicity and long-term morbidity of medical treatment.[64] MCS can be used as temporary circulatory support (TCS) in selected patients as a bridge to recovery, re-evaluation, transplantation, or a permanent implanted left ventricular assist device.[51] They are invasive therapies which are associated with risk to the patient and so should be commenced in centres experienced in their use. See ➤ **Table 5.10** for a guide to TCS devices.[65]

Intra-aortic balloon counter-pulsation using an intra-aortic balloon pump has been the most commonly used TCS, but routine use is no longer recommended in CS as benefit has not been demonstrated.[66] Impella® (Abiomed Inc., Danvers, MA, US) uses a microaxial blood pump which supports the left ventricle. TandemHeart® (LivaNova, London, UK) uses a centrifugal pump to deliver blood flows up to 4.0 L/min through a transseptal cannula. Both devices improve haemodynamics but no survival benefit has yet been proved, although trials are ongoing.[57] Venoarterial extracorporeal membrane oxygenation (VA-ECMO) provides biventricular cardiac support using a centrifugal pump to drain blood from the venous side of the circulation to a membrane oxygenator, before returning it, oxygenated, to the arterial side of the circulation. Blood is returned either via the ascending aorta (via central cannulation) or via the iliac artery (peripheral cannulation). VA-ECMO is currently the most common type of TCS although trial evidence

Table 5.10 Guide to TCS devices

	IABP	TamdemHeart®	Impella®	VA-ECMO
Mechanism	Pneumatic	Centrifugal, paracorporeal	Axial, transvalvular	Centrifugal, extracorporeal
Device configuration	Descending aorta via femoral artery	Inflow: LA via trans-septal (or RA) Outflow: femoral artery (or pulmonary artery)	Inflow: LV or (IVC) Outflow: ascending aorta (or pulmonary artery)	Inflow: femoral vein/IVC or internal jugular vein/SVC; Outflow: femoral, axillary/subclavian, or innominate artery
Type of ventricular support	LV	LV or RV	LV or RV	LV or RV
Maximum cardiac support (L/min)	0.5–1	4	2.5–5	>5
Magnitude of LV unloading	+	+++	++/+++[a]	Variable
Afterload effect	–	+++	None	+++
Complexity of implantation	+	+++	++/+++	+
Complexity of management	+	+++	++	+++
Risk of limb ischaemia	+	+++	++	+++[b]
Risk of haemorrhage	+	+++	+++	+++
Gas-exchange support	None	None	None	+++

IABP, intra-aortic balloon pump; IVC, inferior vena cava; LV, left ventricle; LA, left atrium; RA, right atrium; RV, right ventricle; SVC, superior vena cava; VA-ECMO, venoarterial extracorporeal membrane oxygenation. (+) low; (++) moderate; (+++) high; (–) reduced.
[a] Preload is reduced while afterload is increased.
[b] Can be mitigated by use of distal reperfusion cannula.
Reproduced from Abrams D, Garan AR, Abdelbary A, et al; International ECMO Network (ECMONet) and The Extracorporeal Life Support Organization (ELSO). Position paper for the organization of ECMO programs for cardiac failure in adults. Intensive Care Med. 2018 Jun;44(6):717–729. doi: 10.1007/s00134-018-5064-5 with permission from Springer Nature.

to support its use is awaited.[57] About 57% of patients requiring VA-ECMO due to cardiac failure survive the episode.[67] Complications associated with each device are summarized in ➤ Fig. 5.14.

Nursing management of the patient on VA-ECMO

1. Patient assessment, including regular physical assessment of peripheral and tissue perfusion, vital signs, respiratory function, neurological status, pain and sedation levels, kidney function, and skin integrity. A damped or flat arterial waveform, with similar systolic, diastolic, and mean arterial pressures, may be present due to absent or reduced pulsatility. Mean arterial pressure should be maintained at 65 mmHg or greater.
2. ECMO circuit assessment including lines, pump, and oxygenator. Assess for tight circuit connections, integrity of cannulae, tubing (dark red blood on

IABP | Impella | TrademHeart | ECMO

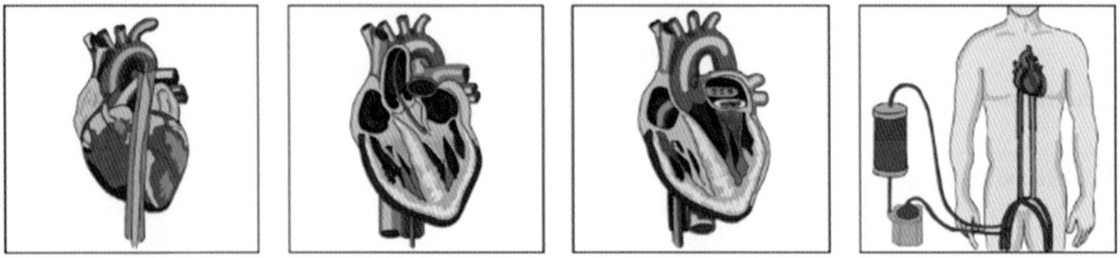

Device-specific complications

IABP
- Spinal cord ischaemia

Impella
- Frequent haemolysis*
- Valvular lesions

TandemHeart
- Air embolism
- Cardiac perforation
- Tamponade
- Residual atrial septal defect
- Massive night atrium to aorta shunt

ECMO
- Air embolism
- Increased left ventricular afterload
- Left ventricular dilation
- Left ventricular blood stasis
- Pulmonary oedema
- Differential oxygenation
- Circuit clots
- Disseminated intravascular or intraoxygenator coagulation
- Oxygenator failure
- Altered drug pharmacokinetics

Common complications

Device insertion site
- Infection
- Bleeding
- Vessel perforation
- Retroperitoneal haematoma
- Limb ischaemia
  - Compartment syndrome
  - Fasciotomy
  - Amputation

Neurological
- CNS haemorrhage
- CNS infarction
- Brain death
- Seizures

Acute kidney injury
- Haemolysis-induced
- Other causes

Haematological
- Haemolysis
- Acquired von Willebrand disease
- Thrombocytopenia
- Hepanin-induced thrombocytopenia
- Venous thromboembolism
- Gastrointestinal or pulmonary bleeding
- Bacteraemia or sepsis

Fig. 5.14 Complications associated with temporary circulatory support devices. ECMO, extracorporeal membrane oxygenation; IABP, intra-aortic balloon pump; TCS, temporary circulatory support. *Severe haemolysis might occur in the case of Impella® pump malposition. Daily Doppler echocardiography is needed to ensure correct positioning of the pump.

Reproduced from Combes A, Price S, Slutsky AS, Brodie D. Temporary circulatory support for cardiogenic shock. Lancet. 2020 Jul 18;396(10245):199–212. doi: 10.1016/S0140-6736(20)31047-3 with permission from Elsevier.

drainage side, bright red blood on return side), and oxygenator (check for signs of clots and/or fibrin), review alarms, circuit pressures, and treatment parameters including revolutions per minute, flow, sweep gas, and fraction of inspired oxygen.

3. Limb perfusion must be monitored hourly by assessing colour, temperature, capillary refill time, and aspect. Near-infrared spectroscopy can be used to monitor perfusion. Peripheral arterial cannulation for VA-ECMO can lead to partial or complete vessel occlusion, compromising blood flow through the limb. An additional perfusion line can be used to guarantee perfusion to the cannulated limb. The perfusion line must be monitored for flow and signs of clots or fibrin.
4. Good fluid management will support haemodynamic stability and ECMO circuit function. Jouncing lines associated with reduction in ECMO flow indicate hypovolaemia. Repeated drops in ECMO flow can lead to formation of clots and fibrin deposits, which can cause circuit failure. Intravenous fluid challenges should be used to counteract this; however, fluid overload should be avoided due to the risk of pulmonary oedema.
5. Left ventricular decompression is sometimes required and strategies include intra-aortic balloon counter-pulsation, Impella®, septostomy, and reconfiguration

of the ECMO circuit.[51] Echocardiography and regular assessment for signs of pulmonary congestion should be employed to guide these strategies.

6. Neurological assessment should be performed hourly and include assessment of pupils (size, shape, reaction) and depth of sedation. In adults, intracranial haemorrhage incidence in patients on ECMO is 2–21%, while acute ischaemic stroke is estimated at 1–33%.[68]
7. Management of anticoagulation and haemostasis using local protocols for titrating anticoagulants (usually administered as continuous infusions to maintain ECMO circuit patency) and blood product transfusion, with regular monitoring of coagulation and full blood count.
8. Assessment and interventions to promote skin and mucous membrane integrity are important due to the high risk of skin and mucous membrane damage. Patients in CS on VA-ECMO are usually immobile, deeply sedated, and require very careful movement to protect cannulae and ECMO flow. Pressure-relieving mattresses, regular repositioning, and regular mouth and eye care should be provided.

Temporary circulatory support—outcomes

TCS should be commenced as a bridge to recovery, transplant, or destination therapy (permanently implanted MCS device). In situations where the patient does not meet the criteria for transplant or permanent MCS, and where CS persists, withdrawal of life-sustaining treatment and palliation is indicated.

Recovery is confirmed through weaning trials: first weaning vasopressor support, then TCS. If TCS can be weaned without compromising haemodynamic stability or requiring high doses of inotropes/vasopressors, the support can be stopped. Patients who are unable to be discontinued from MCS should be considered for long-term options, namely a durable left ventricular assist device or heart transplantation.

Regular discussion should take place during TCS with those close to the patient, and the patient themselves if possible, about prognosis, progress, and goals of care. This should accompany regular discussion by the multidisciplinary team, including palliative care specialists. If continued life-sustaining treatment is no longer considered to be in the patient's best interests, such as following irreversible neurological injury or absence of myocardial recovery with contraindication to a transplant or permanent assist device, the focus of care should move to palliation and withdrawal of TCS. ➤ **Table 5.11** shows the predictors of in-hospital survival after VA-ECMO based on predicting survival after ECMO for refractory CS.[69]

Table 5.11 The predictors of in-hospital survival after VA-ECMO

Risk factors associated with hospital mortality	Chronic renal failure Longer duration of mechanical ventilation prior to ECMO Associated organ failure Pre-ECMO cardiac arrest Congenital heart disease Lower pulse pressure Lower serum bicarbonate
Protective factors	Younger age Weight between 76 and 89 kg Acute myocarditis Post-transplant Refractory ventricular tachycardia/fibrillation High diastolic blood pressure Lower peak inspiratory pressure

Conclusion

In this chapter we described a strategy for the nursing assessment of a cardiovascular patient. We covered the importance of an initial assessment in prioritizing problems and planning timely interventions, especially where urgent action is required. Some tools were presented to facilitate the conduct of an initial assessment. Next, a physical examination of the cardiovascular patient was described with a special focus on the examination of the cardiovascular body system. In addition, we highlighted the importance of track and trigger systems to recognize deterioration in relation to emergency situations and CS. Finally, we reminded nurses entering into cardiovascular care specialization to maintain a holistic approach to assessment and care planning using the functional health patterns framework.

References

1. International Council of Nursing. Definitions of nursing. Available from: https://www.icn.ch/nursing-policy/nursing-definitions.
2. Carnevali DL. The diagnostic reasoning process. In: Carnevali D, Mitchell P, Woods N, Tanner C (Eds),

Diagnostic Reasoning in Nursing. Philadelphia, PA: JB Lippincott; 1984:39–76.
3. Doenges ME, Moorhouse MF, Murr AC. Nursing Care Plans: Guidelines for Individualizing Client Care Across the Life Span. Philadelphia, PA: FA Davis; 2019.
4. Toney-Butler TJ, Unison-Pace WJ. Nursing Admission Assessment and Examination. Treasure Island, FL: StatPearls Publishing; 2019. Available from: https://www.ncbi.nlm.nih.gov/books/NBK493211/.
5. World Health Organization. The ABCDE and SAMPLE history approach. 2018. Available from: https://www.who.int/emergencycare/publications/BEC_ABCDE_Approach_2018a.pdf.
6. Herdman TH, Kamitsuru S. Supplement to NANDA International Nursing Diagnoses: Definitions and Classification, 2018–2020: New Things You Need to Know. New York: Thieme; 2019.
7. Bulechek GM, Butcher HK, Dochterman JM, Wagner CM. Nursing Interventions Classification (NIC). St. Louis, MO: Elsevier; 2019.
8. Astin F, Carroll D, Geest S De, Fernandez-Oliver A-L, Holt J, Hinterbuchner L, et al. A core curriculum for the continuing professional development of nurses working in cardiovascular settings: developed by the Education Committee of the Council on Cardiovascular Nursing and Allied Professions (CCNAP) on behalf of the European Society of C. Eur J Cardiovasc Nurs. 2015;14(2 Suppl):S1–17.
9. Gordon M. Manual of Nursing Diagnosis (13th ed). Burlington, MA: Jones & Bartlett Publishers; 2016.
10. World Health Organization. Commission on Social Determinants of Health. 2016. Available from: https://www.who.int/social_determinants/thecommission/finalreport/en/.
11. Jones DA, Lepley MK. Health Assessment Manual. New York: McGraw-Hill; 1986.
12. Currie K, Rideout A, Lindsay G, Harkness K. The association between mild cognitive impairment and self-care in adults with chronic heart failure: a systematic review and narrative synthesis. J Cardiovasc Nurs. 2015;30(5):382–93.
13. Freddi SG. Cognitive screening tools. Clin Rev. 2013;23(1):12.
14. Ewing JA. Detecting alcoholism: the CAGE questionnaire. JAMA. 1984;252(14):1905–907.
15. Bidwell JT, Lyons KS, Lee CS. Caregiver well-being and patient outcomes in heart failure: a meta-analysis. J Cardiovasc Nurs. 2017;32(4):372.
16. Song H, Fang F, Arnberg FK, Mataix-Cols D, de la Cruz LF, Almqvist C, et al. Stress related disorders and risk of cardiovascular disease: population based, sibling controlled cohort study. BMJ Open. 2019;365:I1255.
17. Piepoli MF, Hoes AW, Agewall S, Albus C, Brotons C, Catapano AL, et al. 2016 European Guidelines on cardiovascular disease prevention in clinical practice: the Sixth Joint Task Force of the European Society of Cardiology and Other Societies on Cardiovascular Disease Prevention in Clinical Practice (constituted by representatives of 10 societies and by invited experts). Developed with the special contribution of the European Association for Cardiovascular Prevention & Rehabilitation (EACPR). Eur Heart J. 2016;37(29):2315–81.
18. McSherry W. Making Sense of Spirituality in Nursing and Health Care Practice: An Interactive Approach. London: Jessica Kingsley Publishers; 2006.
19. Maugans TA. The spiritual history. Arch Fam Med. 1996;5(1):11–16.
20. Lim FA, Brown D V, Jones H. Lesbian, gay, bisexual, and transgender health: fundamentals for nursing education. J Nurs Educ. 2013;52(4):198–203.
21. Caceres BA, Markovic N, Edmondson D, Hughes TL. Sexual identity, adverse life experiences, and cardiovascular health in women. J Cardiovasc Nurs. 2019;34(5):380–89.
22. Taylor C, Lynn P, Bartlett J. Fundamentals of Nursing: The Art and Science of Person-Centered Care. Philadelphia, PA: Lippincott Williams & Wilkins; 2018.
23. Trivedi D. Cochrane review summary: Mini-Mental State Examination (MMSE) for the detection of dementia in clinically unevaluated people aged 65 and over in community and primary care populations. Prim Health Care Res Dev. 2017;18(6):527–28.
24. Newberry L, Barnett GK, Ballard N. A new mnemonic for chest pain assessment. J Emerg Nurs. 2005;31(1):84–85.
25. Stepinska J, Lettino M, Ahrens I, Bueno H, Garcia-Castrillo L, Khoury A, et al. Diagnosis and risk stratification of chest pain patients in the emergency department: focus on acute coronary syndromes. A position paper of the Acute Cardiovascular Care Association. Eur Heart J Acute Cardiovasc Care. 2020;9(1):76–89.
26. Allen E, Williams A, Jennings D, Stomski N, Goucke R, Toye C, et al. Revisiting the pain resource nurse role in sustaining evidence-based practice changes for pain assessment and management. Worldviews Evid Based Nurs. 2018;15(5):368–76.
27. Thim T, Krarup NHV, Grove EL, Rohde CV, Løfgren B. Initial assessment and treatment with the Airway, Breathing, Circulation, Disability, Exposure (ABCDE) approach. Int J Gen Med. 2012;5:117–21.
28. Monsieurs KG, Zideman DA, Alfonzo A, Arntz H-R, Askitopoulou H, Bellou A, et al. European resuscitation council guidelines for resuscitation 2015: section 1. Executive summary. Resuscitation. 2015;95:1–80.
29. do Prado PR, Bettencourt AR de C, de Lima Lopes J. Defining characteristics and related factors of the

nursing diagnosis for ineffective breathing pattern. Rev Bras Enferm. 2019;72(1):221–30.

30. Santos M, Kitzman DW, Matsushita K, Loehr L, Sueta CA, Shah AM. Prognostic importance of dyspnea for cardiovascular outcomes and mortality in persons without prevalent cardiopulmonary disease: the Atherosclerosis Risk in Communities Study. PLoS One. 2016;11(10):e0165111.
31. Jarvis C. Physical Examination and Health Assessment E-Book. St. Louis, MO: Elsevier Health Sciences; 2019.
32. Williams B, Mancia G, Spiering W, Rosei EA, Azizi M, Burnier M, et al. 2018 ESC/ESH Guidelines for the management of arterial hypertension: the Task Force for the management of arterial hypertension of the European Society of Cardiology (ESC) and the European Society of Hypertension (ESH). Eur Heart J. 2018;39(33):3021–104.
33. Kristensen SD, Knuuti J, Saraste A, Anker S, Bøtker HE, Hert S De, et al. 2014 ESC/ESA Guidelines on non-cardiac surgery: cardiovascular assessment and management: the Joint Task Force on non-cardiac surgery: cardiovascular assessment and management of the European Society of Cardiology (ESC) and the European Society of Anaesthesiology (ESA). Eur Heart J. 2014;35(35):2383–431.
34. Thygesen K, Alpert JS, Jaffe AS, Chaitman BR, Bax JJ, Morrow DA, et al. Fourth universal definition of myocardial infarction (2018). Eur Heart J. 2019;40(3):237–69.
35. Montalescot G, Sechtem U, Achenbach S, Andreotti F, Arden C, Budaj A, et al. 2013 ESC guidelines on the management of stable coronary artery disease. Eur Heart J. 2014;35(33):2260–61.
36. Collet JP, Thiele H, Barbato E, Barthélémy O, Bauersachs J, Bhatt DL, et al. ESC Scientific Document Group. 2020 ESC Guidelines for the management of acute coronary syndromes in patients presenting without persistent ST-segment elevation. Eur Heart J. 2020;29:ehaa575.
37. Olson K. Oxford Handbook of Cardiac Nursing. Oxford: Oxford University Press; 2014.
38. Mamas MA, Kwok CS, Kontopantelis E, Fryer AA, Buchan I, Bachmann MO, et al. Relationship between anemia and mortality outcomes in a national acute coronary syndrome cohort: insights from the UK myocardial ischemia national audit project registry. JAMA. 2016;5(11):e003348.
39. Razvi S, Jabbar A, Pingitore A, Danzi S, Biondi B, Klein I, et al. Thyroid hormones and cardiovascular function and diseases. J Am Coll Cardiol. 2018;71(16):1781–96.
40. Zègre-Hemsey JK, Garvey JL, Carey MG. Cardiac monitoring in the emergency department. Crit Care Nurs Clin. 2016;28(3):331–45.
41. Vincent J-L, Einav S, Pearse R, Jaber S, Kranke P, Overdyk FJ, et al. Improving detection of patient deterioration in the general hospital ward environment. Eur J Anaesthesiol. 2018;35(5):325.
42. Zeymer U, Bueno H, Granger CB, Hochman J, Huber K, Lettino M, et al. Acute Cardiovascular Care Association position statement for the diagnosis and treatment of patients with acute myocardial infarction complicated by cardiogenic shock: a document of the Acute Cardiovascular Care Association of the European Society of Card. Eur Heart J Acute Cardiovasc Care. 2020;9(2):183–97.
43. Soar J, Nolan JP, Böttiger BW, Perkins GD, Lott C, Carli P, et al. European resuscitation council guidelines for resuscitation 2015: section 3. Adult advanced life support. Resuscitation. 2015;95:100–47.
44. Andersen LW, Holmberg MJ, Berg KM, Donnino MW, Granfeldt A. In-hospital cardiac arrest: a review. JAMA. 2019;321(12):1200–10.
45. Mebazaa A, Yilmaz MB, Levy P, Ponikowski P, Peacock WF, Laribi S, et al. Recommendations on pre-hospital and early hospital management of acute heart failure: a consensus paper from the Heart Failure Association of the European Society of Cardiology, the European Society of Emergency Medicine and the Society of Academic Emergency Medicine—short version. Eur Heart J. 2015;36(30):1958–66.
46. Truhlář A, Deakin CD, Soar J, Khalifa GEA, Alfonzo A, Bierens JJLM, et al. European Resuscitation Council guidelines for resuscitation 2015: section 4. Cardiac arrest in special circumstances. Resuscitation. 2015;95:148–201.
47. Perkins GD, Olasveengen TM, Maconochie I, Soar J, Wyllie J, Greif R, et al. European Resuscitation Council guidelines for resuscitation: 2017 update. Resuscitation. 2018;123:43–50.
48. National Institute for Health and Care Excellence. Acutely ill patients in hospital: recognition of and response to acute illness in adults in hospital. 2007. Available from: https://www.nice.org.uk/guidance/cg50.
49. Bernstein JA, Cremonesi P, Hoffmann TK, Hollingsworth J. Angioedema in the emergency department: a practical guide to differential diagnosis and management. Int J Emerg Med. 2017;10(1):1–11.
50. Kaufman MB. ACE Inhibitor-related angioedema: are your patients at risk? Pharm Ther. 2013;38(3):170.
51. Chioncel O, Parissis J, Mebazaa A, Thiele H, Desch S, Bauersachs J, et al. epidemiology, pathophysiology and contemporary management of cardiogenic shock: a position statement from the Heart Failure Association (HFA) of the European Society of Cardiology (ESC). Eur J Heart Fail. 2020;22(8):1315–41.
52. Chua WL, See MTA, Legido-Quigley H, Jones D, Tee A, Liaw SY. Factors influencing the activation of the rapid response system for clinically deteriorating patients by

frontline ward clinicians: a systematic review. Int J Qual Health Care. 2017;29(8):981–98.

53. Mancheva L, Dugdale J. Understanding communications in medical emergency situations. In: 2016 49th Hawaii International Conference on System Sciences (HICSS). IEEE; 2016:198–206.
54. Müller M, Jürgens J, Redaèlli M, Klingberg K, Hautz WE, Stock S. Impact of the communication and patient hand-off tool SBAR on patient safety: a systematic review. BMJ Open. 2018;8(8):e022202.
55. Liaw SY, Zhou WT, Lau TC, Siau C, Chan SW. An interprofessional communication training using simulation to enhance safe care for a deteriorating patient. Nurse Educ Today. 2014;34(2):259–64.
56. Harjola VP, Miró O, Vranckx P, Zeymer U. Acute heart failure. 2016. Available from: https://www.escardio.org/static-file/Escardio/Medias/associations/acute-cardiovascular-care-association/AcuteCVDays/Acut%20Heart%20Failure%20Chapter%204.pdf.
57. de Chambrun MP, Donker DW, Combes A. What's new in cardiogenic shock? Intensive Care Med. 2020;46(5):1016–19.
58. EuroShock. Homepage. Available from: http://www.euroshock-study.eu/about-euroshock1.html.
59. Combes A, Price S, Slutsky AS, Brodie D. Temporary circulatory support for cardiogenic shock. Lancet. 2020;396(10245):199–212.
60. Ponikowski P, Voors AA, Anker SD, Bueno H, Cleland JGF, Coats AJS, et al. 2016 ESC Guidelines for the diagnosis and treatment of acute and chronic heart failure: the Task Force for the diagnosis and treatment of acute and chronic heart failure of the European Society of Cardiology (ESC). Developed with the special contribution of the Heart Failure Association (HFA) of the ESC. Eur Heart J. 2016;37(27):2129–200.
61. Menon V, Slater JN, White HD, Sleeper LA, Cocke T, Hochman JS. Acute myocardial infarction complicated by systemic hypoperfusion without hypotension: report of the SHOCK trial registry. Am J Med. 2000;108(5):374–80.
62. Baran DA, Grines CL, Bailey S, Burkhoff D, Hall SA, Henry TD, et al. SCAI clinical expert consensus statement on the classification of cardiogenic shock: this document was endorsed by the American College of Cardiology (ACC), the American Heart Association (AHA), the Society of Critical Care Medicine (SCCM), and the Society of Thoracic Surgeons (STS) in April 2019. Catheter Cardiovasc Interv. 2019;94(1):29–37.
63. Jentzer JC, van Diepen S, Barsness GW, Henry TD, Menon V, Rihal CS, et al. Cardiogenic shock classification to predict mortality in the cardiac intensive care unit. J Am Coll Cardiol. 2019;74(17):2117–28.
64. Thiele H, Jobs A, Ouweneel DM, Henriques JPS, Seyfarth M, Desch S, et al. Percutaneous short-term active mechanical support devices in cardiogenic shock: a systematic review and collaborative meta-analysis of randomized trials. Eur Heart J. 2017;38(47):3523–31.
65. Abrams D, Garan AR, Abdelbary A, Bacchetta M, Bartlett RH, Beck J, et al. Position paper for the organization of ECMO programs for cardiac failure in adults. Intensive Care Med. 2018;44(6):717–29.
66. Neumann F-J, Sousa-Uva M, Ahlsson A, Alfonso F, Banning AP, Benedetto U, et al. 2018 ESC/EACTS guidelines on myocardial revascularization. Eur Heart J. 2019;40(2):87–165.
67. Extracorporeal Life Support Organization. ELSO registry. 2020. Available from: https://www.elso.org/Registry.aspx.
68. Sutter R, Tisljar K, Marsch S. Acute neurologic complications during extracorporeal membrane oxygenation: a systematic review. Crit Care Med. 2018;46(9):1506–13.
69. Schmidt M, Burrell A, Roberts L, Bailey M, Sheldrake J, Rycus PT, et al. Predicting survival after ECMO for refractory cardiogenic shock: the survival after veno-arterial-ECMO (SAVE)-score. Eur Heart J. 2015;36(33):2246–56.

6 Care of the patient with coronary artery disease

VALENTINO ORIOLO, MARGARET CUPPLES, NEIL ANGUS, SUSAN CONNOLLY, AND FELICITY ASTIN

CHAPTER CONTENTS

In this chapter, a brief overview of the epidemiology and pathophysiology of coronary artery disease and coronary risk factors is presented. The main focus of the chapter is the management and nursing care of patients with coronary artery disease manifesting as acute coronary syndromes. A series of case studies of acute coronary syndromes illustrates the key stages in patient management and nursing care. For completeness, a brief outline of the key features and management priorities for patients diagnosed with chronic coronary syndromes and other clinical conditions associated with atherosclerosis is included.

KEY MESSAGES

- Atherosclerosis is a disease of ageing that causes coronary heart disease.
- Coronary artery disease can manifest as acute or chronic coronary syndromes.
- Rapid and accurate risk stratification and assessment of patients presenting with chest pain improves patients' outcomes.
- There is no single diagnostic test for acute coronary syndromes.

- Accurate interpretation of the patient's history and presenting symptoms, electrocardiogram changes, and biomarkers form the foundation of clinical decision-making.
- Patients and those close to them need emotional support to help them through what can be a life-threatening experience.
- Tailored information and cardiovascular prevention and rehabilitation are needed to help patients to recover and self-manage their medications and lifestyle to optimize health and well-being.
- The coronavirus disease 2019 (COVID-19) pandemic has necessitated rapid changes in the way cardiovascular services are configured.

Introduction

The terms coronary artery disease (CAD), ischaemic heart disease, and coronary heart disease all describe the condition in which epicardial arteries that supply the heart with oxygenated blood become narrowed or blocked by atherosclerotic plaque accumulation. For the purpose of this chapter, we will use the term CAD. CAD remains a major cause of morbidity and mortality in Europe and worldwide.[1,2] Coronary atherosclerosis is a disease of ageing that develops over a lifetime. It typically leads to cardiovascular disease including CAD. By middle age, most people will have some degree of atherosclerosis. During the early stages people are often asymptomatic, but in later life progressive atherosclerosis may lead to the clinical manifestations of conditions categorized either as chronic coronary syndromes (CCS)[3] or acute coronary syndromes (ACS).[4,5]

ACS is a generic term that describes syndromes caused by decreased blood flow to the myocardium leading to ischaemia, injury, and necrosis.[4,5] CCS was previously known as stable CAD. This terminology has fallen out of favour because the nomenclature does not reflect current clinical practice.[3] CAD is a dynamic, rather than a stable, condition and the underlying atherosclerotic process and altered arterial function can be modified by environmental and lifestyle factors as well as pharmacological therapies.

The clinical outcomes for patients presenting with the manifestations of CAD have improved considerably with the advent of new treatments and advances in non-invasive diagnostic testing. Cardiovascular nurses need to be equipped to support both the physical and psychological well-being of patients with CAD, as well as those close to them. It is important that nurses understand how and why CAD develops as well as the characteristics of different clinical presentations and their associated management.

A comprehensive account of the management and care of patients presenting across the full continuum of CAD is beyond the scope of this chapter. To develop a more comprehensive understanding of the care of a patient diagnosed with CAD, the material in this chapter can be supplemented by cross-referencing to information contained elsewhere in this textbook:

- Chapter 4 ('Anatomy and physiology of the healthy heart'): this chapter describes the mechanisms of electrical conduction in the heart, the characteristics of a normal electrocardiogram (ECG), and a step-by-step approach to ECG analysis which can be applied to the case studies in this chapter.
- Chapter 5 ('Nursing assessment and care planning in the context of cardiovascular care'): this chapter describes the steps involved in a comprehensive health assessment and a focused cardiovascular assessment. Content about clinical deterioration and cardiogenic shock is also included.
- Chapter 7 ('Care of the patient with cardiac arrhythmias'): this chapter provides a detailed description of common arrhythmias, some of which are referred to in the case studies within this chapter.
- Chapter 11 ('Cardiovascular prevention and rehabilitation'): this chapter provides details on the cardiac rehabilitation process which starts in hospital and continues on into early recovery. A range of patient-reported outcome measures are also described which are relevant to the care of a patient with CAD.
- Chapter 12 ('Pharmacology for cardiovascular nurses'): this chapter describes the common medications used in the care of a patient with CAD and addresses some common challenges such as non-adherence.
- Chapter 13 ('Patient education and communication'); this chapter provides details on therapeutic patient education and communication techniques that can be applied in clinical practice and highlights the importance of health literacy and the provision of accessible health information.

Epidemiology

CAD remains the leading single cause of mortality, responsible for 862,000 deaths (19% of all deaths) among men and 877,000 deaths (20%) among women each year, with mortality rates generally higher in Central and Eastern Europe than in Northern, Southern, and Western Europe.[6] Although mortality rates have declined since the 1960s (more significantly in high-income countries than in middle-income countries) due to both improvements in treatments and declines in risk factors (e.g. smoking, high blood pressure), there has been a slowing of the reduction in the past few years. Moreover, data from the UK have recently shown a rise in mortality from cardiovascular disease for the first time in 50 years in those under 75 years in 2017.[7] The reasons for this increase are not yet fully understood but the obesity/diabetes epidemic is thought to be a contributory factor. What is not yet known is whether this trend is also occurring more widely across Europe as the last published statistics relate to 2016 data.[6]

European-level data on the various diagnoses that constitute CAD are not yet available although registries for ACS (both ST-segment elevation myocardial infarction (STEMI) and non-ST-segment elevation myocardial infarction (NSTEMI)) are in development under the auspices of the European Society of Cardiology (ESC) EURObservational Research Programme (EORP). In the UK, data from the Myocardial Ischaemia National Audit Project (MINAP) registry would suggest that the ratio of STEMIs to NSTEMIs is approximately 40:60 although this figure may be skewed as not all NSTEMIs are recorded on the registry. Data from the large SWEDEHEART registry in Sweden have shown a decline in the 1-year case fatality rate from both STEMI (from 21% to 14%) and NSTEMI (from 26% to 15%) between 1995 and 2014, principally due to improved implementation of evidence-based treatments (revascularization strategies and pharmacotherapy).[8,9] The advent of the high-sensitivity troponin (hs-Tn) assay has likely led to a decrease in the reported incidence of unstable angina (UA) because cases previously diagnosed as UA (with normal creatinine kinase levels) are now diagnosed as ACS (or non-ST-segment elevation (NSTE-ACS[5]) with the additional finding of elevated hs-Tn levels.[5] Troponin is a protein involved in both musculoskeletal and cardiac muscle contraction. It is classified into three subtypes—troponin C, troponin I, and troponin T—with troponin I and troponin T described as being more cardiac specific.[10] The hs-Tn test is the latest generation of cardiac enzyme testing that allows for detection of very low levels of troponin.

The epidemiology of angina is not well understood as attention has largely focused on ACS and there have been few population studies of incident angina. This is somewhat surprising as these studies suggest that angina pectoris (the term that describes the chest pain/discomfort associated with CAD) is the most common presentation of ischaemic heart disease. A population-wide study in Finland[9] using primary care electronic records for the whole country estimated the annual incidence of angina, based on (1) new nitrate prescription and (2) test positivity (either stress test or invasive coronary angiography). Findings showed that the total annual incidence was approximately 2 per 100 population and several times higher than the incidence of non-fatal myocardial infarction (MI). It also clearly demonstrated that angina is not a benign disease, with significantly higher standardized mortality ratios for CAD in the angina cases observed in both sexes (test positive > nitrate positive) compared to the general population, with a strong graded inverse relationship with age.[11]

Another factor influencing population data is the impact of the coronavirus disease 2019 epidemic. While comprehensive data are not yet available, the COVID-19 pandemic could increase CAD mortality rates through several mechanisms. Patients with pre-existing health conditions, such as CAD, who contract COVID-19, are known to have poorer outcomes and COVID-19 itself can trigger cardiovascular comorbidities such as ACS and arrhythmia.[12] The cessation of elective cardiology services during the COVID-19 pandemic combined with patient-related delays in presentation with ACS at accident and emergency departments will also impact epidemiological trends.

Pathophysiology

The association between thrombotic coronary artery occlusion and MI has been apparent for many years, but far less was known about the underpinning pathophysiology and clinical features until relatively recently.[13] The heart muscle, or myocardium, requires a supply of oxygenated blood so that it can contract rhythmically and effectively to fulfil the metabolic demands of all parts of the body. This function depends both on the patency of the coronary arteries, allowing carriage of a sufficient blood flow, and on the extraction of nutrients from the blood by the myocytes. The major vessels supplying the myocardium (the right coronary artery and the left main coronary artery dividing into the left anterior descending and circumflex coronary arteries) and their main branches lie on the epicardial surface of the heart while smaller branches enter into the depths of the muscle (see Chapter 4 for more detail). These smaller arteries and arterioles are the main sites of cellular transfer of nutrients to the myocardium.

Atherosclerosis is caused by an inflammatory process. The initial stage in atherosclerosis development occurs when the normal functioning of endothelial cells which allow smooth flow of blood along the vessel is disrupted. The trigger is an inflammatory response, with release of cytokines and cell surface adhesion molecules such as VCAM-1, causing monocytes and T lymphocytes to adhere to the endothelium. A change in shape of the endothelial cells increases the permeability of the arterial wall, allowing lymphocytes and lipoprotein particles, especially low-density lipoprotein (LDL), to enter the intima. Once under the endothelial surface, monocytes differentiate into macrophages, take up oxidized LDL, and become lipid-laden 'foam cells' which eventually die, but the lipid accumulates forming fatty streaks which evolve over time into atherosclerotic plaques. These plaques, composed of a lipid core surrounded by smooth muscle cells and connective tissue fibres, may undergo calcification. In the initial stages of the development of coronary atherosclerosis, the diameter of the arterial lumen remains unaffected as there is expansion of the media and the external elastic membrane during atheroma development (known as positive remodelling).

Ultimately, however, plaque progression/growth will start to impact luminal size (negative remodelling) and start to cause clinical manifestations of CCS such as stable angina or ACS. Coronary atherosclerosis/plaque formation is a dynamic process and plaque stability depends on multiple factors[13] including their composition, size, location, and the strength of their cap. Stable plaques causing greater than 70% occlusion of the coronary arteries tend to cause the symptoms of stable angina, whereas ACS typically arise from the rupture/erosion of non-obstructive vulnerable plaques that tend to be lipid rich, have a thin cap, and a high concentration of inflammatory cells (➤ Fig. 6.1).[14] Plaque rupture results in the exposure of thrombogenic plaque components such as tissue factor in the coronary circulation which leads to the activation of the coagulation cascade with thrombus formation and acute myocardial ischaemia.

The thrombus can be fibrin rich, fully occluding the arterial lumen and causing a STEMI (ST-segment elevation-ACS). Platelet-rich thrombi can cause more transient luminal occlusion and result in UA or NSTE-ACS.

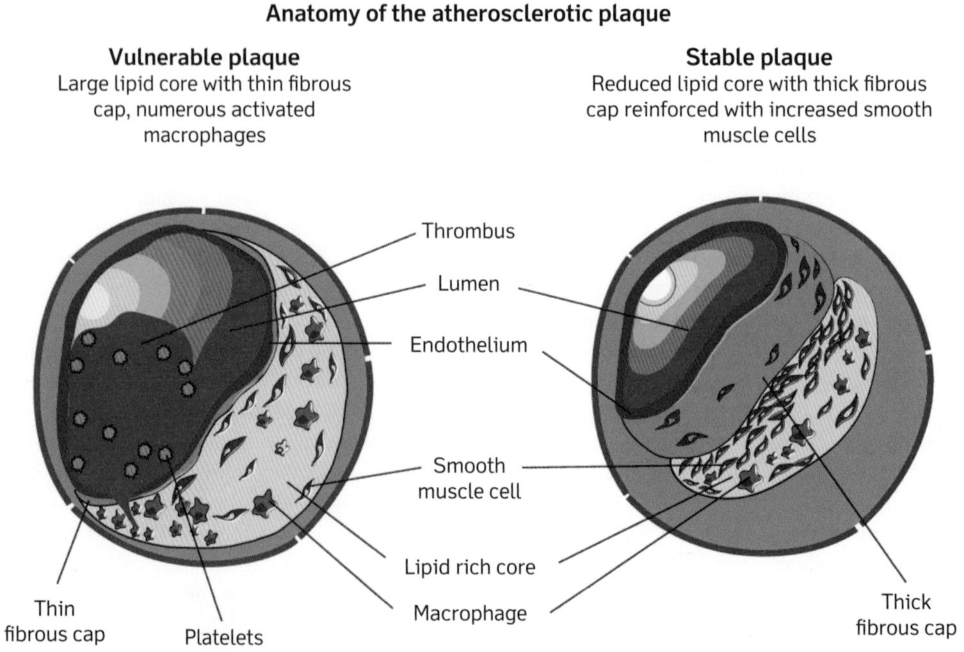

Fig. 6.1 Characteristics of a vulnerable rupture-prone atherosclerotic plaque compared with a stable plaque.

Reproduced from Landmesser U, Koenig W. From risk factors to plaque development and plaque destabilization. In The ESC Textbook of Preventive Cardiology. Ed: Gielen S, De Backer G, Piepoli M, Wood D. Oxford, UK , European Society of Cardiology. 2015 with permission from Oxford University Press.

Risk factors for coronary atherosclerosis

Many causative factors are involved in the development of atherosclerosis (see Chapter 1 and Chapter 11). Various risk factors modulate the impact of causative mechanisms which include the effects of chronic inflammation and infection on the arterial wall and implicate the role of the immune system and genetics.[15] The INTERHEART case–control study showed that just nine potentially reversible risk factors and health behaviours (smoking, dyslipidaemia, hypertension, diabetes, obesity, psychosocial factors, diet, alcohol, and sedentary lifestyle) account for greater than 90% of the population attributable risk of MI in all regions of the world.[16] Of all these risk factors, hypertension is quantitatively the leading contributor to ischaemic CAD morbidity and mortality, given its prevalence in the global population. Of note, the risk of ischaemic CAD among people with hypertension is often increased by coexisting morbidities (e.g. dyslipidaemia, diabetes, obesity). ➤ Table 6.1 shows the principal risk factors for coronary atherosclerosis (both modifiable and non-modifiable).

Mechanisms by which various risk factors impact the development of atherosclerosis have been identified. The increased pressure on blood vessel walls associated with hypertension can cause mechanical injury, stimulating the inflammatory process described previously and promoting formation of atherosclerotic plaques. Smoking causes vascular damage, mediated by nicotine and other chemicals contained within tobacco smoke, which can result in vasoconstriction, raised fibrinogen levels, increased plasma viscosity, and thrombosis. Cigarette smoking is also associated with dyslipidaemia, with higher levels of LDL and lower levels of high-density lipoprotein cholesterol. Hypercholesterolaemia promotes subendothelial uptake of cells and particles and LDL oxidation, with consequent deposition of atherosclerotic plaques in arterial walls. In diabetes, the products of disturbed glucose metabolism may themselves directly cause endothelial damage, provoking an inflammatory reaction. Chronic renal disease, a contributory cause of hypertension and diabetes, and of other metabolic abnormalities, has also been identified as increasing the risk of developing atherosclerosis through the processes of abnormal cellular function.

The impact of psychosocial stressors (stress at work or home, financial stress, recent major life events, and depression) is attributed to a combination of biological and behavioural effects, including increased sympathetic nervous system output and adverse lifestyle behaviours (smoking, poor diet, alcohol, physical inactivity), which contribute to the development of hypertension and dyslipidaemia.[17]

The mediation pathways for the impact of physical inactivity in promoting atherosclerosis have been largely attributed to changes in inflammatory biomarkers, including fibrinogen, lipids, and blood pressure.

It is clear that many of the important risk factors for CAD are lifestyle-related behaviours that are potentially modifiable. As CAD is a chronic condition, the adoption of healthy lifestyle changes and the cessation of harmful ones can help to prevent the development of atherosclerosis. In patients with established CAD, atherosclerotic plaque accumulation can potentially be stabilized or potentially reversed by healthy lifestyle changes.

Table 6.1 Risk factors for coronary atherosclerosis

Non-modifiable risk factors	Modifiable risk factors
Age	Hyperlipidaemia/raised LDL cholesterol
Sex	Hypertension
Family history	Diabetes
Ethnicity	Smoking
	Diet
	Overweight/obesity
	Physical inactivity
	Excess alcohol consumption
	Psychosocial stress, depression
	Substance misuse e.g. cocaine

Clinical manifestations of coronary artery disease

CAD is a dynamic and chronic condition and the way in which it manifests can be very different across individuals. The reduction or cessation of blood flow through the coronary arteries that supply the myocardium can cause to myocardial ischaemia which can lead to tissue injury and necrosis. The way in which CAD manifests depends upon the underlying characteristics of the atherosclerotic plaque and coronary circulation. Myocardial ischaemia may be caused by atherosclerotic plaque accumulation in the coronary arteries, acute coronary artery thrombosis, or microvascular or vasospastic disease. Pathologically sustained myocardial ischaemia disrupts myocyte (cardiac cell) metabolism and the

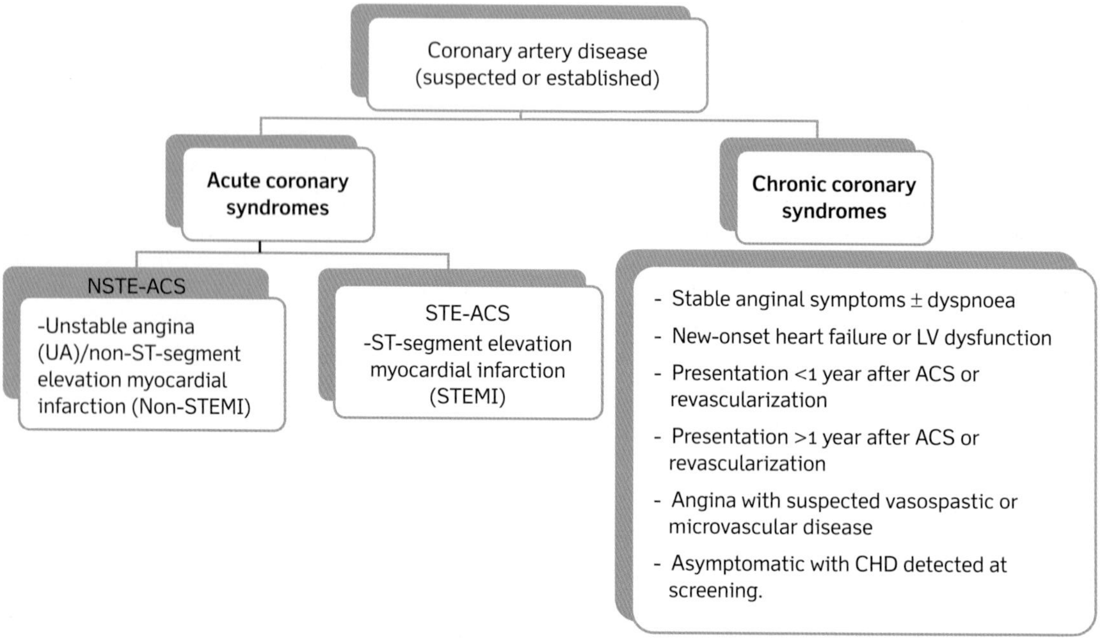

Fig. 6.2 An overview of acute and chronic coronary syndromes. CHD, coronary heart disease; LV, left ventricular.

Source data from 2019 ESC Guidelines for the diagnosis and management of chronic coronary syndromes: The Task Force for the diagnosis and management of chronic coronary syndromes of the European Society of Cardiology (ESC) Knuuti J, Wijns W, Saraste A et al., ESC Scientific Document Group, 2017 ESC Guidelines for the management of acute myocardial infarction in patients presenting with ST-segment elevation: The Task Force for the management of acute myocardial infarction in patients presenting with ST-segment elevation of the European Society of Cardiology (ESC), European Heart Journal, Volume 39, Issue 2, 07 January 2018, Pages 119–177, https://doi.org/10.1093/eurheartj/ehx393; Collet JP, Thiele H, Barbato E, ESC Scientific Document Group, 2020 ESC Guidelines for the management of acute coronary syndromes in patients presenting without persistent ST-segment elevation: The Task Force for the management of acute coronary syndromes in patients presenting without persistent ST-segment elevation of the European Society of Cardiology (ESC), European Heart Journal, ehaa575, https://doi.org/10.1093/eurheartj/ehaa575.

contractile structures of affected cells. MI results from the death (necrosis) of myocytes.[18] At the outset, myocardial ischaemia arises due to an imbalance between myocardial oxygen supply and demand. Sudden cardiac death occurs in about half of patients with ACS before they reach hospital.[19]

Depending on the clinical presentation, CAD can be categorized as CCS[3] or ACS.[4,5] However, in reality, these categories may not be mutually exclusive. This is because many patients with CCS may have also had an episode of ACS (➤ **Fig. 6.2**). Each individual will have their own unique trajectory. The risk of a future cardiac event will vary considerably due to the dynamic nature of CAD and the associated functional alterations in the coronary circulation. ➤ **Fig. 6.2** provides an overview of CCS and ACS in the context of CAD including the revised subcategories of clinical presentations within CCS.

MI is a condition that falls within the classification of ACS but can present with several different underlying causes. The Fourth Universal Definition of Myocardial Infarction differentiates between myocardial injury and acute MI and provides a useful classification system describing the range of clinical presentations of acute MI.[20]

Myocardial ischaemia may be obvious clinically or detected by acute ECG alterations. When accompanied by changes in the concentration of cardiac troponin (cTn), a diagnosis of acute MI is established.

If there are changes in cTn levels without clinical evidence of myocardial ischaemia then a diagnosis of acute myocardial injury can be determined. Myocardial injury requires evidence of raised cTn, with at least one value exceeding the 99th percentile of the upper reference limit (URL), that is, the 99th percentile URL (14 ng/L) is the upper reference range for the biomarker and therefore the majority of people will have a value that falls below the upper reference range of that sample.

Myocardial injury is considered acute if a rise and/or fall of cTn is detected. Myocardial injury is associated with adverse clinical outcomes for patients and is a prerequisite for a diagnosis of MI. Myocardial injury can also be caused by non-ischaemic cardiac conditions such as myocarditis and non-cardiac conditions including renal failure.

Acute MI describes the circumstance in which there is evidence of acute myocardial injury combined with clinical evidence of myocardial ischaemia.[20,21] Thus, for a diagnosis of MI, at least one of the following features (additional to myocardial injury) must be present:

- Symptoms of myocardial ischaemia (typically chest pain).
- New ischaemic ECG changes and/or development of pathological Q waves on the ECG.
- Imaging evidence indicating new loss of viable myocardium.
- Regional myocardial wall motion abnormalities or identification of coronary thrombus by angiography or at autopsy.

In clinical practice, patients with chest pain, or other ischaemic symptoms, and who develop new ST-segment elevation in two contiguous ECG leads, or new left bundle branch block, are considered to have a STEMI. In contrast, clinical presentations that do not include ST-segment elevation are designated as NSTE-ACS. The pathological correlate at the myocardial level is cardiomyocyte necrosis (NSTEMI) or, less frequently, myocardial ischaemia without cell damage (UA).[5] In addition to these categories, MI presentations can be classified into various subtypes dependent on clinical, pathological, and prognostic differences.[21–23]

A consistent and clear classification system for MI is important from regulatory and scientific perspectives and also in clinical practice in order to determine the most appropriate and evidence-based patient management strategy. The following subtypes are outlined in the Fourth Universal Definition of Myocardial Infarction[20]:

- *MI type 1*: results spontaneously from the disruption of an atherosclerotic plaque (rupture, ulceration, fissuring, dissection, or erosion) in one or more coronary arteries accompanied by thrombus formation. In combination, these events decrease myocardial blood flow and result in myocyte necrosis. In this dynamic situation, the relative contribution of plaque and thrombus may vary and thrombus can embolize resulting in myocyte destruction downstream from the primary lesion.
- *MI type 2*: when a condition, other than coronary artery plaque instability, contributes to a mismatch between myocardial oxygen supply and demand. This may occur in patients known to have a CCS (e.g. angina pectoris) who develop an intercurrent illness or acute physiological stress such as gastrointestinal bleeding resulting in a sudden and precipitous reduction in the oxygen-carrying capacity of haemoglobin. Sustained bradyarrhythmias and tachyarrhythmias can also result in myocardial ischaemia and injury causing a type 2 MI. Each of these physiological insults leads to insufficient coronary blood flow, myocardial ischaemia, and an inability to respond to increased myocardial oxygen demands brought about by an intercurrent condition.
- *MI type 3*: describes sudden cardiac death from a suspected MI when biomarkers were not available or obtained prior to death. The patient may have presented acutely with features typical of myocardial ischaemia or infarction, new ECG changes, or life-threatening arrhythmias such as ventricular fibrillation. In some instances, the MI may be reclassified following a postmortem examination.
- *MI type 4*: occurs as a complication of percutaneous coronary intervention (PCI) or stent thrombosis. Myocardial injuries can occur perioperatively or later due to complications arising from the use of devices such as intracoronary stents. The occurrence of procedure-related myocardial injury is determined by the measurement of cTn prior to the procedure and repeated 3–6 hours later. Arbitrarily, a cTn rise of more than five times the 99th percentile URL in patients with normal baseline values is diagnostic.
- *MI type 5*: associated with coronary artery bypass graft (CABG) procedures. A range of factors may result in myocardial injury during CABG procedures. These include processes relating to perioperative cardiac preservation (e.g. cardiopulmonary bypass) as well as traumatic injury to the myocardium during surgery. Increases in cTn are generally expected during CABG procedures; however, the guidance suggests that a type 5 MI should be diagnosed only when cTn levels exceed more than ten times the 99th percentile URL in the first 48 hours following surgery from a normal baseline measure. ECG, angiographic, or imaging

evidence, signalling new myocardial ischaemia/new myocardial injury, should also accompany biomarker measurement.

- *Myocardial infarction with non-obstructive coronary arteries (MINOCA)*: a subtype of MI that is recognized.[23] This refers to patients with a MI in the absence of angiographically defined CAD (narrowing >50% diameter stenosis of a major epicardial vessel). MINOCA is a condition in which an ischaemic mechanism is the cause of myocyte injury. The prevalence of MINOCA may account for 6–8% of patients with MI. This condition is more common in women and patients who present with NSTEMI rather than STEMI. It is thought that atherosclerotic plaque disruption and coronary thrombosis may be a cause of MINOCA (i.e. type 1 MI). However, coronary spasm and spontaneous dissection may also be implicated (i.e. type 2 MI). In such instances, it can be difficult to determine the pathological basis for MI.

From this classification, it is clear that the aetiology of myocardial ischaemia is varied. In patients presenting with symptoms suggestive of decreased coronary blood flow (e.g. chest pain), the healthcare professional should adopt a systematic approach. The assessment of the presenting complaint and associated signs and symptoms are important steps in the assessment process (see Chapter 5 for more detail).

Clinical presentation

The assessment of chest pain and or dyspnoea is an important aspect of a focused cardiovascular assessment (refer to Chapter 5 for a detailed account of a focused cardiovascular assessment). Angina is a presenting complaint for many patients with CAD.

Angina

Angina pectoris is a medical term that refers to the symptoms of chest pain or discomfort that occur during periods of myocardial ischaemia. The term is derived from the Latin meaning a strangling feeling in the chest. Several factors can cause a mismatch between the oxygen supply and myocardial tissue demand leading to myocardial ischaemia: coronary artery stenosis, coronary artery spasm, hypotension, tachyarrhythmias, severe anaemia, thyrotoxicosis, hypertensive emergencies, or severe aortic valve stenosis.[5]

Angina may be classified as being 'typical', 'atypical', or 'non-anginal' chest pain. Typical angina has three characteristics: patients report constricting discomfort in the front of the chest, in the neck, jaw, shoulder or arm, precipitated by physical exertion, and relieved by rest or nitrates within 5 minutes.[3] Atypical angina is suspected if two of the aforementioned characteristics are noted, and non-anginal chest pain if only one, or none, of the characteristics are present.[3]

Interestingly, the majority of patients with suspected CAD present with atypical angina. A smaller proportion present with typical angina symptoms (10–15%).[3] Patients with acute MI presenting with no symptoms tend to have worse clinical outcomes compared to those who do exhibit symptoms.[24] There are several potential causes of acute chest pain, as shown in ➤ **Table 6.2**. The majority of patients presenting with acute chest pain will not have ACS.

Stable angina typically develops when there is a fixed lesion in a coronary artery that causes a 70% stenosis of the lumen of a major epicardial coronary vessel (e.g. left anterior descending, circumflex, or right coronary artery) or a 50% stenosis of the left main coronary artery. The symptoms indicative of stable angina are somewhat predictable, have a trigger such as physical exertion, and resolve within a few minutes. Stable angina falls within the category of CCS.[3]

The Canadian Cardiovascular Society developed a useful classification system, shown in ➤ **Table 6.3**. The framework classifies angina severity into four classes depending on the description of angina symptoms.[25]

The Canadian Cardiovascular Society Grading Scale is recommended as a tool to evaluate the severity of exertional angina that is a feature of CCS.[25]

Assessment and management of patients with suspected acute coronary syndromes

The rapid assessment and risk stratification of patients with suspected ACS saves lives and is central to effective management and care. The overarching treatment goals are to improve myocardial perfusion to minimize myocardial ischaemia, injury, or infarction, minimize complications, and prevent adverse cardiovascular events.[4,5] A significant number of patients who develop ACS do not survive.[5] Restoring the patency of coronary arteries improves survival rates in patients with ACS, but to

Table 6.2 Differential diagnoses of ACS in the setting of acute chest pain

Cardiac	Pulmonary	Vascular	Gastro-intestinal	Orthopaedic	Other
Myopericarditis	**Pulmonary embolism**	**Aortic dissection**	**Oesophagitis,**	**Musculoskeletal**	**Anxiety**
Cardiomyopathies[a]	(Tension)-pneumothorax	Symptomatic aortic	Peptic ulcer, gastritis	Chest trauma	Herpes zoster
Tachyarrhythmias	Bronchitis, pneumonia	Stroke	Pancreatits	Muscle injury/ inflammation	Anaemia
Acute heart failure	Pleuritis		Cholecystitis	Costochondritis	
Hypertensive emergencies				Cervical spine pathologies	
Aortic valve stenosis					
Takotsubo syndrome					
Coronary spasm					
Cardiac trauma					

Bold = common and /or important differential diagnoses.
[a]Diated, hypertrophic and restrictive cardiomyopathies may cause angina or chest discomfort.
Collet JP, Thiele H, Barbato E, et al; ESC Scientific Document Group. 2020 ESC Guidelines for the management of acute coronary syndromes in patients presenting without persistent ST-segment elevation. Eur Heart J. 2020 Aug 29:ehaa575. doi: 10.1093/eurheartj/ehaa575 © The European Society of Cardiology. Reprinted by permission of Oxford University Press.

maximize the potential benefit this must be done as soon as possible.[4]

Pre-hospital delay time has been recognized as an important factor in predicting poor patient outcome. Despite the development of several interventions designed to reduce patient delay times, only about half of these interventions are effective.[26] The way that health services are configured also influences the time taken from symptom onset to restoring coronary blood flow. For example, access to effective pre-hospital care and

Table 6.3 Canadian Cardiovascular Society grading scale for angina severity

Class	Description of angina severity	
I	Angina only with strenuous exertion	Presence of angina during strenuous, rapid, or prolonged ordinary activity (walking or climbing the stairs).
II	Angina with moderate exertion	Slight limitation of ordinary activities when they are performed rapidly, after meals, in cold or windy weather conditions, in response to emotional stress, or on wakening, but also walking uphill, climbing more than one flight of ordinary stairs at a normal pace and in normal conditions. .
III	Angina with mild exertion	Having difficulties walking one or two blocks, or climbing one flight of stairs, at normal pace and conditions.
IV	Angina at rest	No exertion needed to trigger angina.

Reproduced from Campeau L. Letter: Grading of angina pectoris. Circulation. 1976 Sep;54(3):522–3 with permission from Wolters Kluwer.

cardiac catheterization laboratories that are open 24/7 are factors that can influence the survival outcomes of patients presenting with ACS.

The initial assessment is based on the integration of low-likelihood and/or high-likelihood features derived from the clinical setting (i.e. symptoms, vital signs), the 12-lead ECG, and the cTn concentration determined at presentation to the emergency department and serially thereafter.[5] The history of the presenting complaint, the typicality of the anginal pain, and the coronary risk factor profile are also important when assessing patients with suspected ACS. These data will assist in the diagnosis of patients presenting with ACS such as STEMI. Biomarkers such as troponin allow risk stratification and subsequent diagnosis in patients presenting with NSTE-ACS. Troponin results during serial sampling should be interpreted as a quantitative marker: the higher the level at initial testing (0-hour level) or the absolute change during serial sampling, the higher the likelihood for the presence of MI. (See Chapter 5 for an account of a focused cardiovascular assessment.)

The algorithm shown in ➤ Fig. 6.3 provides a useful guide when assessing a patient presenting with cardiac-sounding chest pain; history, clinical findings, and presentation should be considered amid the patient's comorbidities and risk factors for CAD.

Triage decisions are made based upon a rapid rule-in or rule-out framework. The advent of the COVID-19 pandemic requires the additional assessment of infective status for patients and the use of personal protective equipment to protect staff.[12]

The distinction between UA and non-STEMI can only be made retrospectively on the basis of serial cTn measurements. Both conditions fall under the umbrella of NSTE-ACS. In UA, the cardiac biomarkers remain normal or only very minimally elevated.

The key features of management are to restore coronary blood flow as soon as possible through the administration of medicines such as antiplatelet agents (aspirin and P_2Y_{12} inhibitors such as clopidogrel, prasugrel, or ticagrelor) and injectable anticoagulants (such as Xa inhibitors).[12] In conjunction with interventions to restore coronary blood flow, intravenous opioids are administered to relieve pain and anxiolytics, such as benzodiazepines, help to relieve high levels of anxiety. Oxygen is no longer routinely administered but titrated if arterial oxygen saturation is less than 94%.[27]

Primary percutaneous coronary intervention (PPCI) remains the reperfusion treatment of choice for patients with STEMI, ideally within 120 minutes from diagnosis of STEMI based on the history and presenting complaint.[4] If PPCI is not achievable within 120 minutes from diagnostic ECG, perhaps because the patient is unable to access a centre capable of 24/7 PPCI, the patient should be considered for fibrinolytic therapy. Patients who receive fibrinolytic therapy should subsequently undergo routine PCI 2–4 hours after successful lysis. ➤ Fig. 6.4 illustrates the optimal reperfusion times in patients presenting with STEMI.

In patients presenting with STEMI, the aims are (➤ Fig. 6.4):

- To minimize the delay between first medical contact and diagnosis of STEMI to 10 minutes or less.
- To minimize diagnosis to reperfusion time to 120 minutes or less if patient presenting to a non-PPCI centre:
  - In a non-PPCI centre, aim for transfer to a PPCI centre in 30 minutes or less and reperfusion in 90 minutes or less (total time ≤120 minutes).
  - If PPCI is not achievable in 120 minutes or less, aim for fibrinolysis strategy.
- To minimize diagnosis to reperfusion time to 60 minutes or less if patient presents directly to a PPCI centre.

The patient pathway for NSTE-ACS is shown in ➤ Fig. 6.5 and focuses upon risk assessment. Patients at very high risk should undergo invasive therapy within 2 hours of diagnosis. Patients at high risk should be considered for early invasive therapy, ideally within 24 hours of diagnosis; patients at low risk should ideally be considered for selective invasive strategy ischaemic testing prior to invasive therapy. These patients should be managed as per the 2019 ESC Guidelines for the diagnosis and management of CCS.[5]

In patients presenting with NSTE-ACS, the reperfusion timings will be dependent on a number of variables. Similar to the STEMI pathway, the timing for reperfusion is critical in patients with very high-risk or high-risk features (➤ Fig. 6.5). A reperfusion time of 2 hours or less and 24 hours or less should be aimed for in patients with very high and high risk, respectively.[5] Patients with very high-risk features presenting to non-PCI centres should be immediately transferred to a PCI centre for immediate invasive strategy. Patients with high-risk features presenting to non-PCI centres should be transferred to a PCI centre on the same day, aiming for invasive management within 24 hours of NSTE-ACS diagnosis.[5]

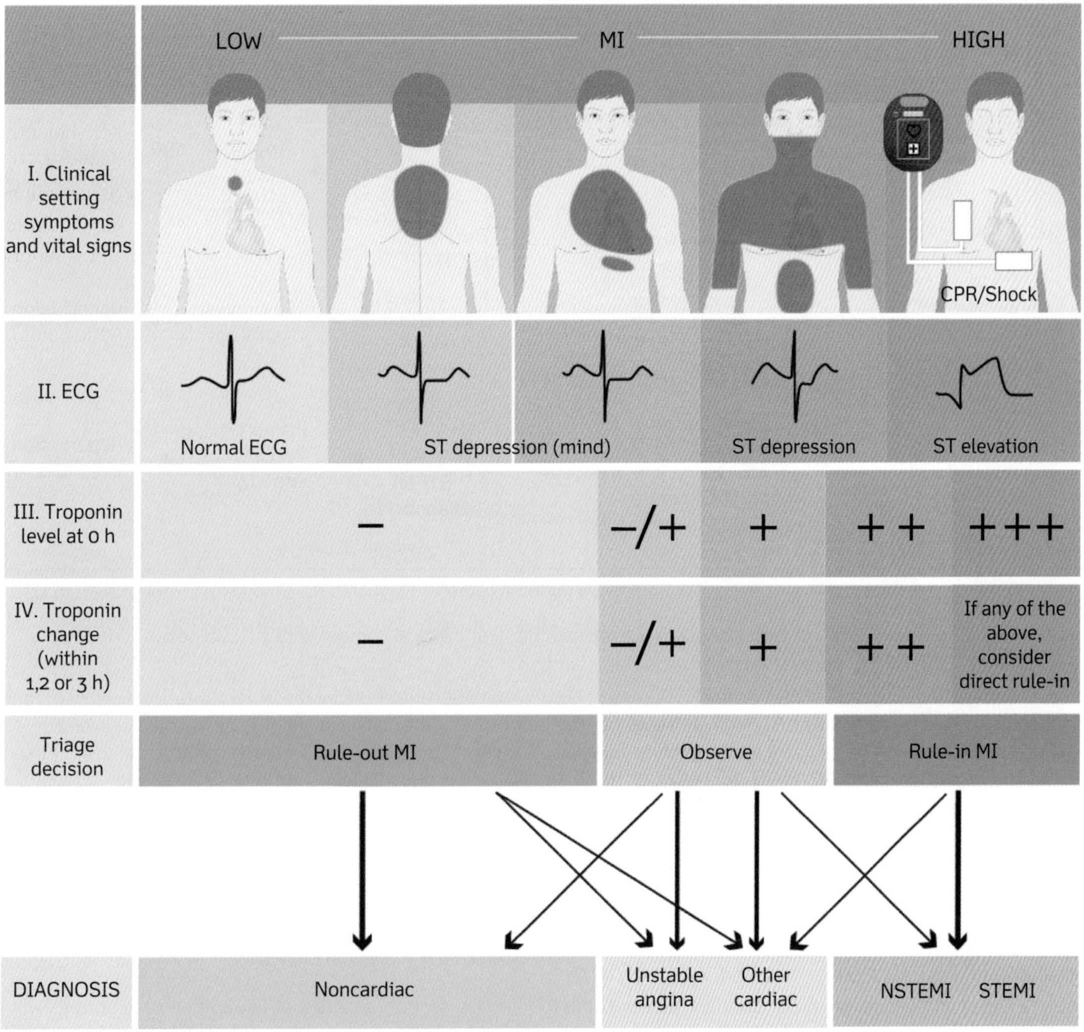

Fig. 6.3 Diagnostic algorithm and triage in acute coronary syndromes. CPR, cardiopulmonary resuscitation; ECG, electrocardiogram/electrocardiography; MI, myocardial infarction; NSTEMI, non-ST-segment elevation myocardial infarction; STEMI, ST-segment elevation myocardial infarction.

Collet JP, Thiele H, Barbato E, et al; ESC Scientific Document Group. 2020 ESC Guidelines for the management of acute coronary syndromes in patients presenting without persistent ST-segment elevation. Eur Heart J. 2020 Aug 29:ehaa575. doi: 10.1093/eurheartj/ehaa575 © The European Society of Cardiology. Reprinted by permission of Oxford University Press.

Coronary artery bypass graft

CABG can be considered as an alternative reperfusion strategy to PCI in patients with stable CAD. The risk of surgical mortality should be assessed using a validated risk score such as the European System for Cardiac Operative Risk Evaluation (EuroSCORE II)[28,29] and the Society of Thoracic Surgeons (STS) score.[30–32]

Clinical characteristics that favour surgical intervention include, but are not limited to, diabetes, reduced left ventricular function, contraindication to dual antiplatelet therapy, and recurrent in-stent restenosis. Additionally, the anatomical complexity and technical difficulty should be evaluated. The SYNTAX score supports the decision-making process when considering CABG over PCI.[32]

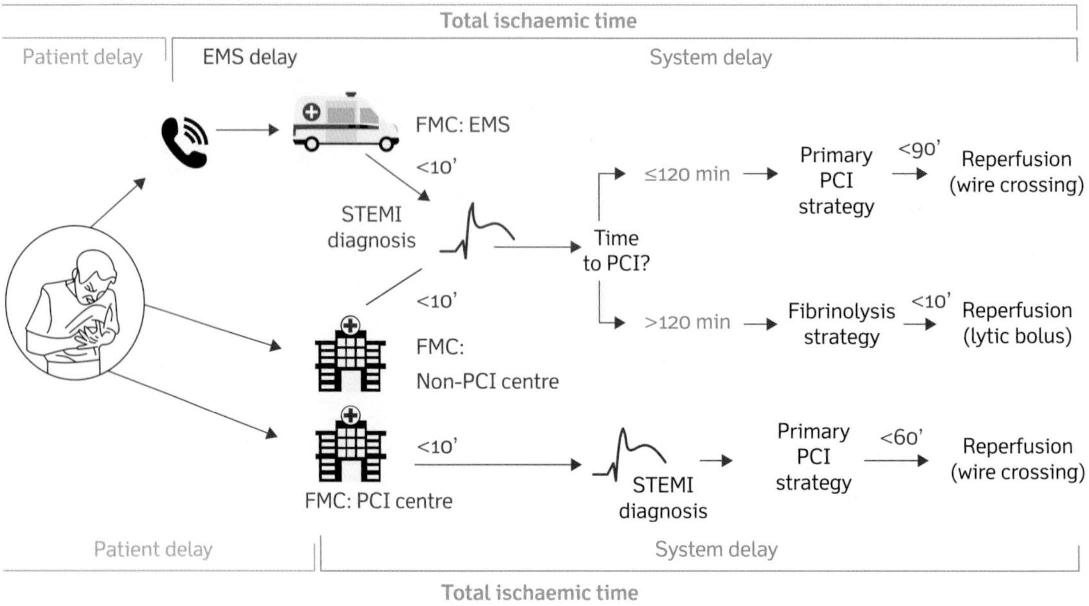

Fig. 6.4 STEMI pathway. EMS, emergency medical system; FMC, first medical contact; PCI, percutaneous coronary intervention; STEMI, ST-segment elevation myocardial infarction.

Ibanez B, James S, Agewall S, et al; ESC Scientific Document Group. 2017 ESC Guidelines for the management of acute myocardial infarction in patients presenting with ST-segment elevation: The Task Force for the management of acute myocardial infarction in patients presenting with ST-segment elevation of the European Society of Cardiology (ESC). Eur Heart J. 2018 Jan 7;39(2):119–177. doi: 10.1093/eurheartj/ehx393. PMID: 28886621. © The European Society of Cardiology. Reprinted by permission of Oxford University Press.

By combining a number of parameters (e.g. the number of lesions, the length of segment, and the aetiology of the occlusion) a numerical score is obtained. A high SYNTAX score (≥33) is indicative of more complex disease and CABG should be considered as an option over PCI due to its mortality benefit.[33] CABG is also the preferred strategy in patients requiring concomitant interventions (e.g. patients with aortopathy and valvular disease requiring surgical intervention). ➤ **Fig. 6.6** summarizes factors to be considered during the decision-making process regarding revascularization approaches. Patients' preferences should also be considered.

In summary, myocardial revascularization should be performed to improve coronary perfusion, symptoms of myocardial ischaemia, and prognosis. In patients presenting with ACS, PPCI/PCI should be completed in a timely fashion. CABG should be considered in patients with multivessel CAD, significant comorbidities, in-stent restenosis, and high SYNTAX score.[34]

Illustrative case studies for acute coronary syndromes

In this section, a series of illustrative case studies will be presented to outline the assessment and management of patients with suspected ACS. A diagnosis of ACS is primarily based on patient history and presenting complaints as well as serial ECGs and cardiac biomarkers, such as hs-TnT; hs-TnT, is used to measure any potential heart damage[19] and diagnose MI. A hs-TnT value above the 99th percentile is considered indicative of MI.[19]

Case study 1. A patient diagnosed with NSTE-ACS: UA

UA is defined as myocardial ischaemia at rest or on minimal exertion in the absence of acute cardiomyocyte injury/necrosis.[5] It is caused by a platelet-rich thrombus causing transient luminal occlusion.

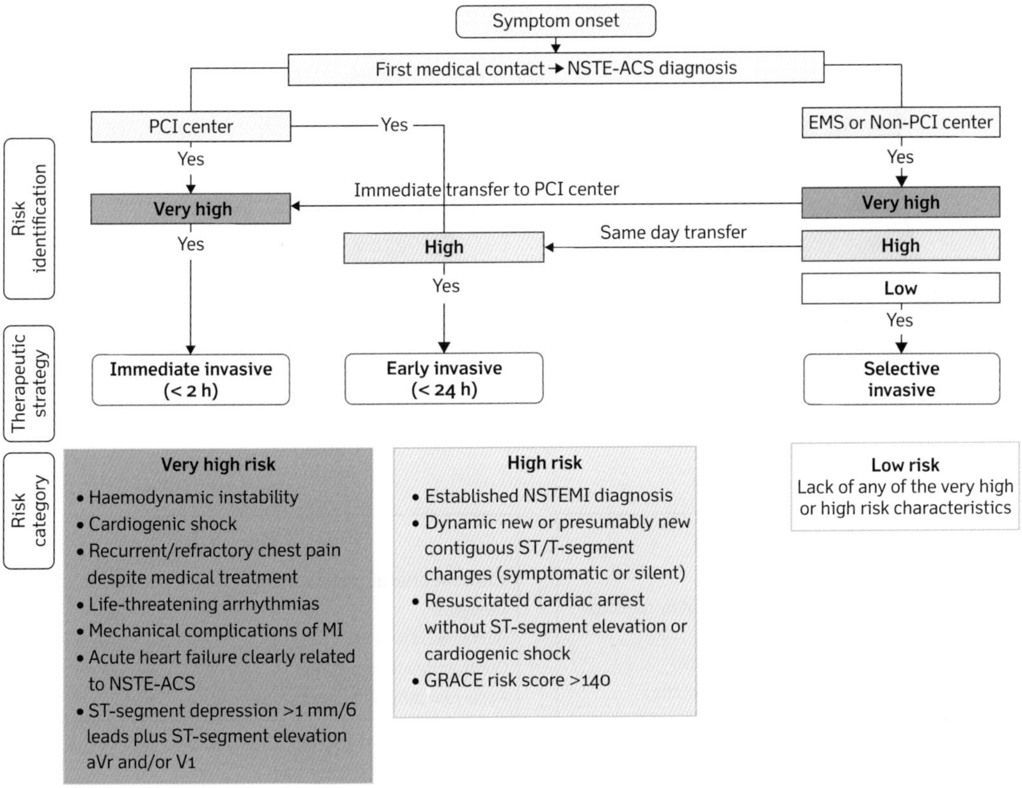

EMS = emergency medical services; GRACE = Global Registry of Acute Coronary Events; MI = myocardial infarction; NSTE-ACS = non-ST-segment elevation acute coronary syndrome; NSTEMI = non-ST-segment elevation myocardial infarction; PCI = percutaneous coronary intervention.
Collet JP, Thiele H, Barbato E, Barthélémy O, Bauersachs J, Bhatt DL, Dendale P, Dorobantu M, Edvardsen T, Folliguet T, Gale CP, Gilard M, Jobs A, Jüni P, Lambrinou E, Lewis BS, Mehilli J, Meliga E, Merkely B, Mueller C, Roffi M, Rutten FH, Sibbing D, Siontis GCM, ESC Scientific Document Group, 2020 ESC Guidelines for the management of acute coronary syndromes in patients presenting without persistent ST-segment elevation: The Task Force for the management of acute coronary syndromes in patients presenting without persistent ST-segment elevation of the European Society of Cardiology (ESC), European Heart Journal, ehaa575, https://doi.org/10.1093/eurheartj/ehaa575

Fig. 6.5 NSTE-ACS pathway. EMS, emergency medical services; GRACE, Global Registry of Acute Coronary Events; MI, myocardial infarction; NSTE-ACS, non-ST-segment elevation acute coronary syndrome; NSTEMI, non-ST-segment elevation myocardial infarction; PCI, percutaneous coronary intervention.

Collet JP, Thiele H, Barbato E, et al; ESC Scientific Document Group. 2020 ESC Guidelines for the management of acute coronary syndromes in patients presenting without persistent ST-segment elevation. Eur Heart J. 2020 Aug 29:ehaa575. doi: 10.1093/eurheartj/ehaa575 © The European Society of Cardiology. Reprinted by permission of Oxford University Press.

Presenting complaint

Mr Ali is a 38-year-old male Asian taxi driver, who presents to the emergency department with chest pain.

History of the presenting complaint

Mr Ali describes noticing a decreased exercise tolerance over the previous 4 weeks with an associated feeling of 'discomfort in his chest'. He also noticed that during stressful situations (e.g. during 'rush hour') he becomes sweaty and clammy and at times experiences a sensation of a 'fist on his chest'. These episodes have increased in frequency and occurred on two separate occasions while at rest.

Baseline assessment

A cardiovascular assessment was performed. Mr Ali's blood pressure was elevated (168/93 mmHg), but equal bilaterally, pulses were equal, and heart rate was in the normal range (60 beats per minute (bpm)). Mr Ali's ECG demonstrated sinus rhythm with no evidence of

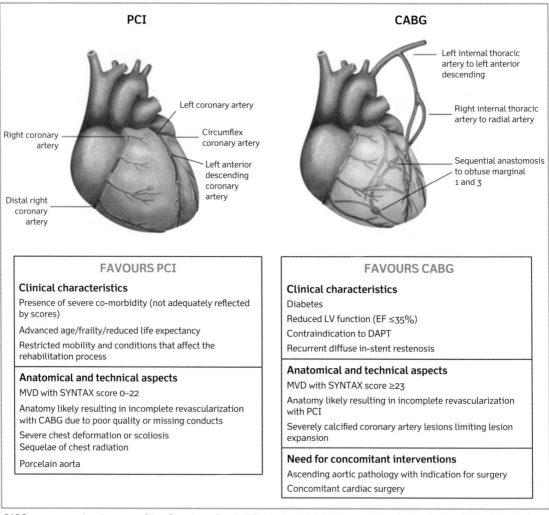

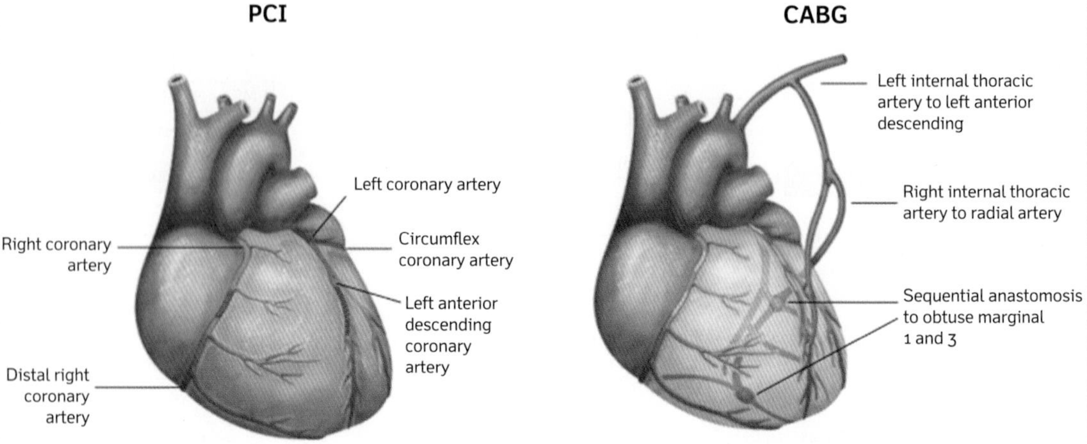

FAVOURS PCI

Clinical characteristics

Presence of severe co-morbidity (not adequately reflected by scores)

Advanced age/frailty/reduced life expectancy

Restricted mobility and conditions that affect the rehabilitation process

Anatomical and technical aspects

MVD with SYNTAX score 0–22

Anatomy likely resulting in incomplete revascularization with CABG due to poor quality or missing conducts

Severe chest deformation or scoliosis

Sequelae of chest radiation

Porcelain aorta

FAVOURS CABG

Clinical characteristics

Diabetes

Reduced LV function (EF ≤35%)

Contraindication to DAPT

Recurrent diffuse in-stent restenosis

Anatomical and technical aspects

MVD with SYNTAX score ≥23

Anatomy likely resulting in incomplete revascularization with PCI

Severely calcified coronary artery lesions limiting lesion expansion

Need for concomitant interventions

Ascending aortic pathology with indication for surgery

Concomitant cardiac surgery

CABG = coronary artery bypass grafting; Cx = circumflex; DAPT = dual antiplatelet therapy; EF = ejection fraction; LAD = left anterior descending coronary artery; LIMA = left internal mammary artery; LV = left ventricular; MVD = multivessel coronary artery disease; PCI = percutaneous coronary intervention; PDA = posterior descending artery; RA = radial artery; RIMA = right internal mammary artery; SYNTAX = Synergy between Percutaneous Coronary Intervention with TAXUS and Cardiac Surgery.
[a]consider no-touch off-pump CABG in case of porcelain aorta.

2018 ESC/EACTS Guidelines on myocardial revascularization, European Heart Journal, Volume 40, Issue 37, 1 October 2019,Page 3096, https://doi.org/10.1093/eurheartj/ehz507

Fig. 6.6 Percutaneous coronary intervention versus coronary artery bypass graft.

Neumann FJ, Sousa-Uva M, Ahlsson A, et al; ESC Scientific Document Group. 2018 ESC/EACTS Guidelines on myocardial revascularization. Eur Heart J. 2019 Jan 7;40(2):87–165. doi: 10.1093/eurheartj/ehy394. Erratum in: Eur Heart J. 2019 Oct 1;40(37):3096. © The European Society of Cardiology. Reprinted by permission of Oxford University Press.

ST-segment abnormality (see ➤ **Fig. 6.7** for ECG and analysis) and a hs-TnT value was reported at 6 hours from the onset of pain as 16 ng/L (reference range: normal value <14 ng/L; indeterminate 15–30 ng/L; positive >30 ng/L).

Discussion

The history of the presenting complaint identifies some features ('red flags') that are of concern. There is a noticeable pattern of a gradual decrease in exercise tolerance. Mr Ali also reports symptoms developing during stressful

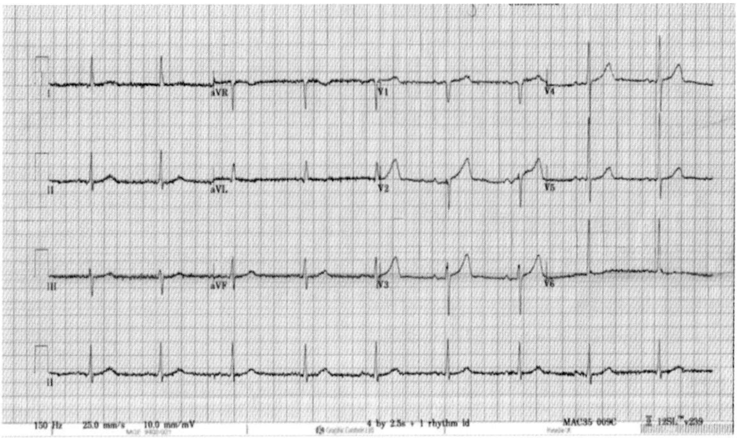

Fig. 6.7 Mr Ali's 12-lead ECG.

situations, with progressively earlier onset. This pattern of angina is often referred to as crescendo angina,[5] also known as UA, and is indicative of atherosclerotic plaque progression. Left untreated, this will lead to atherosclerotic plaque rupture with subsequent inflammatory response leading to thrombus formation.

Thrombus formation will decrease coronary artery flow, both on exertion and at rest, causing the symptoms reported by the patient; UA is classified as an ACS. The symptoms reported by the patient are suggestive of typical anginal pain[3]: a constricting discomfort in the chest lasting approximately 15–20 minutes, with the presence of autonomic features such as nausea and sweating, precipitated by exertion and sometimes relieved by rest.

A cardiovascular focused history is critical when assessing patients presenting with chest pain. In this case, there is a significant coronary risk factor profile. Mr Ali is Asian and has comorbidities of poorly controlled hypertension and type 2 diabetes (tablet controlled). Mr Ali smokes 20 cigarettes per day and has done for 18 years and has attempted to quit in the last 6 months. Mr Ali has a strong family history of premature CAD (his father had a STEMI at 54 years of age). Of all of the coronary risk factors, family history is unmodifiable and hence most significant, but often overlooked. When evaluating coronary risk factors, details about the family history can help to stratify the likelihood of a coronary event.

Management

Mr Ali's presentation is suggestive of UA. The nursing management will focus upon monitoring the recurrence of symptoms, cardiovascular stability (by monitoring baseline observations—blood pressure, pulse, heart rate, and respiration rate), and regular serial ECG recordings. During each interaction with the patient, a simple 'end-of-bed assessment' can be useful in identifying signs and symptoms of distress and 'clues' or indicators of clinical deterioration (see Chapter 5 for details about clinical deterioration and cardiogenic shock). For example, is the patient frightened, pale, and clammy? Is the work of breathing laboured, fast, or irregular? Performing a brief initial assessment can often be sufficient to highlight any 'red flags' in the patient presentation.

A 12-lead ECG should be performed at first medical contact with a maximum target delay of 10 minutes. Serial ECGs should be recorded every 15 minutes if symptoms continue, after 30 minutes of absence of symptoms, and hourly (for 4 hours) after symptoms are alleviated. Lead placement is critical and this should not change between procedures as this can result in lead misplacement and inaccurate ECG recording. Potential ECG changes may be caused by operator error and not a change in the patient's condition (see Chapter 4 for details of how to record an accurate ECG). The nurse plays an important role in the interpretation of the ECG and it is important to use a structured approach (see Chapter 4 for a detailed description of ECG analysis and also Chapter 7 for care of the patient with a cardiac arrhythmia).

Each element of Mr Ali's ECG (➤ Fig. 6.7) is examined individually and then an interpretation made based on the analysis. The specific parameters measured include the following:

- Heart rate (bpm).
- Axis (normal, left, right, extreme, or indeterminate).
- Conduction (rhythm and regular or irregular).

- P waves (lead II gives the best view of P waves. Look at PR interval, P-wave duration, amplitude, and morphology).
- Intervals: PR interval, QT/QTc intervals.
- QRS (duration, amplitude, morphology, in particular amplitude of R waves).
- ST segments (amplitude, morphology, in particular ST elevation or depression in contiguous leads).
- T waves (amplitude, morphology).

When applying this framework to Mr Ali's ECG, the following findings can be described:

- Heart rate (bpm): 60 bpm.
- Axis (normal, left, right, extreme, or indeterminate): normal.
- Conduction (rhythm and regular or irregular): regular sinus rhythm.
- P waves (duration, amplitude, morphology): normal duration, amplitude, and morphology (see Chapter 4).
- Intervals: PR interval, QT/QTc intervals: PR interval 180–200 milliseconds, QTc 400 milliseconds.
- QRS (duration, amplitude, morphology, in particular amplitude of R waves): QRS duration 100 milliseconds (two small squares) of normal morphology and good R-wave progression. R-wave amplitude suggestive of left ventricular hypertrophy.
- ST segments (amplitude, morphology, in particular ST elevation or depression): no evidence of ST-segment depression or elevation.
- T waves (amplitude, morphology): hyperacute T waves in precordial leads.

This informs an understanding of the underlying pathophysiological process at the time of the ECG. Mr Ali's ECG demonstrates normal sinus rhythm at a rate of 60 bpm which is regular. The axis is normal and the PR interval, QRS width, and QTc are within normal ranges. There is good R-wave progression and a suggestion of left ventricular hypertrophy on the leads that represent the left ventricle (V5, V6, I, and aVL, see Chapter 5). There is no evidence of ST-segment changes but the T waves appear to be slightly hyperacute. This ECG meets diagnostic voltage criteria for left ventricular hypertrophy—a condition in which the left ventricle of the heart becomes thickened in response to pressure overload due to conditions such as hypertension or aortic stenosis.

For patients presenting with an UA, oral dual antiplatelet therapy, subcutaneous anticoagulant, beta-blockers, angiotensin-converting enzyme (ACE) inhibitors, and statins are recommended.[17] Dual antiplatelet therapy will inhibit platelet activity and aggregation; anticoagulants will inhibit the coagulation cascade and fibrin clot formation; beta-blockers will inhibit autonomic response and reduce myocardial oxygen demand; ACE inhibitors will decrease preload and afterload, and inhibit cardiac remodelling; and statins will decrease cholesterol formation (see Chapter 12 for more details). A structured approach to diagnostic decision-making (➤ Table 6.4) supports the critical analysis and evaluation of patient data collected when assessing patients presenting with chest pain of suspected cardiac origin. Completing each stage of the process will support critical thinking and guide the diagnosis. Mr Ali has a diagnosis of UA and will require a selective invasive strategy to evaluate his coronary circulation and assess the degree of coronary artery stenosis.

Prior to discharge, the patient and family should be counselled about the implications of this event. The patient should be reminded about the importance of aggressive lifestyle modification including smoking cessation and blood pressure and diabetes control.

It is important to include a discussion about exercise regimens (including intimate personal relations) and the use of glyceryl trinitrate (GTN). The patient should be given a 'GTN protocol' to refer to and instructions on when to call for help.

Case study 2. A patient diagnosed with Prinzmetal angina

Prinzmetal angina, also known as variant angina, is a form of angina manifesting with chest pain and transient ECG changes caused by coronary artery spasm.[35]

Presenting complaint

Miss Taylor is a 28-year-old female white British office worker, who presents to the emergency department after one episode of palpitations and chest tightness.

History of the presenting complaint

Miss Taylor, who is not from the surrounding area, attended a friend's party, during which she consumed a significant amount of alcohol (approximately 30 units)-containing high-energy drinks and approximately 2 g of cocaine. During the early hours of the morning, Miss Taylor attempted to use the toilet but felt dizzy, her heart was racing, and she had a 'funny feeling in the chest'. Unable to walk to the toilet, she decided to consume an additional gram of cocaine to aid her attempt to reach the toilet. When the patient arrived at the bathroom, she had a presyncopal episode with worsening palpitations and

Table 6.4 Mr Ali: diagnostic decision-making framework

History of the presenting complaint	Is there a clear pattern? E.g. are the symptoms associated with physical exertion, or emotional stress? Are the symptoms occurring more frequently in response to less physical effort?	Decreased exercise tolerance over the previous 4 weeks with associated feeling of a 'discomfort on his chest'. Mr Ali also noticed that the symptoms occurred during stressful situations (e.g. during 'rush hour'). These episodes have increased in frequency and occurred on two separate occasions while Mr Ali was at rest
Typicality of symptoms	Is the pain in the chest radiated and/or exertional?	Mr Ali reports discomfort in the chest which is non-radiating and now occurring at rest
'Red flags'	Is there symptom progression? E.g. are the symptoms occurring at an earlier stage of a walk? Are the symptoms now occurring at rest?	Initial decreased exercise tolerance with increasing symptom frequency during emotional distress and now occurring at rest
Coronary risk factors	Sex, age, ethnic background, smoker, high blood pressure, high cholesterol, diabetes, family history of CAD	Male 38-year-old Asian taxi driver with multiple coronary risk factors both modifiable and unmodifiable
'End-of-bed assessment'	Does the patient look unwell? Diaphoretic? Does the patient feel clammy? Is the patient reporting nausea and vomiting? Does the patient feel as if they are going to die?	Mr Ali was comfortable at rest
Cardiovascular assessment	Are baseline observations (blood pressure, heart rate, respiratory rate, pulse oximetry, and temperature) within normal ranges? Is the blood pressure equal in both arms? Are peripheral pulses equally palpable bilaterally? What does the ECG show? Is it sinus rhythm? Is it regular/irregular? Is the rate fast or slow (>100 bpm or <60 bpm)? Is there a P wave? Is there a QRS after each P wave? Is the PR interval in normal range (<200 milliseconds/ 5 small squares)? Is the QRS width in normal range (<120 milliseconds/3 small squares)? Is the ST segment levelled with the isoelectric baseline (e.g. is there ST-segment elevation/depression)?	A cardiovascular assessment was performed. Blood pressure was elevated (168/93 mmHg), but equal bilaterally, pulses were equal, and heart rate was in normal range (60 bpm). The ECG demonstrated sinus rhythm (Fig. 6.7). No sign of abnormalities in the ST segment
hs-TnT	Is the hs-TnT value above normal level? The term myocardial injury should be used when there is evidence of elevated cTn values with at least one value above the 99th percentile URL. The myocardial injury is considered acute if there is a rise and/or fall of cTn values[16]	A hs-TnT value was reported at 6 hours from the onset of pain as 16 ng/L (reference range: normal value <14 ng/L; indeterminate 15–30 ng/L; positive >30 ng/L)
Diagnosis	Cardiac chest pain? Stable angina? ACS?	NSTE-ACS: UA

subsequent chest tightness. A concerned friend called the emergency services and Miss Taylor was taken to the emergency department.

Baseline assessment

Miss Taylor looked anxious, tachypnoeic (respiratory rate >20 breaths per minute), diaphoretic (sweating heavily), and was still intoxicated. A cardiovascular assessment revealed significantly increased systolic and diastolic blood pressure (190/120 mmHg), equal bilaterally. Pulses were equal, fast, and irregular (120–150 bpm). Miss Taylor's ECG showed a fast, irregularly irregular heart rate with no clearly visible P waves (➤ **Fig. 6.8**). Miss Taylor had no history of modifiable or unmodifiable coronary risk factors.

Discussion

Miss Taylor presented with several 'red flags' in the history of the presenting complaint. She had consumed large quantities of alcohol and high-energy drinks in the preceding 24 hours. Miss Taylor also admitted taking illicit drugs: cocaine. A combination of high-energy drinks containing stimulants such as caffeine combined with cocaine use (an adrenoceptor agonist) resulted in hypertension, a rapid, irregular heart rate, and subsequent chest pain.

Adrenoceptors (including alpha, beta 1, and beta 2) are receptors on cells in the body that mediate physiological responses to hormones such as catecholamines. Through this mechanism, adrenoreceptors mediate physiological parameters such as blood pressure, heart rate, and bronchial dilatation/constriction. When the adrenoceptors are overstimulated, as in Miss Taylor's case, an 'overdrive effect' occurs which causes the presenting symptoms. The chest pain is likely to be resulting from a supply–demand mismatch and/or coronary artery spasm. Miss Taylor is tachycardic (i.e. her heart rate is >100 bpm). A rapid heart rate affects the timing of the cardiac cycle; ventricular relaxation (diastole) is when the coronary arteries fill with oxygenated blood. A rapid heart rate can lead to a shorter ventricular diastole which can decrease coronary circulation causing myocardial ischaemia leading to chest pain (supply–demand mismatch). Additionally, cocaine can accelerate atherosclerotic plaque formation, causing coronary spasm with subsequent platelet activation. This can cause chest pain and, in some cases, MI.[36]

Management

Miss Taylor's presentation is suggestive of Prinzmetal angina. The nursing care of Miss Taylor should include reassurance, repetition of baseline observations, until heart rate and blood pressure have returned to normal parameters, and ECG monitoring as previously described. Patients presenting with cocaine-induced palpitations and chest pain are often diagnosed as having Prinzmetal angina. The symptoms are caused by a temporary increase in coronary vascular tone (vasospasm) causing a marked, but transient reduction in coronary artery diameter and decreased coronary perfusion.[5]

A hs-TnT was measured at 21 ng/L which falls within the indeterminate range (normal value <14 ng/L; indeterminate 15–30 ng/L; positive >30 ng/L). TnT can be useful in determining any cardiac myocyte death. Patients should be treated with antiplatelets, nitrates (sublingual or intravenous), and oral benzodiazepines. Beta-blockade should not be administered in the first 24–48 hours after cocaine use as this can cause rebound hypertension.[36] Beta-blockers will block beta-receptors (part

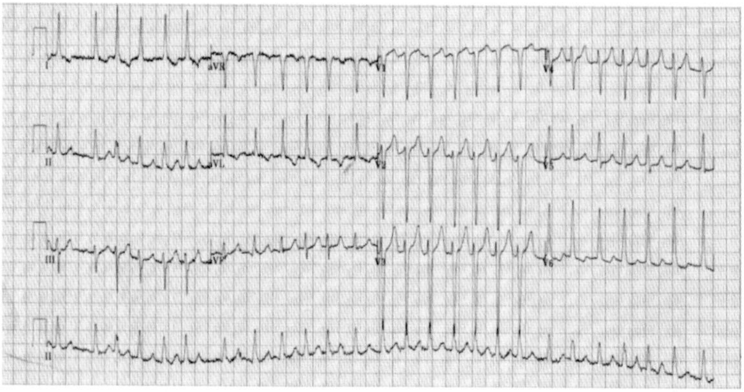

Fig. 6.8 Miss Taylor's 12-lead ECG.

of the adrenoceptors). This will subsequently result in overstimulation of alpha-receptors with significant vasoconstriction and a rise in blood pressure. Miss Taylor has been diagnosed with Prinzmetal angina; she may, or may not, undergo coronary angiogram, as the aetiology of the symptoms appears to be evident.

Using the decision aid framework (➤ Table 6.5), a summary of the cardiovascular assessment highlights the high-risk behaviour of Miss Taylor. The holistic care of this patient should include a discussion of lifestyle change, behaviour modification, and referral to further supportive resources such drug and rehabilitation teams or equivalent (this will vary based on location).

Table 6.5 Miss Taylor: diagnostic decision-making framework

History of the presenting complaint	Is there a clear pattern? E.g. are the symptoms associated with exertion, or emotional situation? Are the symptoms occurring more frequently and require less effort?	Palpitations and chest tightness after consuming approximately 30 units of alcohol, high-energy drinks, and approximately 2 g of cocaine
Typicality of symptoms	Is the pain in the chest radiated and/or exertional?	Chest pain and palpitations with presyncope (feeling faint)
'Red flags'	Is there symptom progression? E.g. are the symptoms occurring at an earlier stage of a walk? Are the symptoms now occurring at rest?	Symptoms onset after consumption of stimulants, alcohol, and illicit drugs
Coronary risk factors	Sex, age, ethnic background, smoker, high blood pressure, high cholesterol, diabetes, family history of CAD	Female 28-year old white British office worker with no coronary risk factors
'End-of-bed assessment'	Does the patient look unwell? Diaphoretic? Does the patient feel clammy? Is the patient reporting nausea and vomiting? Does the patient feel as if they are going to die?	Miss Taylor looked anxious, tachypnoeic, diaphoretic, and was intoxicated
Cardiovascular assessment	Are baseline observations (blood pressure, heart rate, respiratory rate, pulse oximetry and temperature) in normal ranges? Is the blood pressure equal in both arms? Are peripheral pulses equally palpable bilaterally? What does the ECG show? Is it sinus rhythm? Is it regular/irregular? Is the rate fast or slow (>100 bpm or <60 bpm)? Is there a P wave? Is there a QRS after each P wave? Is the PR interval in normal range (<200 milliseconds/5 small squares)? Is the QRS width in normal range (<120 milliseconds/3 small squares)? Is the ST-segment levelled with the isoelectric baseline (e.g. is there ST-segment elevation/depression)?	A cardiovascular assessment revealed significantly increased systolic and diastolic blood pressure (190/120 mmHg), equal bilaterally. Pulses were equal, fast, and irregular (100–150 bpm). ECG was fast, irregularly irregular, with no clear visible P waves and lateral ST-segment depression (Fig. 6.8)
hs-TnT	Is the hs-TnT value above normal level? The term myocardial injury should be used when there is evidence of elevated cTn values with at least one value above the 99th percentile URL. The myocardial injury is considered acute if there is a rise and/or fall of cTn values[16]	A hs-TnT value was measured at 21 ng/L suggestive of myocardial injury (reference range: normal value <14 ng/L; indeterminate 15–30 ng/L; positive >30 ng/L)
Diagnosis	Cardiac chest pain? Stable angina? ACS?	Prinzmetal angina

Using the systematic approach to the ECG analysis, the following can be described:

- Heart rate (bpm): 120–150 bpm.
- Axis (normal, left, right, extreme, or indeterminate): normal.
- Conduction (rhythm and regular or irregular): irregularly irregular.
- P waves (duration, amplitude, morphology): unable to identify clear P waves.
- Intervals: PR interval, QT/QTc intervals: unable to calculate PR interval, QTc approximately 410–500 milliseconds.
- QRS (duration, amplitude, morphology, in particular amplitude of R waves): QRS duration 100 milliseconds (two small squares) of normal morphology and fair R-wave progression.
- ST segments (amplitude, morphology, in particular ST elevation or depression): ST-segment depression V6 (likely related to the rapid heart rate).
- T waves (amplitude, morphology): T-wave inversion in leads I and aVL.

The ECG (➤ **Fig. 6.8**) demonstrates a fast, irregularly irregular rhythm, with normal axis and a heart rate of approximately 120–150 bpm. There are no clearly identifiable P waves, thus the PR interval cannot be calculated. The QRS is normal in width, there is ST-segment depression in V6, and TWI in leads I and aVL. These changes are indicative of myocardial ischaemia and are likely to be secondary to a supply–demand mismatch due to the rapid heart rate. Given the irregularly irregular tachycardia and absence of clearly visible P waves, this ECG meets diagnostic criteria for atrial fibrillation. The troponin rise is indicative of myocardial injury secondary to a supply–demand mismatch, giving a diagnosis of type 2 MI.[20]

Case study 3. A patient presenting with NSTE-ACS: NSTEMI

NSTEMI is defined as angina caused by partial occlusion of an epicardial coronary artery leading to myocardial death/necrosis in the absence of diagnostic criteria for STEMI.

Presenting complaint

Mr Baker, a 51-year-old white British businessman, presents to the emergency department with one episode of severe chest pain.

History of presenting complaint

Two weeks prior to his attendance, Mr Baker experienced severe chest pain, lasting approximately 2 hours. He described the pain as a 'vice-like' sensation and reported feeling 'sweaty, clammy, and nauseous'. Mr Baker decided not to investigate symptoms because of the COVID-19 pandemic. Since the episode of chest pain, he has been experiencing increasing shortness of breath and a feeling of heaviness on minimal exertion, radiating to his jaw and left arm. Prior to attending the emergency department, Mr Baker visited his general practitioner who performed a 12-lead ECG and called an ambulance on seeing the results.

Baseline assessment

On arrival at the emergency department, Mr Baker looked pale, diaphoretic, and had ongoing symptoms of chest pain. On further enquiry, Mr Baker explained that he had a significant family history of premature CAD; both parents suffered an MI in their late 50s. He also reported being a type 2 diabetic but was not consistently adherent to c his prescribed medication. Additional coronary risk factors included untreated hypertension, elevated cholesterol, living alone, clinical depression, and a high alcohol consumption (approximately 40 units per week).

On initial assessment, Mr Baker's blood pressure was significantly raised (187/99 mmHg) and his heart rate was regular (75 bpm). The ECG (➤ **Fig. 6.9**) demonstrated electrical activity with correlated atrial and ventricular activity. The QRS was abnormal, and the heart rate was measured at 75 bpm. A deep TWI was present in the anterior leads (V1–V4).

Discussion

The history of the presenting complaint is typical for acute atherosclerotic plaque rupture (type 1 MI). The patient suffered an episode of severe central chest pain lasting approximately 2 hours and associated with autonomic features. An atherosclerotic plaque rupture causes an inflammatory response with subsequent platelet activation and aggregation, leading to an increased level of thrombin. This can in turn activate the coagulation cascade and ultimately lead to a fibrin clot formation. A fibrin clot will cause coronary stenosis causing the symptoms experienced by the patient.

The 'red flags' are evident during the 'end-of-bed assessment'. Mr Baker has ongoing symptoms of chest pain and is diaphoretic and clammy. Moreover, Mr Baker has multiple coronary risk factors and has been non-adherent with his medications.

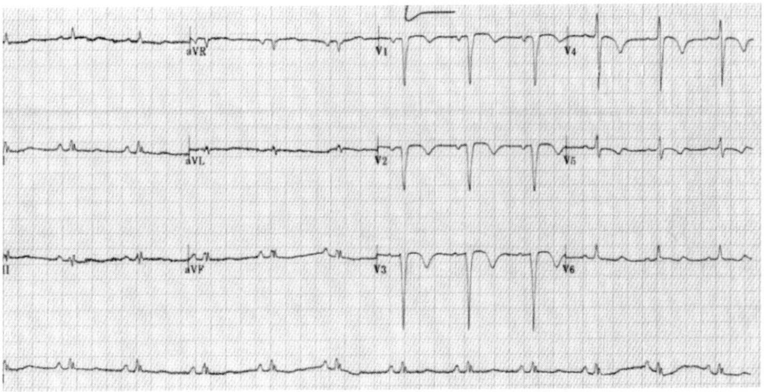

Fig. 6.9 Mr Baker's 12-lead ECG.

A hs-TnT was measured at 1200 ng/L (reference range: normal value <14 ng/L; indeterminate 15–30 ng/L; positive >30 ng/L). This, in addition to the history of the presenting complaint, coronary risk factor profile, and ECG, led to a diagnosis of a NSTEMI. A NSTEMI is characterized by symptoms suggestive of cardiac chest pain, with raised hs-TnT value and absence of ST-segment elevation on the ECG. Mr Baker's ECG demonstrates a deep T wave inversion in the anterior leads (➤ **Fig. 6.9**). This is often referred to as Wellens' syndrome. This is highly specific for a critical stenosis of the left anterior descending artery. Patients diagnosed with NSTEMI should receive oral dual antiplatelet therapy, subcutaneous anticoagulant, and should undergo an angiogram with potential PCI within 24 hours of diagnosis.[4]

Management

Mr Baker's presentation is suggestive of NSTEMI. The nursing care for Mr Baker should include sublingual nitrates and analgesia, if ongoing symptoms, regular ECG, baseline observations.

Using the decision aid framework (➤ **Table 6.6**), ACS is highly likely. The typicality of symptoms, the coronary risk factor profile, and the 'end-of-bed assessment' reinforce the likelihood of the diagnosis. While a cardiovascular assessment highlights high blood pressure as a significant finding, the ECG and hs-TnT assay confirm the diagnosis of NSTEMI.

Prior to discharge, the patient and family should be counselled about the implications of this event. Cardiovascular prevention and rehabilitation, health education, and lifestyle changes should be discussed at this early stage and prior to discharge, with emphasis on exploring the reasons for non-adherence to prescribed medications. It is important to include a discussion about resumption of physical activity and exercise including intimate relations and the use of GTN.

Using the systematic approach to the ECG analysis, the following can be described:

- Heart rate (bpm): 75 bpm.
- Axis (normal, left, right, extreme, or indeterminate): normal.
- Conduction (rhythm and regular or irregular): regular.
- P waves (duration, amplitude, morphology): P-wave morphology, amplitude, and duration, normal.
- Intervals: PR interval, QT/QTc intervals: PR interval 160 milliseconds, QTc 580 milliseconds. QTc should be interpreted with caution. In this instance, it is prolonged because of the T-wave abnormality rather than an arrhythmogenic aetiology.
- QRS (duration, amplitude, morphology, in particular amplitude of R waves): QRS duration 100–120 milliseconds with morphology suggestive of a conduction delay. R-wave progression is poor.
- ST segments (amplitude, morphology, in particular ST elevation or depression): evidence of subtle ST-segment depression in V5 and V6.
- T waves (amplitude, morphology): deep TWI in V1–V5, suggestive of myocardial ischaemia (Wellens' syndrome).

The ECG (➤ **Fig. 6.9**) demonstrates normal sinus rhythm with a rate of 75 bpm and a normal axis. The PR interval is in the normal range but the QTc is prolonged. An abnormal T-wave morphology can affect the QTc, so this finding requires further investigation and careful interpretation. There is subtle ST-segment depression in V5 and V6, suggestive of cardiac ischaemia in those leads.

Table 6.6 Mr Baker: diagnostic decision-making framework

History of the presenting complaint	Is there a clear pattern? E.g. are the symptoms associated with exertion, or emotional situation? Are the symptoms occurring more frequently and require less effort?	Mr Baker presented to the emergency department with one episode of severe chest pain. Two weeks prior to his attendance, he had experienced severe chest pain, lasting approximately 2 hours
Typicality of symptoms	Is the pain in the chest radiated and/or exertional?	Pain was described as a 'vice-like' sensation and patient reports feeling 'sweaty, clammy, and nauseous'
'Red flags'	Is there symptom progression? E.g. are the symptoms occurring at an earlier stage of a walk? Are the symptoms now occurring at rest?	Since the episode of chest pain, he has been experiencing increasing shortness of breath, feeling of heaviness on minimal exertion, radiated to jaw and left arm
Coronary risk factors	Sex, age, ethnic background, smoker, high blood pressure, high cholesterol, diabetes, family history of CAD	Male 51-year-old white businessman with both parents having suffered a MI in their late 50s. He also reported being a type 2 diabetic but was taking his medication inconsistently. Additional risk factors included untreated high blood pressure and cholesterol, living alone, clinical depression, and high alcohol consumption (approximately 40 units per week)
'End-of-bed assessment'	Does the patient look unwell? Diaphoretic? Does the patient feel clammy? Is the patient reporting nausea and vomiting? Does the patient feel as if they are going to die?	Mr Baker looked pale, diaphoretic, with ongoing symptoms of chest pain
Cardiovascular assessment	Are baseline observations (blood pressure, heart rate, respiratory rate, pulse oximetry and temperature) in normal ranges? Is the blood pressure equal in both arms? Are peripheral pulses equally palpable bilaterally? What does the ECG show? Is it sinus rhythm? Is it regular/irregular? Is the rate fast or slow (>100 bpm or <60 bpm)? Is there a P wave? Is there a QRS after each P wave? Is the PR interval in normal range (<200 milliseconds/5 small squares)? Is the QRS width in normal range (<120 milliseconds/3 small squares)? Is the ST segment levelled with the isoelectric baseline (e.g. is there ST-segment elevation/depression)?	On initial assessment, Mr Baker's blood pressure was significantly raised (187/99 mmHg) and the heart rate was regular (75 bpm). The ECG (Fig. 6.9) demonstrated a heart rate of 75 bpm. The QRS was abnormal, and a deep TWI was present in the precordial leads (V1–V6)
hs-TnT	Is the hs-TnT value above normal level? The term myocardial injury should be used when there is evidence of elevated cTn values with at least one value above the 99th percentile URL. The myocardial injury is considered acute if there is a rise and/or fall of cTn values[16]	A hs-TnT value was measured at 1200 ng/L (reference range: normal value <14 ng/L; indeterminate 15–30 ng/L; positive >30 ng/L)
Diagnosis	Cardiac chest pain? Stable angina? ACS?	NSTE-ACS, NSTEMI

Given the history of the presenting complaint, the coronary risk factor profile, and the significant TnT rise, this ECG meets the diagnostic criteria for NSTEMI.

Case study 4. A patient diagnosed with STEMI

Angina is caused by occlusion of an epicardial coronary artery often caused by plaque rupture leading to coronary thrombosis with myocardial death/necrosis.

Presenting complaint

Mr Wright, a 53-year-old Afro-Caribbean male, employed as a university researcher, presents to the emergency department with central crushing chest pain.

History of presenting complaint

Mr Wright called an ambulance following an onset of crushing central chest pain, which radiated to his left jaw and arm. Mr Wright had used his GTN spray twice with no relief. He described the pain as 'severe and crushing ... almost as if someone was sitting on my chest'. Mr Wright recognized the pain as something he should report urgently as he had previously had a MI.

Baseline assessment

On arrival at the emergency department, the patient was complaining of ongoing 'severe chest pain and heaviness' and looked pale, diaphoretic, and apprehensive. He was normotensive (131/84 mmHg) and his heart rate was within the normal limits (70–75 bpm). The patient was known to be a type 2 diabetic, hypertensive, and a tobacco smoker. Mr Wright had previously had a MI and PCI. His ECG (➤ **Fig. 6.10**) demonstrated normal sinus rhythm with P and QRS correlation and of normal interval. The heart rate was regular. The ECG revealed ST-segment elevation in leads II, III, and aVF with reciprocal changes in leads I and aVL and the precordial leads.

Discussion

The history of the presenting complaint, the coronary risk factor profile, 'end-of-bed assessment', and ECG are all significant 'red flags' which when combined suggest a diagnosis of STEMI (➤ **Table 6.7**). Patients presenting with a STEMI should be managed as a medical emergency and should undergo immediate PPCI.[5] Waiting for a hs-TnT assay is not required to aid diagnosis. These patients need to undergo PPCI as soon as feasible to aid coronary reperfusion (➤ **Fig. 6.4**) and decrease myocardial necrosis.[4] In patients with ST-segment elevation, the atherosclerotic plaque rupture instigates an inflammatory response with platelet activation. Subsequently, due to the significant injury, activation of the coagulation cascade leads to fibrin clot formation with a total occlusion of the coronary artery. Total occlusion of the coronary artery leads to a loss of coronary flow, cardiac myocyte death, and ultimately heart failure, if not treated promptly.[5]

PPCI provides a rapid and effective access to the coronary circulation to evaluate the severity of the coronary occlusion. Once the culprit occlusion is identified, a PCI is attempted to restore flow to the affected area. A prompt coronary flow restoration prevents significant cardiac myocyte death and decreases the likelihood of ventricular dysfunction.

Management

Mr Wright's presentation is suggestive of STEMI. Mr Wright should be transferred to the catheterization

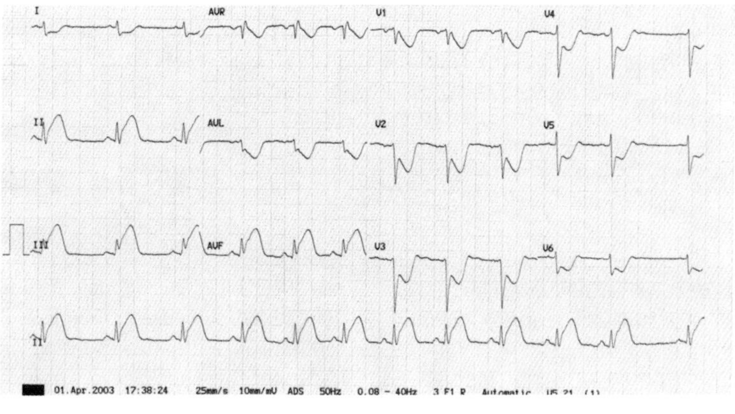

Fig. 6.10 Mr Wright's 12-lead ECG.

Table 6.7 Mr Wright: diagnostic decision-making framework

History of presenting complaint	Is there a clear pattern? E.g. are the symptoms associated with exertion, or emotional situation? Are the symptoms occurring more frequently and require less effort?	Sudden onset of crushing central chest pain. Pain described as 'severe and crushing ... almost as if someone was sitting on my chest'. Patient recognized pain as previously had a MI
Typicality of symptoms	Is pain in the chest, radiated and exertional?	Central chest pain, radiated to left jaw and arm
'Red flags'	Is there symptom progression? E.g. are the symptoms occurring at an earlier stage of a walk? Are the symptoms now occurring at rest?	'Severe and crushing ... almost as if someone was sitting on my chest'. Typical anginal pain, with previous MI
Coronary risk factors	Sex, age, ethnic background, smoker, high blood pressure, high cholesterol, diabetes, family history of CAD	Male 53-year-old Afro-Caribbean with type 2 diabetes, high blood pressure, high cholesterol, and previous MI
'End-of-bed assessment'	Does the patient look unwell? Diaphoretic? Does the patient feel clammy? Is the patient reporting nausea and vomiting? Does the patient feel as if they are going to die?	Clammy, diaphoretic, and apprehensive
Cardiovascular assessment	Are baseline observations (blood pressure, heart rate, respiratory rate, pulse oximetry and temperature) in normal ranges? Is the blood pressure equal in both arms? Are peripheral pulses equally palpable bilaterally? What does the ECG show? Is it sinus rhythm? Is it regular/irregular? Is the rate fast or slow (>100 bpm or <60 bpm)? Is there a P wave? Is there a QRS after each P wave? Is the PR interval in normal range (<200 milliseconds/5 small squares)? Is the QRS width in normal range (<120 milliseconds/3 small squares)? Is the ST segment levelled with the isoelectric baseline (e.g. is there ST-segment elevation/depression)?	Mr Wright was normotensive (131/84 mmHg) and his heart rate was within the normal limits (70–75 bpm). The patient was known to be diabetic (type 2), hypertensive, having previously had a MI and PCI. His ECG (Fig. 6.10) demonstrated normal sinus rhythm with P and QRS correlation and of normal interval. The heart rate was regular. The ECG revealed ST-segment elevation in leads II, III, and aVF with reciprocal changes in lead I, lead aVL, and precordial leads
hs-TnT	Is the hs-TnT value above normal level? The term myocardial injury should be used when there is evidence of elevated cTn values with at least one value above the 99th percentile URL. The myocardial injury is considered acute if there is a rise and/or fall of cTn values[16]	hs-TnT value not measured as not a priority in this presentation. Diagnosis guided by history taking, clinical examination, and ECG
Diagnosis	Cardiac chest pain? Stable angina? ACS?	ACS: STEMI

laboratory for PPCI with continuous cardiac monitoring, a defibrillator, and emergency drugs. Patients diagnosed with STEMI are at high risk for arrhythmias such as ventricular tachycardia or ventricular fibrillation (see Chapter 7). The nursing care prior to PPCI should include reassurance, analgesia, and antiemetic as required, a focused cardiovascular assessment, and serial ECGs. Patients presenting with STEMI are at risk of cardiogenic shock, severe bradycardia, and atrioventricular block and should be carefully monitored.

Cardiogenic shock is characterized by a persistent hypotension, with a systolic blood pressure less than 90 mmHg, despite adequate intravascular volume. It manifests in 6–10% of all STEMIs[22] and remains the leading cause of death in this patient population with an estimated mortality rate of approximately 50%. The aetiology of cardiogenic shock should be identified promptly and treated accordingly. This may include hypovolaemia or drug-induced hypotension and arrhythmias. The nursing care of patients prior to PPCI should focus on continuous cardiovascular monitoring and effective recognition and management of imminent clinical deterioration (see Chapter 5 for details on cardiogenic shock).

Sinus bradycardia can be common in inferior STEMI because the right coronary artery provides oxygenated blood to the sinoatrial node. Type 1 second-degree block (Mobitz I) is also associated with inferior wall MI but rarely causes haemodynamic instability. Should the patient become haemodynamically compromised, intravenous atropine should be given or pacing considered.[34] Type 2 second-degree block (Mobitz II) or complete atrioventricular dissociation (third-degree heart block) are indications for cardiac pacing.

Post PPCI, the patient should be closely monitored. The nursing care for patients post PPCI and/or permanent pacemaker insertion should include access site and wound management. Monitoring of the access site will be dependent on the operator approach. Radial artery access for PCI is the preferred site where possible as it is associated with fewer complications than a femoral artery PCI.[5] However, in patients with cardiogenic shock, an intra-aortic balloon pump may be inserted via the femoral artery. The nursing management of the femoral access site will reflect local guidelines and the availability of closure devices (see Chapter 5 for details on cardiogenic shock and an introduction to intra-aortic balloon pumps and other types of circulatory support).

Wound management post permanent pacemaker insertion is another key aspect of the nursing care. The ability to identify signs of infection and/or sepsis will improve patients' outcomes and hospital discharge times.[37] In a wound infection, the skin will be hot and tender to touch with localized swelling. Systemic signs of sepsis include tachypnoea, tachycardia, hypotension, and fever.

Before discharge from hospital, Mr Wright should start cardiovascular rehabilitation with advice given about his recovery and about how he can modify his lifestyle and adhere to his prescribed medication to improve his heart health and health-related quality of life.

Using the systematic approach to the ECG analysis, the following can be described:

- Heart rate (bpm): 70–75 bpm.
- Axis (normal, left, right, extreme, or indeterminate): normal.
- Conduction (rhythm and regular or irregular): regular with sinus arrhythmia.
- P waves (duration, amplitude, morphology): P-wave morphology, amplitude, and duration, normal.
- Intervals: PR interval, QT/QTc intervals: PR interval 160 milliseconds, QTc 432–447 milliseconds.
- QRS (duration, amplitude, morphology, in particular amplitude of R waves): QRS duration 100 milliseconds. R-wave progression is poor.
- ST segments (amplitude, morphology, in particular ST elevation or depression): evidence of significant ST-segment depression in inferior leads and leads II, III, and aVF with reciprocal change (ST-segment depression) in lead I, lead aVL, and precordial leads.
- T waves (amplitude, morphology): hyperacute inferior T-wave morphology deep T wave inversion with ST-segment depression in V1–V6.

The ECG (➤ **Fig. 6.10**) demonstrates normal sinus rhythm with a normal axis and a rate of 70–75 bpm. The P-wave morphology, PR interval, and QRS duration are in the expected range and the QTc is normal. There is significant ST-segment elevation in the anterior leads with reciprocal changes in lead I, lead aVL, and precordial leads with hyperacute T waves. This ECG meets the diagnostic criteria for STEMI.

In summary, when caring for patients presenting with symptoms suggestive of myocardial ischaemia, a systematic approach will facilitate patient assessment. Subsequently, adequate risk stratification will dictate the pharmacological and invasive management (e.g. PCI) of patients presenting with an ACS. Although PCI and PPCI have become the revascularization strategy of choice for the management of ACS, in patients with stable CAD, CABG can also be considered as an alternative reperfusion strategy.[34]

Priorities for nursing care

The general principles of nursing care for patients with suspected ACS are similar, but obviously the treatments will vary according to ACS classification as per the illustrative case studies. The patient's experience of healthcare is an important indicator of care quality.

1. *Care coordination and teamwork*: the nurse plays a crucial role in the wider team by coordinating, managing, and delivering prescribed treatments and interventions in a timely manner for patients with ACS. This is vital given the association between prompt treatment and positive patient outcomes. Missed and delayed medicines are a common cause of medication error which can lead to adverse patient outcomes.[38] Administering treatments such as medication and oxygen (if prescribed) in a timely manner is very important. The nurse may also play a role in the instigation of other diagnostic tests and assessments such as 12-lead ECG recording and serial troponins.
2. *Assessment of signs and symptoms*: a key priority in the management of patients with suspected ACS is to assess, monitor, and relieve chest discomfort/pain associated with myocardial ischaemia. Chest pain may be evidenced by verbal and non-verbal signs as well as changes in vital signs such as pulse and blood pressure (Chapter 5 provides an overview of pain assessment scales that can be used to assist patients in describing and quantifying any discomfort/pain that they are experiencing). It is important that assessment data are accurately documented so that the effectiveness of any pain relief can be evaluated. A 12-lead ECG measures the heart's electrical activity and shows the progression of depolarization and repolarization and cardiac rhythm; recordings during and after episodes of chest pain are important to assess for signs of myocardial ischaemia (see case studies and Chapter 4 for details about ECG analysis). It is important that relevant diagnostic findings are communicated to the cardiology team in a timely way to guide decision-making about treatment. Following the administration of narcotics for pain relief, blood pressure, respiratory rate, and oxygen saturation should be closely monitored. (Chapter 12 provides an overview of medicines commonly used in cardiovascular care such as analgesics, antianginals, beta-blockers, anxiolytics, antiplatelet agents, anticoagulants, thrombolytics, and diuretics. The potential complications that may also arise from their use are also described.) The nurse plays an important role in evaluating the effectiveness of prescribed medications and looking out for any potential adverse effects.
3. *Timely recognition, critical thinking, and management of clinical deterioration*: nurses play a vital role in rapid recognition of clinical deterioration. Cardiac monitoring, with appropriately set alarms, will provide ongoing continuous ECG data and other haemodynamic and respiratory parameters. This is important for ACS patients as a way of maintaining haemodynamic stability; recognizing signs and symptoms of clinical deterioration, taking appropriate action, and informing senior staff in a timely way is vital. Many healthcare organizations have automated early warning score systems used in ward areas which are useful but not foolproof.[39] An overreliance on such systems is not recommended as, ultimately, experienced nurses' perceptions of a patient's potential for clinical deterioration are more accurate than most published warning scores.[40] It is important to call for help if you are concerned and cannot get help through your rapid response system as per your local protocol.

   Patients with ACS are at risk from decreased cardiac output, excess fluid volume, and ineffective tissue perfusion (see Chapter 4 and Chapter 5 for a more detailed explanation). The nurse needs to understand how physiological parameters interact to enable them to interpret the significance of any changes in vital signs and effectively recognize and manage clinical deterioration. Advanced practitioners will develop the skills to assess jugular venous pressure and auscultate heart and breath sounds to provide additional clinical data which can be indicative of changes in circulating fluid volume (see Chapter 5 for more detail). The nurse will also support the patients through a wide range of potential invasive and non-invasive diagnostic tests which provide important data from which physiological parameters are monitored and interventions planned. For example, serial ECGs and biomarkers, electrolytes, arterial blood gases, clotting times, chest X-rays, echocardiography, and coronary angiography.
4. *Creating a healing environment and promoting sleep, rest, and well-being*: in high-technology areas such as critical care, there is often an emphasis on the technological aspects of patient care. An important and often overlooked part of the nurse's role is to promote patient comfort and make the care environment as conducive to healing as possible. Sleep is an important biological function that supports patient healing but ward inpatients often report poor sleep quality and quantity as hospital environments are very noisy.[41] Care processes such as recording observations and taking bloods should be bundled together as far as possible to minimize night-time sleep disturbance. Offering patients ear plugs or eye masks, or asking them to bring in their own if they

are not available, is one approach that can improve the quality and quantity of inpatient care.[42] Patients also report noise from the built environment, staff, and other patients as sources of night-time sleep disturbance.[41]

5. *Reduced mobility and physical activity limitations*: guidelines vary, but a short period of bed rest to reduce myocardial workload is recommended for patients recovering from ACS. It is important that the patient is positioned comfortably with sufficient pillows and blankets as per their preference. The patient can be positioned in a semi-upright position to maximize lung inflation if they are haemodynamically stable. To avoid complications associated with immobility such as thromboembolic events, the nurse can advise the patients about leg exercises and help them with the application and removal of antiembolic stockings. As recovery progresses, the level of activity will be gradually increased, or decreased, in response to changes in physiological parameters such as pulse, blood pressure, and presence of dyspnoea.

   Basic hygiene needs are important to the well-being of patients. Ensuring that a patient's skin is kept clean and free from pressure injury is an important goal of nursing care. Some patient groups are particularly prone to pressure injury. In cardiology settings, a reduced left ventricular ejection fraction predicts in-hospital pressure ulcer development in patients recovering from MI.[43] Patients will also appreciate the opportunity to clean their teeth regularly and wash their hands after using a commode.

6. *Nutrition and elimination*: small nutritious meals at regular intervals are advised for patients with ACS. A nutritional assessment may be indicated particularly in elderly patients. Nutritional status is reported to be an independent predictor of long-term mortality in septuagenarian patients of the same magnitude as the GRACE score.[44] Recording an accurate fluid balance is important to detect signs of haemodynamic instability and acute kidney injury. The administration of analgesics may lead to constipation which should be avoided as straining at stool, also known as Valsalva manoeuvre, can induce bradycardia.

7. *Psychological support for patients and significant others*: psychological support for the patients with ACS and those close to them is very important as depression and anxiety among survivors and spouses is common. Fear, anxiety, denial, hostility, and grief are common emotions experienced by patients diagnosed with ACS and represent a normal response to a life-threatening event. However, if negative emotions are sustained in the longer term, intervention may be warranted. Each patient will respond differently and it is important to be accepting and supportive of their responses during hospitalizations, but reinforcing denial should be avoided if at all possible. It is important to ask the patient about how they are feeling and to listen actively to their responses (see Chapters 11 and 13). Your behaviour and manner will also convey a non-verbal message to the patient and their family. When information about diagnosis and prognosis is communicated, it is preferable to have significant others present for support as patients often cannot remember verbal information. It may be helpful to use non-pharmacological interventions to reduce psychological distress and some relaxation techniques have been shown to be beneficial in cardiology settings.[4]

8. *Cultural and spiritual care*: an important part of person-centred care is to recognize an individual's needs and preferences for their healthcare. Cultural and religious practices are an important part of an individual's identity and healthcare provision should reflect these. Spirituality is not necessarily connected with religion; patients will have different ways of meeting their own spiritual needs which may be associated with feeling hope, gratitude, a sense of belonging or purpose, to name a few.

9. *Patient education and discharge processes*: patients diagnosed with ACS are often discharged after a short hospital admission and there is a need for nurses, and other members of the multidisciplinary team, to provide timely advice and support. This begins in the peri-infarct phase and extends throughout cardiovascular prevention and rehabilitation. The key aims are always to facilitate a return to health and as normal a life as possible while minimizing the potential for recurrent cardiac events.

   Patients and relatives have a variety of educational, lifestyle, physical, and psychological needs and questions following an ACS. Typical questions relate to causation, what patients can or should be doing now and in the future, and medicine management. Ideally, a cardiac liaison nurse or a member of the cardiovascular prevention and rehabilitation team should be involved at an early stage to address such concerns. This type of approach has been demonstrated to positively influence subsequent uptake of rehabilitation programmes.[45] The initial focus of information is on what has occurred and what will happen next regarding cardiovascular prevention and rehabilitation and medical follow-up. Medicines need to be discussed in sufficient detail to ensure their purpose is understood. Information about when and how to take medicines and their potential side effects should also be included. At the time of hospital discharge, it is important to advise who can be contacted if problems arise. Provision of supplementary printed or digital literature is also useful at a time when there can be so much new information to absorb. This should be in a form that is both accessible and understandable. An immediate discharge summary should be provided with key information for primary health and cardiovascular prevention and rehabilitation teams as well as patients and relatives. Suggested content is listed in ➤ Box 6.1.

The early post-discharge period involves ongoing interaction between hospital, primary care, and cardiovascular prevention and rehabilitation services and good coordination and communication are essential. Attendance at and completion of an exercise-based cardiovascular prevention and rehabilitation programme is of demonstrated benefit in reducing cardiovascular mortality and subsequent hospital admission rates and access is a prominent recommendation of both European[46] and UK clinical guidelines[47] (see Chapter 11 for additional details). This should begin as soon as possible after admission and before discharge from hospital. An invitation to attend an out-patient cardiac rehabilitation session should ideally be received within 10 days of discharge from hospital but it is known that this often takes longer and overall uptake of cardiovascular prevention and rehabilitation remains suboptimal.

Beyond the initial rehabilitation period, continuing emphasis should be given to secondary prevention including optimization of medication, health education, behaviour change, lifestyle and risk factor management, and psychological health. Depending on local arrangements, a hospital follow-up consultation 1 year after the index event can provide an ideal opportunity to reinforce the need for lifestyle improvements, encourage medicine adherence, and implement changes to antiplatelet regimens if this is indicated. Patients with CAD and their partners are prone to anxiety and depression. A range of patient-reported outcome measures are completed as part of cardiovascular prevention and rehabilitation (see Chapter 11 for additional details). Successful cardiovascular prevention and rehabilitation following ACS is crucially dependent on effective multidisciplinary working in partnership with patients and their relatives at all stages.

Box 6.1 Discharge summary content

1. Hospital identification number.
2. Contact details for responsible hospital team/ discharging professional.
3. Medical diagnosis.
4. Discharge medication—including dose, duration (especially antiplatelet therapy), and titration needs (beta-blockers and ACE inhibitors).
5. Agreed targets for blood pressure, weight, smoking cessation, cholesterol, and alcohol consumption.
6. Information: physical activity including resumption of sex, return to work, driving, travel/holidays, and other relevant activities.
7. Follow-up: out-patient appointments and cardiovascular prevention and rehabilitation arrangements.
8. Information on psychological support needs for patients and significant others.

Chronic coronary syndromes

In considering CCS, there are at least six potential clinical presentations for this group of conditions: (1) suspected CAD and 'stable' anginal symptoms, and/or dyspnoea; (2) new onset of heart failure or left ventricular dysfunction and suspected CAD; (3) asymptomatic or with stabilized symptoms less than 1 year after ACS, or revascularization; (4) asymptomatic or symptomatic greater than 1 year after initial diagnosis or revascularization; (5) angina and suspected vasospastic or microvascular disease; and (6) asymptomatic, with CAD detected at screening.[3] Each clinical presentation is associated with a different level of risk for a future cardiovascular event such as death or MI.[3] Those without ACS will be assessed for pre-test probability and clinical likelihood of coronary heart disease.[3] The main diagnostic pathways for patients presenting with CCS are shown in ➤ Fig. 6.11.

To establish a diagnosis of obstructive CAD in patients with a low to intermediate pre-test probability of CAD, an anatomical test such as coronary computed tomography angiography will be conducted. Functional tests such as exercise ECG or nuclear stress testing may also be used.

Priorities for nursing care

The nurse plays an important role in caring for patients undergoing invasive or non-invasive tests from

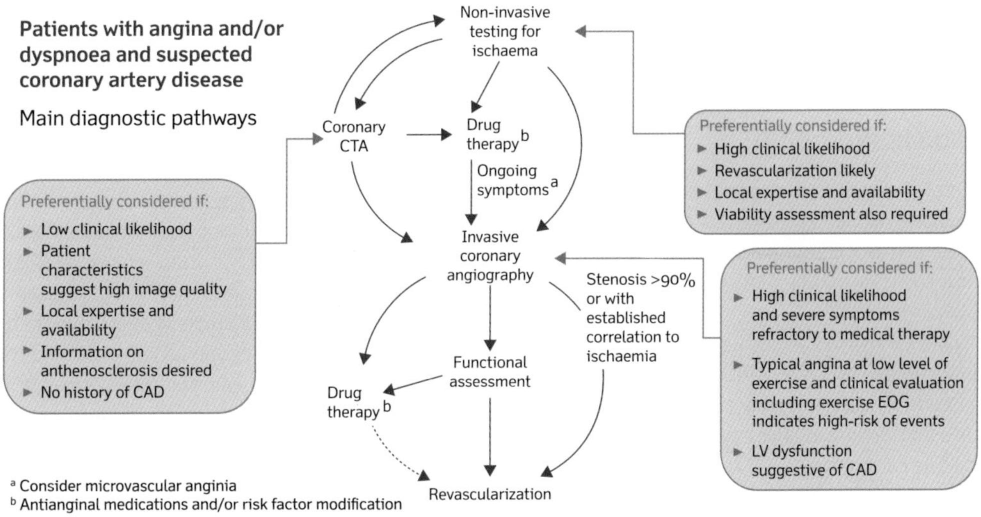

Fig. 6.11 Diagnostic and management pathways for patients with angina/dyspnoea and suspected CAD.

Collet JP, Thiele H, Barbato E, et al; ESC Scientific Document Group. 2020 ESC Guidelines for the management of acute coronary syndromes in patients presenting without persistent ST-segment elevation. Eur Heart J. 2020 Aug 29:ehaa575. doi: 10.1093/eurheartj/ehaa575 © The European Society of Cardiology. Reprinted by permission of Oxford University Press.

taking a patient history, seeking informed consent, and preparing the patients for the procedure to ensure that the procedure is conducted safely. For many patients, this can be a stressful experience so it is important that the nurse provides reassurance and effective education about aftercare. For the purpose of this section, we will focus upon the management and nursing care of the patient with one clinical presentation, namely stable angina.

The mainstay of treatment is the control of symptoms and the reduction of the risk of adverse events associated with CAD. The optimization of medication therapy is the first-line treatment for patients with stable angina to relieve angina symptoms and reduce the risk of future adverse cardiovascular events. The management priorities for the patient with stable angina are to provide information and support to enable them to self-manage angina symptoms. Health professionals play a key role in supporting patients to manage their medications so that they understand the rationale for the prescription, side effects to look out for, and how to administer them correctly (e.g. nitrate spray/tablets). Recommended drugs include nitrates, calcium channel blockers, beta-blockers, ACE inhibitors, antithrombotic agents (e.g. aspirin or clopidogrel), and lipid-lowering medications. Non-adherence to cardiovascular medications is commonplace and may be intentional or non-intentional; the factors influencing medication adherence are complex and influenced by several factors (see Chapter 12 for details about common cardioprotective medications and non-adherence).

Coronary revascularization may be considered for patients with angina symptoms that are not satisfactorily controlled if optimal medical therapy is not effective.[3] Recent trials have indicated that PCI reduces ischaemic burden in patients with stable CAD but may not necessarily improve survival or reduce risk for recurrent MI compared to optimal medical therapy alone.[48]

Nurses and allied health professions play a key role in providing effective therapeutic patient education and self-management support to patients and those close to them. Effective self-management support promotes healthy lifestyle change (smoking cessation, a heart healthy diet, 30–60 minutes of physical activity most days, and a healthy weight <25 kg/m^2).[3] For patients diagnosed with stable angina, it is important to help them to understand why the symptoms occur and ensure that they know when to seek medical assistance. Patients will also need support to balance periods of physical activity and rest so that they can pace themselves to enable them to manage activities of daily living. These measures in conjunction with the prescription of cardiovascular medications maximize patient health, well-being, and quality of life (see Chapters 11–13).

Other clinical conditions associated with atherosclerosis

Acute aortic syndrome

Atherosclerotic plaque rupture can occur throughout the cardiovascular system. An increased cardiovascular risk factor profile can precipitate plaque formation leading to CAD, acute aortic syndrome (AAS) and peripheral artery disease.

Cardiovascular risk factors include family history of cardiovascular disease (such as CAD, cerebrovascular disease, and aortic aneurysm), early onset of cardiovascular disease in a first-degree relative aged 55 years or younger, and premature cardiovascular-related death. Patients' risk factors include history of high blood pressure, diabetes, hypercholesterolaemia, smoking, kidney disease, poor dietary habits, and sedentary lifestyle.

AAS is caused by a tear in the aorta that allows infiltration of the blood from the cardiovascular lumen into the media.[49] This causes aortic dissection. Aortic dissection has been classified into types I, II, and III or type A and type B.[49,50] It is a life-threatening condition. Patients with aortic dissection are likely to present with sudden and severe onset of chest pain, described as a 'ripping' or 'tearing' which radiates into the interscapular area. In patients presenting with symptoms suggestive of aortic dissection, the likelihood of AAS should be evaluated. This is dependent on several factors: pre-existing conditions (e.g. family history, known existing aortic aneurysm or valve disease, previous aortic surgery, and connective tissue disorders), pain characteristics as previously described, and 'red flag' findings on clinical examination. These include systolic pressure discrepancy, focal neurological deficit, and shock.

A definitive diagnosis is obtained by medical imaging such as a computed tomography scan. Once the diagnosis has been confirmed, patients should undergo immediate emergency surgery. As haemodynamic instability is frequently present, careful monitoring of baseline observation is required. Chest pain caused by AAS is severe: nursing care should be holistic, providing adequate analgesia and comfort to the patient and their relatives.

Peripheral artery disease

Peripheral artery disease encompasses all arterial disease: cerebrovascular disease, upper and lower extremities artery disease, mesenteric artery disease, and renal artery disease.[51] Patients with acute plaque rupture will present with different symptoms, based on the territory affected.

An inflammatory response and thrombus formation in the cerebral circulation may lead to a stroke or transient ischaemic attack. Patients may present with focused neurological symptoms such as unilateral weakness of upper and lower limbs, slurred speech, and blurred vision. The acronym FAST (Facial drooping, Arm weakness, Speech difficulties, Time to call for medical help)[52,53] is used to help with the diagnosis of stroke. Patients presenting with symptoms suggestive of stroke should undergo brain imaging as soon as possible with a non-enhanced computed tomography scan. This will guide the ongoing management of the patient which may include thrombolysis or thrombectomy.[53]

Patients presenting with suspected transient ischaemic attack should receive immediate antiplatelet therapy (aspirin 300 mg, unless contraindicated) with subsequent specialist advice and consideration for magnetic resonance imaging to assess any level of ischaemia or detect any haemorrhage.[53]

The nursing care for patients presenting with symptoms suggestive of stroke should include a baseline assessment of vital signs and continuous monitoring of level of consciousness. Stroke can be a life-changing event and the nursing care of patients with subsequent permanent weakness should include careful physical and psychological support.

Family members should be included in the cardiovascular prevention and rehabilitation programme and this should begin as soon as the patient has overcome the acute presentation.

Other clinical conditions associated with the cardiovascular system are listed in ➤ **Box 6.2**. Many of these are covered in other chapters in this book.

In summary, nurses and allied health professionals play a key role in caring for patients presenting with cardiovascular disease. Early recognition and management of an acute syndrome will improve survival rates.[4,5] A holistic approach to patient care is important to improve care quality and the inpatient hospital experience.

Conclusion

This chapter has presented the anatomy and physiology of the coronary arteries, with associated pathophysiology. The mechanisms involved in the atherosclerotic plaque formation were described and the chapter illustrated how risk factors contribute to atherosclerotic plaque rupture

Box 6.2 Clinical conditions associated with the cardiovascular system

- Upper and lower extremity artery disease.
- Mesenteric artery disease.
- Renal artery disease.
- Diseases of arteries and veins: venous insufficiency and thromboembolism.
- Aortic dissection.
- Hyperlipidaemia.
- Hypertension: primary and secondary.
- Hypotension: dizziness and syncope, and postural.
- Dyspnoea: orthopnoea and paroxysmal nocturnal dyspnoea.
- Palpitations.
- Disorders of heart wall: pericardium, myocardium, and endocardium.
- Valve disease: aortic stenosis, mitral stenosis, and infective endocarditis.
- Shock: impairment of cellular metabolism and organ dysfunction.

and coronary ischaemia. Coronary ischaemia can manifest in several different ways, as illustrated in the case studies, requiring a systematic approach to patient assessment. This approach includes history taking, 'end-of-bed assessment', and nursing and medical management of patients. Each patient with ACS requires angiography: the different options for reperfusion therapy were presented. In patients with STEMI, timing is of the essence and reperfusion should be achieved within 120 minutes of first diagnostic ECG.[4,5] In patients with NSTEMI and UA, timing of reperfusion will depend on risk stratification: ongoing symptoms, ECG changes, and the likelihood of a further event.[4,5]

Finally, other diseases associated with the cardiovascular system were outlined with greater emphasis on AAS[50] and cerebrovascular events.[53] Diagnosis of these life-threatening and life-changing conditions is based on clinical findings and confirmed by computed tomography. Prompt surgical, pharmacological, or invasive intervention will improve survival and quality of life. Other less common conditions that can cause angina include syndrome X—a condition in which microvascular dysfunction causes angina in patients with epicardial coronary arteries that appear to be normal on angiography.

Nurses play a key role in the health professional team providing care to patients and those close to them. The role of the nurse in cardiology settings varies considerably across different countries. An advanced level of technical knowledge is required for nurses working in today's healthcare organizations, which needs to be balanced alongside the provision of empathic and compassionate care.

References

1. Nichols M, Townsend N, Scarborough P, Rayner M. Cardiovascular disease in Europe 2014: epidemiological update. Eur Heart J. 2014;35(42):2950–59.
2. Benjamin EJ, Virani SS, Callaway CW, et al. Heart disease and stroke statistics—2018 update: a report from the American Heart Association. Circulation. 2018;137(12):e67–492.
3. Knuuti J, Wijns W, Saraste A, et al. 2019 ESC Guidelines for the diagnosis and management of chronic coronary syndromes. Eur Heart J. 2020;41(3):407–77.
4. Ibanez B, James S, Agewall S, et al. 2017 ESC Guidelines for the management of acute myocardial infarction in patients presenting with ST-segment elevation: the Task Force for the management of acute myocardial infarction in patients presenting with ST-segment elevation of the European Society of Cardiology (ESC). Eur Heart J. 2018;39(2):119–77.
5. Collet JP, Thiele H, Barbato E, et al. 2020 ESC Guidelines for the management of acute coronary syndromes in patients presenting without persistent ST-segment elevation. Eur Heart J. 2021;42(14):1289–367.
6. Timmis A, Townsend N, Gale CP. EHJ—Quality of Care and Clinical Outcomes: now recommended for MEDLINE listing. Eur Heart J. 2017;38(17):1278.
7. Mitchell J. Heart and circulatory disease deaths in under 75's see first sustained rise in 50 years. British Heart Foundation; 2019. https://www.bhf.org.uk/what-we-do/news-from-the-bhf/news-archive/2019/may/heart-and-circulatory-disease-deaths-in-under-75s-see-first-sustained-rise-in-50-years.
8. Szummer K, Wallentin L, Lindhagen L, et al. Improved outcomes in patients with ST-elevation myocardial infarction during the last 20 years are related to implementation of evidence-based treatments: experiences from the SWEDEHEART registry 1995–2014. Eur Heart J. 2017;38(41):3056–65.
9. Szummer K, Wallentin L, Lindhagen L, et al. Relations between implementation of new treatments and improved outcomes in patients with non-ST-elevation myocardial infarction during the last 20 years: experiences from SWEDEHEART registry 1995–2014. Eur Heart J. 2018;39(42):3766–76.
10. Welsh P, Preiss D, Hayward C, et al. Cardiac troponin T and troponin I in the general population. Circulation. 2019;139(24):2754–64.
11. Hemingway H, McCallum A, Shipley M, Manderbacka K, Martikainen P, Keskimäki I. Incidence and prognostic

implications of stable angina pectoris among women and men. JAMA. 2006;295(12):1404–11.
12. Nishiga M, Wang DW, Han Y, Lewis DB, Wu JC. COVID-19 and cardiovascular disease: from basic mechanisms to clinical perspectives. Nat Rev Cardiol. 2020;17(9):543–58.
13. Ambrose JA, Singh M. Pathophysiology of coronary artery disease leading to acute coronary syndromes. F1000Prime Rep. 2015;7:8.
14. Landmesser U, Koenig W. From risk factors to plaque development and plaque destabilization. In: Gielen S, De Backer G, Piepoli M, Wood D (Eds) The ESC Textbook of Preventive Cardiology. Oxford: Oxford University Press; 2015:26–29.
15. Sitia S, Tomasoni L, Atzeni F, et al. From endothelial dysfunction to atherosclerosis. Autoimmun Rev. 2010;9(12):830–34.
16. Yusuf S, Hawken S, Ounpuu S, et al. Effect of potentially modifiable risk factors associated with myocardial infarction in 52 countries (the INTERHEART study): case–control study. Lancet. 2004;364(9438):937–52.
17. Pedersen SS, von Känel R, Tully PJ, Denollet J. Psychosocial perspectives in cardiovascular disease. Eur J Prev Cardiol. 2017;24(3 Suppl):108–15.
18. Frangogiannis NG. Pathophysiology of myocardial infarction. Compr Physiol. 2015;5(4):1841–75.
19. Adabag AS, Luepker RV, Roger VL, Gersh BJ. Sudden cardiac death: epidemiology and risk factors. Nat Rev Cardiol. 2010;7(4):216–25.
20. Thygesen K, Alpert JS, Jaffe AS, et al. Fourth universal definition of myocardial infarction. Eur Heart J. 2018;40(3):237–69.
21. Anderson JL, Morrow DA. Acute myocardial infarction. N Engl J Med. 2017;376(21):2053–64.
22. Chapman AR, Adamson PD, Mills NL. Assessment and classification of patients with myocardial injury and infarction in clinical practice. Heart. 2017;103(1):10–18.
23. Tamis-Holland JE, Jneid H, Reynolds HR, et al. Contemporary diagnosis and management of patients with myocardial infarction in the absence of obstructive coronary artery disease: a scientific statement from the American Heart Association. Circulation. 2019;139(18):e891–908.
24. Björck L, Nielsen S, Jernberg T, Zverkova-Sandström T, Giang KW, Rosengren A. Absence of chest pain and long-term mortality in patients with acute myocardial infarction. Open Heart. 2018;5(2):e000909.
25. Campeau L. Grading of angina pectoris. Circulation. 1976;54(3):522–23.
26. Farquharson B, Abhyankar P, Smith K, et al. Reducing delay in patients with acute coronary syndrome and other time-critical conditions: a systematic review to identify the behaviour change techniques associated with effective interventions. Open Heart. 2019;6(1):e000975.
27. O'Driscoll BR, Howard LS, Earis J, et al. BTS guideline for oxygen use in adults in healthcare and emergency settings. Thorax. 2017;72(Suppl 1):ii1–90.
28. Roques F, Nashef SA, Michel P, et al. Risk factors and outcome in European cardiac surgery: analysis of the EuroSCORE multinational database of 19030 patients. Eur J Cardiothorac Surg. 1999;15(6):816–22.
29. Roques F, Michel P, Goldstone AR, Nashef SA. The logistic EuroSCORE. Eur Heart J. 2003;24(9):881–82.
30. Nashef SA, Roques F, Sharples LD, et al. EuroSCORE II. Eur J Cardiothorac Surg. 2012;41(4):734–44.
31. Shahian DM, O'Brien SM, Filardo G, et al. The Society of Thoracic Surgeons 2008 cardiac surgery risk models: part 1—coronary artery bypass grafting surgery. Ann Thorac Surg. 2009;88(1 Suppl):S2–22.
32. Shahian DM, O'Brien SM, Filardo G, et al. The Society of Thoracic Surgeons 2008 cardiac surgery risk models: part 3—valve plus coronary artery bypass grafting surgery. Ann Thorac Surg. 2009;88(1 Suppl):S43–62.
33. Zhang YJ, Iqbal J, Campos CM, et al. Prognostic value of site SYNTAX score and rationale for combining anatomic and clinical factors in decision making: insights from the SYNTAX trial. J Am Coll Cardiol. 2014;64(5):423–32.
34. Neumann FJ, Sousa-Uva M, Ahlsson A, et al. 2018 ESC/EACTS Guidelines on myocardial revascularization. Eur Heart J. 2019;40(2):87–165.
35. Rodriguez Ziccardi M, Hatcher JD. Prinzmetal angina. StatPearls; 2020. https://www.ncbi.nlm.nih.gov/books/NBK430776/.
36. Rezkalla SH, Kloner RA. Cocaine-induced acute myocardial infarction. Clin Med Res. 2007;5(3):172–76.
37. NHS England. Second sepsis action plan. 2017. https://www.england.nhs.uk/wp-content/uploads/2017/09/second-sepsis-action-plan.pdf.
38. Cousins DH, Gerrett D, Warner B. A review of medication incidents reported to the national reporting and learning system in England and Wales over 6 years (2005–2010). Br J Clin Pharmacol. 2012;74(4):597–604.
39. Gerry S, Bonnici T, Birks J, et al. Early warning scores for detecting deterioration in adult hospital patients: systematic review and critical appraisal of methodology. BMJ. 2020;369:m1501.
40. Romero-Brufau S, Gaines K, Nicolas CT, Johnson MG, Hickman J, Huddleston JM. The fifth vital sign? Nurse worry predicts inpatient deterioration within 24 hours. JAMIA Open. 2019;2(4):465–70.
41. Astin F, Stephenson J, Wakefield J, et al. Night-time noise levels and patients' sleep experiences in a medical assessment unit in Northern England. TONURSJ. 2020;14(1):80–91.
42. Garside J, Stephenson J, Curtis H, Morrell M, Dearnley C, Astin F. Are noise reduction interventions effective

in adult ward settings? A systematic review and meta-analysis. Appl Nurs Res. 2018;44:6–17.
43. Jaul E, Barron J, Rosenzweig JP, Menczel J. An overview of co-morbidities and the development of pressure ulcers among older adults. BMC Geriatr. 2018;18(1):305.
44. Komici K, Vitale DF, Mancini A, et al. Impact of malnutrition on long-term mortality in elderly patients with acute myocardial infarction. Nutrients. 2019;11(2):224.
45. Cossette S, Frasure-Smith N, Dupuis J, Juneau M, Guertin MC. Randomized controlled trial of tailored nursing interventions to improve cardiac rehabilitation enrollment. Nurs Res. 2012;61(2):111–20.
46. Piepoli MF, Hoes AW, Agewall S, et al. 2016 European Guidelines on cardiovascular disease prevention in clinical practice: the Sixth Joint Task Force of the European Society of Cardiology and Other Societies on Cardiovascular Disease Prevention in Clinical Practice (constituted by representatives of 10 societies and by invited experts). Developed with the special contribution of the European Association for Cardiovascular Prevention & Rehabilitation (EACPR). Eur Heart J. 2016;37(29):2315–81.
47. National Institute for Health and Care Excellence. Secondary Prevention in Primary and Secondary Care for Patients Following a Myocardial Infarction. Clinical Guideline 172. London: National Institute for Health and Care Excellence; 2013. https://www.nice.org.uk/guidance/CG172.
48. Ferraro R, Latina JM, Alfaddagh A, et al. Evaluation and management of patients with stable angina: beyond the ischemia paradigm: JACC state-of-the-art review. J Am Coll Cardiol. 2020;76(19):2252–66.
49. Erbel R, Aboyans V, Boileau C, et al. 2014 ESC Guidelines on the diagnosis and treatment of aortic diseases: document covering acute and chronic aortic diseases of the thoracic and abdominal aorta of the adult. The Task Force for the Diagnosis and Treatment of Aortic Diseases of the European Society of Cardiology (ESC). Eur Heart J. 2014;35(41):2873–926.
50. Sampson UK, Norman PE, Fowkes FG, et al. Global and regional burden of aortic dissection and aneurysms: mortality trends in 21 world regions, 1990 to 2010. Glob Heart. 2014;9(1):171–80.e10.
51. Aboyans V, Ricco JB, Bartelink MEL, et al. 2017 ESC Guidelines on the diagnosis and treatment of peripheral arterial diseases, in collaboration with the European Society for Vascular Surgery (ESVS): document covering atherosclerotic disease of extracranial carotid and vertebral, mesenteric, renal, upper and lower extremity arteries. Endorsed by: the European Stroke Organization (ESO), The Task Force for the Diagnosis and Treatment of Peripheral Arterial Diseases of the European Society of Cardiology (ESC) and of the European Society for Vascular Surgery (ESVS). Eur Heart J. 2018;39(9):763–816.
52. American Stroke Association. Stroke symptoms. https://www.stroke.org/en/about-stroke/stroke-symptoms.
53. National Institute for Health and Care Excellence. 2019 Stroke and transient ischaemic attack in over 16s: diagnosis and initial management. NICE Guideline 128. 2019. https://www.nice.org.uk/guidance/ng128.

7 Care of the patient with cardiac arrhythmias

GERALDINE LEE, NINA FÅLUN, NEIL ANGUS, JEROEN HENDRIKS, TONE M. NOREKVÅL, SELINA KIKKENBORG BERG, AND DONNA FITZSIMONS

CHAPTER CONTENTS

This chapter discusses the care of patients with cardiac arrhythmias. It describes the different types of arrhythmias, their treatment, and nursing priorities for patient care.

KEY MESSAGES

- Cardiac arrhythmia is a common complication of acute coronary syndrome, cardiomyopathy, and inherited cardiac conditions. Other regulatory imbalances such as electrolyte disturbance, thyroid dysfunction, or drug interactions can also predispose to arrhythmias.
- Patients can be asymptomatic, but in many cases palpitations, dyspnoea, chest pain, or syncope are experienced. Some arrhythmias can be life-threatening and require emergency intervention.
- Cardiac monitoring and interpretation of the 12-lead electrocardiogram is the cornerstone of diagnosis.
- The psychosocial impact and lifestyle implications of cardiac arrhythmia can be challenging for patients

and their families and nursing care should focus on education and support to facilitate shared decision-making and adherence to selected therapies.

Introduction

The term cardiac arrhythmia refers to any rhythm that is not sinus rhythm and because the electrical conduction through the heart is affected, they can reduce the cardiac output with serious consequences for the patient. The main types of arrhythmias are:

- Atrial fibrillation (AF).
- Supraventricular tachycardia (SVT).
- Bradycardia (defined as a heart rate <50 beats per minute (bpm)).
- Heart block, where there is a conduction delay or impedance in the atrioventricular (AV) conduction pathway.
- Ventricular fibrillation (VF), which fortunately is rare but can be fatal.

Arrhythmias can present in isolation or with acute events, such as a myocardial infarction, or acute coronary syndrome (ACS) and can originate in the atria or in the ventricles. Depending on their location, they can be deemed asymptomatic/non-urgent (i.e. the person feels unwell, but their cardiac output is not significantly compromised) or life-threatening (i.e. they significantly impact the cardiac output and unless resolved immediately, lead to cardiac arrest). Therefore, early diagnosis is important, especially in the presence of other cardiac-related pathologies and for many, once detected and treated, patients can lead a normal life.

Epidemiology and pathophysiology

Arrhythmias are a common cardiovascular complaint, generally associated with older age and often in those with other cardiovascular conditions such as coronary heart disease or valvular disease.[1] However, they also occur in younger people, in particular SVTs. In the UK, there are approximately 2 million people living with an arrhythmia and although they can affect any age group, they tend to be predominantly in older people, especially in those with coronary heart disease.[1] While historic estimates suggest that up to 90% of patients with ACS will experience an arrhythmia in the peri-infarct period,[2] the incidence of life-threatening arrhythmias in the early period following ACS has decreased in recent decades. This improvement is attributed to widespread availability of effective revascularization strategies, including thrombolysis and percutaneous coronary intervention, as well as increased use of beta-blockers.[3]

The majority of arrhythmias are caused by conduction abnormalities in the AV pathway. These arrhythmias can be as a result of another cardiac condition that causes structural and electrical changes to occur within the heart, or they can be genetic abnormalities, associated with channelopathies and abnormal conduction pathways. Therefore, the management of the arrythmia relies on a thorough history taking, clinical assessment, 12-lead ECG, and other diagnostic tests to confirm the diagnosis and to determine the best possible treatment for each individual. The normal conduction system and heart rhythm have been outlined in Chapter 4.

Clinical presentation

The presentation of an arrhythmia varies depending on the particular rhythm disturbance and whether the patient has a history of coronary heart disease, heart failure, or underlying valvular disease. A patient presenting with an acute myocardial infarction, for instance, may experience heart block and thus obtaining an accurate history, undertaking a thorough clinical assessment, and performing a 12-lead ECG is important in determining the underlying pathology (see also Chapter 4). Some people, especially those with AF or atrial flutter, may have experienced no symptoms and often the detection of the arrhythmia is an incidental finding.

There are key questions to ask at the time of presentation, as shown in ➤ **Fig. 7.1**.

Signs and symptoms

With the tachyarrhythmias described previously (AF, SVT), some people will complain of feeling their heart beating very fast and having chest discomfort. If it is their first time with symptoms, especially of SVTs, many mistakenly believe they are having a heart attack, as they may experience chest pain. Other symptoms include feeling light-headed or breathless, being tired, and feeling nauseated. In terms of signs, people present with tachycardia, hypotension, tachypnoea, polyuria, diaphoresis, and nausea/vomiting. They may be pale and anxious, especially if they have never had symptoms

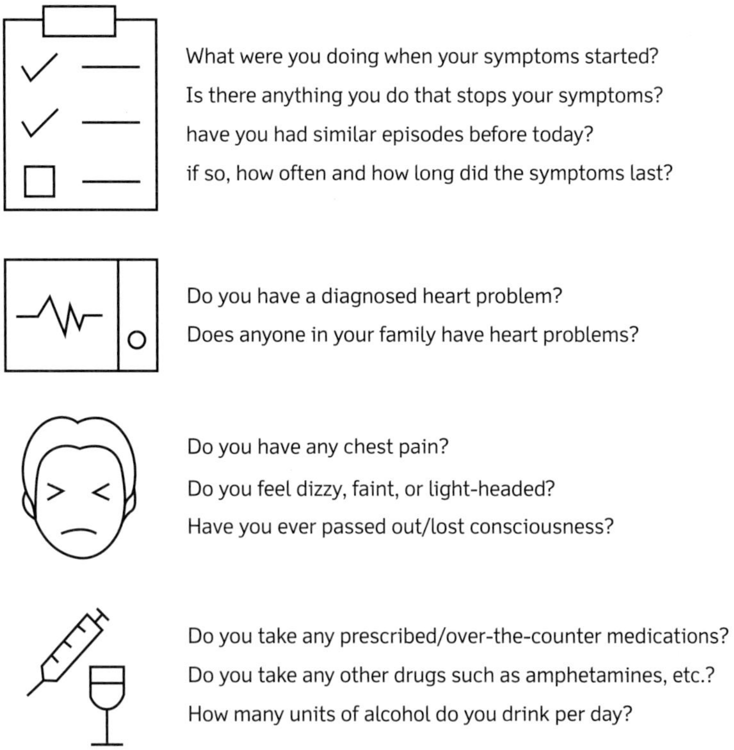

What were you doing when your symptoms started?
Is there anything you do that stops your symptoms?
have you had similar episodes before today?
if so, how often and how long did the symptoms last?
Do you have a diagnosed heart problem?
Does anyone in your family have heart problems?
Do you have any chest pain?
Do you feel dizzy, faint, or light-headed?
Have you ever passed out/lost consciousness?
Do you take any prescribed/over-the-counter medications?
Do you take any other drugs such as amphetamines, etc.?
How many units of alcohol do you drink per day?

Fig. 7.1 Key questions to ask at the time of clinical presentation of an arrhythmia.

before. ➤ **Table 7.1** shows the common, uncommon, and rare symptoms reported by patients with SVTs and Fig. 7.1 is a useful guide when taking a history.

Those experiencing bradycardia or heart block may present with reduced conscious level and feel nauseous/vomiting, fatigued, short of breath, and light-headed. Some patients may present with syncope and it is imperative to determine if the cause is cardiac or non-cardiac (i.e. neurological). As well as recording heart rate, blood pressure, temperature, oxygen saturation, and respiratory rate as part of the clinical assessment, obtaining a 12-lead ECG is important. Taking a thorough clinical history is important and will assist in determining if the rhythm disturbance is due to an underlying cardiac pathology (see also Chapter 4 and Chapter 5).

Diagnostic tests and differential diagnosis

An understanding of the coronary blood supply and the cardiac conduction system and skills in basic ECG interpretation are necessary for the assessment and effective management of arrhythmias in the acute setting (see Chapter 3). Accurate patient evaluation requires awareness of possible presenting signs and symptoms (➤ **Table 7.1**), thorough history taking, clinical assessment, timely review of a 12-lead ECG, and use of additional diagnostic tests (e.g. cardiac troponins) in order to confirm the diagnosis. Evaluation must be followed by prompt and appropriate intervention, based on the patient's haemodynamic status, in order to ensure optimal patient outcomes.

For those with suspected SVTs, a treadmill exercise may be useful to determine if the heart rate and blood pressure are a response to minimal exercise—this is especially valid in those with a reported low level of physical activity. As well as diagnostic testing, blood tests should be routinely considered to ensure there is no underlying pathology contributing to or causing the arrhythmia; these include a complete blood count, fasting blood glucose, and thyroid function screen (especially relevant in AF). To rule out any underlying valvular or structural heart disease, a transthoracic echocardiogram should be performed and this is a recommendation in those with AF as

Table 7.1 Most common symptoms during sustained SVT

Common	Uncommon	Rare
Chest discomfort or pressure	Chest pain	Asymptomatic
Dyspnoea	Diaphoresis	Tachycardiomyopathy
Light-headedness, dizziness, or presyncope	Nausea	Sudden death with WPW syndrome
Palpitations	Syncope	
Polyuria		

WPW, Wolff–Parkinson–White.
Katritsis DG, Boriani G, Cosio FG, et al. European Heart Rhythm Association (EHRA) consensus document on the management of supraventricular arrhythmias, endorsed by Heart Rhythm Society (HRS), Asia-Pacific Heart Rhythm Society (APHRS), and Sociedad Latinoamericana de Estimulación Cardiaca y Electrofisiologia (SOLAECE). Europace. 2017 Mar 1;19(3):465–511. doi: 10.1093/europace/euw301. © The European Society of Cardiology. Reprinted by permission of Oxford University Press.

part of their initial assessment to ensure that the AF is not valvular AF.[5] Electrophysiology studies need to be performed for those with tachycardias where the underlying mechanism is uncertain and in SVTs to determine if the SVT is a sinus node reentrant tachycardia or focal atrial tachycardia.

Electrocardiographic monitoring

ECG monitoring is one of the most valuable diagnostic tools in modern medicine. The main purpose of the monitoring of cardiac patients is to detect and treat adverse arrhythmias.[6] It was introduced to intensive cardiac care units (ICCUs) with specialized monitors and devices in the early 1960s.[7] 'A crucial advance, not only in coronary care but in hospital medicine generally, was giving nurses the responsibility for the detection and treatment of arrhythmias, including defibrillation'[8]. In the mid 1970s, in-hospital telemetries were introduced to European hospitals, and arrhythmia monitoring became less cumbersome. During the last four decades, portable telemetry monitoring has been widely used for in-hospital detection of arrhythmias in a diverse group of medical and surgical patients. Indeed, it is still a cornerstone of care in most critical care settings, but definitive guidance regarding the indications, type and duration of monitoring are required.[9]

In-hospital continuous ECG monitoring

Types of cardiac monitoring and devices used

Continuous bedside monitoring of the ECG is automatic for all patients admitted to ICCUs and nurses bear significant responsibility for their management. While these provide a level of reassurance for the clinical team, the associated wires and noises can be anxiety provoking for the patient and careful education and reassurance is required to ensure patients understand the functionality and limitations of this intervention. The purpose of the continuous monitoring is (1) immediate recognition of sudden cardiac arrest to improve time to defibrillation; (2) to recognize deteriorating conditions that may lead to a life-threatening, sustained arrhythmia; (3) to facilitate management of arrhythmias even if not immediate life-threatening; and (4) to facilitate diagnosis of arrhythmias or cause of symptoms as syncope and palpitations and subsequent guide appropriate management.[10]

ECG transfer from ambulances to hospital

Acquisition of a prehospital 12-lead ECG in patients with suspected ST-elevation myocardial infarction is recommended to detect life-threatening arrhythmias and allow prompt defibrillation if indicated.

Holter monitoring

A Holter monitor is a small, wearable device that keeps track of the patient's heart rhythm for up to 7 days. The main aim of the monitoring is to analyse the electrical activity of the heart outside of the clinical setting. A Holter monitor is most often used when a person experiences transient episodes of symptoms that might be explained by a heart rhythm disturbance.

Implantable loop recorder

An implantable loop recorder is a small electrophysiology device used for long-term monitoring of a patient's heart electrical activity and is recommended when symptoms (e.g. syncope) are sporadic and suspected to be related to arrhythmia and when a symptom–rhythm correlation cannot be established by conventional diagnostic techniques. The implantable loop recorder is inserted just beneath the skin of the patient's chest and can record heart rhythms for up to 3 years. It is continuously looping its memory and has automatic triggers to store recordings. The implantable loop recorder can also be patient activated.

Mobile cardiac telemetry devices

These provide real-time, outpatient pocket ECG monitoring for up to 30 days. ECG data are transmitted automatically via smartphones to a diagnostic laboratory where monitor watchers can notify physicians when significant arrhythmias occur. Mobile cardiac telemetry devices are used when in-hospital telemetry monitoring and/or Holter monitoring have failed to detect arrhythmia. More recent technology using skin patches has shown good preliminary results. There are also new ambulatory devices being trialled to detect AF including photoplethysmography that are worn on the wrist. Use of these new technologies has made detecting arrhythmias easier and faster and therefore has the potential to assist healthcare professionals to instigate the appropriate treatment more efficiently, although ethical issues need to be considered.

Clinical guidelines and practice standards

Diagnostic tools like resting 12-lead ECG, serial ECGs, or Holter monitoring are frequently suggested in European Society of Cardiology (ESC) Guidelines. However, continuous monitoring by telemetry to diagnose complex arrhythmias, detect early warning signals of potentially life-threatening events, or as follow-up after invasive treatment or surgery is rarely included. Overall, most ESC Guidelines do not have clear recommendations for appropriate use of continuous arrhythmia monitoring by in-hospital telemetry, even though telemetry monitoring is widely used in non-critical care wards and the monitoring decreases the need for beds in intensive care units.[9] However, in more recent ESC Guidelines, recommendations are included (➤ Table 7.2).

In order to make evidence-based decisions regarding the appropriate use of scarce resources such as monitoring, clinicians require guidance. In 2004, the American Heart Association (AHA) recognized this challenge and developed a comprehensive set of practice standards for in-hospital cardiac monitoring to help assess which patients were appropriate for admission to non-critical telemetry beds.[11] These were based primarily on expert opinions. Similarly, the 2017 update to the practice standards was developed using limited trial data.[10] The AHA practice standards classify patients as follows: class I (monitoring should be performed), class II (monitoring reasonable to perform/may be considered), and class III (monitoring no benefit/not recommended). These practice standards are not limited to indications for telemetry only, but include recommendations for ST-segment and QT interval monitoring—as well as for patient care issues and recommendations on how telemetry should be organized and integrated into clinical practice. However, these recommendations do not seem commonly implemented in European hospitals.

Inappropriate telemetry monitoring is common in most clinical settings. Lack of guidance, time, and resources may result in non-adherence to guidelines and inadequate arrhythmia surveillance—with both over- and

Table 7.2 ESC Guideline recommendations: indications for in-hospital ECG monitoring

Indication	Recommendations	Class	Level
Syncope[1]	Immediate in-hospital monitoring (in-bed or by telemetry) is indicated in high risk patients	I	C
STEMI[2]	It is indicated that all STEMI patients have ECG monitoring for a minimum of 24 hours	I	C
NSTEMI	NSTEMI at low risk for cardiac arrhythmias ≤24 hours	*ND	*ND
	NSTEMI at intermediate or high risk for cardiac arrhythmias ≥24 hours	*ND	*ND
Atrial fibrillation and stroke[3]	In patients with TIA or ischemic stroke, screening for AF is recommended for short term ECG monitoring (followed by continuous ECG monitoring for at least 72 hours)	I	B

*ND, not defined.
1: 2018 ESC Guidelines for the diagnosis and management of syncope
2: 2017 ESC Guidelines for the management of acute myocardial infarction in patients presenting with ST-segment elevation
3: 2016 ESC Guidelines for the management of atrial fibrillation

under-monitoring. Often, concern for clinical deterioration rather than a concern for development of arrhythmias influences telemetry ordering and guidelines adherence.[12] This may cause inconsistent monitoring, which has the potential to compromise patient safety and care outcomes.

Monitor stations and electronic ordering systems

Management of patients at risk of serious arrhythmias is a joint collaboration between nurses and physicians in ICCUs and in medical and surgical wards. The monitor station is usually located in intensive care units and administrated by dedicated monitor watchers. Intensive care and cardiac nurses are key professionals who respond to device alarms and manage central monitor stations. Alarms released from multiple telemetry units must be recognized, interpreted, and used to guide appropriate treatment in a timely manner. Accordingly, calling the central ICCU monitor station regarding ward interventions when complex arrhythmias are reported is important feedback.[13] It is debatable whether it is advantageous to use dedicated monitor watchers. Using dedicated monitor watchers is resource demanding and it is unknown whether it improves patient outcomes. However, when nurses fail to interpret ECG monitoring data, it may cause inconsistent monitoring, which also potentially compromises patient safety.[9] Telemetry is a powerful tool for real-time monitoring of a patient's heart rhythm. Nevertheless, the number of telemetries available is a limited resource in most hospitals. Computerized order entry systems, usually based upon hospital-driven protocols derived from the AHA practice standards, are increasingly used to reduce inappropriate telemetry surveillance. To order telemetry, physicians must select an indication for monitoring. This order must be revised within predefined timeframes for each telemetry indication. Giving nursing staff assessment tools to discontinue telemetry when appropriate, the average numbers of patients monitored by telemetry is proven to be decreased with up to 70% and the average length of stay on telemetry to be reduced from 58 to 31 hours.[14]

Arrhythmia monitoring

Most common arrhythmias observed by in-hospital tele-metry are AF or atrial flutter, and non-sustained VF. Patients pre-diagnosed with heart failure, arrhythmias, chest pain, and syncope of suspected cardiac origin at hospital admission have the most frequent event rate.[13] Arrhythmias of any kind are revealed in 24–33% of patients monitored by telemetry, of which up to 10% are potentially life-threatening events.[15] The mortality rate in monitored patients is low, as 1.7–4.0% of the monitored population dies before hospital discharge. Nevertheless, in-hospital telemetry monitoring is proven to be an independent and strong predictor of survival of cardiac arrest before hospital discharge.[16] Arrhythmia detection is reported to affect clinical change of management in 7–18% of all patients monitored.[13] Compliance with recommendations for length of stay on telemetry according to the AHA practice standards is inconsistent, and both over- and under-monitoring is frequently reported.

Accurate electrode positioning is a crucial skill in cardiovascular nursing (➤ Fig. 7.2). Ensuring consistent lead placement over time is crucial to avoid changing the QRS

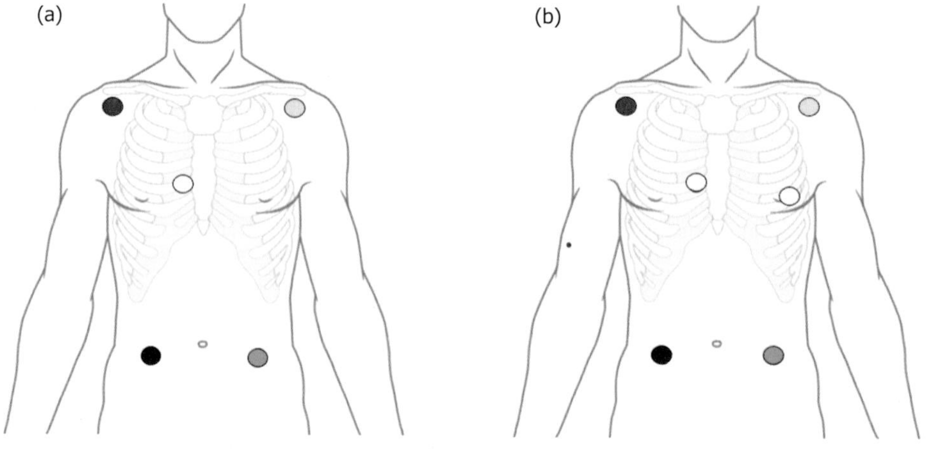

Fig. 7.2 (a) ECG standard five-lead placement. (b) ECG standard/HEXAD six-lead placement.

morphology and thereby cause a potential misdiagnosis. In a critical care unit, the bedside cardiac monitor (oscilloscope) provides a continuous display of the patient's heart rhythm. It is important to select the correct monitoring leads for arrhythmia identifications, usually lead II to diagnose atrial activity and measure heart rate. At the monitor station, two leads will be screened, usually lead II and a second lead, V2 or V5, to distinguish between arrhythmias and artefacts and to track variation in ST-segment elevation. The Mason–Likar ECG configuration includes limb position (shoulders and hips) and one or two precordial electrodes (V1 and/or V5) (➤ **Fig. 7.2**). Mispositioned arm electrodes attached closer to the heart or sternum, or mispositioned precordial leads (V) attached closer to the heart, may change QRS morphology resulting in misdiagnosis of arrhythmias and ischemia.[13] Both the limb electrodes and the V electrodes are frequently mispositioned. Overall, 26–38% of the electrodes are reported to be mispositioned incorrectly in clinical practice.[6,14,17]

Cardiac nurses also raise the quality of arrhythmic surveillance by properly preparing the skin in male patients and thorough hair clipping at electrode sites. Low adherence to this recommendation can be a major problem, since electrically noisy signals due to poor electrode attachment produce artefacts that can simulate ventricular tachycardia (VT) and lead to subsequent inappropriate treatment.[11] Changing electrodes every 48 hours at a minimum, or as recommended by the manufacturer, is important. It is a class IC recommendation in the 2017 update to the AHA practice standards. Cleaning the electrode area with soap and water to remove skin oils and debris and drying it prior to electrode placement has a class IB recommendation. A non-adherence practice might affect telemetry monitoring. Electrodes may dry out or be disconnected from the patient, increasing electrical impedance, in turn reducing signal quality. Standardization of skin preparation procedures improves electrical conduction, reduces artefacts, and leads to fewer false alarms.[9,10]

Medical equipment shared between different wards and patients is a potential source of nosocomial infections. Telemetry units are frequently shared among different wards and patients. Therefore, disposable protection covers it is crucial for decreasing potential contamination. Disposable ECG lead wires are also recommended. Usually, nurses spend an average of 20 minutes per patient per day on telemetry maintenance, including changing batteries, addressing alarms, and notifying clinicians.[12] Nurses must have a high level of knowledge of and skill in telemetry monitoring to respond appropriately when arrhythmias occur. In many countries, master's degree programmes in cardiac or intensive care nursing education include heart rhythm interpretation in their curriculum. However, there is a paucity of in-hospital educational programmes in cardiac monitoring.

Alarm fatigue

Alarm fatigue is defined as being immune and desensitized by the noise caused by technical support and devices within hospital units.[18] In the last decade, the number of devices with alarms in hospital settings has increased exponentially. Alarms are released from equipment as monitors, ventilators, infusion pumps, feeding pumps, and pulse oximeters. The audible alarm burden for one bed in an ICCU is estimated to 187 per day. ECG monitors are identified as the alarm source in 37% of all alarms in an ICCU.[19] Alarms were intentionally created to enhance patient safety, but now alarms have become an urgent patient safety issue themselves. The overwhelming numbers of false alarms contributes to alarm fatigue and thereby create safety issues. Nurses might ignore alarm signals, turn down the volume, adjust the alarm setting, or deactivate alarms, compromising patient safety. Monitor alarms are intentionally set for high sensitivity, with numerous false alarms as a result, causing alarm fatigue. Eliminating unnecessary telemetry monitoring in patients and discontinuing monitoring when it is no longer clinically indicated might decrease this alarm burden and reduce serious events related to alarm fatigue. The sensory overload when nurses are exposed to excessive numbers of alarms might lead to both desensitization and missed alarms and challenge patient safety. Implementing off-site central monitoring by monitoring technicians may reduce the high alarm burden related to on-site monitoring of non-critically ill patients.

Patient information and support

It has long been recognized that most patients monitored consider non-invasive devices and telemetries as a source of discomfort and anxiety, and up to 60% do not receive any explanation on in-hospital monitoring.[20] It is important to inform the patient that the monitor is only reading their heart rate and they must inform the cardiac nurses if they experience symptoms including chest pain, palpitations, or breathlessness. Some patients might find the arrhythmia surveillance quite daunting. Placing a telemetry unit with associated wires on a patient's chest is reported to cause sleep disturbances and to exacerbate a patient's delirium.[21] Accordingly, information should be tailored to the needs of the patient's age, hearing ability, and cognitive level.[6] Several factors have been identified that disrupt the proper flow of information in a healthcare setting, thus affecting optimal delivery of the information patients need. Often, telemetry monitoring is initiated as the patient arrives in the coronary care unit. The environment at arrival is typically hectic, with multiple interruptions as nurses are multitasking to meet the needs of all patients in their care. This may lead to inadequate delivery and receipt of important information. Furthermore, failure in communicating relevant and sufficient information at patient handover between shifts may reduce the quality of information given to patients.

Nurses play a key role in the monitoring and diagnosis of cardiac arrhythmia. In ➤ **Table 7.3** we provide an overview of common cardiac arrhythmias with associated rhythm strips, characteristics of diagnosis, symptoms, and potential treatments. These will be expanded in more depth later in the chapter. The primary aim of arrhythmia management is to restore normal sinus rhythm when possible, although patients displaying signs of haemodynamic compromise or circulatory collapse will require immediate intervention with the aim of controlling ventricular rate and optimizing cardiac output.[22] A range of pharmacological and electrical interventions including synchronized cardioversion, cardiac pacing, and defibrillation may be indicated. In the acute setting, patients with arrhythmias may be completely asymptomatic with uncompromised cardiac output. However, arrhythmia onset may in some instances lead to significant reductions in cardiac output and result in a high risk of life-threatening patient deterioration (see also Chapter 5).

Bradyarrhythmias—diagnosis, treatment, care, and prevention

Bradycardia is defined as a heart rate less than 50 bpm and occurs in up to 18% of patients with ACS.[23] Patients with bradycardia are often asymptomatic and normotensive and no treatment is required. Furthermore, endurance athletes often have a resting heart rate less than 50 bpm with no clinical sequalae noted. However, slow heart rates resulting from myocardial infarction or ischaemia may require prompt pharmacological or electrical intervention particularly if signs of haemodynamic compromise are evident.

Sinus bradycardia

In the acute cardiac patient, sinus bradycardia is seen most often in inferior myocardial infarction, as it is the right coronary artery that provides the sinoatrial (SA) node blood supply in most people. This rhythm disturbance is often transient, occurring in the first few hours of an infarct and typically resolving in the first 24 hours. An increase in vagal tone due to nausea and pain may contribute to sinus bradycardia, so these symptoms should be adequately treated as a priority. If a patient has received beta-blockers, calcium channel blockers, or digoxin in the pre-infarct period this may also explain sinus bradycardia, so it is important to obtain and carefully evaluate the patient's medication history. When there is evidence of haemodynamic compromise, with symptoms such as dyspnoea, dizziness, hypotension (systolic blood pressure <90 mmHg), or if ischaemic ECG changes are noted, then sinus bradycardia can be treated initially by judicious administration of intravenous atropine in small doses (0.5–1 mg).[24] This may be sufficient to improve symptoms and atropine can be administered, in repeated doses, up to a maximum total of 3 mg. It should be noted that atropine administration may cause reflex tachycardia thereby increasing myocardial oxygen demand and intensifying any underlying ischaemia. If bradycardia and associated haemodynamic compromise persist despite administration of atropine, then temporary cardiac pacing may occasionally be indicated.

Junctional rhythm

If the SA node fails to generate the impulses needed to stimulate cardiac contraction, then cells in the atrioventricular (AV) node area may assume the role of pacemaker. Cardiac rhythms originating in the AV node region are described as junctional rhythms. AV nodal impulses may be conducted in a retrograde (backwards) or antegrade (forwards) direction through the ventricular bundle branches. When retrograde conduction occurs, inverted P waves may be seen immediately following QRS complexes, the reverse of normal conduction. On occasion, QRS complexes may mask P waves. Junctional rhythms typically have a rate of around 50 bpm and QRS complexes are narrow.

Idioventricular rhythm

Idioventricular rhythm (IVR) occurs when an area other than the SA or AV node takes over as pacemaker. Widened QRS complexes are visible on the ECG. IVR is referred to as an 'escape' rhythm in which contractile impulses originate at ventricular level. IVR is typically of short duration and associated with a heart rate of 40 bpm or less. As with other bradyarrhythmias, treatment is determined by consideration of the underlying cause and assessment of any associated symptoms. In the acute setting,

Table 7.3 Arrhythmia types

Type of arrhythmia	Characteristics of diagnosis	Symptoms	Treatment
Sinus bradycardia 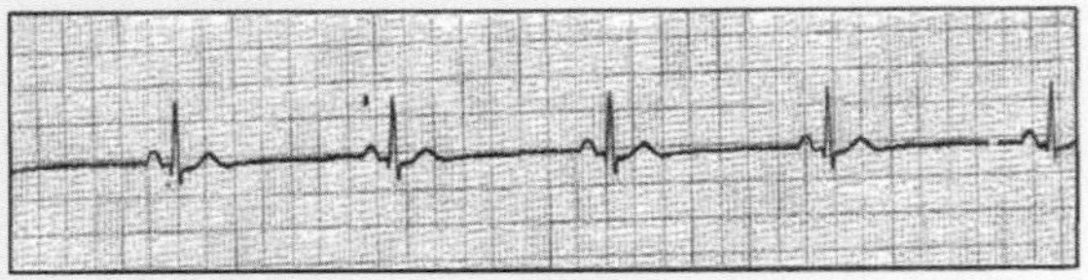 (1)	Regular bradycardia with resting ventricular rate <50 bpm P waves with constant morphology precede every QRS complex P waves positive in limb lead II	Increase in vagal tone due to nausea and pain Dyspnoea Dizziness Hypotension	Administration of 0.5–1 mg of intravenous atropine, up to a maximum of 3 mg
Junctional rhythm 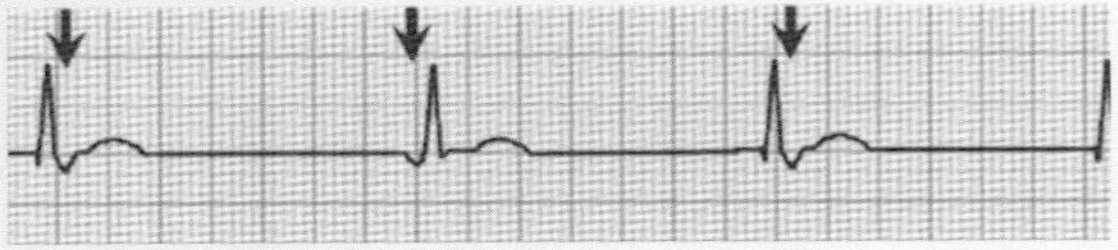 (2)	Rate of around 50 bpm QRS complexes are narrow AV node impulses may be conducted in retrograde (backwards) or antegrade (forwards) Retrograde—inverted P waves may be seen immediately following QRS complexes	Can be due to bradycardia and/or loss of AV synchrony Light-headedness Palpitations Effort intolerance Chest heaviness Dyspnoea	Cardiac pacing in symptomatic patients
Idioventricular rhythm 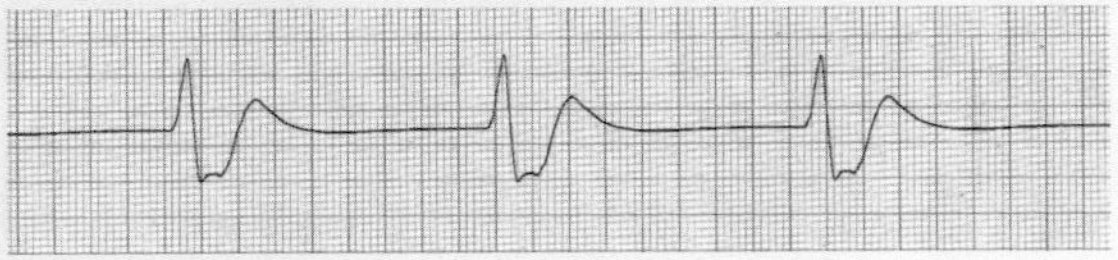 (3) 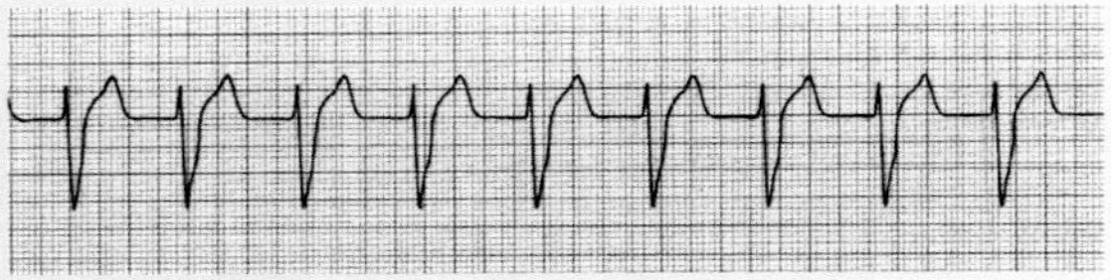 (4)	Widened QRS complexes visible on ECG IVR of short duration Heart rate of ≤40 bpm	Acute setting—accelerate IVR (heart rate 100–120 bpm) may occur	Treatment determined by consideration of the underlying cause and assessment of associated symptoms

(continued)

Table 7.3 Continued

Type of arrhythmia	Characteristics of diagnosis	Symptoms	Treatment
First-degree AV block 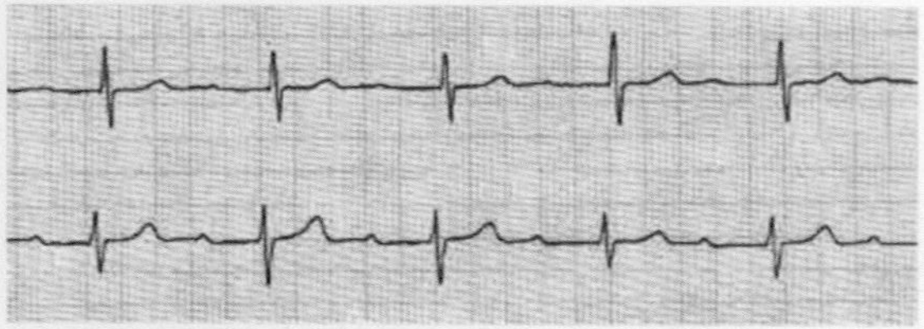 (1)	PR interval is prolonged (>200 ms) Heart rate often normal (60–100 bpm) Conduction of atrial impulses is delayed at the level of the AV node Heart rhythm remains regular, with a QRS complex following each P wave	May be asymptomatic or if ventricular rate is slow may have symptoms of bradycardia	Generally well tolerated and often does not require treatment. If prolongation of the PR is extreme (>440 ms) and patient is symptomatic cardiac pacing may be required Any electrolyte imbalances should be corrected
Second-degree AV block—Mobitz type I 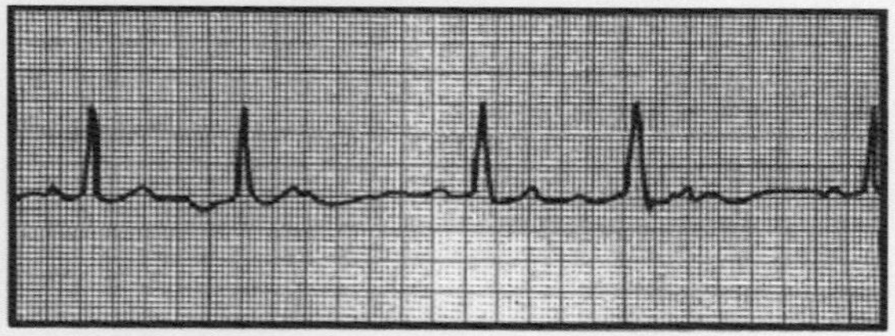 (1)	Progressive lengthening of the PR interval over several cardiac cycles prior to an atrial impulse being completely blocked at the AV node level On the ECG when an atrial impulse is blocked, a P wave is visible but no QRS complex follows Ventricular rate is irregular The heart rate may be low to normal (40–70 bpm)	May be asymptomatic; however, slow or irregular ventricular rates may cause chest pain and symptoms of bradycardia	Tends to be transient and treatment may not be necessary In cases with haemodynamic compromise, administration of intravenous atropine or temporary cardiac pacing may be necessary
Second-degree AV block—Mobitz type II 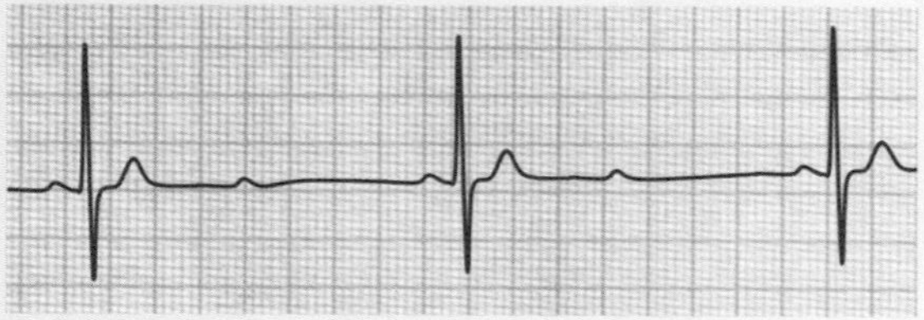 (1)	Variable non-conduction of atrial impulses There is no preceding lengthening of the PR interval Dropped beats may follow a regular or irregular pattern and this block occurs below the level of the AV node in the AV bundle or one or more of its distal branches	Fatigue Dyspnoea Hypotension Reduced cardiac output—pallor, diaphoresis Chest pain Syncope Sudden cardiac arrest	Atropine may be given to increase the heart rate in symptomatic patients Cardiac pacing will be required because of the increased risk of clinical deterioration with progression to complete heart block or asystole
Third degree (complete) AV block 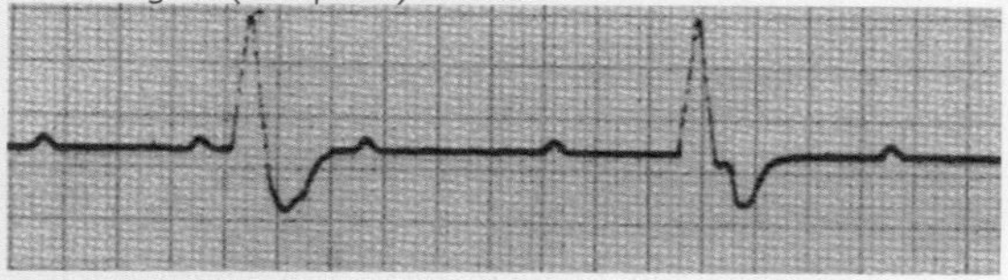 (1)	Effectively no transmission of electrical impulses between atria and ventricles See text for further characteristics depending on the location of the escape rhythm	Symptomatic hypotension Light-headedness Dizziness Syncope Fatigue Chest pain Asystole	In complete AV block (with no ventricular escape rhythm) asystole will occur and the patient will require immediate resuscitation Cardiac pacing is likely to be required Depending on myocardial damage, a permanent pacemaker may be required

Asystole 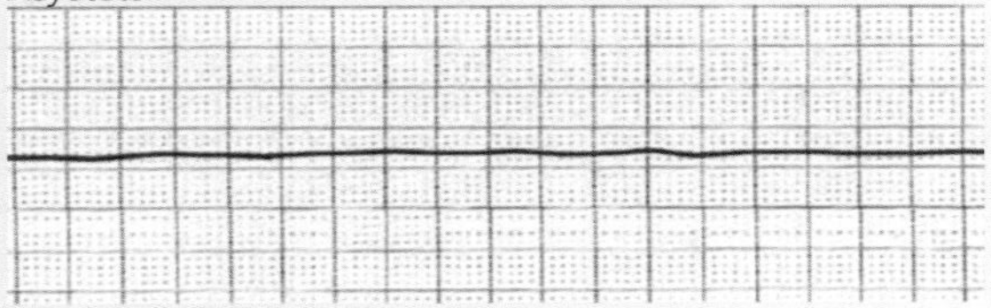 (1)	In asystole, all functional myocardial activity has ceased In practice, asystole may be preceded by the occurrence of a bradyarrhythmia or a degree of heart block	Possible secondary conditions include hypoxia, hypovolaemia, hypothermia, hyperkalaemia or hypokalaemia, metabolic disorders, thrombosis, tension pneumothorax, cardiac tamponade, and toxins	In patients with viable myocardium, it may be possible to establish effective cardiac pacing via transcutaneous, transoesophageal, or endocardial routes—though clinical outcomes in this patient group are generally very poor
Temporary cardiac pacing 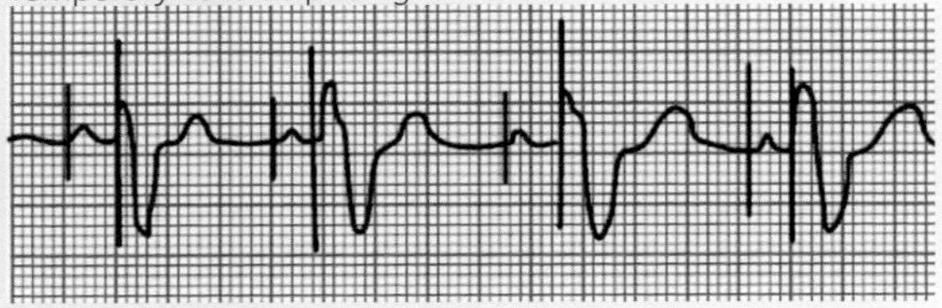 (5)	Probably better omitted as not an arrhythmia but a treatment for other arrhythmias	Probably better omitted as not an arrhythmia but a treatment for other arrhythmias	Probably better omitted as not an arrhythmia but a treatment for other arrhythmias
Sinus tachycardia 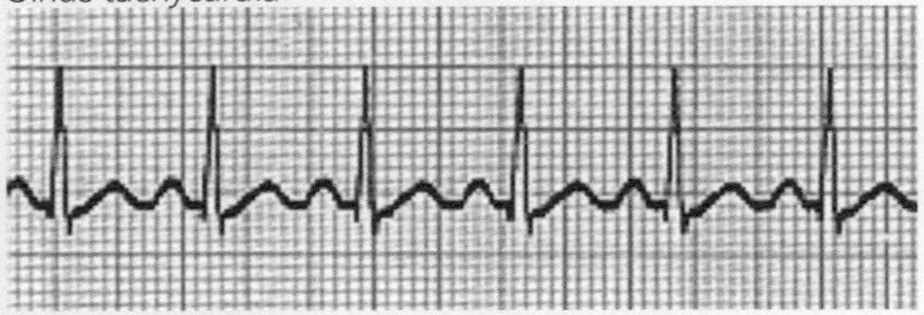 (1)	Increase in sympathetic nervous system activity caused by pathological stressors such as myocardial ischaemia and low cardiac output	Hypotension Shock Dyspnoea Signs of pulmonary congestion or heart failure	Beta-blockers or calcium channel blockers to heart slow rate Ablation procedures if inappropriate and persistent
Supraventricular tachycardia 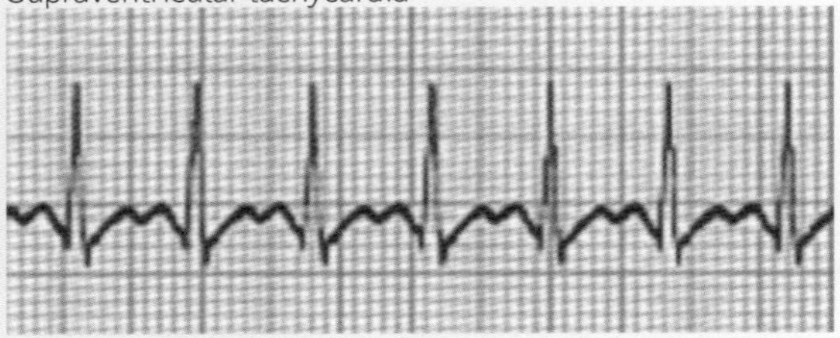 (1)	QRS complexes are usually narrow (0.04–0.12 sec) SVT often has a rapid, regular rhythm although this may be irregular if AF or atrial flutter is present	Palpitations Sensation of rapid, racing heart Dizziness Chest pain Dyspnoea Diaphoresis Syncope	Carotid sinus pressure Vagal manoeuvres Cardioversion Medicines—adenosine, beta-blockers, calcium channel blockers, antiarrhythmic agents

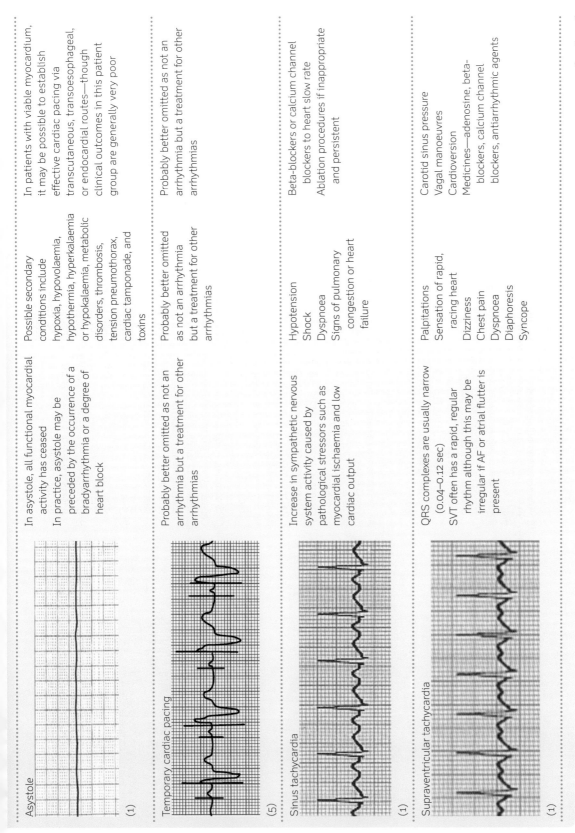

(continued)

Table 7.3 Continued

Type of arrhythmia	Characteristics of diagnosis	Symptoms	Treatment
Paroxysmal atrial tachycardia 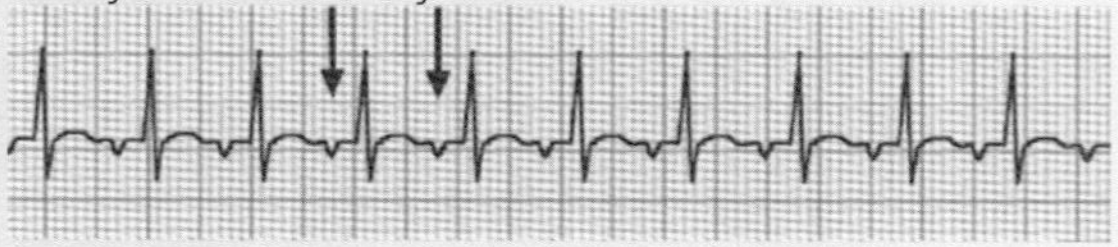 (2)	Rapid heart rate of 160–220 bpm P waves are usually regular and identical in shape, suggesting a single point of origin, but on examination of the ECG these may be inverted on lead II signalling an abnormal atrial origin	Dizziness Palpitations Chest pain Dyspnoea	If the patient is stable, vagal stimulation may be successful in terminating the arrhythmia Adenosine may be given to try and terminate the arrhythmia In more persistent and troublesome cases, antiarrhythmic medication or ablation therapy may be indicated
Atrial fibrillation 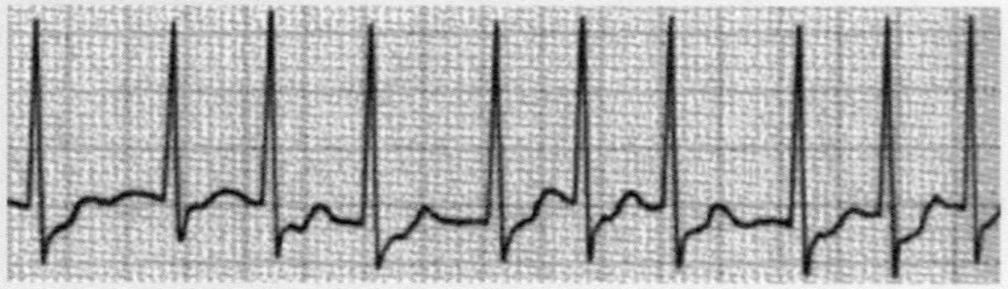 (1)	AF can present as a narrow complex tachycardia Heart rhythm is always irregularly irregular If there is aberrant conduction AF will present as a broad complex tachycardia Rapid heart rate No discernible P waves are visible on the ECG	Irregularly, irregular pulse Palpitations Fatigue Dyspnoea Hypotension Chest pain	Complex management covering five treatment domains. See main text for details
Broad complex tachycardia 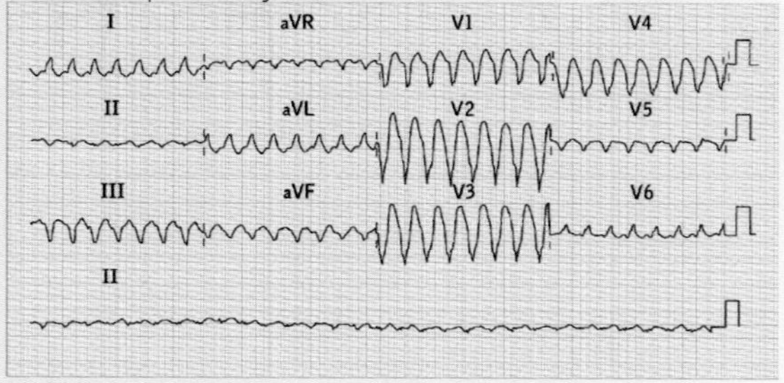 (6)	QRS complex >120 ms Caused by ventricular conducting system not functioning (bundle branch block) or AV node dysfunction. May be supraventricular or ventricular in origin	Depend on the haemodynamic consequences of arrhythmia rather than its origin. May cause: Dizziness Palpitations Chest pain Heart failure Syncope	If patient is unstable: Life support as appropriate Identify/treat reversible causes Synchronized direct current shocks Amiodarone

Ventricular tachycardia 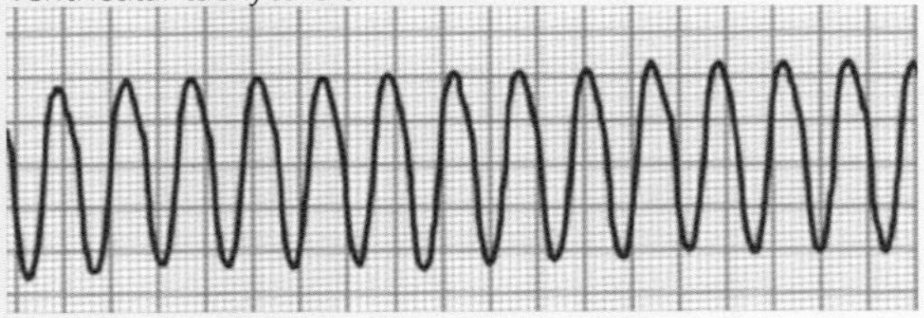 (1)	VT should be strongly suspected if the ventricular rate exceeds 100 bpm (often higher) and QRS complexes are widened with an abnormal shape or when there is dissociation between atrial and ventricular activity or when fusion beats are present	Dramatically reduced cardiac output Altered or lost consciousness Risk of developing pulmonary oedema, heart failure, and cardiogenic shock	If there is loss of consciousness due to reduced cardiac output, immediate defibrillation is indicated Haemodynamically stable patients may be treated with intravenous antiarrhythmic agents with amiodarone being the drug of choice Patients may require cardioverter defibrillator implantation
Torsades de pointes 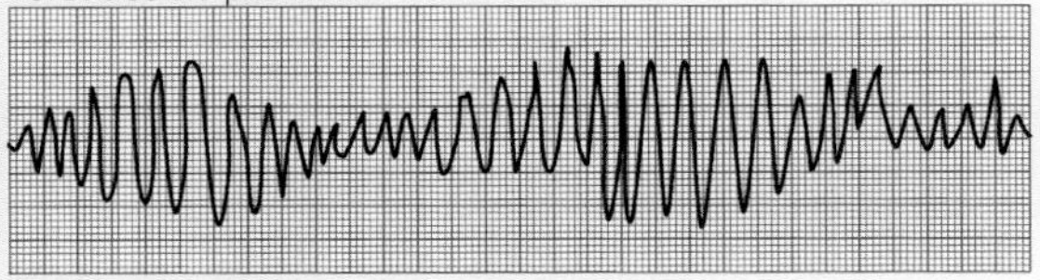 (5)	Polymorphic QRS complexes that move about the isoelectric baseline of the ECG producing a spindle-shaped pattern Often associated with a prolonged QT interval	Palpitations Dizziness Nausea Diaphoresis Chest pain Dyspnoea Hypotension Syncope	Intravenous magnesium administration A beta-blocker, not sotalol as it increases the QT interval, or cardiac pacing may also be beneficial Antiarrhythmics must be avoided as they tend to prolong the QT interval and may worsen the condition
Ventricular fibrillation 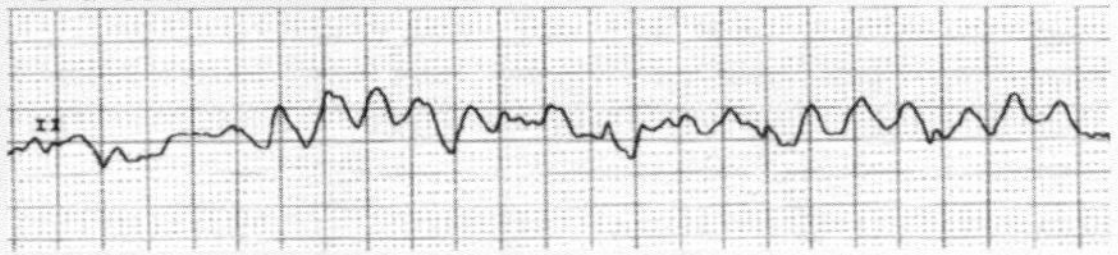 (1)	VF is characterized by chaotic and irregular ventricular activity with deflections of variable height and width visible on the ECG No QRS complexes are identifiable Myocardial muscle contraction is absent Cardiac output ceases	Rapid loss of consciousness Pulseless	Application of basic and advanced life support Early defibrillation

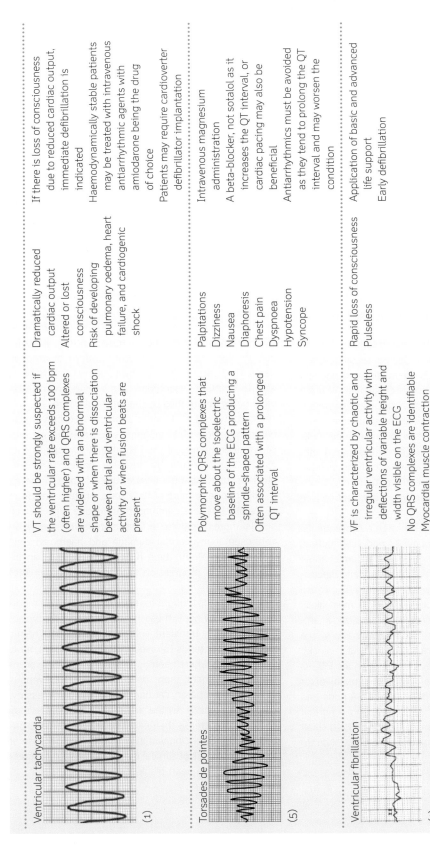

(1) Reproduced from Creed, F., & Spiers, C. (Eds.), Care of the Acutely Ill Adult: An essential guide for nurses. Oxford, UK: Oxford University Press 2010 with permission from Oxford University Press.
(2) Reproduced from Myerson, S., Choudhury, R., & Mitchell, A. (Eds.), Emergencies in Cardiology. Oxford, UK: Oxford University Press 2009 with permission from Oxford University Press.
(3) Courtesy of Mahmoud Sakr. Attribution-ShareAlike 3.0 Unported (CC BY-SA 3.0).
(4) Reproduced from Ghuran AV, Camm AJ. Ischaemic heart disease presenting as arrhythmias. Br Med Bull. 2001;59:193–210. doi: 10.1093/bmb/59.1.193 with permission from Oxford University Press.
(5) Reproduced from Thomas, J., & Monaghan, T. The cardiovascular system. In Oxford Handbook of Clinical Examination and Practical Skills. Oxford, UK: Oxford University Press 2014, with permission from Oxford University Press.
(6) Reproduced from Wilkinson, I., Raine, T., Wiles, K., Goodhart, A., Hall, C., & O'Neill, H. Oxford Handbook of Clinical Medicine. Oxford, UK: Oxford University Press 2017 with permission from Oxford University Press.

typically in the first 24 hours following myocardial infarction, accelerated IVR (heart rate 100–120 bpm) may occur. This is thought to be the result of reperfusion of ischaemic myocardial tissue. It is generally transient and well tolerated by patients.[25]

Atrioventricular (heart AV) block

In healthy people, electrical impulses produced by the SA node spread across the atria resulting in depolarization and contraction of the atrial muscle. Thereafter, impulses are conveyed via the AV node and bundle branches and result in coordinated ventricular depolarization and contraction. AV block occurs when there is a delay or failure in the conduction of electrical impulses needed to stimulate ventricular contraction. This can occur at the level of the AV node or further down the conduction system. It may be transient or permanent. The epidemiology of AV block, otherwise known as heart block, is much harder to quantify and many cases are undiagnosed until the patient presents with another, often related complaint. There are several types including first-degree, second-degree, and third-degree heart block; in addition, congenital heart block, where the incidence of congenital AV block has been reported at between 1 in 15,000 and 1 in 20,000 births.[26] For some patients, there are no symptoms and it is thought that a percentage of the population has first-degree heart block. However, for those associated with cardiovascular conditions such as coronary heart disease, heart failure, or valvular disease, the patient may be extremely symptomatic and require urgent intervention (see Chapters 6, 8, and 10).

In the acute setting, AV block may be a consequence of medicines that slow or impair AV node conduction, for example, beta-blockers, digoxin, or calcium channel blockers. Myocardial ischaemia, infarction, and electrolyte imbalances such as hyperkalaemia may also cause AV block. In inferior infarction, AV block is most likely to arise at the level of the AV node. In anterior infarction, the development of AV block is generally at the level of the AV bundle or branches (fascicular block). When assessing AV block, the PR interval on the ECG is measured. The PR interval represents the time taken for electrical impulses to travel between the SA node and the ventricles prior to ventricular contraction. A normal PR interval is between 0.12 and 0.2 seconds (3–5 small squares on the ECG). Prolongation of the PR interval indicates AV block.

First-degree AV block

In first-degree block, the PR interval is prolonged (>200 milliseconds) although the heart rate is often normal (60–100 bpm). Conduction of atrial impulses is delayed at the level of the AV node. The heart rhythm remains regular with a QRS complex following each P wave. First-degree block is generally benign and well tolerated by patients; however, in the acute context, the patient should be continuously monitored as there is a risk of progression to second- or third-degree block.

Second-degree AV block

Second-degree block has two variants, Mobitz type I (Wenckebach) and Mobitz type II AV block, each with distinctive characteristics. In Mobitz type I block there is progressive lengthening of the PR interval over several cardiac cycles prior to an atrial impulse being completely blocked at the AV node level. On the ECG, when an atrial impulse is blocked a P wave is visible but no QRS complex follows. The ventricular rate is irregular but usually follows a predictable pattern of dropped beats. The heart rate may be low to normal (40–70 bpm) with the patient's symptoms and haemodynamic stability being determined by the ventricular rate.

Mobitz type II AV block is characterized by variable non-conduction of atrial impulses. There is no preceding lengthening of the PR interval. Dropped beats may follow a regular or irregular pattern and this block occurs below the level of the AV node in the AV bundle or one or more of its distal branches. This form of AV block is less common than Mobitz type I block but is more likely to be associated with extensive anteroseptal myocardial damage and haemodynamic instability. In Mobitz type II AV block, there is an increased risk of progression to third-degree (complete) heart block.

If the cause is thought to relate to the action of medicines on the AV node, these can be stopped. This type of block is usually transient, with minimal haemodynamic impairment. It tends to resolve within a few days; however, in cases where haemodynamic compromise or instability is evident, then administration of intravenous atropine or temporary cardiac pacing may be necessary. For Mobitz type II, in the acute setting atropine may be given to increase the heart rate in symptomatic patients. Cardiac pacing will also be required because of the increased risk of clinical deterioration with progression to complete heart block or asystole.

Third-degree (complete) AV block

In complete heart block, there is effectively no transmission of electrical impulses between atria and ventricles. If a focus (or foci) near the AV node takes over as pacemaker, the resulting escape rhythm may sustain adequate ventricular contraction and cardiac output with a heart rate in the range of 40–60 bpm. If the escape rhythm originates from a location in the nodal region, then ventricular depolarization will look normal on the ECG and QRS complexes will be narrow. If the escape rhythm originates lower in the conduction system, this will be a less reliable pacemaker, with a slower heart rate. The associated QRS complexes will be broad indicating aberrant conduction through the ventricular myocardium. Complete heart block is unlikely to be well tolerated by acute patients who may develop symptomatic hypotension and cardiac pacing is likely to be required.

Decisions about whether to implant a permanent pacemaker depend on the primary cause and assessment of the patient's underlying cardiac rhythm after the acute phase of illness has passed. In acute inferior infarction, complete heart block is often transient and may resolve in the first week making permanent pacing unnecessary. Conversely, in anterior infarction, complete heart block is more likely to be persistent and to indicate substantial myocardial damage. This is associated with poorer clinical outcomes and is likely to require implantation of a permanent pacemaker.

In complete AV block with no ventricular escape rhythm, ventricular standstill (asystole) will occur and the patient will require immediate resuscitation. The ECG may show a normal regular pattern of atrial depolarizations (P waves); however, QRS complexes are absent.

Asystole

Some secondary conditions may precipitate asystole in acute illness. These conditions include hypoxia, hypovolaemia, hypothermia, hyperkalaemia or hypokalaemia, metabolic disorders, thrombosis, tension pneumothorax, cardiac tamponade, and toxins.[27] It is essential that these are excluded or treated when attempting to resuscitate an asystolic patient.

It may be possible in asystolic patients with viable myocardium to establish effective cardiac pacing via transcutaneous, transoesophageal, or endocardial routes; however, clinical outcomes in this patient group are generally very poor.[28]

Tachyarrhythmias—diagnosis, treatment, care, and prevention

Tachyarrhythmias are disturbances of heart rhythm with an inappropriately fast heart rate (>100 bpm) and are classified by their ECG morphology (shape) as narrow or broad complex, and by their origin as supraventricular or ventricular. In the acute context, patients with tachyarrhythmias are often symptomatic with varying degrees of haemodynamic instability, in some instances requiring urgent intervention. Ventricular tachyarrhythmias are an important cause of cardiac arrest and sudden cardiac death in acute cardiac patients. Persistent tachycardia is undesirable in patients with myocardial ischaemia and infarction as when the heart rate is rapid, the diastolic phase of the cardiac cycle is shortened. This has multiple negative effects including decreased time within the cardiac cycle to allow adequate atrial and ventricular filling, increased myocardial oxygen demand, and a reduction in coronary blood flow. Cumulatively, these effects reduce coronary and tissue perfusion, cardiac output, and blood pressure. Furthermore, normal compensatory mechanisms to adjust coronary blood flow in situations of increased myocardial demand are unlikely to be effective in the ACS patient (see Chapter 6).

Sinus tachycardia

Sinus tachycardia occurs in up to 30% of acute myocardial infarction patients[29] due to an increase in sympathetic nervous system activity caused by pathological stressors such as myocardial ischaemia and low cardiac output evidenced by hypotension and shock. Sinus tachycardia is commonly seen at presentation and tends to reduce as pain, nausea, and initial anxiety are relieved. However, in a proportion of patients, especially those with extensive anterior infarctions, sinus tachycardia may persist and signal significant left ventricular impairment. The occurrence of persistent or late sinus tachycardia is therefore an adverse prognostic indicator associated with substantial increases in morbidity and early mortality.[30] It is important in such patients to optimize care to limit further myocardial damage and ensure the best possible clinical outcomes. Most patients receive early beta-blockade as part of the routine management of acute myocardial infarction; however, caution is required in patients with sinus tachycardia who may have large infarctions, symptomatic hypotension, and signs of pulmonary congestion or heart failure.

Supraventricular tachycardia

SVT is sometimes referred to as 'narrow complex tachycardia', occurring when the heart rate at rest increases to over 100 bpm (see ➤ Table 7.5 at the end of the chapter for a case study example). The term groups together tachyarrhythmias that originate from abnormal foci above the level of the AV node. Unfortunately, there is a paucity of data on SVT population epidemiology,[4] with one estimate from the US, suggesting there are 89,000 new cases annually, and 570,000 patients with paroxysmal SVT. Across Europe, the incidence of SVT is approximately 35 cases per 100,000 patients with a prevalence of 2.25 cases per 1000 in the general population and females have a greater risk of paroxysmal SVT compared to males.[4] In terms of age at presentation, lone paroxysmal SVT occurs in younger people (mean age 37 years) compared to those with underlying cardiovascular disease (mean age 67 years). The younger patients also had a faster paroxysmal SVT heart rate (mean 186 vs 155 bpm) and were more likely to have presented to the emergency department with their SVT.[31]

In SVT, myocardial depolarization proceeds normally after atrial impulses are conducted to the AV node and therefore QRS complexes are usually narrow (0.04–0.12 seconds). SVT often has a rapid, regular rhythm although this may be irregular if AF or atrial flutter is present. It can, on occasions, be difficult to differentiate between SVT with aberrant ventricular conduction and VT. Symptoms can be rare (i.e. once a year) or frequently (several times a day) and often resolve without treatment after a few minutes. However, for others, their SVT can last several hours, and they may attend their local emergency department for treatment. The precipitants of SVT are related to age, sex, and associated comorbidities with two distinct subsets of patients identified—those with other cardiovascular disease and those with lone paroxysmal SVT. SVTs are also reported in pregnancy; there is limited data on incidence of arrhythmias in pregnancy, although there is some evidence that first presentations are often seen in pregnant women with no previous history of palpitations.[32]

Paroxysmal atrial tachycardia

Paroxysmal atrial tachycardia is a 'reentrant arrhythmia' resulting from the presence of abnormal electrical connections in the cardiac conduction system. This can be congenital or acquired and atrial tachycardia is particularly associated with non-ischaemic heart disease and pulmonary conditions. It is usually episodic (paroxysmal) and patients may present acutely with a rapid heart rate between 160 and 220 bpm. P waves are usually regular and identical in shape, suggesting a single point of origin, but on examination of the ECG these may be inverted on lead II, signalling an abnormal atrial origin.

If a patient with a regular narrow complex tachycardia is stable, then vagal stimulation may be successful in terminating it. This can be achieved by use of Valsalva manoeuvres or carotid sinus massage. The latter should only be attempted when the presence of carotid bruits has been excluded. If these measures are unsuccessful in terminating the arrhythmia, then adenosine may be given to try and terminate the arrhythmia. To be effective, adenosine has to be given rapidly due to its very short half-life. In more persistent and troublesome cases, antiarrhythmic medication or ablation therapy may be indicated.

Irregular narrow complex tachycardias

Irregular narrow complex tachycardias are most likely to be due to atrial flutter with variable block or to AF.

Atrial fibrillation (AF)

AF[33] is the most common arrythmia and it is thought that, worldwide, 33 million people live with this arrhythmia.[34] It is associated with irregular impulses within the atria causing the atria to fibrillate and fire irregularly at rates of between 80 and 200 bpm. There are certain conditions associated with it including hyperthyroidism, mitral valve disease, and other metabolic disorders. AF is associated with an increased risk of thromboembolic complications such as ischaemic stroke and transient ischaemic attack, complications such as heart failure, cognitive impairment, reduced quality of life, and an elevated risk of mortality. AF poses a substantial burden on the healthcare system, with AF-related hospitalizations as the main cost driver.

In 2010, approximately 33.5 million individuals globally were affected with AF, higher prevalence rates were seen in low- to middle-income countries.[34] Estimates have indicated that this number will rise tremendously and by 2050 there will be 15.9 million individuals with AF in the US alone.[35] Individuals with AF have a fivefold higher risk of stroke compared to those without AF. Moreover, AF is independently associated with increased mortality rates: a twofold increased risk of all-cause mortality in women and a 1.5-fold increase in men.[5] AF occurs due to the discharge of very high numbers of electrical impulses from multiple ectopic sites in the atria of the heart. No discernible P waves are visible on the ECG and as high numbers of atrial impulses continually bombard the AV node, it becomes refractory to further stimulation and impulses are variably conveyed to the ventricular system. The net effect is an irregularly, irregular cardiac rhythm often associated with a rapid heart rate. In ACS, new-onset AF commonly occurs in the first 72 hours and is an important prognostic indicator often associated with severe damage to the left ventricle and heart failure leading to increased short- and longer-term mortality.[36]

AF is considered a progressive condition which may start with short episodes that in due course may occur more frequently and episodes may be more persistent. Factors such as ageing and cardiovascular conditions such as hypertension and diabetes, as well as exposure to risk factors such as obesity, induce structural and electrical remodelling in the atria of the heart, predisposing to the development or worsening of AF. Structural remodelling leads to electrical dissociation, which favours the process of reentry. AF episodes often initiate by rapid focal activity around the pulmonary veins, but can also be induced by reentrant wavefronts. AF-induced electrical remodelling refers to the fact that the atrial myocardium responds to a high rate of the fibrillation atria, by shortening the atrial refractoriness and atrial action potential. Due to the related increased repolarization, AF keeps itself alive, which has been expressed as 'AF begets AF'.[37]

Types of AF

AF is a chronic condition, which commences in short episodes, advancing to longer and more recurrent episodes. If untreated, it is likely that AF will result in a permanent arrhythmia. AF may be found in patients with severe symptoms and limited in their daily activities as well as patients being completely asymptomatic (see ➤ Table 7.4 at the end of the chapter for a case study example). Based on the presentation, duration, and termination of the arrhythmia, the following types of AF have been identified:

- *First diagnosed AF*: has not been diagnosed before, evidence for the arrhythmia is recorded on ECG.
- *Paroxysmal AF*: self-terminating AF, mostly within 48 hours, although some episodes may last for up to 7 days. Note: episodes that are converted within 7 days should be considered paroxysmal.[5]
- *Persistent AF*: AF continuing longer than 7 days, including episodes that have been terminated by cardioversion after at least 7 days.
- *Permanent AF*: AF that is accepted by the patient and the treating physician. This means that the aim to achieve sinus rhythm is abandoned and a rate control strategy is pursued, to prevent potential complications and to reduce symptoms.

Table 7.4 CHA_2DS_2-VASc score and individual determinants

CHA_2DS_2-VASc risk factor	Points
Congestive heart failure Signs/symptoms of heart failure or objective evidence of reduced left ventricular ejection fraction	+1
Hypertension Resting blood pressure > 140/90 mmHg on at least two occasions or current antihypertensive treatment	+1
Age 75 years or older	+2
Diabetes mellitus Fasting glucose >125 mg/dL (7 mmol/L) or treatment with oral hypoglycaemic agent and/or insulin	+1
Previous stroke, Transient Ischaemic Attack, or Thromboembolism	+2
Vascular disease Previous myocardial infarction, peripheral artery disease, or aortic plaque	+1
Age 65–74 years	+1
Sex category (female)	+1

Kirchhof P, Benussi S, Kotecha D, et al. 2016 ESC Guidelines for the management of atrial fibrillation developed in collaboration with EACTS. Eur J Cardiothorac Surg. 2016 Nov;50(5):e1–e88. doi: 10.1093/ejcts/ezw313.

Thromboembolic complications

AF is associated with an increased risk of thromboembolic complications such as stroke or transient ischaemic attack. It is therefore crucial to determine the available risk factors that may elevate the risk of stroke in individuals with AF and calculate the yearly risk of stroke accordingly, in order to initiate appropriate stroke prevention (Table 7.4).

AF diagnosis

At the initial assessment, comprehensive medical evaluation is warranted and includes the assessment of medical history and concomitant conditions, as well as clinical examination. In symptomatic patients with suspected AF, the arrhythmia needs to be documented via a 12-lead

ECG, which is considered the gold standard to confirm AF diagnosis, demonstrating an irregular ventricular rate and absence of discernible P waves. Prolonged monitoring via Holter recording (24-hour or 7-day period) or implanted loop recorder in certain cases, aims to capture heart rate and rhythm and any irregularities. A transthoracic echocardiogram is recommended in all patients with AF to identify structural diseases such as valvular disease, and assess left ventricular size and function and other parameters of the heart. An exercise stress test should take place in those patients with symptoms of myocardial ischaemia, testing the cardiac capacity in responding to exercise. Kidney and thyroid function, serum electrolytes, and a full blood count should be evaluated.[5]

Silent AF and screening

Before the diagnosis of AF is set, patients may have symptoms that trigger screening for an irregular heart rhythm. However, many patients will be asymptomatic, meaning an absence of symptoms or complaints. Silent or undetected AF is common, especially in the elderly[38] and may lead to disabling consequences such as stroke or mortality. Recording of an ECG is considered an effective method to document AF,[39] although in cases of paroxysmal episodes this may not be effective. However, novel technology for prolonged monitoring or screening is evolving. Nevertheless, detection of AF is crucial in order to prevent worsening of the arrhythmia and prevention of complications. Therefore, opportunistic screening is recommended in patients over 65 years of age, by pulse taking or an ECG.[5] Once the recording of AF on an ECG has been established, the diagnosis of AF can be confirmed.

Wearables for detection of AF

The proportion of incident AF yielded by opportunistic screening is relatively low, and paroxysmal AF is often missed. The Apple watch, which was recently evaluated in the Apple Heart Study, demonstrated that wearable technology can safely identify heart rate irregularities confirmed to be AF.[40] Such devices can have an important role in the detection and management of AF and prevention of complications such as stroke but further research is needed on their efficacy. However, a 12-lead ECG should still be in place to confirm the findings and is the cornerstone in commencing AF treatment.[41]

Treatment/management

The management of AF is complex and should cover five treatment domains, as outlined in ➤ **Fig. 7.3**:[33,42]

1. *In the acute phase, it is crucial to apply rate and/or rhythm control strategies* aiming to improve symptoms and restore haemodynamic stability. A combination of these strategies may apply. In the acute setting, the preferred pharmacological rate control strategy includes beta-blockers and diltiazem or verapamil.[43,44] Acute restoration of sinus rhythm can be achieved with electrical or pharmacological cardioversion. Pharmacological cardioversion may be effective in 50% of cases and does not require fasting or sedation.[45] Electrical cardioversion has demonstrated better results (e.g. restoration of sinus rhythm and less hospitalization)[46,47] and is recommended over pharmacological cardioversion in the acute setting. Agents such as flecainide or propafenone are effective but cannot be used in patients with structural heart disease. Alternatively, ibutilide, vernakalant (in patients with mild heart failure), or amiodarone may be considered. Patient characteristics and underlying conditions will guide the choice of medication.
2. *Identification and treatment of precipitating factors* is necessary to reduce the cardiovascular risk profile and associated AF risk burden. These may include underlying cardiovascular conditions as well as modifiable risk factors. Exposure to these risk factors may lead to the development or worsening of AF and their management should be integrated in the AF management approach. The attention on obesity as a risk factor for AF[42] and potentially for ischaemic stroke, thromboembolism, and death in patients with AF[48] has increased significantly over time. Specialized risk factor clinics with a focus on intensive weight reduction alongside management of other risk factors has demonstrated significant reduction of AF recurrences and symptom burden.[49,50] Moreover, long-term sustained weight reduction is associated with significantly improved maintenance of sinus rhythm.[51] It is therefore crucial that weight loss, as well as management of other risk factors in obese patients with AF, should be considered as an integral part of AF management.[5]
3. *Assessment of stroke risk and determine the necessity to initiate oral anticoagulation therapy* to prevent thromboembolic complications. It is recommended that this assessment is guided by the CHA_2DS_2-VASc score (➤ **Table. 7.4**),[52] which is a point system to determine the yearly risk of stroke in patients with AF. The score assesses the presence of conditions which increase the risk of stroke in patients with AF, such as congestive heart failure (1 point); hypertension (1 point); age 65–74 years (1 point) or above 75 years (2 points); diabetes mellitus (1 point); previous stroke, transient ischaemic attack (TIA), or thromboembolism (2 points); vascular disease (1 point); and female

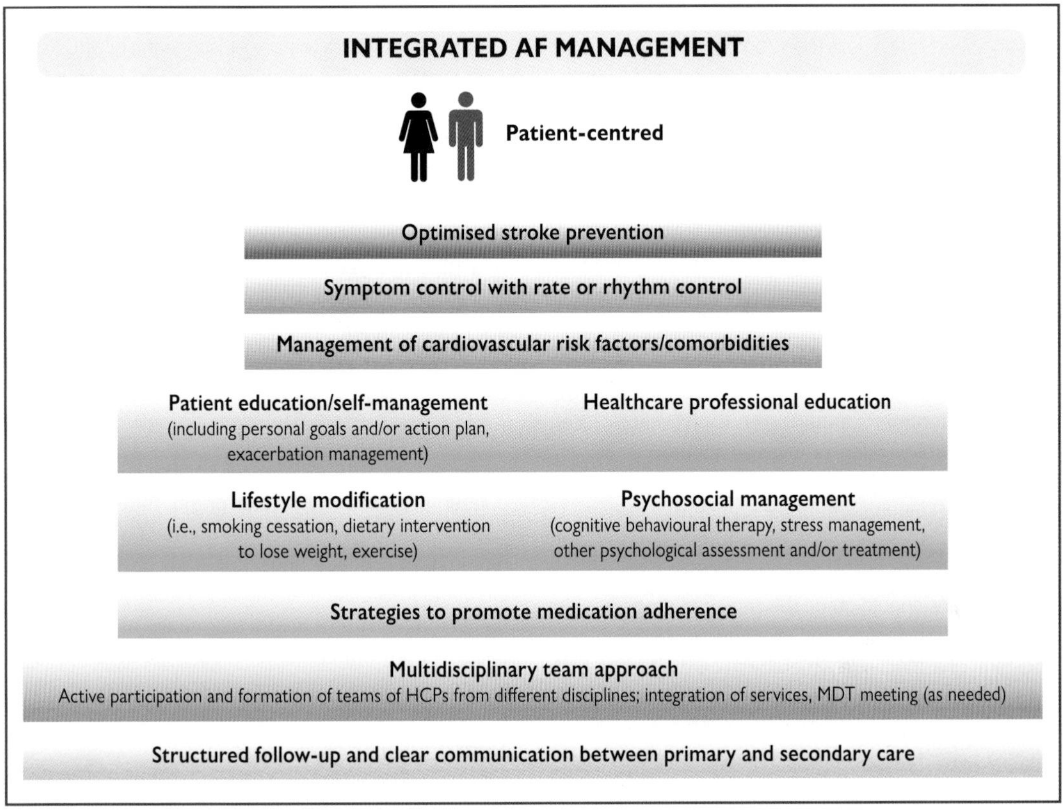

Fig. 7.3 Components of integrated AF management. AF = atrial fibrillation; HCP = healthcare professional;MDT = multidisciplinary team.

Hindricks G, Potpara T, Dagres N, et al; ESC Scientific Document Group. 2020 ESC Guidelines for the diagnosis and management of atrial fibrillation developed in collaboration with the European Association for Cardio-Thoracic Surgery (EACTS): The Task Force for the diagnosis and management of atrial fibrillation of the European Society of Cardiology (ESC) Developed with the special contribution of the European Heart Rhythm Association (EHRA) of the ESC. Eur Heart J. 2021 Feb 1;42(5):373–498. doi: 10.1093/eurheartj/ehaa612. © The European Society of Cardiology. Reprinted by permission of Oxford University Press.

sex (1 point). Patients without stroke risk factors (CHA_2DS_2-VASc score = 0), do not need anticoagulant therapy. As a class I recommendation, men and women with 2 or more points on the score need to be treated with oral anticoagulation therapy. In those patients with only 1 point on the score, the class IIa recommendation is that oral anticoagulation should be considered, taking contraindications and patient preferences into account. Even though female sex yields a CHA_2DS_2-VASc score of 1, in the absence of additional stroke risk factors, this does not qualify for anticoagulation therapy to be considered.[5] Anticoagulation therapy can be provided by means of a vitamin K antagonist (VKA) which requires monitoring of the international normalized ratio, or a non-vitamin K antagonist oral anticoagulant (NOAC). Large trials have demonstrated safety and effectiveness of the NOACs and there is a clear preference in the use of NOACs compared to VKAs, supported by ESC guidelines[5] (see also Chapter 12).

4. *Evaluation of the heart rate to consider a rate control strategy*, which aims to reduce the heart rate to improve symptoms and preserve left ventricular function. Rate control is an essential aspect of AF management to improve AF-related symptoms without applying a rhythm control strategy. The optimal heart rate target in patients with AF remains variable. The Rate Control Efficacy in Permanent AF (RACE II) study compared patients with a strict heart rate target of less than 80 bpm at rest, or a lenient heart rate of less than 110 bpm, demonstrating no significant differences in a composite outcome of cardiovascular mortality or

clinical conditions requiring hospitalization.[53] Therefore, a resting heart rate of less than 100 bpm can be considered as an appropriate heart rate target in a rate control strategy. In general, beta-blockers, digoxin, diltiazem, or verapamil are recommended medications to apply a rate control strategy in patients with AF with a left ventricular ejection fraction (LVEF) greater than 40%. Given that diltiazem and verapamil may have a negative inotropic effect in patients with heart failure, beta-blockers and digitalis are recommended in patients with AF with LVEF less than 40%.[5]

5. *Assessment of AF-related symptoms and determination of the need for a rhythm control strategy* by means of long-term antiarrhythmic pharmacological treatment, cardioversion, or invasive ablation procedures. Applying a rhythm control strategy aims to improve AF-related symptoms and to maintain sinus rhythm. A rigorous assessment of underlying cardiovascular conditions is important and safety considerations should guide the choice of drug. The spectrum of a rhythm control strategy ranges from long-term pharmaceutical therapy to cardioversion and invasive ablation procedures. In some cases, a 'pill-in-the-pocket approach' will be applied. This means that selected patients with infrequent paroxysmal episodes of symptomatic AF will be instructed to self-administer a single dose of flecainide or propafenone to restore sinus rhythm. This approach has been proven effective, is practical, and may be more convenient for patients.[54] In general, the following recommendations should be considered when applying a long-term rhythm control strategy in patients with AF[5]:
   - Aim to improve symptoms, and restore and maintain sinus rhythm. In patients with permanent AF (i.e. accepted AF), the priority is a rate control strategy and no longer to achieve sinus rhythm.
   - Cardioversion of AF is recommended in symptomatic patients with persistent or long-standing persistent AF and as part of a rhythm control strategy.
   - The choice between electrical and pharmaceutical cardioversion should be guided by clinical aspects such as haemodynamic instability, as well as patient and physician preferences.
   - In haemodynamically unstable patients, electrical cardioversion is recommended to restore cardiac output.
   - In patients without a history of ischaemic or structural heart disease, pharmacological cardioversion by means of flecainide, propafenone, or vernakalant is recommended. However, in those patients with a history of ischaemic or structural heart disease, amiodarone is the recommended agent for cardioversion of AF.
   - The choice of an antiarrhythmic drug requires careful evaluation of underlying cardiovascular conditions, as well as potential side effects, patient preferences, and symptom burden.
   - Structured evaluation of patients on antiarrhythmic drugs should be in place to confirm their suitability for treatment.

Broad complex tachycardia

As noted previously, broad complex tachycardias can occur due to SVT or AF with aberrant ventricular conduction or from a ventricular origin. In order to differentiate between these, careful analysis of a 12-lead ECG is required. In acute settings, if there is obvious and severe circulatory collapse then management should proceed on the assumption of a ventricular cause as the risk to the patient of an untreated ventricular tachycardia is much greater.

Ventricular tachycardia (VT)

Ventricular tachyarrhythmias are among the most life-threatening in acute cardiac patients and often occur early following ACS onset. VT occurs when three or more ventricular extra systoles occur consecutively. VT may be intermittent or sustained and is caused by an ectopic focus in the left or right ventricle discharging electrical impulses at a rate in the range of 120–250 bpm independently of the normal conduction system. In the acute cardiac patient, VT may arise from a single area of enhanced electrical automaticity thereby producing abnormal but identical QRS complexes (monomorphic VT) or from several areas of ectopic activity when consecutive QRS complexes will look different (polymorphic VT). ECG criteria for determining VT are not absolute but it should be strongly suspected if the ventricular rate exceeds 100 bpm (often higher) and QRS complexes are widened with an abnormal shape or when there is dissociation between atrial and ventricular activity or when fusion beats are present. Fusion beats occur when there is a collision between antegrade atrial and retrograde ventricular depolarization. In instances of very rapid ventricular rates, there are multiple risks to patients including dramatically reduced cardiac output, with altered or loss of consciousness and potential deterioration to VF. A modest reduction in cardiac output and coronary blood flow may be tolerated in the short term, but the risk of developing pulmonary oedema, heart failure, and cardiogenic shock are greatly increased.

Acute management of VT requires identification and management of reversible causes; however, if there is loss of consciousness due to reduced cardiac output, immediate defibrillation is indicated. Patients with sustained VT who are haemodynamically stable may be treated with intravenous antiarrhythmic agents with amiodarone being the drug of choice. It is also important to assess and correct any detectable electrolyte abnormalities including hypokalaemia (low serum potassium) and hypomagnesaemia (low serum magnesium) in this patient group. If sinus rhythm is not restored, synchronized cardioversion or overdrive pacing may be attempted. Patients who remain at high risk of further ventricular arrhythmias may also require pharmacological maintenance therapy and cardioverter defibrillator implantation.

Ventricular fibrillation (VF)

VF causes cardiac arrest and untreated will lead to death. VF is characterized by chaotic and irregular ventricular activity with deflections of variable height and width visible on the ECG. No QRS complexes are identifiable. In the absence of coordinated ventricular depolarization, myocardial muscle contraction is absent and cardiac output ceases with a resulting rapid loss of consciousness. VF most commonly occurs in the early hours following myocardial infarction and is thought to be the primary mechanism of pre-hospital sudden cardiac death in patients with ACS. VF may be preceded by an episode of VT or precipitated by the occurrence of ventricular ectopic beats during the repolarization phase of the cardiac cycle ('R on T' ectopic). The probability of a successful clinical outcome in VF is enhanced by early recognition, effective application of basic and advanced life support, and early defibrillation.

Torsade de pointes

Torsade de pointes or 'twisting of the points' is a recognized variant of VT. It is characterized by a distinctive ECG pattern in which polymorphic QRS complexes that move about the isoelectric baseline of the ECG produce a spindle-shaped pattern. This arrhythmia, which can be congenital or acquired, is often associated with a prolonged QT interval. In the acute context, this may be caused by myocardial ischaemia or infarction and can result in loss of consciousness and progression to VF with a risk of death.

Management includes intravenous magnesium administration. This is often effective in terminating the arrhythmia. A beta-blocker (but not sotalol as it increases the QT interval) or cardiac pacing may also be beneficial.[55] Antiarrhythmics must be avoided as they tend to prolong the QT interval and may worsen the condition.

Patient experience of living with an arrhythmia

While the diagnosis and treatment of cardiac arrhythmia is an acute priority, it is crucial that individualized patient experiences of living with an arrhythmia are understood by healthcare professionals, as well as being considered when determining a treatment/management plan. The importance of patient- and family-centred care has been highlighted in ESC Guidelines, particularly in patients with ventricular arrhythmias who are at risk of sudden cardiac death.[56] In general, arrhythmias have a significant psychosocial impact on patients, affecting many facets of a normal life—such as sporting activities,[57] the ability to drive,[58] and sleep quality.[59] Additionally, such conditions also often have a negative impact on sexual relations, with cardiac patients frequently reporting at least one sexual problem after a cardiac event.[60] Such problems are commonly associated with being male,[60] possibly due to erectile dysfunction—which was reported by patients with an implantable cardioverter defibrillator (ICD) as an area of significant concern, along with lack of interest in sex and an overprotective partner.[61] Sexual issues may also be linked to body image concerns, which are particularly common in female patients with an ICD under the age of 50 years.[62] Many of the issues discussed here are prevalent in patients with an ICD, which is likely linked to the shock-related anxiety and fear[63] that are often experienced in this population (see Chapter 10 and Chapter 14). These sections also discuss further psychosocial effects of having an ICD and the issues surrounding deactivation discussions. Taking patients with AF as a further example, a qualitative study of 25 patients showed these individuals to suffer both discomfort and limitations in their daily life.[64] Specifically, patients reported impacts including anxiety, emotional concerns, that symptoms were affected by distress/exertion, and a lack of knowledge and security regarding AF.

Patient experience can be improved by nursing interventions that focus on how the patient's arrhythmia impacts their everyday life and addressing any potential concerns; as well as through initiatives such as multimedia educational resources[65] and nurse-led clinics. Taking AF clinics as an example, these have been shown to be cost-effective, reduce mortality rates, and improve medication adherence.[66] However, more research into patient perspectives of these clinics is necessary, as findings related to patient knowledge and satisfaction were mixed.[66]

Individualized and more systematic efforts to improve patient knowledge, ability to manage, and overall experience with their arrythmia are critical. For example, patients with AF who had high illness acceptance levels were shown to have significantly better quality of life.[67] Later in this chapter, an example of a patient-centred and integrated approach to follow-up and outpatient care for patients with AF is provided (see 'Example—follow-up and outpatient care of patients with atrial fibrillation'). Interestingly, the aforementioned study also showed female sex to be a predictor of worse quality of life in AF,[67] while women have also been shown to delay access to medical help after a cardiac event when compared to men[68] and be more psychosocially impacted by having an ICD.[69] These issues, along with the previously mentioned body image concerns in female patients with an ICD, may indicate that the efforts of healthcare providers need to be tailored based on sex—as well as being specific to each individual patient.

Catheter ablation

For SVTs and AF, catheter ablation may be beneficial. In SVT, ablating part of the conduction pathway by radiofrequency waves or, less frequently, freezing, cryoablation, has been shown to reduce symptoms and stop (i.e. ablate) the rhythm disturbance.[70] However, the efficacy of ablation varies with rates for SVT ablation showing very modest long-term clinical success ranging from 23% to 83%.[4]

In the case of AF, ablation aims to isolate the pulmonary veins from the body of the left atrium. This is done to prevent the electrical signals that originate between the entrance of the pulmonary vein and the left atrium triggering AF and producing a line of scar around each vein and thus reducing frequency of AF. The procedure is often referred to as pulmonary vein isolation and the efficacy of the procedure is mixed, with some patients experiencing symptoms within a few months of their procedure and sometimes requiring repeat procedures.[71] One study found the earlier patients reported symptoms after the procedure, the greater the likelihood that the procedure had not been successful.[72] With ventricular disturbances, radiofrequency ablation is the method used, especially in those with structural heart disease such as heart failure and cardiomyopathy.[73] From a nursing perspective, it is important that the patient is fully aware of the variable success rate of the procedure and they may require lifelong medication for their AF.

Temporary cardiac pacing

When the conduction system of the heart fails at the level of the SA node, sites lower in the conduction system may assume the role of pacemaker. Cardiac rhythms arising from sites other than the SA node have slower heart rates and are less reliable as pacemakers. Cardiac pacemakers can be inserted to treat symptomatic bradycardia (heart rate <40 bpm) or heart block that has resulted in a low systolic blood pressure or when there is a risk of ventricular asystole. The risk of asystole is greatly increased in patients with second-degree (Mobitz type II) or complete heart block. Temporary cardiac pacing requires direct electrical stimulation of the myocardium by artificial means. This is usually achieved by placement of an endocardial lead (electrode) introduced percutaneously via a large central vein such as the right internal jugular, right subclavian, or femoral vein. The lead is advanced, under continuous X-ray screening, into the right atrium and across the tricuspid valve into the right ventricular apex. After placement the lead is connected to an external pulse generator (battery) in order to stimulate myocardial contraction and control the heart rate. Following positioning, the location and stability of the pacing lead is confirmed by asking the patient to take deep breaths or cough and by X-ray. The threshold voltage required to stimulate myocardial depolarization (capture) is also confirmed before setting the pacing device to a suitable level in excess of the minimum voltage required. During the period that a patient is pacemaker dependent, the underlying heart rate and rhythm and capture threshold must be regularly reviewed.

Endocardial pacing requires specialist expertise and equipment and if this is not immediately available, and the clinical need is pressing, a transcutaneous pacing device may be utilized as a bridge measure. This non-invasive method of pacing is most suitable when used as an emergency treatment until endocardial pacing can be established. It applies a pacing stimulus to the heart directly via electrodes placed on the thoracic wall. Although less reliable than endocardial pacing, this intervention offers a rapidly deployable option for non-specialists that may be sufficient to maintain an adequate circulation until endocardial pacing can be established. The main disadvantage of transcutaneous pacing is the discomfort that may be experienced by alert patients who may consequently require a sedation.

Permanent cardiac pacing

If a patient is at continuing risk of life-threatening arrhythmias, or their underlying heart rhythm is inadequate to maintain an effective circulation, or symptoms persist beyond the acute phase of cardiac illness, then a permanent pacemaker is required. This process, requiring a local anaesthetic, places an endocardial pacing lead(s) via the venous system and connects this/these to a pulse generator (battery) located in a subcutaneous pouch created in the chest wall.

Implantable cardioverter defibrillators (ICD)

Type of device

ICDs have been used in patients for more than 30 years. The efficiency of the ICD has been shown superior to medical treatment, with an early meta-analysis demonstrating a reduction in arrhythmic mortality of 50%. In the early era, the ICD was placed in the abdomen and implanted surgically via thoracotomy with epicardial leads fixed to the ventricles. Later, a complete transvenous system was introduced, and is still the standard. The main component of the ICD system is a defibrillation lead, advanced into the right ventricle over either the cephalic vein or the subclavian vein, and connected to the device that is placed subcutaneously in the left pectoral region. The ICD consists of the battery and an electronic system detecting and storing arrhythmia episodes, and delivering therapy. Efficacy testing of the device during the implantation procedure was standard practice for many years, but availability of high-energy devices in parallel with technical developments changed clinical practice and this is now rarely done.[74] A recent development is a completely subcutaneously implantable ICD system which consists of a subcutaneous device connected to a subcutaneous lead that is placed along the left side of the sternum. One of the main advantages of the subcutaneous ICD system is the prevention of device-related endocarditis (see Chapter 8) that causes significant complications in patients with the conventional transvenous ICD systems. However, the subcutaneous device is not suitable for patients who require bradycardia pacing, patients who need cardiac resynchronization therapy, or patients suffering from tachyarrhythmia that can be easily terminated by antitachycardia pacing.[55] A wearable external defibrillator has also been developed consisting of electrode pads, leads, and a defibrillator attached to a vest. This wearable device may be considered as a bridge to implantation or in patients with poor left ventricular systolic function who are at risk of sudden cardiac death for a limited period, but who are not candidates for an ICD. For patients with LVEF less than 35% and left bundle branch block, cardiac resynchronization is indicated provided there has been at least 3 months of optimal pharmacological therapy.[55] The cardiac resynchronization therapy defibrillator has leads placed in the right atrium and ventricle and in the left ventricle through the coronary sinus vein. The device is programmed to treat heart failure by synchronizing the function of the left and right ventricles and act on ventricular arrhythmias (see Chapter 10).

Indications

Patients are treated with an ICD for the prevention of sudden cardiac death on two main indications:

- Primary prevention: in individuals who are at risk of but have not yet had an episode of sustained VT, VF, or resuscitated cardiac arrest.
- Secondary prevention: individuals who have survived a prior sudden cardiac arrest or patients with haemodynamically not tolerated or recurrent sustained VT after myocardial infarction.

ICD therapy is also recommended in patients with symptomatic heart failure (New York Heart Association class II–III) and LVEF less than 35% after more than 3 months of optimal medical therapy.

Types of therapy

The ICD can be programmed to a whole range of therapies depending on the detected heart rates and cycle length. Cardiac defibrillation aims to return abnormally fast or disorganized rhythm with an electric shock. A shock is applied when very fast heart rates are detected, while antitachycardia pacing is administered first in slower VT in order to avoid shock if possible. A vast number of VTs are non-sustained and terminated spontaneously. The ICD also has a brady pacing function. ICDs may cause complications including inappropriate shocks (20%), lead failure (17%), and, as mentioned, device-related infection (6%).[75] Often patients with an ICD are treated with medications in order to minimize both appropriate and inappropriate ICD therapy. In secondary prevention (patients post myocardial infarction and in patients with heart failure), amiodarone reduces the occurrence of ventricular arrhythmias.[55,76] Patients with an ICD have significantly reduced ICD interventions when prescribed amiodarone, particularly when combined with beta-blockers.[55] However, nurses should be knowledgeable about the side effects of both these drugs, and amiodarone in particular (see Chapter 12). Follow-up of patients is mandatory and has traditionally been performed in the outpatient clinic at regular intervals. However, increasingly patients are followed up by remote monitoring. This is convenient for patients in rural areas, and also has a health economic advantage. The face-to-face meeting with the cardiologist and nurse is still important, and remote monitoring should be coupled with the possibility of telephone contact.

Restrictions

Arrhythmias can affect many areas in the lives of patients and families, such as ability to drive, intimate relations, sleep quality, body image concerns (particularly in younger women), and participation in organized sports (particularly in children and adolescents).[55] Some of these areas are affected by ICD therapy as well. The ICD device is built with protective shields so that the majority of items will not affect the device. However, electromagnetic fields may temporarily cause disturbances, depending on the distance to the ICD and strength of the electromagnetic field. Items not in good working order may also cause electrical current into the body. If the patient is feeling dizzy, light-headed, has a change in heart rate, or receives a shock while using a device, he or she should be advised to move away from it. Any temporary effect is unlikely to cause reprogramming or damage to the ICD, but the specialist centre should be contacted in due course (or immediately if symptoms persist). Special considerations should be made regarding certain household items (induction hob on a cooker/stove, electronic weighing scales, metal detectors, electric fence), tools (boat engines, gasoline powered tools, welding equipment, jumper cables), and communication equipment (amateur radio/walkie talkie), and a recommended distance of 30 cm should be kept. Items with a minimal risk, but which should be kept at a distance of at least 15 cm, include mobile phones, tablets, wireless communication devices, electric drills, hedge trimmers, hair dryers, electric shavers, toothbrush charging bases, and magnets in the wheels of exercise bikes. An exhaustive list can be obtained from the ICD manufacturer. Anti-theft detectors and airport security systems are most likely safe if the person walks normally through and does not stop and linger. Handheld wands should not be held over the device. Patients should be advised to carry their ICD identification card on their person. Certain medical procedures can also affect the ICD. Patients should be advised to inform their treating physician or dentist that they have an ICD. Modern ICD devices are compatible with magnetic resonance imaging procedures under certain conditions and patients can safely undergo magnetic resonance imaging scans. Transcutaneous electrical nerve stimulation and therapeutic ultrasound (often performed by physiotherapists), radiation therapy, and external defibrillation are acceptable with precautions and distance to the ICD. In order to maximize the derived benefit of the ICD, these issues need to be addressed in the care and counselling of patients. Importantly, the ICD-related information should be tailored to the needs of the patient taking age, sex, and comorbidities into consideration.

Surgical procedures

In the case of tachyarrhythmias with underlying structural heart disease, surgical ablation is beneficial. It is usually undertaken on patients who need to have cardiac surgery for other pathologies, such as valve replacement/repair, and therefore the procedure can be done as one operation. It is commonly known as the maze procedure.[77] In terms of AF, the biatrial Cox–Maze procedure has an approximately 90% success rates for all types of AF.[78] The main risk factor associated with surgical procedures is stroke but a recent long-term follow-up of the Maze procedure reported good outcomes for patients with reduced AF burden and a low incidence of stroke.[79]

Evaluation, discharge home, and follow-up

Example—follow-up and outpatient care of patients with atrial fibrillation

In most patients, regular follow-up is needed to ensure continued management and should warrant the implementation and/or modification of the initial, integrated management plan. A structured follow-up implies review on a regular basis, in particular when initiating or adjusting pharmacotherapeutic therapy, in order to monitor adherence, side effects, and adverse effects. Also, continuous patient education as well as coordination of care and communication among the different care providers involved, is crucial. An integrated approach to manage the care for AF[33] patients has demonstrated significant improvements in clinical outcomes[80] and is the recommended AF management approach by international guidelines.[42,81] Such an integrated care approach consists of four major fundamentals[42]:

1. *Patient-centred care*: patients should be placed in a central role in their care process and should be actively involved in decision-making. Continuous patient education covering aspects such as AF as a condition, symptom recognition, potential complications, and treatment options, is crucial and aims to empower patients to undertake self-management and lifestyle activities which may result in improved adherence and willingness to be involved in shared/informed decision-making.
2. *Multidisciplinary team approach*: the management of AF has become complex and a multidisciplinary AF team approach (e.g. specialized AF-Clinic) may be warranted rather than the delivery of care by one single healthcare professional alone. Such an approach encourages integration and collaboration between primary and secondary healthcare services,

and creates important opportunities for nurses and allied health professionals in educating patients and coordinating care, while closely collaborating with a medical specialist in an interdisciplinary way.

3. *Technology tools*: smart technology tools can be used to provide patient education and support self-management and therapy adherence, but also to support decision-making in the treatment team. Such tools have the potential to improve communication within the AF team as well as to enhance the delivery of evidence-based care and consequently improve outcomes.[33] Examples may include web-based interfaces, smartphone technology, as well as computerized tools (see also Chapter 11 and Chapter 13).
4. *Comprehensive management and access to all treatment options*: comprehensive treatment is required in which all facets of AF management (e.g. rate and rhythm control, prevention of thromboembolic complications, risk factor management, and lifestyle modification) will be covered and a diversity of specialists should be involved. Complex cases, such as patients requiring complex invasive procedures, or those patients with recurrent bleeding, could be underpinned by a dedicated AF Heart Team.[82]

Stroke prevention in atrial fibrillation

To determine the yearly risk of stroke in patients with AF, it is recommended to follow a risk stratification scheme such as the CHA_2DS_2-VASc score (see 'Treatment/management' in the 'Atrial fibrillation' section of this chapter and ➤ **Table. 7.4**). The ESC Guidelines for the management of AF provide clear recommendations on when anticoagulation should be administered.

Vitamin K antagonists and non-vitamin K antagonist oral anticoagulants

The first anticoagulants used in the prevention of thromboembolic complications in the management of AF were warfarin and other VKAs. These anticoagulants have demonstrated positive effects in reducing thromboembolic risk and complications. VKAs have a narrow therapeutic interval, which requires patients to be regularly monitored and dose adjustments to achieve an adequate time in therapeutic range.[5] Also, these are currently the only anticoagulation treatment in patients with AF with mechanical heart valve prosthesis and mitral valve disease.[83]

More recently, NOACs have been introduced (also see Chapter 8 and Chapter 12). Although these products have a shorter half-life compared to VKAs (in some cases a twice-daily dose is required), they have a predictable effect and regular monitoring is not required. Therefore, strict adherence to the prescribed treatment regimen is crucial. Caution is required in patients with chronic kidney disease and application of adjusted doses may be required. The NOACs include the direct thrombin inhibitor dabigatran and the factor Xa inhibitors apixaban, edoxaban, and rivaroxaban. Large phase III trials have been performed and demonstrated safety and effectiveness in terms of important clinical endpoints such as mortality, stroke or systemic embolism, and major bleeding.[84–87]

Antiplatelets

Antiplatelet (aspirin) cannot be used as an alternative to oral anticoagulants. Monotherapy is not recommended for stroke prevention in AF management nor as an addition to VKAs or NOACs.[5] Large trials have demonstrated better effects in terms of preventing strokes compared to single or dual antiplatelet therapy (i.e. aspirin and clopidogrel).[88] Moreover, antiplatelet therapy carries a greater risk of bleeding.[89] See Chapter 12.

Alternative treatment approaches

Left atrial appendage occlusion or exclusion may be considered for stroke prevention in those patients with contraindications to long-term oral anticoagulation therapy.[33] These procedures may be considered in patients with AF undergoing cardiac surgery and the procedure can be performed simultaneously. The Watchman device has been compared to warfarin and demonstrated non-inferiority for the prevention of stroke.[90]

Combined antithrombotic and antiplatelet therapy after a cardiac ischaemic event

Careful consideration of antithrombotic therapy is required in patients with AF suffering a myocardial infarction. Aspects such as the stroke risk, bleeding risk, and risk of ACS should be included in the consideration, given that co-prescription of anticoagulation and antiplatelet therapy increases the risk of major haemorrhage.[91] The ESC Guidelines[42] provide the following recommendations in patients with AF at risk of stroke to prevent recurrent coronary and cerebral ischaemic events (➤ **Fig. 7.4** and ➤ **Fig. 7.5**):

- After elective coronary stenting for stable coronary artery disease, combination triple therapy with aspirin, clopidogrel, and an anticoagulant should be considered for 1 month.
- After an ACS with stent implantation, combination triple therapy with aspirin, clopidogrel, and an oral anticoagulant should be considered for 1–6 months.

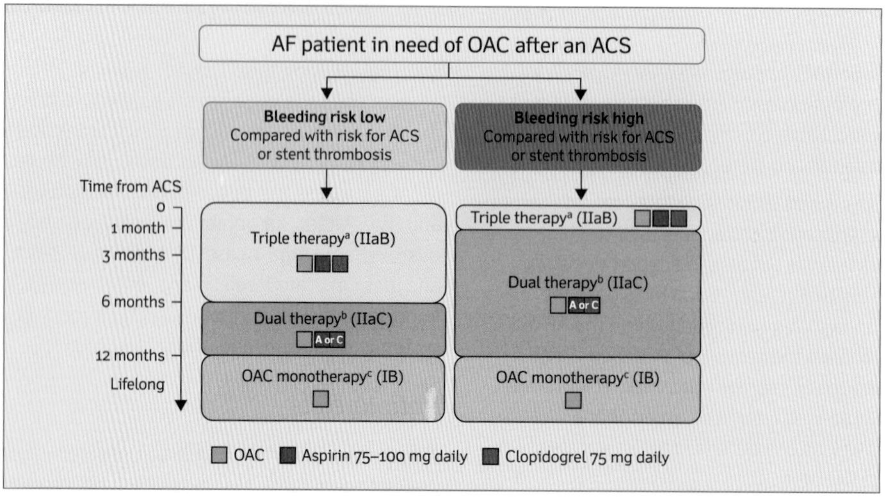

ACS = acute coronary syndrome; AF = atrial fibrillation; OAC = oral anticoagulation (using vitamin K antagonists or non-vitamin K antagonist oral anticoagulants);
PCI = percutaneous coronary intervention.
[a]Dual therapy with OAC and aspirin or clopidogrel may be considered in selected patients, especially those not receiving a stent or patients at a longer time from the index event.
[b]OAC plus single antiplatelet.
[c]Dual therapy with OAC and an antiplatelet agent (aspirin or clopidogrel) may be considered in patients at high risk of coronary events.

Fig. 7.4 Antithrombotic therapy after an acute coronary syndrome in patients with AF requiring oral anticoagulation.
Kirchhof P, Benussi S, Kotecha D, et al. 2016 ESC Guidelines for the management of atrial fibrillation developed in collaboration with EACTS. Eur J Cardiothorac Surg. 2016 Nov;50(5):e1–e88. doi: 10.1093/ejcts/ezw313. © The European Society of Cardiology. Reprinted by permission of Oxford University Press.

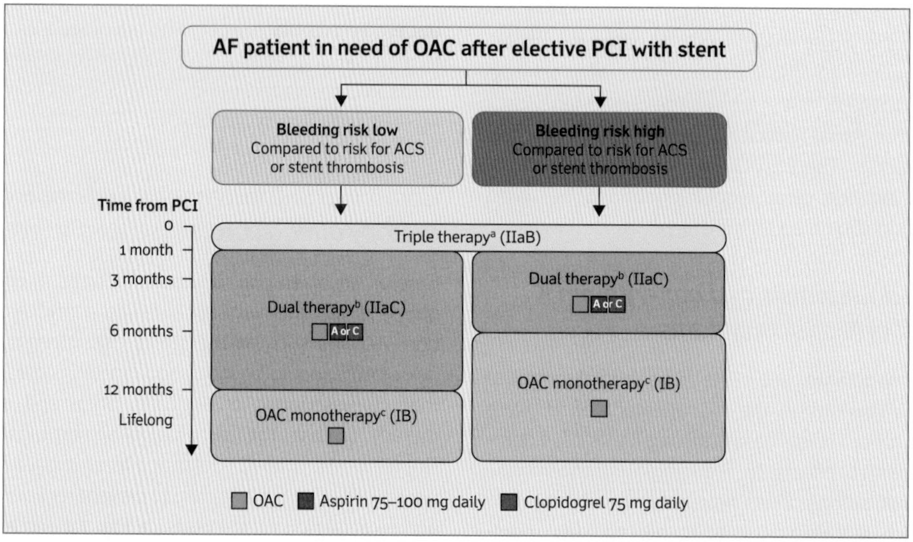

ACS = acute coronary syndrome; AF = atrial fibrillation; OAC = oral anticoagulation (using vitamin K antagonists or non-vitamin K antagonist oral anticoagulants);
PCI = percutaneous coronary intervention.
[a]Dual therapy with OAC and aspirin or clopidogrel may be considered in selected patients.
[b]OAC plus single antiplatelet.
[c]Dual therapy with OAC and an antiplatelet agent (aspirin or clopidogrel) may be considered in patients at high risk of coronary events.

Fig. 7.5 Antithrombotic therapy after elective percutaneous intervention in patients with AF requiring anticoagulation.
Kirchhof P, Benussi S, Kotecha D, et al. 2016 ESC Guidelines for the management of atrial fibrillation developed in collaboration with EACTS. Eur J Cardiothorac Surg. 2016 Nov;50(5):e1–e88. doi: 10.1093/ejcts/ezw313. © The European Society of Cardiology. Reprinted by permission of Oxford University Press.

- After an ACS without stent implantation, dual treatment with an oral anticoagulant and aspirin or clopidogrel should be considered for up to 12 months.
- The duration of the combination antithrombotic therapy should be kept to a limiting period, balancing the estimated risk of recurrent coronary events and bleeding.[5]

Self-care, patient education, and health

Risk factors

For SVTs, alcohol, caffeine, tiredness, or drugs can trigger symptoms and therefore using appropriate communication techniques to make lifestyle enquiries and elicit an accurate history is an important first step. Advising the patient to reduce their caffeine and alcohol intake and to refrain from taking drugs such as amphetamines may be beneficial. For AF, underlying cardiovascular conditions may be present for a long time without causing obvious symptoms for the patient. However, these conditions may cause atrial remodelling, which may have started long before the first episode of AF manifests.[92] Besides genetic factors, numerous cardiovascular markers for the progression of AF have been identified including age, hypertension, heart failure, valvular heart disease, previous stroke/transient ischaemic attack, chronic obstructive pulmonary disease, sleep apnoea, diabetes mellitus, obesity and inactive lifestyle, smoking, and alcohol abuse.

Prevention

For arrhythmias associated with acute presentations, the related risk factors for cardiovascular disease need to be assessed and managed. The common risk factors are the modifiable behavioural-related risk factors that include a diet high in saturated fat and processed food, smoking, lack of physical activity, and excessive alcohol intake as well as the known risk factors such as hypertension, hypercholesterolaemia, diabetes mellitus, sleep apnoea, and obesity. In relation to SVTs, for those who experience symptoms and can identify triggers, they need to be educated in reducing or avoiding the known triggers and these include alcohol, stress, and potentially caffeine, although there is some evidence recently that caffeine plays a minor role in triggering SVTs.[93] There is now evidence that excessive alcohol has a key role in symptoms, especially in AF, and moderate or minimal drinking is associated with a significantly reduced burden of AF symptoms.[94]

Implantable cardioverter defibrillator—education and psychoeducation

Although the ICD is very successful in preventing sudden cardiac death, patients still suffer from the symptoms and awareness of the underlying disease and the knowledge of relying on a life-saving electronic device. Studies have shown most patients live well with their ICD. However, patients living with an ICD can suffer from anxiety, fear of shock, and avoidance of situations, places, and objects that patients associate with shock. About 25% of patients suffer from anxiety and 15% depression.[95] It can lead to social isolation, avoidance of physical activity (including sexual activity), and mood disorders. Patients may also suffer from phantom shocks, a phenomenon of perception of an ICD shock without actually having received a shock.[96] Women are generally more affected by psychosocial outcomes than men.[69] In addition, it has been suggested that negative emotions could be the cause rather than the result of arrhythmia, and that psychological stress can increase the risk of shock. Furthermore, psychosocial status seems to predict mortality.[97] Even though many patients with an ICD have heart failure, their conditions are complicated by their high risk of sudden cardiac death and their mental struggle to live with an implanted device. Furthermore, the ICD population is heterogeneous in those treated with an ICD for secondary prevention. Many of them do not have heart failure but suffer from an arrhythmic disease. These patients might experience greater uncertainty[98] whereas patients treated with an ICD for secondary prevention who have heart failure, might experience lower physical function and quality of life.

Effects of psychoeducation

A few small psychoeducational intervention studies have demonstrated improvements in anxiety, depression, quality of life,[99] physical outcomes,[100] as well as fewer unplanned hospital admissions and calls to healthcare providers.[99,100] Interventions with cognitive behavioural therapy can reduce anxiety in patients with an ICD.[101] Also, ICD-specific cardiac rehabilitation and e-learning seems helpful in improving health outcomes.[102]

Sexuality

Patients may experience sexual dysfunction and a decrease in sexual activity after implantation of an ICD. Sexual dysfunction is common in patients with an ICD and is not limited to erectile dysfunction, but also orgasmic function, desire, intercourse, and overall satisfaction are affected. The ICD implant is often followed by long-term abstinence from sexual activity and/or an emerging fear of having sexual activity after ICD implantation. These experiences are often linked to exercise intolerance, medication side effects, and psychological problems, such as anxiety and depression. The concerns cover fear of the ICD firing during sexual activity, an over-protective partner, erectile dysfunction, and lack of sexual interest. It is reasonable to return to sexual activity after an ICD is implanted, and it is generally safe for those who had the ICD implanted for primary prevention or for secondary prevention, if moderate physical activity does not precipitate arrhythmias. During sexual counselling, it may be reasonable to address the following areas: timing of safe resumption of sexual activity, what to do if a shock occurs during sex, explanation that an ICD shock will not harm their partner, the level of sexual activity that is safe, how to deal with changes in sexual desire or function, and prepregnancy counselling for women who wish to become pregnant. Referral to sexual rehabilitation might be suggested since sexual rehabilitation improves sexual function and exercise capacity.

Cardiovascular prevention and rehabilitation

Implantable cardioverter defibrillator

Outpatient cardiovascular prevention and rehabilitation is indicated in patients receiving an ICD, but the extent to which it impacts shock status of the patient is controversial.[102] A Cochrane review found no documentation for effect of exercise-based cardiac rehabilitation on any outcome (mortality, adverse events, quality of life) except physical capacity, potentially due to small sample sizes in the trials.[103] Patients both with primary and secondary prevention ICDs benefit from exercise training. International policy statements encourage cardiac patients to be active for a minimum of 2.5 hours per week in multiple sessions each lasting at least 10 minutes.[104] Low participation rates in cardiovascular prevention and rehabilitation programmes is a global problem. The literature reports female sex, age, comorbidity, socioeconomic burden, distance, and disbelief in the beneficial effect as the most important barriers to participation. Patients with a primary prevention ICD are less physically active than patients with a secondary prevention ICD. Low physical activity in patients with an ICD might be influenced by fear of exercise-induced shock and low New York Heart Association class (see also Chapter 11).

Palliative care

(See also Chapter 14.)

ICD—deactivation discussions

The use of ICD therapy as patients approach end of life is contentious.[105–107] Terminally ill patients are more likely to develop hypoxia, pain, heart failure, and electrolyte disturbances predisposing them to arrhythmias and thus increasing the frequency of shock therapy from ICDs.[108] It has been found that around 20% of patients with ICDs receive shocks in the final weeks of their lives.[109] Deactivation of the shock function of an ICD in a patient who is dying of a terminal illness, whether cardiac or another condition, prevents the delivery of painful ICD shocks. Individual consideration should be given based on the four ethical principles: respect for patient autonomy, beneficence, non-maleficence, and justice. Honouring both informed consent and informed refusal by the patient to deactivate their device is an integral part of these principles. Cognitively competent patients who wish to have their ICD deactivated to prevent further suffering are entitled to have this performed. If the patient loses capacity and is therefore unable to make an informed decision, an advance directive or next of kin should be consulted. In cases where the clinician refrains from deactivation due to personal beliefs, a second physician willing to carry out the procedure should be involved.[108,109] The ESC Guidelines recommend that professionals discuss end of life issues with all patients before device implantation and at significant points along the illness trajectory.[55]

Discussing deactivation with the patient and family at the end of life is imperative in order to enable choice and prevent undue distress.[110] These discussions should be initiated without delay, and should coincide with the agreement on a 'do not attempt cardiopulmonary resuscitation' order.[105] The patient should also be informed that the decision to deactivate his/her device can be reversed and the patient can choose to reactivate all device functions. The results of the discussion should be noted in medical records, following certain requirements and taking local rules and legislation into account. A multidisciplinary team effort (physicians, nurses, allied health professionals) is important in order to guide the patient through the decision and following procedure. Before, during, and after deactivation, patients should not be left alone, and family support should be encouraged. Deactivation is a procedure achieved by device reprogramming, or application of a magnet directly over the

Box 7.1 Key elements of nursing roles in the care of patients with arrythmias

- Setting up and managing continuous cardiac monitoring to identify and promptly treat arrythmias including defibrillation.
- Discontinuing monitoring when appropriate according to agreed protocols.
- Interdisciplinary working with physicians and other members of the multidisciplinary team.
- Demonstrating understanding and knowledge of drugs used in the care of arrythmia patients.
- Providing education and support to facilitate shared decision-making and adherence to selected therapies.
- Advocating for appropriate management decisions around care, for example, patient awareness of procedure success rates and ICD deactivation.

device. Nurses need to know where the magnet is kept and how to use it. However, placing a magnet on the patient is an intervention depending on a physician's order. In device reprogramming, it may be preferable to suspend only antitachycardia therapies and maintain pacing for bradycardia to avoid symptomatic deterioration. A pacemaker, as opposed to an ICD, will not resuscitate a patient, but can prevent symptomatic bradycardia and worsening of heart failure, and thus improve quality of life of the patient.[106,108] The ESC Guidelines recommend that ICD deactivation should be considered when clinical conditions deteriorate.[110] However, care of patients does not end with device deactivation, and palliative care interventions to minimize symptoms need to be implemented[106,107] (see Chapter 14).

Conclusion

Cardiac arrhythmias are a common cardiovascular complaint which are typically asymptomatic or 'non-urgent', though some can be life-threatening. Given that most patients can lead a normal life once arrythmias are detected and treated, they should always be considered when caring for any patient with a cardiovascular disorder. The cornerstone skill in this area is patient monitoring, through proper ECG technique and interpretation—allowing the various rhythm types to be quickly identified and appropriately treated. However, care should extend beyond solely managing symptoms and should include a focus on the holistic needs of patients and carers. It is crucial that patients are supported through changes in their everyday life, as well as with anxiety, emotional issues, and changes

Table 7.5 Case studies—arrhythmic heart disease

	Atrial fibrillation	Supraventricular tachycardia
1. Patient population and medical history	Ronan is an 83-year-old widower who lives alone in the same town as his daughter and grandchildren. Ronan lost his wife 8 years ago, but has an active social life and has adapted well to living alone. His previous medical history includes a history of hypertension, smoking, diabetes, and aortic valve replacement 5 years ago that was complicated by renal failure. For the past month, he has felt increasingly short of breath and easily fatigued	Sarah is a 17-year-old student in her final year of high school. She lives with her parents and two younger siblings. Sarah has no pre-existing medical conditions, according to her mother she has always been a very healthy and active child. She is on the school's basketball team. For the past 2 years Sarah has experienced episodes of tachycardia every other month with a sudden onset and stop. These were accompanied by palpitations, breaking into a sweat, and dizziness and lasted for up to 30 minutes. Sarah could not identify a specific trigger. In the last 3 months, these episodes happen more frequently, once or twice per week, and they last longer. Sarah is scared. She no longer dares to participate in basketball practice and other social activities, always afraid that the next episode might start. She misses interacting with her friends

(continued)

Table 7.5 Continued

	Atrial fibrillation	Supraventricular tachycardia
2. Clinical presentation	Ronan presents to his family doctor who is concerned about his worsening symptoms. He can only walk 1–2 blocks on flat ground without stopping and has great difficulty climbing stairs. The doctor explains that he needs to investigate these symptoms and refers him for an urgent outpatient assessment with the rapid access cardiac team	Now that Sarah's paroxysmal tachycardias happen more frequently, an episode can be documented by Holter monitoring and her physician refers Sarah to an electrophysiologist. He confirms a narrow complex tachycardia with a rate of around 180 bpm. All other tests, including echocardiogram, are normal
3. Evaluation pathway	The rapid access cardiology nurse sees Ronan 3 days later. She undertakes a thorough assessment and orders an ECG and echocardiogram as well as a full range of blood tests. The cardiologist and nurse meet with Ronan to review his case. The doctor states that Ronan has AF which puts him at significant risk for stroke with a CHA_2DS_2-VASc score of 5. The clinic nurse reports that Ronan is independent with all his activities of daily living, is moderately frail, has an alcohol consumption of 20 units per week, and normal body mass index. He is highly motivated to be treated, hoping that his symptoms will improve and restore his quality of life	The electrophysiologist discusses with Sarah and her parents all possible treatment options, including antiarrhythmic medication and catheter ablation. Sarah's perceived psychological strain is high. She misses her social activities and is concerned about the tachycardia occurring during her final exams. She just wants her normal life back as quickly as possible. Therefore, the electrophysiologist recommends an electrophysiological study with possible catheter ablation of the tachycardia which he suspects to be an AV nodal reentry tachycardia. Sarah and her parents agree to this approach
4. Treatment	The nurse discusses Ronan's test results with him and reassures him that his valve is OK. She explains the ECG results including what AF is in simple terms. She discusses how it increases the chance of stroke, offering him an opportunity to ask questions and a patient booklet for advice. Ronan states he wants to maintain his current quality of life and reduce the risk of stroke. He asks if tablets can help him, and is reassured that while the tablets available do not stop AF, they can reduce his risk of stroke. The cardiac team recommends lifestyle modification and beta-blocker therapy as the preferred option for Ronan	Sarah is admitted on the day of her procedure. She undergoes electrophysiological study with percutaneous access through the femoral vein and conscious sedation. An AV nodal reentry tachycardia can be induced and successfully ablated by slow pathway modification. No other arrhythmias are inducible A nurse talks to Sarah about her fears and together they explore some strategies to deal with them including the option of accessing a patient support group for young people with arrhythmia in the region
5. In-hospital nursing care and priorities	Ronan states that he has no problem taking medication and that his pharmacist will add this new tablet to his daily pill box. When the nurse discusses lifestyle modification with Ronan and explains that alcohol consumption increases the risk of AF, Ronan states that he would prefer to reduce his alcohol intake than suffer disability from a stroke. He does not want to abstain from alcohol altogether. Together Ronan and the nurse agree goals of having at least 4 alcohol-free days per week and make a plan to reduce his alcohol intake to 6 units per week. The nurse offers Ronan her card with access to a cardiac helpline for advice and arranges a follow-up call with Ronan in 4 weeks and a clinic review in 12 weeks	Immediately after the procedure, Sarah is transferred to the cardiology ward where the cardiac nurse monitors her to ensure vascular haemostasis, haemodynamic stability, and absence of new arrhythmias. After 6 hours of strict bed rest, Sarah can get up and take care of herself. No complications occur and Sarah can be discharged the next day. Following advice from the nurse, Sarah is referred to a psychologist

Table 7.5 Continued

	Atrial fibrillation	Supraventricular tachycardia
6. Discharge planning and follow-up	At follow-up, Ronan is doing well and not experiencing any problems associated with his new medication. He discloses difficulty maintaining his alcohol-free days and they renegotiate a plan he feels is more realistic, which includes limiting alcohol to 2 units per day	Sarah stays at home for 3 days after the discharge, before she returns to school. She follows the recommendations to refrain from physical exercise and not lift anything heavy for 10 days. Sarah recovers quickly from the procedure. She regains confidence and resumes playing basketball and meeting friends. She perceives that her parents are very protective and feels it useful to discuss these issues with her psychologist. A follow-up Holter monitoring 3 months after the procedure shows no relevant arrhythmia

to their sexual relations. Such support should be patient centred and focus on continuous patient education and comprehensive treatment through a multidisciplinary team approach. In addition to alleviating patient burden, this would also aid in supporting patients to make positive lifestyle adjustments (diet, exercise, alcohol intake, smoking, etc.) and in their adherence to interventions and medical treatments. While quality of life improvements are possible for the majority of patients, palliative care is an important consideration for those with ICDs and deactivation discussions should be considered where appropriate. ➤ Box 7.1 outlines the key nursing priorities identified in this chapter in the care of patients with arrythmias. In addition, ➤ Table 7.5 provides two case study examples.

References

1. Schnabel RB, Yin X, Gona P, Larson MG, Beiser AS, McManus DD, et al. 50 year trends in atrial fibrillation prevalence, incidence, risk factors, and mortality in the Framingham Heart Study: a cohort study. Lancet. 2015;386(9989):154–62.
2. Thompson DR, Webster RA. Caring for the Coronary Patient. Oxford: Butterworth-Heinemann; 2004.
3. Askari AT, Shishehbor MH, Kaminski MA, Riley MJ, Hsu A, Lincoff AM, GUSTO-V Investigators. The association between early ventricular arrhythmias, renin-angiotensin-aldosterone system antagonism, and mortality in patients with ST-segment-elevation myocardial infarction: insights from Global Use of Strategies to Open coronary arteries (GUSTO) V. Am Heart J. 2009;158(2):238–43.
4. Katritsis DG, Boriani G, Cosio FG, Hindricks G, Jaïs P, Josephson ME, et al. European Heart Rhythm Association (EHRA) consensus document on the management of supraventricular arrhythmias, endorsed by Heart Rhythm Society (HRS), Asia-Pacific Heart Rhythm Society (APHRS), and Sociedad Latinoamericana de Estimulación Cardiaca y Electrofisiologia (SOLAECE). Europace. 2017;19(3):465–511.
5. Kirchhof P, Benussi S, Kotecha D, Ahlsson A, Atar D, Casadei B, et al. 2016 ESC Guidelines for the management of atrial fibrillation developed in collaboration with EACTS. Eur Heart J. 2016;37(38):2893–962.
6. Pettersen TR, Fålun N, Norekvål TM. Improvement of in-hospital telemetry monitoring in coronary care units: an intervention study for achieving optimal electrode placement and attachment, hygiene and delivery of critical information to patients. Eur J Cardiovasc Nurs. 2014;13(6):515–23.
7. Day HW. History of coronary care units. Am J Cardiol. 1972;30(4):405–407.
8. Julian DG. The history of coronary care units. Br Heart J. 1987;57(6):497–502.
9. Fålun N, Moons P, Fitzsimons D, Kirchhof P, Swahn E, Tubaro M, Norekvål TM. Practical challenges regarding in-hospital telemetry monitoring require the development of European practice standards. Eur Heart J Acute Cardiovasc Care. 2018;7(8):774–76.
10. Sandau KE, Funk M, Auerbach A, Barsness GW, Blum K, Cvach M, et al. Update to practice standards for electrocardiographic monitoring in hospital settings: a scientific statement from the American Heart Association. Circulation. 2017;136(19):e273–344.
11. Drew BJ, Funk M. Practice standards for ECG monitoring in hospital settings: executive summary and guide for implementation. Crit Care Nurs Clin North Am. 2006;18(2):157–68, ix.

12. Najafi N, Auerbach A. Use and outcomes of telemetry monitoring on a medicine service. Arch Intern Med. 2012;172(17):1349–50.
13. Fålun N, Nordrehaug JE, Hoff PI, Langørgen J, Moons P, Norekvål TM. Evaluation of the appropriateness and outcome of in-hospital telemetry monitoring. Am J Cardiol. 2013;112(8):1219–23.
14. Dressler R, Dryer MM, Coletti C, Mahoney D, Doorey AJ. Altering overuse of cardiac telemetry in Non–Intensive Care Unit settings by hardwiring the use of American Heart Association guidelines. JAMA Intern Med. 2014;174(11):1852–54.
15. Funk M, Fennie KP, Stephens KE, May JL, Winkler CG, Drew BJ, PULSE Site Investigators. Association of implementation of practice standards for electrocardiographic monitoring with nurses' knowledge, quality of care, and patient outcomes: findings from the practical use of the latest standards of electrocardiography (PULSE) trial. Circ Cardiovasc Qual Outcomes. 2017;10(2):e003132.
16. Cleverley K, Mousavi N, Stronger L, Ann-Bordun K, Hall L, Tam JW et al. The impact of telemetry on survival of in-hospital cardiac arrests in non-critical care patients. Resuscitation. 2013;84(7):878–82.
17. Fålun N, Oterhals K, Pettersen T, Brørs G, Olsen SS, Norekvål TM, TELMON-NOR investigators. Cardiovascular nurses' adherence to practice standards in-hospital telemetry monitoring. Nurs Crit Care. 2020;25(1):37–44.
18. Drew BJ, Harris P, Zègre-Hemsey JK, Mammone T, Schindler D, Salas-Boni R, et al. Insights into the problem of alarm fatigue with physiologic monitor devices: a comprehensive observational study of consecutive intensive care unit patients. PLoS One. 2014;9(10):e110274.
19. Sendelbach S, Funk M. Alarm fatigue: a patient safety concern. AACN Adv Crit Care. 2013;24(4):378–86.
20. Squires A, Ciecior D. Teaching patients about telemetry. Dimens Crit Care Nurs. 2000;19(6):36–39.
21. Chen S, Palchaudhuri S, Johnson A, Trost J, Ponor I, Zakaria S. Does this patient need telemetry? An analysis of telemetry ordering practices at an academic medical center. J Eval Clin Pract. 2017;23(4):741–46.
22. Gorenek B, Blomström Lundqvist C, Brugada Terradellas J, Camm AJ, Hindricks G, Huber K, et al. Cardiac arrhythmias in acute coronary syndromes: position paper from the joint EHRA, ACCA, and EAPCI task force. EuroIntervention. 2015;10(9):1095–108.
23. Trappe HJ. Tachyarrhythmias, bradyarrhythmias and acute coronary syndromes. J Emerg Trauma Shock. 2010;3(2):137–42.
24. Scheinman MM, Thorburn D, Abbott JA. Use of atropine in patients with acute myocardial infarction and sinus bradycardia. Circulation. 1975;52(4):627–33.
25. Riera ARP, Barros RB, de Sousa FD, Baranchuk A. Accelerated idioventricular rhythm: history and chronology of the main discoveries. Indian Pacing Electrophysiol J. 2010;10(1):40–48.
26. Bordachar P, Zachary W, Ploux S, Labrousse L, Haissaguerre M, Thambo JB. Pathophysiology, clinical course, and management of congenital complete atrioventricular block. Heart Rhythm. 2013;10(5):760–66.
27. Truhlář A, Deakin CD, Soar J, Khalifa GE, Alfonzo A, Bierens JJ, et al. European Resuscitation Council. European Resuscitation Council Guidelines for resuscitation 2015: section 4. Cardiac arrest in special circumstances. Resuscitation. 2015;95:148–201.
28. Meaney PA, Nadkarni VM, Kern KB, Indik JH, Halperin HR, Berg RA. Rhythms and outcomes of adult in-hospital cardiac arrest. Crit Care Med. 2010;38(1):101–108.
29. Mann DL, Zipes DP, Libby P, Bonow R (Eds). Braunwald's Heart Disease: A Textbook of Cardiovascular Medicine (10th ed). Philadelphia, PA: Saunders; 2014.
30. Patel PJ, Borovskiy Y, Killian A, Verdino RJ, Epstein AE, Callans DJ, et al. Optimal QT interval correction formula in sinus tachycardia for identifying cardiovascular and mortality risk: findings from the Penn atrial fibrillation Free study. Heart Rhythm. 2016;13(2):527–35.
31. Orejarena LA, Vidaillet H, DeStefano F, Nordstrom DL, Vierkant RA, Smith PN, Hayes JJ. Paroxysmal supraventricular tachycardia in the general population. J Am Coll Cardiol. 1998;31(1):150–57.
32. Rosenfeld LE. Pregnancy and arrhythmias. In: Cha TM, Lloyd MA, Birgersdotter-Green UM (Eds), Arrhythmias in Women: Diagnosis and Management. Oxford: Oxford University Press; 2014:227–42.
33. Freedman B, Hindricks G, Banerjee A et al. World Heart Federation Roadmap on Atrial Fibrillation - A 2020 Update Global Heart 2021;16(1):41. DOI:http://doi.org/10.5334/gh.1023
34. Chugh SS, Havmoeller R, Narayanan K, Singh D, Rienstra M, Benjamin EJ, et al. Worldwide epidemiology of atrial fibrillation: a Global Burden of Disease 2010 Study. Circulation. 2014;129(8):837–47.
35. Miyasaka Y, Barnes ME, Gersh BJ, Cha SS, Bailey KR, Abhayaratna WP, et al. Secular trends in incidence of atrial fibrillation in Olmsted County, Minnesota, 1980–2000, and implications on the projections for future prevalence. Circulation. 2006;114(2):119–25.
36. González-Pacheco H, Márquez MF, Arias-Mendoza A, Álvarez-Sangabriel A, Eid-Lidt G, González-Hermosillo A, et al. Clinical features and in-hospital mortality associated with different types of atrial fibrillation in patients with acute coronary syndrome with and without ST elevation. J Cardiol. 2015;66(2):148–54.
37. Camm AJ, Lüscher TF, Maurer G, Serruys PW (Eds). The ESC Textbook of Cardiovascular Medicine. Oxford: Oxford University Press; 2009.

38. Davis RC, Hobbs FD, Kenkre JE, Roalfe AK, Iles R, Lip GY, Davies MK, et al. Prevalence of atrial fibrillation in the general population and in high-risk groups: the ECHOES study. Europace. 2012;14(11):1553–59.
39. Fitzmaurice DA, Hobbs FD, Jowett S, Mant J, Murray ET, Holder R et al. Screening versus routine practice in detection of atrial fibrillation in patients aged 65 or over: cluster randomised controlled trial. BMJ. 2007;335(7616):383.
40. Turakhia MP, Desai M, Hedlin H, Rajmane A, Talati N, Ferris T, et al. Rationale and design of a large-scale, app-based study to identify cardiac arrhythmias using a smartwatch: the Apple Heart Study. Am Heart J. 2019;207:66–75.
41. Steffel J, Verhamme P, Potpara TS, Albaladejo P, Antz M, Desteghe L, et al. The 2018 European Heart Rhythm Association Practical Guide on the use of non-vitamin K antagonist oral anticoagulants in patients with atrial fibrillation. Eur Heart J. 2018;39(16):1330–93.
42. Hindricks G, Potpara T, Dagres N, Arbelo E, Bax JJ, Blomström-Lundqvist C, et al. ESC Scientific Document Group. 2020 ESC Guidelines for the diagnosis and management of atrial fibrillation developed in collaboration with the European Association for Cardio-Thoracic Surgery (EACTS): The Task Force for the diagnosis and management of atrial fibrillation of the European Society of Cardiology (ESC) Developed with the special contribution of the European Heart Rhythm Association (EHRA) of the ESC. Eur Heart J. 2021 Feb 1;42(5):373-498. doi: 10.1093/eurheartj/ehaa612. Erratum in: Eur Heart J. 2021 Feb 1;42(5):507. Erratum in: Eur Heart J. 2021 Feb 1;42(5):546–547. Erratum in: Eur Heart J. 2021 Oct 21;42(40):4194. PMID: 32860505.
43. Siu CW, Lau CP, Lee WL, Lam KF, Tse HF. Intravenous diltiazem is superior to intravenous amiodarone or digoxin for achieving ventricular rate control in patients with acute uncomplicated atrial fibrillation. Crit Care Med. 2009;37(7):2174–79.
44. Scheuermeyer FX, Grafstein E, Stenstrom R, Christenson J, Heslop C, Heilbron B, et al. Safety and efficiency of calcium channel blockers versus beta-blockers for rate control in patients with atrial fibrillation and no acute underlying medical illness. Acad Emerg Med. 2013;20(3):222–30.
45. Gitt AK, Smolka W, Michailov G, Bernhardt A, Pittrow D, Lewalter T. Types and outcomes of cardioversion in patients admitted to hospital for atrial fibrillation: results of the German RHYTHM-AF Study. Clin Res Cardiol. 2013;102(10):713–23.
46. Cristoni L, Tampieri A, Mucci F, Iannone P, Venturi A, Cavazza M, Lenzi T. Cardioversion of acute atrial fibrillation in the short observation unit: comparison of a protocol focused on electrical cardioversion with simple antiarrhythmic treatment. Emerg Med J. 2011;28(11):932–37.
47. Crijns HJGM, Weijs B, Fairley AM, Lewalter T, Maggioni AP, Martín A, et al. Contemporary real life cardioversion of atrial fibrillation: results from the multinational RHYTHM-AF study. Int J Cardiol. 2014;172(3):588–94.
48. Overvad TF, Rasmussen LH, Skjøth F, Overvad K, Lip GY, Larsen TB. Body mass index and adverse events in patients with incident atrial fibrillation. Am J Med. 2013;126(7):640.e9–17.
49. Abed HS, Wittert GA, Leong DP, Shirazi MG, Bahrami B, Middeldorp ME, et al. Effect of weight reduction and cardiometabolic risk factor management on symptom burden and severity in patients with atrial fibrillation: a randomized clinical trial. JAMA. 2013;310(19):2050–60.
50. Pathak RK, Middeldorp ME, Lau DH, Mehta AB, Mahajan R, Twomey D, et al. Aggressive risk factor reduction study for atrial fibrillation and implications for the outcome of ablation: the ARREST-AF cohort study. J Am Coll Cardiol. 2014;64(21):2222–31.
51. Pathak RK, Middeldorp ME, Meredith M, Mehta AB, Mahajan R, Wong CX, et al. Long-term effect of goal-directed weight management in an atrial fibrillation cohort: a long-term follow-up study (Legacy). J Am Coll Cardiol. 2015;65(20):2159–69.
52. Lip GYH, Nieuwlaat R, Pisters R, Lane DA, Crijns HJ. Refining clinical risk stratification for predicting stroke and thromboembolism in atrial fibrillation using a novel risk factor-based approach: the euro heart survey on atrial fibrillation. Chest. 2010;137(2):263–72.
53. Van Gelder IC, Groenveld HF, Crijns HJGM, Tuininga YS, Tijssen JG, Alings AM, et al. Lenient versus strict rate control in patients with atrial fibrillation. N Engl J Med. 2010;362(15):1363–73.
54. Saborido CM, Hockenhull J, Bagust A, Boland A, Dickson R, Todd D. Systematic review and cost-effectiveness evaluation of 'pill-in-the-pocket' strategy for paroxysmal atrial fibrillation compared to episodic in-hospital treatment or continuous antiarrhythmic drug therapy. Health Technol Assess. 2010;14(31):iii–iv, 1.
55. Priori SG, Blomström-Lundqvist C, Mazzanti A, Blom N, Borggrefe M, Camm J, et al. 2015 ESC Guidelines for the management of patients with ventricular arrhythmias and the prevention of sudden cardiac death: the Task Force for the Management of Patients with Ventricular Arrhythmias and the Prevention of Sudden Cardiac Death of the European Society of Cardiology (ESC). Endorsed by: Association for European Paediatric and Congenital Cardiology (AEPC). Eur Heart J. 2015;36(41):2793–867.
56. Norekvål TM, Kirchhof P, Fitzsimons D. Patient-centred care of patients with ventricular arrhythmias and risk of sudden cardiac death: what do the 2015 European Society of Cardiology guidelines add? Eur J Cardiovasc Nurs 2017;16(7):558–64.
57. Mont L. Arrhythmias and sport practice. Heart. 2010;96(5):398–405.

58. Margulescu AD, Anderson MH. A review of driving restrictions in patients at risk of syncope and cardiac arrhythmias associated with sudden incapacity: differing global approaches to regulation and risk. Arrhythm Electrophysiol Rev. 2019;8(2):90–98.
59. Berg SK, Higgins M, Reilly CM, Langberg JJ, Dunbar SB. Sleep quality and sleepiness in persons with implantable cardioverter defibrillators: outcome from a clinical randomized longitudinal trial. Pacing Clin Electrophysiol. 2012;35(4):431–43.
60. Byrne M, Doherty S, Murphy AW, McGee HM, Jaarsma T. The CHARMS Study: cardiac patients' experiences of sexual problems following cardiac rehabilitation. Eur J Cardiovasc Nurs. 2013;12(6):558–66.
61. Berg SK, Elleman-Jensen L, Zwisler AD, Winkel P, Svendsen JH, Pedersen PU, Moons P. Sexual concerns and practices after ICD implantation: findings of the COPE-ICD rehabilitation trial. Eur J Cardiovasc Nurs. 2013;12(5):468–74.
62. Vazquez LD, Kuhl EA, Shea JB, Kirkness A, Lemon J, Whalley D, et al. Age-specific differences in women with implantable cardioverter defibrillators: an international multicenter study. Pacing Clin Electrophysiol. 2008;31(12):1528–34.
63. Forman J, Baumbusch J, Jackson H, Lindenberg J, Shook A, Bashir J. Exploring the patients' experiences of living with a subcutaneous implantable cardioverter defibrillator. Eur J Cardiovasc Nurs. 2018;17(8):698–706.
64. Ekblad H, Rönning H, Fridlund B, Malm D. Patients' well-being: experience and actions in their preventing and handling of atrial fibrillation. Eur J Cardiovasc Nurs. 2013;12(2):132–39.
65. Boyde M, Song S, Peters R, Turner C, Thompson DR, Stewart S. Pilot testing of a self-care education intervention for patients with heart failure. Eur J Cardiovasc Nurs. 2013;12(1):39–46.
66. Rush KL, Burton L, Schaab K, Lukey A. The impact of nurse-led atrial fibrillation clinics on patient and healthcare outcomes: a systematic mixed studies review. Eur J Cardiovasc Nurs. 2019;18(7):526–33.
67. Jankowska-Polańska B, Kaczan A, Lomper K, Nowakowski D, Dudek K. Symptoms, acceptance of illness and health-related quality of life in patients with atrial fibrillation. Eur J Cardiovasc Nurs. 2018;17(3):262–72.
68. Ruston A, Clayton J. Women's interpretation of cardiac symptoms at the time of their cardiac event: the effect of co-occurring illness. Eur J Cardiovasc Nurs. 2007;6(4):321–28.
69. Spindler H, Johansen JB, Andersen K, Mortensen P, Pedersen SS. Gender differences in anxiety and concerns about the cardioverter defibrillator. Pacing Clin Electrophysiol. 2009;32(5):614–21.
70. Calkins H, Hindricks G, Cappato R, Kim YH, Saad EB, Aguinaga L, et al. 2017 HRS/EHRA/ECAS/APHRS/SOLAECE expert consensus statement on catheter and surgical ablation of atrial fibrillation: executive summary. J Interv Card Electrophysiol. 2017;50(1):1–55.
71. Andrade JG, Macle L, Khairy P, Khaykin Y, Mantovan R, De Martino G, et al. Incidence and significance of early recurrences associated with different ablation strategies for AF: a STAR-AF substudy. J Cardiovasc Electrophysiol. 2012;23(12):1295–301.
72. Gaztañaga L, Frankel DS, Kohari M, Kondapalli L, Zado ES, Marchlinski FE. Time to recurrence of atrial fibrillation influences outcome following catheter ablation. Heart Rhythm. 2013;10(1):2–9.
73. Sapp JL, Wells GA, Parkash R, Stevenson WG, Blier L, Sarrazin JF, et al. Ventricular tachycardia ablation versus escalation of antiarrhythmic drugs. N Engl J Med. 2016;375(2):111–21.
74. Wilkoff BL, Fauchier L, Stiles MK, Morillo CA, Al-Khatib SM, Almendral J, et al. 2015 HRS/EHRA/APHRS/SOLAECE expert consensus statement on optimal implantable cardioverter-defibrillator programming and testing. Heart Rhythm 2016;13(2):e50–86.
75. van der Heijden AC, Borleffs CJW, Buiten MS, Thijssen J, van Rees JB, Cannegieter SC, et al. The clinical course of patients with implantable cardioverter-defibrillators: extended experience on clinical outcome, device replacements, and device-related complications. Heart Rhythm. 2015;12(6):1169–76.
76. Piccini JP, Berger JS, O'Connor CM. Amiodarone for the prevention of sudden cardiac death: a meta-analysis of randomized controlled trials. Eur Heart J. 2009;30(10):1245–53.
77. Doll N, Götte J, Wehbe MS, Weimar T, Merk DR. Correcting arrhythmias: interventional and surgical ablation therapy. Thorac Cardiovasc Surg. 2017;65(Suppl 3):S196–99.
78. Weimar T, Doll KN. Surgical therapy of atrial fibrillation. In: Ziemer G, Haverich A (Eds), Cardiac Surgery: Operations on the Heart and Great Vessels in Adults and Children. Berlin: Springer; 2017:947–63.
79. Ad N, Holmes SD, Massimiano PS, Rongione AJ, Fornaresio LM. Long-term outcome following concomitant mitral valve surgery and Cox maze procedure for atrial fibrillation. J Thorac Cardiovasc Surg. 2018;155(3):983–94.
80. Gallagher C, Elliott AD, Wong CX, Rangnekar G, Middeldorp ME, Mahajan R, et al. Integrated care in atrial fibrillation: a systematic review and meta-analysis. Heart. 2017;103(24):1947–53.
81. NHFA CSANZ Atrial Fibrillation Guideline Working Group, Brieger D, Amerena J, Attia J, Bajorek B, Chan KH, et al. National Heart Foundation of Australia and the Cardiac Society of Australia and New Zealand:

Australian Clinical Guidelines for the Diagnosis and Management of Atrial Fibrillation 2018. Heart Lung Circ. 2018;27(10):1209–66.

82. Kotecha D, Breithardt G, Camm AJ, Lip GYH, Schotten U, Ahlsson A, et al. Integrating new approaches to atrial fibrillation management: the 6th AFNET/EHRA Consensus Conference. Europace. 2018;20(3):395–407.

83. Eikelboom JW, Connolly SJ, Brueckmann M, Granger CB, Kappetein AP, Mack MJ, et al. Dabigatran versus warfarin in patients with mechanical heart valves. N Engl J Med. 2013;369(13):1206–14.

84. Connolly SJ, Ezekowitz MD, Yusuf S, Eikelboom J, Oldgren J, Parekh A, et al. Dabigatran versus warfarin in patients with atrial fibrillation. N Engl J Med. 2009;361(12):1139–51.

85. Granger CB, Alexander JH, McMurray JJV, Lopes RD, Hylek EM, Hanna M, et al. Apixaban versus warfarin in patients with atrial fibrillation. N Engl J Med. 2011;365(11):981–92.

86. Patel MR, Mahaffey KW, Garg J, Pan G, Singer DE, Hacke W, et al. Rivaroxaban versus warfarin in nonvalvular atrial fibrillation. N Engl J Med. 2011;365(10):883–91.

87. Giugliano RP, Ruff CT, Braunwald E, Murphy SA, Wiviott SD, Halperin JL, et al. Edoxaban versus warfarin in patients with atrial fibrillation. N Engl J Med. 2013;369(22):2093–104.

88. ACTIVE Writing Group of the ACTIVE Investigators C, Connolly S, Pogue J, et al. Clopidogrel plus aspirin versus oral anticoagulation for atrial fibrillation in the Atrial fibrillation Clopidogrel Trial with Irbesartan for prevention of Vascular Events (ACTIVE W): a randomised controlled trial. Lancet. 2006;367(9526):1903–12.

89. ACTIVE Investigators, Connolly SJ, Pogue J, Hart RG, Hohnloser SH, Pfeffer M, et al. Effect of clopidogrel added to aspirin in patients with atrial fibrillation. N Engl J Med 2009; 360(20):2066–78.

90. Holmes DR, Kar S, Price MJ, Whisenant B, Sievert H, Doshi SK, et al. Prospective randomized evaluation of the Watchman Left Atrial Appendage Closure device in patients with atrial fibrillation versus long-term warfarin therapy: the PREVAIL trial. J Am Coll Cardiol. 2014;64(1):1–12.

91. Dans AL, Connolly SJ, Wallentin L, Yang S, Nakamya J, Brueckmann M, et al. Concomitant use of antiplatelet therapy with dabigatran or warfarin in the Randomized Evaluation of Long-Term Anticoagulation Therapy (RE-LY) trial. Circulation. 2013;127(5):634–40.

92. Cosio FG, Aliot E, Botto GL, Heidbüchel H, Geller CJ, Kirchhof P, et al. Delayed rhythm control of atrial fibrillation may be a cause of failure to prevent recurrences: reasons for change to active antiarrhythmic treatment at the time of the first detected episode. Europace. 2008;10(1):21–27.

93. Voskoboinik A, Kalman JM, Kistler PM. Caffeine and arrhythmias: time to grind the data. JACC Clin Electrophysiol. 2018;4(4):425–32.

94. Voskoboinik A, Wong G, Lee G, Nalliah C, Hawson J, Prabhu S, et al. Moderate alcohol consumption is associated with atrial electrical and structural changes: insights from high-density left atrial electroanatomic mapping. Heart Rhythm. 2019;16(2):251–59.

95. Berg SK, Rasmussen TB, Thrysoee L, Lauberg A, Borregaard B, Christensen AV, et al. DenHeart: differences in physical and mental health across cardiac diagnoses at hospital discharge. J Psychosom Res. 2017;94:1–9.

96. Berg SK, Moons P, Zwisler AD, Winkel P, Pedersen BD, Pedersen PU, Svendsen JH. Phantom shocks in patients with implantable cardioverter defibrillator: results from a randomized rehabilitation trial (COPE-ICD). Europace. 2013;15(10):1463–67.

97. Berg SK, Rasmussen TB, Mols RE, Thorup CB, Borregaard B, Christensen AV, et al. Both mental and physical health predicts one year mortality and readmissions in patients with implantable cardioverter defibrillators: findings from the national DenHeart study. Eur J Cardiovasc Nurs. 2019;18(2):96–105.

98. Carroll SL, Arthur HM. A comparative study of uncertainty, optimism and anxiety in patients receiving their first implantable defibrillator for primary or secondary prevention of sudden cardiac death. Int J Nurs Stud. 2010;47(7):836–45.

99. Dunbar SB, Langberg JJ, Reilly CM, Viswanathan B, McCarty F, Culler SD, et al. Effect of a psychoeducational intervention on depression, anxiety, and health resource use in implantable cardioverter defibrillator patients. Pacing Clin Electrophysiol. 2009;32(10):1259–71.

100. Lewin RJ, Coulton S, Frizelle DJ, Kaye G, Cox H. A brief cognitive behavioural preimplantation and rehabilitation programme for patients receiving an implantable cardioverter-defibrillator improves physical health and reduces psychological morbidity and unplanned readmissions. Heart. 2009;95(1):63–69.

101. Maia ACCO, Braga AA, Soares-Filho G, Pereira V, Nardi AE, Silva AC. Efficacy of cognitive behavioral therapy in reducing psychiatric symptoms in patients with implantable cardioverter defibrillator: an integrative review. Braz J Med Biol Res. 2014;47(4):265–72.

102. Berg SK, Pedersen PU, Zwisler AD, Winkel P, Gluud C, Pedersen BD, Svendsen JH. Comprehensive cardiac rehabilitation improves outcome for patients with implantable cardioverter defibrillator. Findings from the

COPE-ICD randomised clinical trial. Eur J Cardiovasc Nurs. 2015;14(1):34–44.

103. Nielsen KM, Zwisler AD, Taylor RS, Svendsen JH, Lindschou J, Anderson L, et al. Exercise-based cardiac rehabilitation for adult patients with an implantable cardioverter defibrillator. Cochrane Database Syst Rev. 2019;2(2):CD011828.

104. Piepoli MF, Corrà U, Adamopoulos S, Benzer W, Bjarnason-Wehrens B, Cupples M, et al. Secondary prevention in the clinical management of patients with cardiovascular diseases. Core components, standards and outcome measures for referral and delivery: a policy statement from the cardiac rehabilitation section of the European Association for Cardiovascular Prevention & Rehabilitation. Endorsed by the Committee for Practice Guidelines of the European Society of Cardiology. Eur J Prev Cardiol. 2014;21(6):664–81.

105. Hill L, McIlfatrick S, Taylor BJ, Dixon L, Cole BR, Moser DK, Fitzsimons D. Implantable cardioverter defibrillator (ICD) deactivation discussions: reality versus recommendations. Eur J Cardiovasc Nurs. 2016;15(1):20–29.

106. Jaarsma T, Beattie JM, Ryder M, Rutten FH, McDonagh T, Mohacsi P, et al. Palliative care in heart failure: a position statement from the palliative care workshop of the Heart Failure Association of the European Society of Cardiology. Eur J Heart Fail. 2009;11(5):433–43.

107. Hjelmfors L, Strömberg A, Friedrichsen M, Sandgren A, Mårtensson J, Jaarsma T. Using co- design to develop an intervention to improve communication about the heart failure trajectory and end-of-life care. BMC Palliat Care. 2018;17(1):85.

108. Padeletti L, Arnar DO, Boncinelli L, Brachman J, Camm JA, Daubert JC, et al. EHRA Expert Consensus Statement on the management of cardiovascular implantable electronic devices in patients nearing end of life or requesting withdrawal of therapy. Europace. 2010;12(10):1480–89.

109. Wright GA, Klein GJ, Gula LJ. Ethical and legal perspective of implantable cardioverter defibrillator deactivation or implantable cardioverter defibrillator generator replacement in the elderly. Curr Opin Cardiol. 2013;28(1):43–49.

110. Hill L, McIlfatrick S, Taylor BJ, Jaarsma T, Moser D, Slater P, et al. Patient and professional factors that impact the perceived likelihood and confidence of healthcare professionals to discuss implantable cardioverter defibrillator deactivation in advanced heart failure: results from an International Factorial Survey. J Cardiovasc Nurs. 2018;33(6):527–35.

8 Care of the patient with valvular heart disease

TONE M. NOREKVÅL, BRITT BORREGAARD, TINA B. HANSEN, TRINE B. RASMUSSEN, AND SANDRA B. LAUCK

CHAPTER CONTENTS

This chapter covers the care of patients with valvular heart disease. It addresses the principles of interdisciplinary working of members of the Heart Team and identifies the nursing priorities for patient care.

KEY MESSAGES

- The natural history of valvular heart disease is associated with significant mortality and morbidity, increased symptoms, and poor quality of life, as well as high rates of hospital readmission and healthcare utilization.

- In the past decade, there has been a paradigm shift in the management of valvular heart disease with the rapid emergence of minimally invasive transcatheter options for patients with varying surgical risk profiles and valve diseases.
- Acquired valvular heart disease is primarily a disease of ageing. A comprehensive understanding of frailty, including the pathophysiology, screening, and clinical implications, is a core competency of cardiovascular nurses who provide care to patients with complex valvular heart disease.
- The multidisciplinary Heart Team for the provision of comprehensive, collaborative care to patients with valvular heart disease guides the assessment pathway and treatment recommendations. This team-based approach aims to leverage the strengths and skills of its members to optimize the safety and quality of patient care.
- Endocarditis is an infection of the endocardial surface involving the heart valves and/or surrounding structures typically caused by bacteria. Close monitoring for early signs of disease progression, inadequate infection control, and complications is essential to prevent clinical deterioration.
- Patients recovering from infective endocarditis will often have been physically inactive for weeks or months due to diagnostic delay, their symptom burden, long-term hospitalization, and possible postsurgical restrictions.
- The implications of changes in haemodynamics, the trajectory of heart failure, and the variation in clinical presentation across age groups and pathologies create unique challenges to optimize outcomes and support patients and their family.

Introduction

Degenerative valvular disease is the next cardiovascular epidemic in developed countries. Prevalence rises markedly with age, from less than 2% in patients under the age of 65 years, to 8.5% in those aged 65–75 years, and 13.2% after the age of 75 years.[1] The natural history of valvular heart disease is associated with significant mortality and morbidity, increased symptoms, and poor quality of life, as well as high rates of hospital readmission and healthcare utilization. The complexity of the care of patients with valvular heart disease is compounded by the impact of concomitant conditions including heart failure, the multisystem impact of impaired cardiac output, and age-associated frailty. In addition, patients present with significant variation in clinical status depending on aetiology, disease progression, and treatment decisions. Cardiovascular nurses require foundational knowledge about the pathology and clinical presentation of valvular heart disease, the unique assessment findings and diagnostic modalities, and the treatment management options. The spectrum of these conditions encompasses multiple disease processes associated with individual or combined heart valves. The focus of this chapter is restricted to the acquired valvular heart diseases most frequently seen in cardiovascular nursing practice: aortic valve disease, mitral regurgitation, and infective endocarditis.

Epidemiology

The prevalence of valvular heart disease is challenging to quantify due to the variation in clinical presentation and often latent disease progression, the absence of systematic disease surveillance and delay to diagnosis, and the compounded effect of comorbidities. Epidemiological considerations include distinct groups that experience high rates of valvular heart disease in Europe including the elderly, the heart failure population, people living with cardiac devices and/or at high risk of blood-borne infections, and people originally from countries with higher rates of rheumatic heart disease. Of these, the ageing population represents the single most important driver of disease prevalence. For example, according to a population-based study in Norway that spanned over 14 years, aortic stenosis was prevalent in 0.2% of people in the 50- to 59-year-old cohort, 1.3% in the 60- to 69-year-old cohort, 3.9% in the 70- to 79-year-old cohort, and 9.8% in the 80- to 89-year-old cohort.[2] This pattern is similarly seen in the setting of mitral valve disease, which follows closely the epidemic of heart failure.

The incidence of infective endocarditis has also been rising in middle and high income countries (industrialized is a dated term) countries, while the epidemiological profile has evolved significantly in the past decade. This increase is associated with the growing prevalence in degenerative valvular disease in the elderly population, increasing use of prosthetic valves and implantable cardiac devices in cardiac treatment, exposure to invasive procedures and nosocomial bacteraemia, and the devastating effects of the epidemic of addiction and high-risk intravenous drug use.[3,4] More than one-third of affected patients are over 70 years old in higher-income countries due to the increased vulnerability of older people to infection and the higher likelihood of invasive treatments; men outpace women at a ratio of approximately 2:1.[3] The incidence of endocarditis is reported to be between 3 and 10 per 100,000 person-years; as many cases are either not identified, or diagnosed postmortem, prevalence is higher than documented.[3,4] Although improvements in diagnostic tools, novel antibiotics, and changes in treatment regimens have improved survival since the 1960s, prognosis remains devastatingly poor, with 10–25% in-hospital and 20–40% 1-year mortality. Risk factors for poor outcome in the setting of endocarditis include heart failure, renal failure, advanced age and involvement of the central nervous system, most often cerebral embolisms, and social determinants of health.

Pathophysiology

The impaired function of heart valves to respond to intracardiac pressure changes to open and close appropriately in a carefully timed sequence may be the result of multiple mechanisms and pathologies (see also Chapter 4). Importantly, the lack of regulation of haemodynamic flow associated with restricted or regurgitant valves can have deleterious effects on cardiac function and cardiac output, and can be a trigger and accelerator of the cascade of heart failure. Central to the pathophysiology of most valvular heart diseases, the following concepts are essential:

- Stenosis: narrowing, thickening, or vegetations restrict forward blood flow resulting in the inability of the valve leaflets to adequately open.
- Regurgitation or insufficiency: inability of the valve leaflets to close appropriately to prevent backward flow, resulting in leaking from an area of higher pressure to lower pressure.
- Pressure gradient: the difference in pressure (measured in mmHg) between two chambers and/or vessels. The pressure gradient is a measurement of the grade of haemodynamic significance of valvular heart disease.

Aortic stenosis

Aortic stenosis occurs when the orifice of the aortic valve is reduced, preventing the valve from opening fully and reducing blood flow from the left ventricle into the aorta. There are three known causes of aortic stenosis: rheumatic disease, calcific disease, and congenital valve disease. In North America and Europe, calcific disease of a native trileaflet valve or a congenitally bicuspid valve remains the most common cause of aortic stenosis.

The mechanism of calcification is due to an inflammatory process caused by mechanical stress, lipid deposition, and some characteristics similar, but not entirely, to arterial atherosclerosis. These changes are known to occur earlier in bicuspid valves than in normal tricuspid valves, presumably attributed to increased mechanical stress and earlier initiation of the inflammatory process in the asymmetrical bicuspid valve.

Aortic stenosis can be viewed on a continuum from aortic sclerosis to severe aortic stenosis. Aortic sclerosis is characterized by calcification or focal leaflet thickening of the valves with preserved normal function. As aortic stenosis develops, the leaflets thicken, calcium nodules form, new blood vessels appear, and blood flow through the left ventricular outflow tract is increasingly obstructed. Left ventricular output is initially maintained by adaptation of the increasingly hypertrophic left ventricle. This compensation mechanism serves to normalize the left ventricle wall stress.

Progression of aortic stenosis produces a reduction in valve area and an increased pressure gradient across the valve. As the aortic leaflets thicken and calcify, antegrade velocity initially remains normal until the orifice area reaches less than half of the normal valve area of about 3–4 cm^2 in adults. As aortic stenosis becomes increasingly haemodynamically significant, there is rising pressure overload on the left ventricle which decompensates with a decline in cardiac output and a rise in pulmonary artery pressure. In advanced stages of the disease, secondary pulmonary hypertension may result in right-sided heart failure.

Aortic regurgitation

Aortic regurgitation occurs when blood flows backwards across the aortic valve from the aorta into the left ventricle during diastole due to an incompetent valve. In chronic aortic regurgitation, the left ventricle enlarges to maintain a normal cardiac output. Increased afterload is compensated for by left ventricular hypertrophy, but decompensation and systolic left ventricular dysfunction may gradually develop. Acute aortic regurgitation is a sudden haemodynamically significant aortic incompetence which causes an abrupt increase in end-diastolic pressure, decreased cardiac output, and heart failure which can progress to cardiogenic shock (see also Chapter 5). The most common causes of chronic aortic valve regurgitation are diseases of the aortic leaflets or the aortic root. Aortic leaflet conditions include degenerative leaflet calcifications, a bicuspid aortic valve, damaging processes such as infective endocarditis, or rheumatic fever. In contrast, aortic root conditions comprise idiopathic root dilatation, aortic dissection, Marfan syndrome, collagen vascular disease, and syphilis.

Mitral stenosis

The primary cause of mitral stenosis is rheumatic heart disease, which accounts for approximately 98% of clinical presentations; prevalence, morbidity, and mortality are highest predominantly in developing or economically marginalized countries. Patients can present at all ages, and may have concomitant valvular heart disease. In contrast, degenerative calcific mitral stenosis is mostly seen in elderly patients.

Rheumatic valvular heart disease causes thickening of the valve leaflets by fibrous distortion, which, combined with increasingly rigid cusps, results in narrowing of the valve. Over time, the mitral valve area decreases and the left atrial pressure increases to exert force and eject blood into the left ventricle. A pressure gradient develops between the left atrium and the left ventricle to help assist the diastole. The elevated left atrial pressures are transmitted to the pulmonary veins and the right side of the heart. On exertion, as cardiac output and jet velocity across the mitral valve increase, the transmitted pressure gradient becomes exponentially larger, and pulmonary oedema can occur.

Mitral regurgitation

Mitral regurgitation results from the incomplete closure of the mitral valve and a pressure gradient between the left ventricle and the left atrium, which leads to abnormal systolic backward flow of blood from the left ventricle to the left atrium. Mitral regurgitation causes left ventricle volume overload. Due to the increased volume, left atrial pressure rises, leading to compensatory left atrial enlargement.

As mitral regurgitation worsens and the stress on the left ventricle increases, left ventricular hypertrophy develops to maintain normal left ventricular pressures. Eventually, systolic heart failure ensues. In chronic mitral regurgitation, symptoms may be delayed for years due to the adaptation of the left ventricle. In acute mitral regurgitation, the left ventricle is unable to compensate properly, causing patients to experience significant haemodynamic instability.

Mitral regurgitation can arise either due to disease of the mitral valve apparatus known as organic mitral regurgitation (primary), or due to left ventricular disease or remodelling due to idiopathic cardiomyopathy or coronary artery disease known as functional mitral regurgitation (secondary or ischaemic cardiomyopathy). The causes of organic mitral regurgitation comprise degenerative mitral regurgitation (including leaflet prolapse, mitral annular calcification, and myxomatous changes), rheumatic heart disease, and infective endocarditis which can result in leaflet perforation and chordal rupture.

Infective endocarditis

Endocarditis is an infection of the endocardial surface involving the heart valves and/or surrounding structures. The infection may involve the native heart valves, but also implanted cardiac devices/implants, such as pacemakers (see also Chapter 7) and heart valve prostheses. Endocarditis can be non-infectious, although typically it is an infection caused by bacteria or, more rarely, fungi. Bacteria may invade and damage the tissue causing heart valve destruction, and leading to acute heart failure (30–50%). Bacterial vegetations can dislodge into the vascular circulation, resulting in thromboembolic events (20–30%), including stroke (15–20%) and more peripherally, commonly to the spleen.[3,4] Approximately 70% of all cases of endocarditis involve native heart valve tissue, 20% heart valve prosthesis, and 10% cardiac devices. Due to a higher flow across the left-sided valves, the higher risk of lesions, and bacterial growth, the left-sided heart valves are more frequently affected, accounting for 80–85% of cases; the aortic and mitral valves are equally affected in 10% of these cases.[3,4] Right-sided and device-related endocarditis remain rare, although growing numbers of device endocarditis have been reported; this may be due to the increase in, and complexity of, cardiac device treatment. Once the valvular apparatus is critically diseased, pathophysiological processes are similar to those described previously in the case of aortic or mitral regurgitation.

The triggering event of an endocardial infection is epithelial damage of the heart valves or endocardium in combination with bacteraemia. The natural defence system of the endothelium against infection is reduced once the damage occurs and bacteria may attach to its flawed surface. Groups at risk include people with congenital heart disease, degenerative heart valve disease, and intracardiac devices and prosthesis, and individuals who are subject to blood-borne infections and septicaemia through the use of intravenous drugs. In addition, haemodialysis catheters, dental infections, and colonic polyps present additional routes of microbial entry. The most common pathogens are staphylococci and streptococci, which together account for more than 70% of all cases of infective endocarditis, whereas enterococci infection is seen in increasing numbers in the elderly population. The pathogen creates solid vegetations or masses consisting of bacteria, white blood cells, fibrin, and platelets that invade and destroy the surrounding tissue. The vegetations may dislodge into the circulation, and can cause harmful and potentially deadly complications, particularly cerebral and other embolic events.

Clinical presentation

Aortic stenosis

Aortic stenosis has a prolonged asymptomatic latent period that creates unique challenges for a timely diagnosis and treatment plan. The compensatory mechanisms described earlier coupled with the potential patient perception that changes in health status may be the result of normal ageing can defer diagnostic investigations. The onset of symptoms of aortic stenosis marks a pivotal delineation in the determination of prognosis: left untreated, the risk of sudden death for severe aortic stenosis ranges from 8% to 34% after the onset of symptoms, and survival is limited to 1–3 years.

At their earliest stage of diagnosis, patients are likely to present with a decrease in exercise tolerance, fatigue, and/or dyspnoea on exertion. On examination, a slow rate of increase in the carotid pulse, a mid to late peaking intensity of a systolic murmur, and a reduced intensity of the second heart sound are consistent with signs of severe aortic stenosis. Advanced disease is characterized by the onset of one or more of the triad of manifestations of aortic stenosis—heart failure, angina, and/or syncope (see more information on these conditions in Chapters 6, 7, and 10)—which can be explained by the following mechanisms:

- Heart failure: left ventricular pressure overload increases when aortic stenosis becomes more haemodynamically compromising; the increased wall stress leads to left ventricular hypertrophy and the subsequent cascade of left ventricular diastolic dysfunction, increased end-diastolic pressure, and pulmonary congestion. Exertional symptoms are caused by impaired cardiac output.
- Angina: in the absence of concomitant coronary artery disease, angina in the setting of left ventricular dysfunction is the result of decreased coronary supply due to diastolic dysfunction, left ventricular hypertrophy, and mechanical compression.
- Syncope/presyncope: decreased cerebral perfusion and peripheral vascular resistance can cause patients to experience syncope or presyncope, especially in the most advanced stages of aortic stenosis.

Aortic regurgitation

Once symptomatic, patients with aortic regurgitation typically present with signs of left-sided heart failure, including dyspnoea on exertion, orthopnoea, and fatigue. Patients may experience angina in the absence of arteriosclerotic disease due to decreased aortic diastolic pressure and increased oxygen demand. Acute aortic regurgitation rapidly leads to dyspnoea or pulmonary oedema and/or cardiogenic shock due to the rapid elevation of end-diastolic pressures in the left ventricle. Some patients even with severe chronic aortic regurgitation may remain asymptomatic for a long time. In this setting and when left ventricular function is preserved, the probability of adverse events is low. In contrast, when the left ventricular end-systolic diameter is 50 mm or larger, the probability of death, symptoms, or left ventricular dysfunction is reported to be 19% per year.[5] In symptomatic patients with severe chronic aortic regurgitation, mortality without surgical treatment may be as high as 10–20% per year.[5] In acute presentations, haemodynamic instability is associated with a poor prognosis in the absence of treatment.

Mitral stenosis

Symptoms usually appear gradually over years, with patients first reporting dyspnoea on exertion triggered by infection, stress, pregnancy, or atrial fibrillation. Atrial fibrillation often begins in paroxysms and eventually becomes chronic with high risk of left atrial thrombus formation. Progression of disease with increasing left atrial and pulmonary venous pressures will cause progressive dyspnoea and heart failure. At more advanced stages, patients may experience fatigue due to low cardiac output, weakness, or, when right ventricular failure is present, abdominal discomfort due to hepatomegaly.

Severe rheumatic mitral stenosis is commonly observed in teenagers or young adults, although most patients usually do not experience symptoms until the second to fourth decade of life. Survival in asymptomatic patients with rheumatic mitral stenosis is generally good, however, depending on country. Symptomatic patients have a poor prognosis with a 5-year survival of only 44%.[6]

Mitral regurgitation

Similar to aortic stenosis, patients with chronic mitral regurgitation may be asymptomatic for years as compensatory mechanisms are activated. Initial signs include exercise intolerance, dyspnoea, orthopnoea, palpitations, new atrial arrhythmias, and lower extremity oedema. The gradual onset of symptoms may cause patients to seek medical care for subacute and vague symptoms, including fatigue and inability to sleep. Auscultation reveals a holosystolic murmur which is best heard at the apex. In moderate to severe mitral regurgitation, a third heart sound gallop is audible because of the high diastolic flow into the ventricle; in acute mitral regurgitation, the non-compliance of the left chambers can be manifested in a fourth heart sound gallop. Left ventricular dilatation can cause patients to have a left laterally displaced point of maximal impulse in advanced disease.

As disease progresses, left-sided heart failure and symptoms related to low cardiac output intensify. Patients can further develop right-sided heart failure due to increased pressures from the left heart affecting the right ventricle.

In contrast, symptoms progress rapidly in acute presentations as compensatory mechanisms fail to maintain the balance of oxygen supply and demand; tachycardia in response to reduced forward stroke volume, severe dyspnoea due to pulmonary congestion and oedema, and signs of left or biventricular failure due to pulmonary hypertension require immediate medical attention. Anxiety, diaphoresis, and decreased breath sounds can manifest worsening decompensation. In patients with severe chronic mitral regurgitation who are asymptomatic, the 5-year all-cause mortality rate is estimated at 22%, while cardiovascular mortality rate is 14%.[7] Acute mitral regurgitation carries a poor prognosis in the absence of intervention.

Infective endocarditis

The rate of symptom development and clinical deterioration in the setting of infective endocarditis depends on the pathogen and patients' overall health vulnerabilities. The initial symptoms often resemble those of other infections such as influenza or pneumonia and may include unspecific symptoms like fever, chills, fatigue, muscle pain, loss of appetite, and general discomfort. Consequently, patients may be misdiagnosed and treatment may be delayed. Given the potential rapid onset of septicaemia and haemodynamic instability, this delay in diagnosis can result in debilitating or fatal complications.

The most common objective clinical findings of endocarditis are fever and a new heart murmur corresponding to heart valve insufficiency. Signs and symptoms of microembolization and immunological responses such as petechiae (tiny purple or red spots on the skin, whites of the eyes, or inside the mouth), splinter haemorrhages (thin, red to reddish-brown lines of blood under the nails), Janeway lesions (red spots on the soles of the feet or the palms of the hands), Osler nodes (red, tender spots under the skin of the fingers or toes), and Roth spots (red spots with white or pale centres on the retina) may be present. The diagnosis of infective endocarditis is based on the modified Duke criteria, of which the most decisive ones are positive blood cultures with typical endocarditis pathogens and evidence of endocardial involvement with positive echocardiography or other imaging modalities.[3,4]

Assessment pathway

The assessment pathway for valvular heart disease is complex; it requires a multimodality and multidisciplinary approach to develop a comprehensive understanding of the patient's disease state and to develop a tailored treatment plan. In addition to the central importance of detailed physical assessment described elsewhere in this text (see Chapter 5), cardiac imaging, additional considerations in the setting of endocarditis, and functional and frailty assessment are particularly salient to the management of complex valvular heart disease.

Cardiac imaging and other diagnostic tests

Transthoracic echocardiography remains the most critical diagnostic modality for assessing the presence and severity of valvular heart disease. This non-invasive imaging provides images of calcified or flailed leaflets, mobility, valve structure, and anatomy. Measurement of left ventricular mass, ejection fraction, and transvalvular pressure gradients, velocity, and areas provide important diagnostic information. In many situations, transoesophageal echocardiography is required to perform a precise diagnosis both of the disease pathology and mechanism of valve disease. This information is furthermore important for assessment of surgical timing and detailed surgical planning.

Computed tomography (CT) is emerging as a powerful diagnostic tool, particularly in the setting of procedure planning for transcatheter treatment options. CT can determine annulus size and shape, risk of annular injury and coronary occlusion in the setting of aortic valve deployment, and provide imaging guidance in advance of angiographic procedures.

Other useful diagnostic modalities include 12-lead electrocardiography (ECG) to screen for left ventricular hypertrophy, chest radiography to assess for signs of heart failure, including cardiomegaly, prominent ascending aorta, and/or pulmonary venous congestion. Left and right cardiac catheterization and coronary angiography can augment haemodynamic assessment and identification of concomitant coronary artery disease. Measurement of plasma concentration of B-type natriuretic peptide (BNP) and N-terminal pro-BNP may be useful to document disease progression.

Additional considerations for infective endocarditis

Initial diagnostic procedures include investigations to confirm or deny the Duke criteria (➤ Fig. 8.1) and include a thorough medical history to identify predisposing factors and bacterial port of entry; auscultation; bloodwork including cultures to identify pathogen, biochemical infection response, and organ function; transoesophageal (and transthoracic) echocardiography; ECG investigating possible atrioventricular conduction disturbances; and, particularly in suspected prosthetic endocarditis, also positron emission tomography CT.[3,4] Screening in relation to weight loss and nutritional status, risk of pressure ulcers, falls assessment, functional capacity and frailty assessment are also relevant investigations at the time of hospital admission serving as a baseline for nursing strategies during a lengthy treatment.

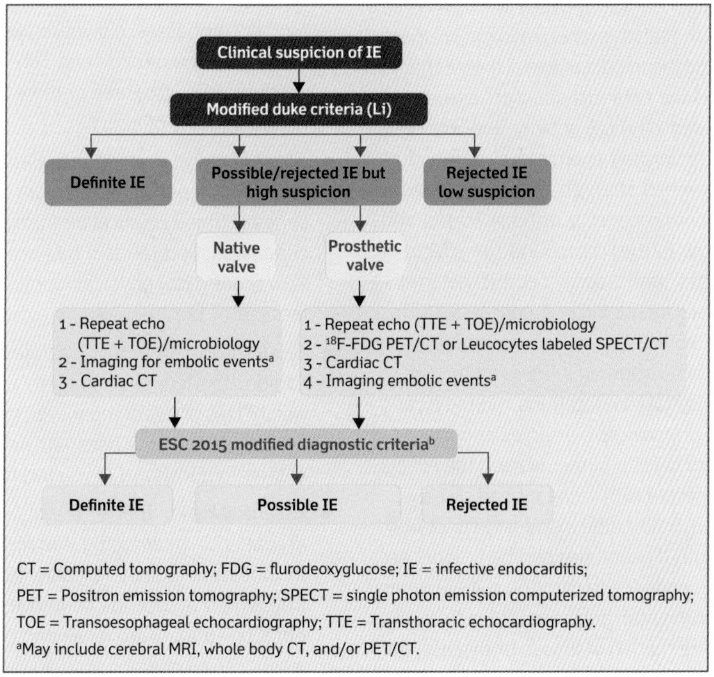

Fig. 8.1 Modified Duke criteria for the diagnosis of infective endocarditis (IE).

Habib G, Lancellotti P, Antunes MJ, et al; ESC Scientific Document Group. 2015 ESC Guidelines for the management of infective endocarditis: The Task Force for the Management of Infective Endocarditis of the European Society of Cardiology (ESC). Endorsed by: European Association for Cardio-Thoracic Surgery (EACTS), the European Association of Nuclear Medicine (EANM). Eur Heart J. 2015 Nov 21;36(44):3075–3128. doi: 10.1093/eurheartj/ehv319 © The European Society of Cardiology. Reprinted by permission of Oxford University Press.

Functional assessment and frailty

Acquired valvular heart disease is primarily a disease of ageing. The assessment of physical, mental, and social functional status and frailty is essential to determine patients' health status and support treatment decisions. A comprehensive understanding of frailty, including the pathophysiology, screening, and clinical implications, is a core competency of cardiovascular nurses who provide care to patients with complex valvular heart disease.

What is frailty?

Frailty is different from ageing and helps explain the heterogeneity of older adults. Frailty is a complex health state, often defined as an age-related, multisystem syndrome that increases health vulnerabilities and risks of adverse events (e.g. significant decline, functional impairment, death) when exposed to stressors (e.g. hospitalization, illness), compared with patients of the same age. Clinically, frailty can be conceptualized as a continuous spectrum of impaired resilience.[8] The challenge for patients with valvular heart disease is to maintain the fragile balance between their physical, mental, and social health status reserve; manage their accumulation of deficits and the impact of social determinants of health; and withstand the potential stressors associated with treatment. Decreased physical activity and impaired walking performance, diminished energy level and endurance (e.g. fatigue), weakened strength and balance, poor cognition, depressed mood, impaired nutritional status, and unintentional weight loss further compound the effects of comorbidities, disabilities, and socioeconomic determinants of health (e.g. social support, income, education).[9] This reduced reserve affects multiple organ systems and is associated with increased risks, including longer length of stay, delirium and other in-hospital complications, morbidity, and mortality.[10] The loss of physiological reserves and the progressive accumulation of deficits further worsen the effects of the cycle of frailty in people with valvular heart disease.

Although interrelated, frailty differs and is distinct from disability and comorbidity. Disabilities can be broadly defined as difficulty or dependency in carrying out activities of daily living or instrumental activities of daily living. Comorbidity refers to the burden of illness or disease, defined by the total burden of physiological dysfunction that affects patients' reserve. Frailty can worsen as a result of both disabilities and comorbidities.[11]

Why measure frailty?

The predictive value of frailty continues to be highlighted in multiple clinical trials and national registries. There is a widespread clinical consensus that the assessment of frailty augments the comprehensive evaluation of patients, informs treatment decision and early discharge planning, and supports individualized care to mitigate risks and optimize outcomes.[12] There is increasing evidence that the devastating effects of frailty can be attenuated by exercise and nutrition interventions to improve physical functioning after valvular heart disease treatment.[13]

How is frailty measured?

The absence of consensus surrounding assessment tools, the unstandardized measurements employed in research and clinical care, and the lack of validation in the valvular heart disease population continue to be significant barriers to the incorporation of frailty measurement in practice. The following are among the most consistently used instruments:[14]

- *Fried Scale*: this is the most frequently cited frailty scale and has been demonstrated to predict mortality and disability in patients with cardiac disease. The scale captures the core phenotypic domains of frailty and encompasses slowness, weakness, low physical activity, exhaustion, and shrinking (unintentional weight loss), with three or more of five criteria required for a diagnosis of frailty.
- *Short Physical Performance Battery*: the scale captures slowness, weakness, and balance and is measured by a series of timed physical performance tests—gait speed, chair rises, and tandem balance; each is scored 0 to 4 (low score = low physical function). A total score of 5 or less out of 12 is required for a diagnosis of frailty.
- *Study of Osteoporotic Fractures Index*: the index is a composite score of three frailty criteria to predict risk—weight loss of 5% or more over 3 years; ability to perform five sequential chair rises with arms folded on chest; and answer to question 'Do you feel full of energy?'
- *Essential Frailty Toolset*: the scale was recently validated in patients undergoing aortic valve replacement. It includes four indicators: ability to perform five chair rises in less than 15 seconds; cognitive status measured by the MiniCog (three-word recall and clock test drawing); and recent serum haemoglobin and albumin (➤ Fig. 8.2).

Comprehensive management plan

The following section provides an overview of multidisciplinary approaches to patient management, nursing

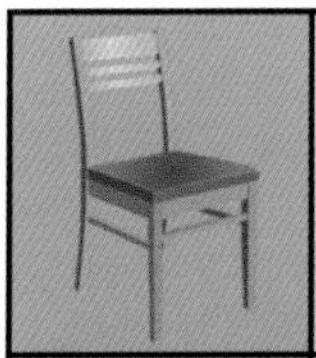	Five chair rises <15 seconds		0 points
	Five chair rises ≥15 seconds		1 points
	Unable to complete		2 points
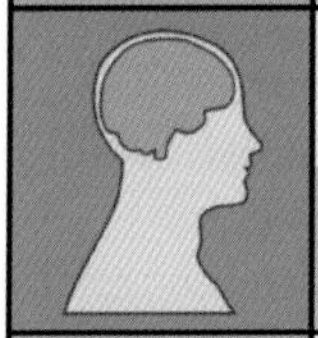	No cognitive impairment		0 points
	Cognitive impairment		1 point
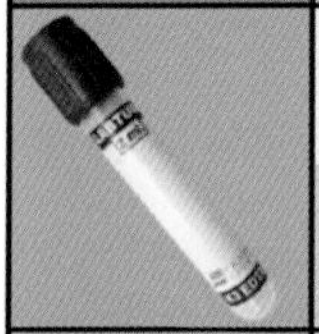	Hemoglobin	≥13.0 g/dL ♂ ≥12.0 g/dL ♀	0 points
	Hemoglobin	<13.0 g/dL ♂ <12.0 g/dL ♀	1 point
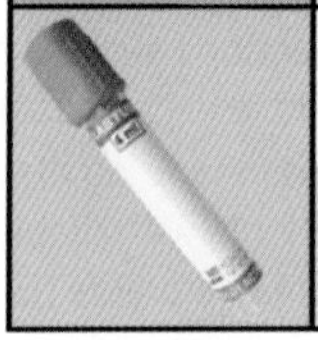	Serum albumin	≥3.5 g/dL	0 points
	Serum albumin	<3.5 g/dL	1 point

Fig. 8.2 The Essential Frailty Toolset measurements and scoring.[14]

Reproduced from Lauck SN, TM. Frailty, quality of life, and palliative approach. In: Transcatheter Aortic Valve Replacement Program Development: A Guide for the Heart Team. New York 2019 with permission from Wolters Kluwer.

care, and treatment options, including surgical and minimally invasive procedures, and recommendations about integrating a palliative approach among patients with different valve diseases will be given and are summarized in ➤ Box 8.1. This information augments the foundational recommendations provided in the European Society of Cardiology (ESC) and other guidelines.[3,15]

The Heart Team approach and specialized care

The concept of a multidisciplinary Heart Team for the provision of comprehensive, collaborative care to patients with valvular heart disease has emerged across regions and guidelines as a standard of care to guide the assessment pathway and treatment recommendations. This team-based approach aims to leverage the strengths and skills of its members to optimize the safety and quality of patient care (see also Chapter 3). The Heart Team comprises core and extended members who collectively provide care across the continuum (➤ Fig. 8.3). Although the foundation of the team may be the cardiothoracic surgeon and interventional cardiologist, each additional member provides value. Discussions centred on treatment options (e.g. surgical repair or replacement, percutaneous option, or medical management) are strengthened by the contributions of surgeons, cardiologists, imaging specialists, nurses, and other stakeholders. This team is best suited to discuss the management of concomitant conditions (e.g. the need for coronary revascularization) and individualized procedure planning. Mortality risk models including the EuroScore and the Society of Thoracic Surgeons (STS) score, are commonly used to assess and predict outcomes after surgery in terms of survival and major complications.[15] These risk scores can help guide the multidisciplinary team's evaluation of risk and benefits, and provide individualized treatment recommendations.

There are multiple layers of responsibility across multiple specialities, roles, and training. The formal responsibilities in patient assessment, treatment decisions, and procedural planning vary across valvular heart disease programmes, but all play pivotal roles in shepherding patients on the pathways of diagnosis, treatment, and follow-up. Although the distinct benefits associated with the Heart Team approach have yet to be fully evaluated, the aim is to provide high-quality, patient-centred care. Continuity is established and maintained from the time of initial consultation, procedure, and follow-up, which, in

Box 8.1 Key elements of nursing roles in the care of patients with valvular heart disease

1. Care coordination, patient and family education, early and ongoing discharge planning, and case management as part of the heart care interdisciplinary team.
2. Comprehensive understanding of frailty and its implications for patients with complex valvular heart disease.
3. Capacity to conduct a comprehensive face-to-face or telephone assessment to ascertain health status (e.g. shortness of breath, palpitation, syncope, change in physical condition, nutritional status, sleep patterns, mental health, and impact of comorbidities) in the outpatient clinic setting.
4. Exceptional communication skills applied to both patients families and the healthcare team.
5. Clinical observations of patients' haemodynamic condition immediately following valve surgery: rapid changes in condition, observation of fluids and monitoring of cardiac rate and rhythm, and appropriate use of vasoactive agents and fluid management.
6. Educating patients to observe for signs of wound infections after discharge for valve surgery.
7. Detection, treatment, and identification of the underlying causes of delirium.
8. Supporting the patient with delirium: decreasing visual and auditory stimuli, resuming day/night circadian rhythm, family support, and therapeutic communication skills.
9. Following nursing protocols or care standards for care of patients having TAVI: recovery from sedation/anaesthesia, vascular access haemostasis, cardiac rhythm monitoring, neurological status, readiness for mobilization, and renal function.
10. Special roles in the care of patients with infective endocarditis:
    a. Careful and comprehensive baseline assessment for nursing strategies addressing a long treatment duration.
    b. Specialist care coordination: role as the cross-disciplinary contact.
    c. Managing complications related to antimicrobial treatment: opportunistic infections such as oral or genital candidiasis, drug fever, skin rashes, and diarrhoea.
    d. Understanding of complex care needs for patients with diabetes, haemodialysis, and stroke sequelae (patient population with a high comorbidity burden).
    e. Development of a strong therapeutic relationship to address adherence given the length of treatment (see Chapter 12 and 13).
    f. Nurse-led follow-up clinics post discharge to monitor symptoms and provide education to support self-care.

similar specialities, has been found to affect the overall patient experience. Barriers to the development of a Heart Team approach include the absence of a valve programme coordinator (e.g. nurse), effective communication, scheduling and coordination, and 'programme culture' that is not conducive to interdisciplinary practice, also referred to as 'multidisciplinary' in the literature on the management of valvular heart disease. The pivotal role of cardiovascular nurses in the continuum of care of this complex patient group is increasingly noted in American and Canadian guidelines but currently absent from the ESC guidelines. The recognition of nurses is in the value of care coordination, patient and family education, early and ongoing discharge planning, and case management.

Nursing competencies in the outpatient clinic setting centre on the capacity to conduct a comprehensive in-person or telephone assessment to ascertain health status (e.g. shortness of breath, palpitation, syncope, change in physical condition, nutritional status, sleep patterns, mental health, and impact of comorbidities), and exceptional communication skills applied to both patients and the healthcare team.

In addition, specialized clinics in high-volume referral centres provide access to multidisciplinary expertise, integrated care processes for surveillance and follow-up, and the provision of multiple treatment options. In particular, the ongoing monitoring of cardiac echocardiography findings is essential to guide treatment, and contribute to the early recognition of disease progression.

Further, the emergence of multiple treatment options is an opportunity for the Heart Team to promote shared decision-making and the use of decision aids to incorporate patients' values and priorities. By this, the team can strengthen a patient-centred approach[16]—including ensuring that patients and families are informed and participate fully in their treatment plan—and optimize risk-stratified procedure planning to tailor care to individual needs.[17]

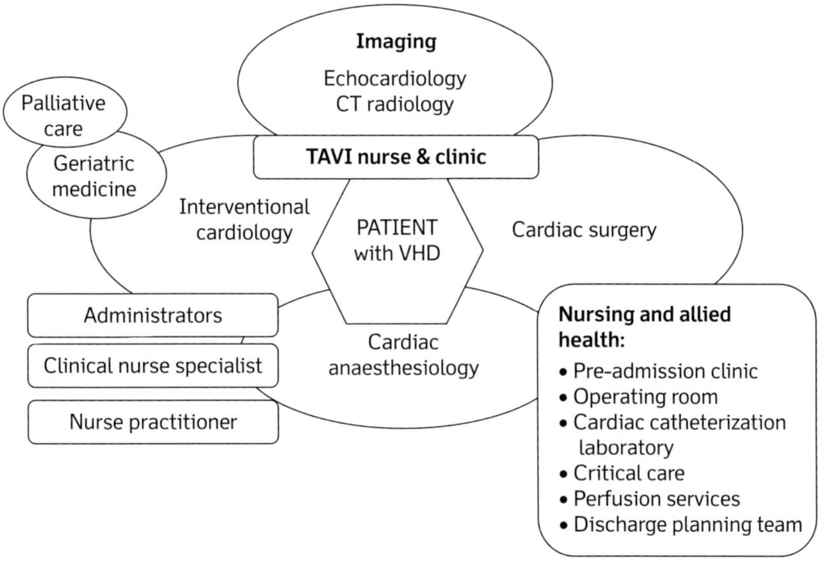

Fig. 8.3 The Heart Team approach in the management of valvular heart disease (VHD).

Although the Heart Team approach has been promoted primarily in the setting of the treatment of aortic stenosis and mitral regurgitation, a similar philosophy and approach is recommended as best practices in the management of infective endocarditis. In particular, coordinated and expert interdisciplinary care is essential as patients may require various treatment modalities, can have uneven recovery trajectories, are subject to significant complications, and may be transferred between and within institutions at various timepoints of treatment. Multidisciplinary endocarditis teams are recommended in the treatment/management and include consultants in cardiology with specialist competencies in echocardiography of valve disease, cardiac surgery, infectious diseases and/or medical microbiology, and radiology, as well as cardiac care nurses with specialist competencies (see also Chapter 3) in caring for patients with endocarditis and who will often function as the cross-disciplinary contact.[3]

Medical management

Valve replacement or repair is the primary treatment strategy for most valvular heart diseases as disease progression cannot be otherwise treated. The careful consideration of timing of intervention, risks and benefits, symptom burden, and patient preference are essential to developing a comprehensive management plan.

The concomitant presence of heart failure symptoms is particularly salient to patient management. Existing guidelines provide detailed recommendations to treat volume overload and other manifestations of decompensating cardiac function. Similarly, treatment with angiotensin-converting enzyme inhibitors, angiotensin receptor blockers, and beta-blockers are useful in patients with heart failure or hypertension.[15] In acute mitral regurgitation, treatment with nitrates and diuretics is recommended to reduce filling pressures. Specific clinical guidelines to further optimize the medical treatment for symptoms and comorbidities should be included, as appropriate.[15]

Special considerations: medical management of infective endocarditis

The medical management of infective endocarditis merits further discussion. The treatment of bacteraemia entails an average of 4–6 weeks of high-dosage intravenous antibiotic therapy in accordance with current guidelines.[1,2] Identifying and treating the infection site is a crucial part of the treatment to prevent infection exacerbation or recurrence. Additional prophylaxis may include tooth extractions, removal of intestinal polyps, and harm reduction strategies for intravenous drug users. Various outpatient antimicrobial treatment options have been found to be effective, including partial oral treatment at home,[18] and may be a treatment alternative for some patients.

During the course of illness, patients will often suffer considerable weight loss and depleted muscle mass, as a result of reduced appetite and/or physical activity. Other physical complications and discomforts, such as arrhythmia, heart failure symptoms, sleep disturbances, nausea and vomiting, pain, and skin itching, are also characteristic of infective endocarditis. Given the potentially poor prognosis, patients may struggle with concerns about survival, recovery, family, and work.[6]

An integral part of the management of patients with infective endocarditis is specialized care. Close monitoring for early signs of disease progression, inadequate infection control, and complications is essential to prevent clinical deterioration. This entails routine surveillance of bloodwork and ECG, observations for immunological and thromboembolic manifestations, and signs and symptoms of complications. Factors that may affect recovery and that should be assessed and addressed as part of qualified care for patients with endocarditis also include nutritional therapy, physical activity initiatives, mental health management, sleep quality management, and interventions aimed at risk reduction for people struggling with addictions.

Complications related to antimicrobial treatment include the management of opportunistic infections such as oral or genital candidiasis, drug fever, skin rashes, and diarrhoea. As the comorbidity burden in this patient population is relatively high, complex care for patients with diabetes, haemodialysis, and stroke sequelae are important competencies for cardiovascular nursing. Given the length of treatment and the need for adherence to treatment, a strong therapeutic relationship with patients and their caregivers is essential to ensure a good outcome.

Surgical valve replacement and repair

Understanding the basics

Surgical valve replacement or repair usually requires a sternotomy incision (a vertical line incision along the sternum) and the use of cardiopulmonary bypass, although minimally invasive surgical techniques (e.g. ministernotomy) are also available for selected patients.

In patients with aortic stenosis, valve replacement remains the dominant strategy, although newer solutions involving valve repair are gaining some attention. When replacing the aortic valve, the surgeon excises the diseased valve and replaces it with either a biological or a mechanical valve, based on clinical indication and patient preference. As biological valves degenerate over time, they may need to be replaced, and are most commonly offered to patients over the age of 65 years. Below this age, current recommendations include the selection of a mechanical valve, where the degeneration is a lesser issue. Importantly, living with a mechanical valve requires lifelong anticoagulation to prevent valve thrombosis.[15]

In patients with mitral regurgitation, treatment depends on disease severity, and anatomical considerations. Valve repair is the recommended strategy to optimize outcomes. Mitral valve repair includes patching holes in the valve, reconnecting valve leaflets, removing excess valve tissue to improve closing of the valve, and replacing cords. Commonly, the surgeon tightens or reinforces a ring around the valve (annulus), a procedure known as valve annuloplasty. If a repair is not feasible, valve replacement may be necessary. As with replacements of the aortic valve, both mechanical and biological replacements are prosthesis options.

Treatment considerations and recommendations depending on the valve affected can be reviewed more thoroughly in current clinical guidelines.[15]

Priorities of care

- The main focus in the immediate postoperative period is the patient's haemodynamic condition. Clinical observations performed by critical care nurses include rapid changes of the condition, observation of fluids, and monitoring of cardiac rate and rhythm, with the appropriate use of vasoactive agents and fluid management.
- Sternal precautions are performed to prevent separation and dehiscence of the sternal bone by avoiding excessive tension on the surgical incision. Sternal precautions also reduce pain and help prevents infections. These include:
  - Not lifting more than 2 kg in each hand (local variations might occur).
  - Not pushing or pulling with the arms.
  - Not reaching behind the back or reach both arms to the side.
  - Not reaching both arms over the head.
- Postoperative mobilization begins on the first postoperative day and supports the patient to recover and helps to prevent atelectasis. When mobilizing the patient, sternal precautions are part of the daily routine, and require ongoing reminders and coaching.
- As with postsurgical care in general, nutritional status, fluid intake and output balance, and prevention of constipation should be considered and included in the care of the patient.

- Wound care is an important part of postoperative care; local guidelines on bandages/dressings should be followed. The wound should be inspected daily during admission and after removal of the dressing. The nurse must teach the patient how to observe for signs of infections after discharge. Although not a common complication, 1–4% of all patients experience deep sternal wound infections after cardiac procedures. This serious complication is associated with increased morbidity and mortality. Similarly, among patients with a concurrent coronary artery bypass graft procedure, wound care of the incision of the leg (or arm) must be performed thoroughly.
- Another potential area of awareness is the patient's overall health status. In addition to the functional decline immediately after surgery, patients might also experience impaired mental health.[19,20] The underlying heart valve disease and the stress of undergoing heart valve surgery can affect quality of life and mental health.[21] Patients may also experience non-specific symptoms, including anxiety, depression, and pain (see also Chapter 11).[20]
- Discharge planning begins at admission by including both the patient and caregivers in what to expect when going home. The patients might need help resuming activities of daily living, and adhering and adapting to sternal precautions when resuming normal activities.

Potential complications

In the early recovery period, common complications include atrial fibrillation and other arrhythmias, heart failure, bleeding, and pleural and pericardial effusions. Furthermore, chest pain and pain management due to sternal discomfort are essential areas of awareness.

Postoperative delirium is a potentially devastating complications that occurs in a significant proportion of patients undergoing open heart surgery. Delirium is a disturbance of awareness with a reduced capacity to focus, sustain, or change focus.[19] The onset of delirium affects both the patient and family caregivers.[22] Older age, pre-existing psychological disorders, alcohol use, high comorbidity burden, low serum albumin, medical treatment with antidepressant agents, opioids, and benzodiazepines are known risk factors. Several screening tools are available to assess and monitor delirium, including the Confusion Assessment Method (CAM)[23] which has been used in patients after aortic valve replacement and demonstrated a prevalence of delirium of 60% after surgery.[10] Nurses play an essential role in both detecting, treating, and identifying the underlying causes of delirium. To support the patient with delirium, recommendations include decreasing visual and auditory stimuli, the use of a quiet room, resumption of day/night circadian rhythm (e.g. use of clocks, calendar, natural light/darkness), the use of usual hearing aid and glasses, family support, and therapeutic communication skills (see also Chapter 13).[19] Patients may have long-lasting memories of their delirium; thus, nursing competency in the management of this complication is essential for patient safety and optimal outcomes.[22]

Transcatheter valve replacement and repair

In the past decade, there has been a paradigm shift in the management of valvular heart disease with the rapid emergence of minimally invasive transcatheter options for patients with varying surgical risk profiles and valve diseases. These procedures share similar features that include transfemoral or minimally invasive alternative vascular access, catheter-based delivery of the valve replacement or repair device, and the possibility of a rapid recovery given the avoidance of thoracotomy and cardiopulmonary bypass. This field of practice is advancing rapidly. The following is limited to two established treatment options that are now widely available across regions: transcatheter aortic valve implantation (TAVI) and transcatheter mitral valve repair using percutaneous mitral leaflet plication.

Transcatheter aortic valve implantation

In 2010, the findings of the Placement of Aortic Transcatheter Valve (PARTNER) clinical trial first established TAVI as the standard of care for inoperable patients. Subsequently, recent research has supported the increasing use of TAVI as a safe and effective treatment also for lower-risk patients.[15,24,25] The care of TAVI patients is rapidly becoming a core competency of cardiovascular nursing in cardiac centres.

Understanding the basics

TAVI is a minimally invasive valve implantation procedure that uses a catheter and expandable stent technology to deliver a device within the native or failed bioprosthetic surgical aortic valve. Original calcified valve leaflets are displaced by the TAVI valve using balloon-, self-, or mechanically expandable mechanisms to seat the device within the diseased orifice. For most patients, vascular access is usually through the femoral artery; in the setting of excessive arterial calcification and/or tortuosity, an alternative minimally invasive surgical approach—for example, the subclavian artery, the ascending aorta, or the cardiac apex—can be selected.

In earlier years, TAVI was often performed under protocols similar to cardiac surgery, including under general anaesthesia, with the use of multiple invasive lines, and in an operating room, while most patients recovered in a critical care unit and remained in the hospital for more than 5 days. Increasingly, TAVI programmes have adapted their processes of care to better match the procedure and technology, and mitigate the risks associated with the extended admission of frail elderly. In most cases, TAVI can be safely performed under local anaesthesia, without a central venous line or urinary catheter, and in a hybrid suite or a cardiac catheterization laboratory, with minimal requirements for critical care recovery and a length of stay of 1–2 days.[17] However, this minimal length of stay is still to be implemented in most clinical practices in Europe.

Priorities of care

Early recovery focuses on the rapid return to baseline status, the careful monitoring for potential complications, and preparation for discharge and safe transition home. Nursing protocols or care standards ought to highlight (1) recovery from sedation/anaesthesia, (2) vascular access haemostasis, (3) cardiac rhythm monitoring, (4) neurological status, (5) readiness for mobilization, and (6) renal function. In addition, vigilant scrutiny of mental status and infection can assist in the early recognition of delirium and sepsis, and help mitigate known risks that elderly patients face during hospital admission. An example of a nursing care pathway that was evaluated in a multicentre study is provided in ➤ Table 8.1.[26]

Potential complications

Outcomes in contemporary TAVI continue to improve, and most patients have excellent results. Nevertheless, cardiovascular nurses must be aware of potential adverse events that warrant monitoring, early recognition, and intervention. These outcomes are collectively grouped and defined by the Valve Academic Research Consortium (VARC2)[27] and include the following with some highlighted aetiologies:

- Mortality: includes in hospital and up to 30 days post procedure.
- Myocardial infarction: obstruction of coronary blood flow due to leaflet displacement over the ostia.
- Stroke: dislodged calcium from the diseased valve leaflets.
- Bleeding (minor and major): vascular injury, internal bleeding (e.g. stroke).
- Acute kidney injury: administration of contrast.
- Vascular access complications (minor and major): puncture, catheter apparatus, and/or closure device injury.
- Conduction disturbances and arrhythmias: implant-related damage to conduction tissue requiring new permanent pacemaker.

In addition, elderly patients are at higher risk for accelerated deconditioning due to periprocedure stressors, impaired mobilization, and delayed resumption of normal hydration, nutrition, and activities of daily living. In the longer term there is also excess risk of prosthetic endocarditis after TAVI as compared to medical treatment.

Transcatheter mitral valve repair (mitral valve leaflet plication)

Building on the legacy of cardiac surgery and the established Alfieri procedure that involves the suturing of mitral valve leaflets, transcatheter mitral valve repair may be indicated for higher surgical risk patients who present with primary (e.g. degenerative) or secondary (e.g. functional) mitral regurgitation.

Understanding the basics

Mitral valve leaflet plication is a minimally invasive procedure that involves vascular access in the femoral vein, and advancing a delivery catheter across the intra-atrial septum to the diseased mitral valve. Guided primarily by transoesophageal echocardiography, the operator grasps the valve leaflets and deploys one or more clips, thus joining the leaflets and reducing the valve orifice area. Transoesophageal echocardiography imaging is used to confirm the decrease in regurgitant flow across the mitral valve.

Mitral valve leaflet plication is routinely performed in a hybrid suite or in a cardiac catheterization laboratory through a transfemoral route under general anaesthesia because of the need for transoesophageal echocardiography and the variable procedure times. Patients usually remain haemodynamically stable throughout the procedure and have minimal critical care requirements in the early recovery period. Most patients spend 1–2 days in hospital.

Table 8.1 TAVI post-procedure protocol

Interventions/ component of care	0–6 hours	6–12 hours	12–18 hours	18–24 hours	24–36 hours
Goal of care #1: return to baseline haemodynamic and neurological status					
Vital signs	Q15 min × 4 Q1 h × 3	Q4 hours			
Neuro vital signs and Cincinnati Stroke Scale assessment	Q15 min × 4 Q30 min × 2 Q1 hour × 3	Q4 hours			
Goal of care #2: vascular access haemostasis					
Vascular access monitoring	Q15 min × 4 Q1 hour × 3	Q4 hours			
Diagnostic tests	CBC			CBC	
Pain assessment	Assess and treat access sites and/or back/postural pain discomfort as required. Avoid opioids and sedative hypnotics to minimize risk of delirium. Communicate abnormal findings early				
Goal of care #3: absence of new conduction delay					
Cardiac rhythm monitoring	Continuous monitoring. Analyse PR interval and cardiac rhythm with each set of vital signs				
Diagnostic tests	12-Lead ECG				
Communication	Inform physician of any new intraventricular conduction delay				
Goal of care #4: removal of invasive monitoring devices					
Peripheral/central vascular access	If goal of care #1 achieved, remove central venous and peripheral arterial catheters	Apply saline lock to peripheral intravenous access			Remove saline lock before discharge
Goal of care #5: early mobilization and return to baseline elimination, hydration, and nutrition					
Mobilization and activity	Head of bed flat ×2 hours, then ↑ 30° Total bedrest ×4 hours then stand at side of bed	Mobilize short distance Up in chair		Facilitate uninterrupted sleep Encourage self-care behaviour	Mobilize for 5–10 min every 4–6 hours

(continued)

Table 8.1 Continued

Interventions/ component of care	0–6 hours	6–12 hours	12–18 hours	18–24 hours	24–36 hours
Elimination—avoid urinary catheterization	Monitor eGFR ×1 Mobilize to commode and/or standing position when bedrest completed	Mobilize to toilet Anticipate low urine output in the early recovery period until return to baseline hydration status eGFR POD 1			
Hydration and nutrition	NPO until haemostasis and confirmed clinical stability IV infusion 50–75 mL/hour	If LVEF ≥50%: encourage fluids If LVEF <50%: encourage fluids within limit of any pre-procedure fluid restrictions Up in chair for meals Encourage nutritional intake and preferred foods			
Goal of care #6: readiness for next-day discharge					
Patient and family education	Teaching about maintaining vascular access haemostasis	Teaching about importance of return to baseline status (e.g. motivation for mobilization) Begin discharge teaching		Complete discharge teaching	
Discharge planning		Confirm discharge plan with patient and family		Assess readiness for discharge	Confirm discharge criteria

CBC, complete blood count; eGFR, estimated glomerular filtration rate; ECG, electrocardiogram; IV, intravenous; LVEG, left ventricular ejection fraction; min, minutes; NPO, nothing by mouth; POD, postoperative day; Q, every.

Priorities of care

In the early recovery period, priorities include (1) recovery from general anaesthesia and (2) vascular access haemostasis. Given the heart failure burden associated with mitral regurgitation, close monitoring of cardiac function may be warranted.

Potential complications

The procedure is generally well tolerated. Venous access reduces the risk of severe vascular injury; nevertheless, bleeding following arterial or ventricular access remains one of the most frequent major complications. Rates of pericardial tamponade and clip-specific complications (e.g. embolization and/or detachment) are low.[28]

Surgical treatment of infective endocarditis

In patients with infective endocarditis, surgery has two primary objectives: removal of the infected tissues and reconstruction of the cardiac morphology, as well as replacement or repair of the affected valve(s). The primary focus of the infection responsible for the infective endocarditis should preferably be treated before surgery is performed.[3] The timing of surgery depends on the consideration of haemodynamic impairment, the benefits of sufficient infection control, and risks of embolism and other complications. Patient care is consistent with the priorities and potential complications described in previous sections.

In the setting of endocarditis related to an implanted device, complete hardware extraction in addition to the antibiotic regimen are essential. At that time, the clinical team and the patient may re-evaluate the indication for device treatment and reimplantation as the risk of repeat infection is high. In some cases, lifelong antibiotics may be an appropriate strategy, particularly among older and more frail patients to mitigate further risks.

Medical management: integrating a palliative approach

The treatment of patients who are dying 'with' valvular heart disease but not 'from' valvular heart disease does little to modify the poor prognosis associated with comorbidities, excessive frailty, and disability. The futility of treatment in patients with excessive comorbidities, functional and cognitive decline, and/or frailty is well established. The adoption of a palliative approach can help improve continuity of care and support patients' transition to a focus on symptom management.

Palliative approach and valvular heart disease programmes

The advanced age and health vulnerabilities of valvular heart disease patients, their procedure-focused clinical trajectories, the complexities of the referral patterns, and the involvement of multiple medical specialities combine to form a 'perfect storm' for potentially failing to attend to the important end of life requirements of patients presenting with severe aortic stenosis. When there is not a treatment option with a likelihood of significant benefit of improved quantity and quality of life, programmes ought to provide an alternative care plan for patients for whom a valve intervention has been deemed clinically futile.

A palliative approach is a way of caring for those with life-limiting illnesses that focuses on improving patients' and families' quality of life. This holistic, needs-based perspective aims to assess and improve symptom management, communication, advanced care planning, and psychosocial and spiritual needs regardless of prognosis. The focus is on meeting a person's and his/her family's full range of needs at all stages of a life-limiting illness.[29] The integration of a palliative approach can be a parallel process to the pursuit of curative care so that if and when an intervention is not an option, the patient, family, and healthcare team can change the focus of discussions to match the changing health trajectory.[30]

Integrating best practices

There can be barriers to adopting a palliative approach in valvular heart disease programmes: clinicians may perceive that discussions about end of life may remove hope, cause increased confusion, or be incongruent with previous discussions. The complexity of treatment decisions, prognostic uncertainty, lack of knowledge about palliative care, and confidence to initiate or pursue discussions about end of life further contribute to a lack of clarity of the responsibility of the multidisciplinary team.

To overcome these barriers, the following steps are recommended to identify patients who would benefit from a palliative approach:

- Ask yourself: 'Would I be surprised if this patient died in the next 6–12 months?'
- Look for one or more general clinical indicators (e.g. limited self-care, in chair or bed >50% of the day, multiple hospitalizations in the past 6 months, and/or the requirement for extensive home or residential care).
- Look for two or more cardiac disease indicators (e.g. New York Heart Association functional class III or

IV, renal impairment, cardiac cachexia, two or more episodes needing intravenous furosemide, and/or inotropes in the past 6 months).

- Asking simple questions such as 'Tell me what you understand about your illness', 'Tell me what you expect by having the valve procedure', or 'What is most important to you?' can help inform patients' goals of care and help improve outcomes and patients' experiences.[31]

The decision of appropriate treatment (medical/surgical treatment or a palliative approach) should always be reached through a process of shared decision-making with the patients and by including perspectives of the family. As older age and high comorbidity burden increase the risk of interventions and, thus, might have a negative impact on life expectancy and quality of life, an appropriate risk assessment is needed, especially in the elderly patient.

The complexity of valvular heart disease—irrespective of aetiology and treatment options—highlights the central importance of nurses' role in optimizing patients' capacity for self-care during their health trajectories. Promotion of physical, mental, and social health status hinges on education tailored to the unique needs of patients and their families (see also Chapter 13), awareness of potential complications and risk for deterioration (see also Chapter 5), and partnerships to support adherence to treatment are nurse-led strategies that can improve outcomes and patient experiences. These components of care are illustrated in ➤ **Table 8.2** which outlines two case studies focused on aortic stenosis and infective endocarditis.

After a heart valve procedure: follow-up

Facilitating safe transition home

The early period after returning home from the hospital can be particularly challenging for patients and their families. The evidence concerning patient experiences solely after heart valve surgery is scant, but in the few studies that do exist, patients report experiencing tiredness and deconditioning, worry about symptoms, and concerns about returning to their usual way of life.[20,32–34] In general, altered bodily awareness, symptom burden, and the increased risk of complications in the early postoperative period may postpone the overall recovery process.[32]

Similarly, the risk of readmission should be considered before discharge, as emerging evidence shows high readmission rates after both surgical procedures and TAVI, especially in the early period after discharge.[35] Thus, discharge planning should include an assessment of the readmission risk, including data on clinical symptoms, possible effusions, and frailty status.[36] In combination, this information can inform an individualized, early follow-up including symptom management in the early postoperative period, patient education, and awareness-raising concerning mental health—and is therefore suggested.[20,32,36]

Patients recovering from infective endocarditis will often have been physically inactive for weeks or months due to diagnostic delay, their symptom burden, long-term hospitalization, and possible postsurgical restrictions. Though the area of research seems largely unexplored, patients report slow physical and mental recovery.[37,38] Qualitative findings describe patient experiences of physical weakness and extreme fatigue, but also identify emotional instability, including anxiety and depression as major themes.[39] Although the rate of recurrence of endocarditis is fairly low (2–6%), high readmission rates of 65% within the first year have been reported and up to 35% of previously employed patients have been reported not returning to work within 1 year post discharge.[3,38,40] This indicates that the burden of the disease, both for the patient and the healthcare system, potentially continues to be substantial following a successful treatment. For patients having undergone heart valve surgery, possible complications include those similar to other valve surgery patients.

Surveillance and monitoring

As with the clinical assessment before treatment, monitoring and surveillance in the period after discharge should ideally be performed in multidisciplinary heart valve clinics. The monitoring should include observations aimed at detecting deterioration of the valve and the overall condition of the patient.[15] Nurses play an essential role in the follow-up and symptom monitoring during follow-up.

Surveillance after completion of medical therapy for endocarditis includes patients' self-monitoring as well as follow-up visits according to local guidelines.[3,4] Investigations at follow-up include a physical examination, bloodwork and cultures, and possibly transthoracic echocardiogram. Patients should be educated to observe for signs of recurrent infection and of heart failure indicative of valve dysfunction. Other health issues may persist

Table 8.2 Clinical case studies on aortic stenosis and infective endocarditis

	Aortic stenosis	Infective endocarditis
1. Patient population and medical history	Margaret is an 84-year-old widow who lives alone in the same town as her daughter and grandchildren. Margaret lost her husband the previous year, and has found it difficult to live alone. Her previous medical history includes a history of hypertension, smoking, dyslipidaemia, previous hip replacement, myocardial infarction, and coronary artery bypass 12 years ago. For the past 6 months, she has felt increasingly short of breath and easily fatigued	John is a 43-year-old carpenter who is married and the father of two young boys. John has previously been in good health and has rarely sought medical care. Over the past 2 months, he has felt increasingly unwell and tired, has experienced intermittent fevers, and lost nearly 10 kg. His wife encourages him to see their family physician, who treats him with a short course of antibiotics for a likely diagnosis of mild pneumonia
2. Clinical presentation	Margaret's family doctor is concerned about her worsening symptoms. She can only walk 2 blocks without stopping and has difficulties climbing stairs. He refers her for an echocardiogram which reveals a significantly reduced valve area of 0.8 cm^2 and a high transvalvular gradient of 42 mmHg. Her left ventricular function is preserved, but she has mild mitral insufficiency	John's condition deteriorates and one night he wakes up feeling very short of breath and anxious. He is pale, his skin is clammy, and his ankles are swollen. John's wife drives him to the emergency department. On admission, his temperature is 38.5°C, blood pressure 130/80 mmHg, pulse regular at 110 beats per minute. A chest X-ray shows signs of congestion, and a systolic heart murmur is audible. After undergoing an echocardiogram, the cardiologist tells John that she is worried he might have bacterial endocarditis
3. Evaluation pathway	The Heart Team meets to review Margaret's presentation. The surgeon states that Margaret has significant risks for open surgery, including previous sternotomy and newly diagnosed moderate renal impairment. The heart valve clinic nurse reports that Margaret is independent with her activities of daily living, is moderately frail, but experiences good quality of life. She is motivated to be treated and hopes that her symptoms will improve. Her coronary angiogram and CT scan are unremarkable. The Heart Team recommends TAVI as the preferred option for Margaret	The transoesophageal echocardiogram reveals mitral valve endocarditis with vegetations on the anterior leaflet. Blood cultures are positive for *Staphylococcus aureus*, and further confirm John's diagnosis. The cardiologist consults with an infectious disease specialist to review the findings and develop a treatment plan
4. Treatment	Margaret is admitted on the day of her procedure, and undergoes TAVI with percutaneous vascular access through the femoral artery. The procedure is done with local anaesthesia and light sedation	John requires a 4-week regimen of in-hospital intravenous antibiotics and telemetry monitoring to control the infection. His hospitalization is complicated by poor sleep, loss of appetite, low mood, and stress associated with family and financial concerns. Upon clearance from the infectious disease consultant, John undergoes surgical mitral valve repair

(continued)

Table 8.2 Continued

	Aortic stenosis	Infective endocarditis
5. In-hospital nursing care and priorities	Immediately following the procedure, the cardiac nurse monitors Margaret to ensure vascular haemostasis, haemodynamic stability, and absence of new conduction delay. To present any deconditioning, the nurse assists Margaret to ambulate 4 hours after her procedure, and to resume normal hydration, nutrition, and elimination as soon as possible. The next day, she is transferred to the cardiology ward where she is encouraged to walk and to take care of herself. With the absence of complications and a discharge plan in place, Margaret is ready to return home 2 days after her procedure	In the cardiac surgery intensive care unit, the nurse follows the local postoperative nursing care standard. The priorities of care include monitoring for any complications, ensuring appropriate cardiac output, and providing supportive care. John is rapidly extubated, and transferred to the cardiac ward the day after his surgery. Nurses teach him about sternal precautions, and the importance of breathing exercises and mobilization. Although he is thankful that his surgery was uncomplicated, his mood remains low and his sleep is easily disrupted. John's recovery is lengthened by a further 2-week course of intravenous antibiotics before he is cleared for discharge
6. Discharge planning and follow-up	As planned prior to the procedure, Margaret's daughter stays with her mother for 3 nights to help her recover. Margaret follows the recommendations to have 2–3 short walks every day, rest, and eat nutritious foods. She sees her family doctor 1 week after discharge, and has a follow-up echocardiogram 1 month after her TAVI. She is pleased to notice that her shortness of breath has improved significantly, and feels a bit stronger every day	John is relieved to return home after so many weeks. He has lost weight and still feels tired. His healthcare team has told him that, although he is cured, it will take up to 6 months for him to return to his normal function. John and his wife are fearful about his health, and still have many questions. John plans to rest, spend time with his family, and start the cardiac rehabilitation programme as soon as possible

after the end of treatment and should be addressed in follow-up care, including nutritional issues, pain management, and mental health problems which could be managed in a nurse-led clinic.

Post-procedure echocardiography

Echocardiography is recommended in existing guidelines as a vital part of the management of the patient after heart valve procedures with specific time points of follow-up after discharge varying, depending on the type of surgery, choice of the prosthesis, and pertinent guidelines.[15] The echocardiography should focus on functioning of the prosthesis, stenosis, regurgitation, paravalvular leakage, and ejection fraction. Furthermore, echocardiography should include assessment of pericardial effusion which commonly occurs within the first month after open heart valve surgery.

Considerations for antithrombotic management

Following surgery, oral anticoagulation is recommended as a lifelong treatment for all patients with mechanical valves (see also Chapter 12). The anticoagulation treatment (warfarin) includes clinical consultations based on individual assessment, close monitoring of international normalized ratio (INR), patient education, and possible self-monitoring among patients capable of this[15] (➤ Box 8.2).

Among patients with bioprostheses or mitral repair, temporary anticoagulation may be recommended depending on the site and type of surgery. Long-term anticoagulation is driven by other considerations, including atrial fibrillation, heart failure, or impaired left ventricular function. The anticoagulation after both surgical treatment and TAVI remains the subject of current studies and recommendations should be checked in the most contemporary guidelines.

Box 8.2 Cardiovascular nurse management of patients on warfarin following valve replacement

Patients who have a surgical mechanical valve replacement are recommended a lifelong treatment with oral anticoagulation, warfarin. In addition, temporary treatment with warfarin should be considered after surgical implantation of a mitral or tricuspid bioprosthesis.[15] Although based on low-level evidence, in patients receiving surgical aortic bioprostheses, low-dose aspirin is favoured as an alternative to postoperative anticoagulant.[15]

Treatment with warfarin requires close monitoring in order to achieve therapeutic levels and reduce the risk of bleeding (see also Chapter 12). The INR should be maintained within a therapeutic range near a median value. The specific values should be assessed according to recent guidelines.[15] Accordingly, the INR target level should be adapted to patient risk factors and the thrombogenicity of the valve prosthesis.

Thromboembolism and anticoagulant-related bleedings are known complications following prosthetic valve procedures, which is why the monitoring remains essential. If the INR falls too low, patients may not have sufficient protection from developing thromboembolism. On the other hand, if the INR is too high, the patient will be at increased risk of bleeding. Also, the high variability of the INR is associated with reduced survival following valve surgery. The risk of major bleeding increases when the INR exceeds 4.5, and an INR greater than 6.0 requires a rapid medical reversal of the anticoagulation.

Oral anticoagulation should be started within the first postoperative days and to ensure sufficient treatment, intravenous unfractionated heparin is commonly added to the treatment until a therapeutic level of INR has been obtained. Thus, regular monitoring is required and much more frequently in the early initiation period. Once the INR is stabilized in the therapeutic range, monitoring can be reduced, but often, the patients are discharged with monitoring twice a week.

Therefore, to ensure patient adherence, patient education is a priority. The patient education should include the following:

1. How warfarin works.
2. The need for self-monitoring for signs of bleeding (e.g. gums, urine, stools, nosebleeds, vomiting blood, and unusual headache).
3. When and how to contact a health professional.
4. Preventing bleeding (e.g. use a soft toothbrush, electric shaver, avoiding falls, and taking care with knives in the kitchen).
5. Interaction of warfarin with alcohol, foods, and medications.

Portable patient self-testing devices and patient self-management systems are available for patients to use at home to test blood and adjust the warfarin dose to keep the INR within the therapeutic range. Allowing patients to self-manage has been shown to significantly reduce mortality and thromboembolic events in addition to increasing patient adherence.[41,42]

In many countries, monitoring INR or teaching patients and/or informal caregivers to do so is performed in nurse-led anticoagulation/warfarin clinics. The specialized nurses in these clinics carry out dose adjustment and patient education for self-monitoring and management and prevention of complications. However, a survey conducted on delegates at the ESC Nurses' Spring meeting in 2014 found that nurses working in cardiovascular care had knowledge deficits relating to anticoagulation with warfarin and dietary and medicinal interactions.[43] In addition, less than half reported that they offered patient self-testing devices and patient self-management systems to their patients, despite their availability.

Endocarditis prophylaxis

Prevention of infections in the prosthetic valve is important, as the risk of developing infective endocarditis is increased after surgery. The evidence regarding endocarditis prophylaxis is sparse and the topic remains contentious among clinicians; most commonly, endocarditis prophylaxis includes a single-dose antibiotic treatment when patients undergo dental procedures, especially bleeding procedures. Impeccable dental hygiene in general is recommended.[3,15] Furthermore, whenever patients experience fever of unknown origin, clinicians should be aware and consider screening for endocarditis prophylaxis.

Patient education and information during follow-up

Patient education during recovery and follow-up may include information on expected physical recovery, sick leave, sexuality and intimacy issues, social functioning, engaging in sports, observation and care of scars, possible insurance issues, patient organizations, and the use of peer support (➤ Table 8.3).

Table 8.3 Patient education during recovery and follow-up

Topic	What to inform patients
Wound care	Patients should inspect the wound every day within the first weeks after surgery to prevent infections Signs to be aware of include redness, heat, swelling, and pain Stitches should be removed after 7–10 days after surgery (local variations might occur) Patients might feel itchy, numb, or tingly around the incisions for the first months
Pain	Patients should be encouraged to perform exercises during the postoperative period—often physiotherapists will guide patients on this during admission—and rehabilitation Most patients experience muscular pain within the first period after surgery If patients experience chest pain/angina, local guidelines on whom to contact should be followed
Sternal precautions	Patients are encouraged to follow sternal precautions (see earlier in this chapter) to help prevent infections and reduce pain
Nutrition	Immediately after the surgery and within the first month after, a diet rich in proteins and calories is recommended. This reduces the catabolic phase and stimulates the anabolic phase (the healing and recovery phase) After the healing period, a heart-friendly diet is recommended among patients undergoing combined valvular and bypass surgery Patients often experience reduced appetite and weight loss within the first month after surgery, but the patients should be encouraged to eat sufficiently
Sleep	Patients often have trouble sleeping and feel more tired and have reduced energy
Exercise	Patients are commonly offered rehabilitation or specific physical exercises by a physiotherapist. In addition, patients should be encouraged to go for daily walks Outdoor bicycling is not recommended in the period of the sternal precautions
Shortness of breath	During the first period after surgery, shortness of breath can occur Beware of patients with low ejection fraction (and/or a diagnosis of heart failure) and patients with known reduced lung capacity
Cognition	It is normal to have mild trouble with short-term memory or to feel confused in the early period after surgery
Mental health	Many patients experience impaired mental health/quality of life. Similarly, mood changes in the early period after surgery are normal As part of the rehabilitation following surgery, patients should be screened for symptoms of anxiety and depression and local guidelines on how to react should be followed
Driving (car)	Driving is not recommended within the 1–2 months after surgery due to sternal precautions (beware of local variation)
Constipation	Constipation due to immobilization and use of pain killers is normal, and patients should be informed about how to prevent this
Sexual activity	Patients can resume sexual activity after discharge, but should be told that sexual activity should be performed with awareness of the sternal bone and sternal precautions. Some medicines and mental health after surgery might influence the sexual response for both men and women
Relatives	Relatives are encouraged to participate in all consultations and to be involved during admission It is important to recognize the need for support to relatives

Mental health

Patients may suffer from symptoms of anxiety and depression in the period after discharge, which may affect adherence to treatment and discharge guidelines, and delay recovery and return to everyday life. Evidence regarding the effect of specific screening tools is lacking; among patients with symptoms of anxiety and depression, a collaboration with/or referral to a general practitioner is recommended. The risk of impaired mental health is increased among both patients treated with valvular diseases in general, and among patients suffering from infective endocarditis (see also Chapter 11).

Physical and cardiac rehabilitation

Although the evidence on the effect of physical rehabilitation following isolated heart valve surgery is sparse,[44] it is still recommended. Rehabilitation should include exercise prescription and training similar to what is recommended among patients undergoing coronary artery bypass grafting.[15] The consideration of unique clinical issues—including the potential occurrence of pleural and/or pericardial effusions, impaired left ventricular function, and arrhythmias—is pivotal to safe cardiac rehabilitation in the setting of valvular heart disease. Cardiac rehabilitation is recommended after the termination of the period of sternal restrictions (6–8 weeks after surgery) (see also Chapter 11).

Currently, there is a gap in research focused on investigating cardiac rehabilitation in patients treated for infective endocarditis. In planning follow-up care and assessing adverse outcomes, clinicians and policymakers, therefore, have little information about referral rates, participation rates, or content and efficacy of any programmes offered. There is, however, mounting evidence that recovery after infective endocarditis is slow and often inadequate. Therefore, the need for providing more effective follow-up care seems evident.

Follow-up: patient-reported outcomes and experiences

The way clinicians, researchers, policymakers, and the general public think about health, healthcare, and the role of patients as partners is changing. Increasingly, multiple stakeholders recognize the importance of physical, mental, and social patient-reported health status, the adverse consequences of illness from patients' perspectives, and that patients are the most important experts of their health and illness[45] (see also Chapter 2). The ESC has strongly endorsed the importance of measuring patient-reported perspectives in practice and research to improve quality of care.[46] This is particularly salient in the management of complex valvular heart disease where the potential risks and benefits can vary greatly; the reporting of mortality and morbidity does not suffice to fully capture patients' experiences of care. To this end, we provide a short introduction to the measurement of health-related quality of life and other patient-centred quality indicators.

Patient-reported outcome and experience measurements (PROMs and PREMs) are umbrella terms used to capture information obtained directly from patients about various aspects of their health and healthcare, including symptoms, functioning, well-being, quality of life, perceptions about treatment, and satisfaction with care received and with their professional communication with clinicians. A PROM is a precise, reliable, valid, and reproducible measure of aspects of patients' health status using questionnaires or other scales. Patient-related outcome data come directly from the patient, without the interpretation of the patient's responses by a physician, nurse, or anyone else.

The purpose of measuring patients' perspectives of their care is to augment conventional indicators of treatment decision and outcome evaluation and to strengthen a patient-centred approach to care. PROMs and PREMs can improve the quality of patient care and the optimization of resource utilization.

The selection of patient-reported instruments should reflect the goals of measurement. The process of PROM and PREM development includes the identification and synthesis of the conceptually driven domains to be measured, followed by validation testing to confirm the robustness of the measures. This rigour is essential to support claims that can be made about outcomes. Instruments can be defined as scientifically valid if the outcomes are conceptually defined and operationalized in questionnaires and if the questionnaires can meet established standards of reliability, validity, responsiveness, and sensitivity and withstand the scrutiny of psychometric evaluation.[45] Equally important, however, is the clinical relevance of the measure. PROMs capture disease-specific (e.g. heart failure) and/or generic (e.g. overall quality of life) domains. PREMs measure patients' perception of their experience with healthcare (➤ **Fig. 8.4**).

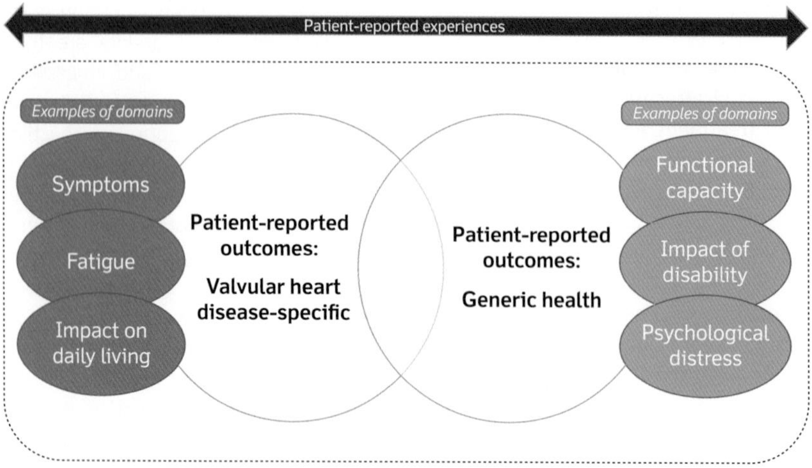

Fig. 8.4 Generic and disease-specific patient-reported outcomes.

Conclusion

Cardiovascular nurses require a comprehensive understanding of the complexity of managing valvular heart disease in a diverse and clinically demanding population. The implications of changes in haemodynamics, the trajectory of heart failure, and the variation in clinical presentation across age groups and pathologies create unique challenges to optimize outcomes and support patients and their family. The rapid advances in technology, procedural approaches, and cardiac imaging make this clinical area particularly exciting for cardiovascular nurses to demonstrate their leadership and unique competencies, and contribute significantly to improving the lives of people living with valvular heart disease.

References

1. d'Arcy JL, Prendergast BD, Chambers JB, Ray SG, Bridgewater B. Valvular heart disease: the next cardiac epidemic. Heart. 2011;97(2):91–93.
2. Eveborn GW, Schirmer H, Heggelund G, Lunde P, Rasmussen K. The evolving epidemiology of valvular aortic stenosis. The Tromso study. Heart. 2013;99(6):396–400.
3. Habib G, Lancellotti P, Antunes MJ, Bongiorni MG, Casalta JP, Del Zotti F, et al. 2015 ESC Guidelines for the management of infective endocarditis: the Task Force for the Management of Infective Endocarditis of the European Society of Cardiology (ESC). Endorsed by: European Association for Cardio-Thoracic Surgery (EACTS), the European Association of Nuclear Medicine (EANM). Eur Heart J. 2015;36(44):3075–128.
4. Baddour LM, Wilson WR, Bayer AS, Fowler VG, Tleyjeh IM, Rybak MJ, et al. Infective endocarditis in adults: diagnosis, antimicrobial therapy, and management of complications: a scientific statement for healthcare professionals from the American Heart Association. Circulation. 2015;132(15):1435–86.
5. Bonow RO, Lakatos E, Maron BJ, Epstein SE. Serial long-term assessment of the natural history of asymptomatic patients with chronic aortic regurgitation and normal left ventricular systolic function. Circulation. 1991;84(4):1625–35.
6. Horstkotte D, Niehues R, Strauer BE. Pathomorphological aspects, aetiology and natural history of acquired mitral valve stenosis. Eur Heart J. 1991;12(Suppl B):55–60.
7. Enriquez-Sarano M, Akins CW, Vahanian A. Mitral regurgitation. Lancet. 2009;373(9672):1382–94.
8. Afilalo J. Frailty in patients with cardiovascular disease: wh y, when, and how to measure. Curr Cardiovasc Risk Rep. 2011;5(5):467–72.
9. Forcillo J, Condado JF, Ko YA, Yuan M, Binongo JN, Ndubisi NM, et al. Assessment of commonly used frailty markers for high- and extreme-risk patients undergoing transcatheter aortic valve replacement. Ann Thorac Surg. 2017;104(6):1939–46.
10. Eide LS, Ranhoff AH, Fridlund B, Haaverstad R, Hufthammer KO, Kuiper KK, et al. Comparison of frequency, risk factors, and time course of postoperative delirium in octogenarians after transcatheter aortic valve implantation versus surgical aortic valve replacement. Am J Cardiol. 2015;115(6):802–809.
11. Afilalo J, Alexander KP, Mack MJ, Maurer MS, Green P, Allen LA, et al. Frailty assessment in the cardiovascular care of older adults. J Am Coll Cardiol. 2014;63(8):747–62.
12. Hawkey MC, Lauck SB, Perpetua EM, Fowler J, Schnell S, Speight M, et al. Transcatheter aortic valve replacement

program development: recommendations for best practice. Catheter Cardiovasc Interv. 2014;84(6):859–67.

13. Afilalo J, Lauck S, Kim DH, Lefèvre T, Piazza N, Lachapelle K, et al. Frailty in older adults undergoing aortic valve replacement: the FRAILTY-AVR Study. J Am Coll Cardiol. 2017;70(6):689–700.
14. Lauck S, Norekvål TM. Frailty, quality of life, and palliative approach. In: Hawkey M, Lauck SB, Perpetua E, Simone A (Eds), Transcatheter Aortic Valve Replacement Program Development: A Guide for the Heart Team. New York: Wolters Kluwer; 2020:116–32.
15. Vahanian A, Beyersdorf F, Praz F, Milojevic M, Baldus S, Bauersachs J, et al. ESC/EACTS Scientific Document Group. 2021 ESC/EACTS Guidelines for the management of valvular heart disease. *Eur Heart J.* 2021 Aug 28:ehab395. doi: 10.1093/eurheartj/ehab395. Epub ahead of print. PMID: 34453165.
16. Coylewright M, Palmer R, O'Neill ES, Robb JF, Fried TR. Patient-defined goals for the treatment of severe aortic stenosis: a qualitative analysis. Health Expect. 2016;19(5):1036–43.
17. Lauck SB, Wood DA, Baumbusch J, Kwon JY, Stub D, Achtem L, et al. Vancouver transcatheter aortic valve replacement clinical pathway: minimalist approach, standardized care, and discharge criteria to reduce length of stay. Circ Cardiovasc Qual Outcomes. 2016;9(3):312–21.
18. Iversen K, Ihlemann N, Gill SU, Madsen T, Elming H, Jensen KT, et al. Partial oral versus intravenous antibiotic treatment of endocarditis. N Engl J Med. 2019;380(5):415–24.
19. Hardin SR, Kaplow R. Cardiac Surgery Essentials for Critical Care Nursing (2nd ed). Burlington, MA: Jones & Bartlett Learning; 2016.
20. Berg SK, Zwisler AD, Pedersen BD, Haase K, Sibilitz KL. Patient experiences of recovery after heart valve replacement: suffering weakness, struggling to resume normality. BMC Nurs. 2013;12(1):23.
21. Thomson Mangnall LJ, Gallagher RD, Sibbritt DW, Fry MM. Health-related quality of life of patients after mechanical valve replacement surgery: an integrative review. Eur J Cardiovasc Nurs. 2015;14(1):16–25.
22. Instenes I, Fridlund B, Amofah HA, Ranhoff AH, Eide LS, Norekval TM. 'I hope you get normal again': an explorative study on how delirious octogenarian patients experience their interactions with healthcare professionals and relatives after aortic valve therapy. Eur J Cardiovasc Nurs. 2019;18(3):224–33.
23. Inouye SK, van Dyck CH, Alessi CA, Balkin S, Siegal AP, Horwitz RI. Clarifying confusion: the confusion assessment method. A new method for detection of delirium. Ann Intern Med. 1990;113(12):941–48.
24. Mack MJ, Leon MB, Thourani VH, Makkar R, Kodali SK, Russo M, et al. Transcatheter aortic-valve replacement with a balloon-expandable valve in low-risk patients. N Engl J Med. 2019;380(18):1695–705.
25. Popma JJ, Deeb GM, Yakubov SJ, Mumtaz M, Gada H, O'Hair D, et al. Transcatheter aortic-valve replacement with a self-expanding valve in low-risk patients. N Engl J Med. 2019;380(18):1706–15.
26. Wood DA, Lauck SB, Cairns JA, Humphries KH, Cook R, Welsh R, et al. The Vancouver 3M (multidisciplinary, multimodality, but minimalist) clinical pathway facilitates safe next-day discharge home at low-, medium-, and high-volume transfemoral transcatheter aortic valve replacement centers: the 3M TAVR Study. JACC Cardiovasc Interv. 2019;12(5):459–69.
27. Kappetein AP, Head SJ, Genereux P, Piazza N, van Mieghem NM, Blackstone EH, et al. Updated standardized endpoint definitions for transcatheter aortic valve implantation: the Valve Academic Research Consortium-2 consensus document. J Thorac Cardiovasc Surg. 2013;145(1):6–23.
28. Puls M, Lubos E, Boekstegers P, von Bardeleben RS, Ouarrak T, Butter C, et al. One-year outcomes and predictors of mortality after MitraClip therapy in contemporary clinical practice: results from the German transcatheter mitral valve interventions registry. Eur Heart J. 2016;37(8):703–12.
29. Jaarsma T, Beattie JM, Ryder M, Rutten FH, McDonagh T, Mohacsi P, et al. Palliative care in heart failure: a position statement from the palliative care workshop of the Heart Failure Association of the European Society of Cardiology. Eur J Heart Fail. 2009;11(5):433–43.
30. Lauck S, Garland E, Achtem L, Forman J, Baumbusch J, Boone R, et al. Integrating a palliative approach in a transcatheter heart valve program: bridging innovations in the management of severe aortic stenosis and best end-of-life practice. Eur J Cardiovasc Nurs. 2014;13(2):177–84.
31. Lauck SB, Gibson JA, Baumbusch J, Carroll SL, Achtem L, Kimel G, et al. Transition to palliative care when transcatheter aortic valve implantation is not an option: opportunities and recommendations. Curr Opin Support Palliat Care. 2016;10(1):18–23.
32. Hansen TB, Zwisler AD, Berg SK, Sibilitz KL, Buus N, Lee A. Cardiac rehabilitation patients' perspectives on the recovery following heart valve surgery: a narrative analysis. J Adv Nurs. 2016;72(5):1097–108.
33. Kirk BH, De Backer O, Missel M. Transforming the experience of aortic valve disease in older patients: a qualitative study. J Clin Nurs. 2019;28(7–8):1233–41.
34. Oterhals K, Fridlund B, Nordrehaug JE, Haaverstad R, Norekval TM. Adapting to living with a mechanical aortic heart valve: a phenomenographic study. J Adv Nurs. 2013;69(9):2088–98.
35. Danielsen SO, Moons P, Sandven I, Leegaard M, Solheim S, Tønnessen T, Lie I. Thirty-day readmissions in surgical and transcatheter aortic valve replacement: a systematic review and meta-analysis. Int J Cardiol. 2018;268:85–91.

36. Borregaard B, Dahl JS, Riber LPS, Ekholm O, Sibilitz KL, Weiss M, et al. Effect of early, individualised and intensified follow-up after open heart valve surgery on unplanned cardiac hospital readmissions and all-cause mortality. Int J Cardiol. 2019;289:30–36.
37. Verhagen DW, Hermanides J, Korevaar JC, Ekholm O, Sibilitz KL, Weiss M, et al. Health-related quality of life and posttraumatic stress disorder among survivors of left-sided native valve endocarditis. Clin Infect Dis. 2009;48(11):1559–65.
38. Rasmussen TB, Zwisler AD, Thygesen LC, Bundgaard H, Moons P, Berg SK. High readmission rates and mental distress after infective endocarditis—results from the national population-based CopenHeart IE survey. Int J Cardiol. 2017;235:133–40.
39. Rasmussen TB, Zwisler AD, Moons P, Berg SK. Insufficient living: experiences of recovery after infective endocarditis. J Cardiovasc Nurs. 2015;30(3):E11–19.
40. Butt JH, Kragholm K, Dalager-Pedersen M, Rørth R, Kristensen SL, Chaudry MS, et al. Return to the workforce following infective endocarditis: a nationwide cohort study. Am Heart J. 2018;195:130–38.
41. Roberts M, Rollason J, Warren S. Safe anticoagulant management for patients taking warfarin. Nurs Times. 2019;115(12):52–55.
42. Heneghan C, Ward A, Perera R, khead C, Fuller A, et al. Self-monitoring of oral anticoagulation: systematic review and meta-analysis of individual patient data. Lancet. 2012;379(9813):322–34.
43. Oterhals K, Deaton C, De Geest S, Jaarsma T, Lenzen M, Moons P, et al. European cardiac nurses' current practice and knowledge on anticoagulation therapy. Eur J Cardiovasc Nurs. 2014;13(3):261–69.
44. Sibilitz KL, Berg SK, Tang LH, Risom SS, Gluud C, Lindschou J, et al. Exercise-based cardiac rehabilitation for adults after heart valve surgery. Cochrane Database Syst Rev. 2016;3:CD010876.
45. Norekval TM, Falun N, Fridlund B. Patient-reported outcomes on the agenda in cardiovascular clinical practice. Eur J Cardiovasc Nurs. 2016;15(2):108–11.
46. Anker SD, Agewall S, Borggrefe M, Calvert M, Jaime Caro J, Cowie MR, et al. The importance of patient-reported outcomes: a call for their comprehensive integration in cardiovascular clinical trials. Eur Heart J. 2014;35(30):2001–2009.

9 Care of the patient with inherited cardiac conditions and congenital heart diseases

JODIE INGLES, TOOTIE BUESER, PASCAL MCKEOWN, PHILIP MOONS, AND DONNA FITZSIMONS

CHAPTER CONTENTS

This chapter is focused on inherited cardiac conditions in terms of their diagnosis, management, and holistic nursing care. The purpose is to provide an overview of the genetic basis of these conditions and an understanding of the care required for people with inherited cardiac conditions and the congenital heart diseases most commonly seen in clinical practice.

KEY MESSAGES

- The inherited basis of certain cardiac conditions is a rapidly expanding area of knowledge development and future innovations in care pathways are anticipated.
- The population of patients with congenital heart disease is growing, which results in an increased demand for efficient diagnosis and evidence informed nursing care.
- While treatment options have improved in many cases, the impact of inherited cardiac conditions and congenital heart diseases is multifaceted and lifelong.
- Caring for patients with these conditions requires a distinct patient- and family-centred approach to care from all professionals in the multidisciplinary team.

Introduction

A significant proportion of cardiovascular diseases have an underlying genetic basis, as a result of chromosomal abnormalities, disease-causing changes in single genes, and the interaction of minor genetic changes (polymorphisms) with environmental factors. It is estimated that the burden of inherited cardiovascular conditions is greater than cancer.[1]

There is a huge drive for personalized medicine in cardiovascular care as advances in molecular genetics and therapeutics develop. Furthermore, advances in cardiovascular imaging and diagnostic techniques, as well as increased knowledge about inherited conditions, have resulted in more patients and family members identified from this patient group. It is, therefore, of great importance that cardiovascular nurses and allied health professionals have a basic grounding in genetic principles as they will soon encounter more patients with these conditions in both specialist and general settings, and will be expected to facilitate the delivery of personalized medicine in the future.

Further, cardiovascular nurses and allied health professionals will increasingly encounter patients with congenital heart disease (CHD). Given the dramatic improvement of life expectancy in childhood, more than 90% of children with CHD will reach adulthood. However, in the fourth and fifth decades of life, many patients present with long-term complications of the structural defect. Cardiovascular nurses need to understand the features of the different heart defects and be attuned to the changing needs of the patient and family across the lifespan, including the provision of palliative and supportive care as appropriate.

Genetic principles and cardiac genetic testing

Understanding the genetic basis of diseases can have significant benefit. There are many cardiovascular diseases that are known to be caused by genetic variants, affecting all aspects of the heart. Some may be inherited as Mendelian traits, where there is a direct and sizeable risk to relatives. Usually these can be discovered by genetic testing to identify and quantify the risk involved. Other diseases including coronary artery disease[2] and atrial fibrillation,[3] have a more complex underlying aetiology, being due to a combination of genetic and environmental factors. Genetic risk of complex diseases can be derived from the presence of hundreds to thousands of genetic variants, and the cumulative risk of disease for an individual can be expressed as a polygenic risk score. At present, polygenic risk scores are not often used in mainstream cardiology, although this is likely to evolve in coming years as our knowledge increases.

Basic principles of genetics

Our bodies are made up of millions of cells which contain all the genetic information that determines many of our attributes and health. We have approximately 22,000 genes and these encode proteins that perform specific tasks in our body. Inherited diseases are those caused primarily due to a change in the DNA code in a gene, impacting the function of a specific protein it encodes. We have two copies of every gene, one which is inherited from our mother and the other from our father. The sex chromosomes include XX (female) and XY (male). The DNA sequence is a series of nucleotides, including adenine (A), guanine (G), cytosine (C), and thymine (T). Nucleotides are read in groups of three, and the order will determine the resulting amino acid. Therefore, a single change, like a spelling mistake, will result in a different amino acid being substituted into the protein sequence. This is known as a missense change. These changes can result in errors in the protein structure and/or function. Other changes can result in a loss of function, for example, a small insertion or deletion of a nucleotide(s) which causes a shift in the reading frame and eventually a premature truncation. Where the change is so drastic that the protein may become truncated or radically altered, the cells are capable of 'mopping up' the dysfunctional protein (known as nonsense-mediated decay) and the result is overall lower levels of normal protein (known as haploinsufficiency). Changes to the DNA sequence are called variants. Not all variants cause disease, and in fact rare variation in our genetic make-up is common. This becomes a challenge when trying to determine whether a specific genetic change is causative of disease or not.

Comprehensive three-generation family history

A comprehensive three-generation family history is a key aspect of the clinical assessment of families with known or suspected inherited cardiac conditions (ICCs). Communicating effectively at this stage can be useful to develop rapport and gain a better understanding of the social circumstances in the family, for example, who is in contact, where relatives reside, and how family communication is likely to proceed. Importantly, it may also shed light on the inheritance pattern in the family, allowing inheritance risk information to be passed on to at-risk family members.

The family history is a valuable tool (➤ **Fig. 9.1**). In drawing this, circles denote females, and squares males. Typically, those with clinical evidence of disease are represented as black filled-in symbols, while unfilled symbols are unknown or unaffected clinical status. As there are two copies of most alleles, the notation +/– represents an individual with one affected allele, as would be sufficient to cause autosomal dominant disease (➤ **Fig. 9.1**). Alternatively, recessive inheritance requires both alleles to be affected, therefore those expressing clinical disease will be +/+ while their carrier parents will be +/–. Other inheritance patterns are explained in more detail later in the chapter. Family members who are deceased will be shown with a diagonal line through their symbol, and typically at least three-generations should be recorded.

Inherited diseases can follow different modes of inheritance, and in many cases this information can be gleaned from the family history (➤ **Fig. 9.1**). These include:

- Autosomal dominant: one gene copy is affected resulting in disease, known as a heterozygous change. There is a one in two risk of passing on the disease to offspring.
- Autosomal recessive: both gene copies are affected resulting in disease. This can be the same variant

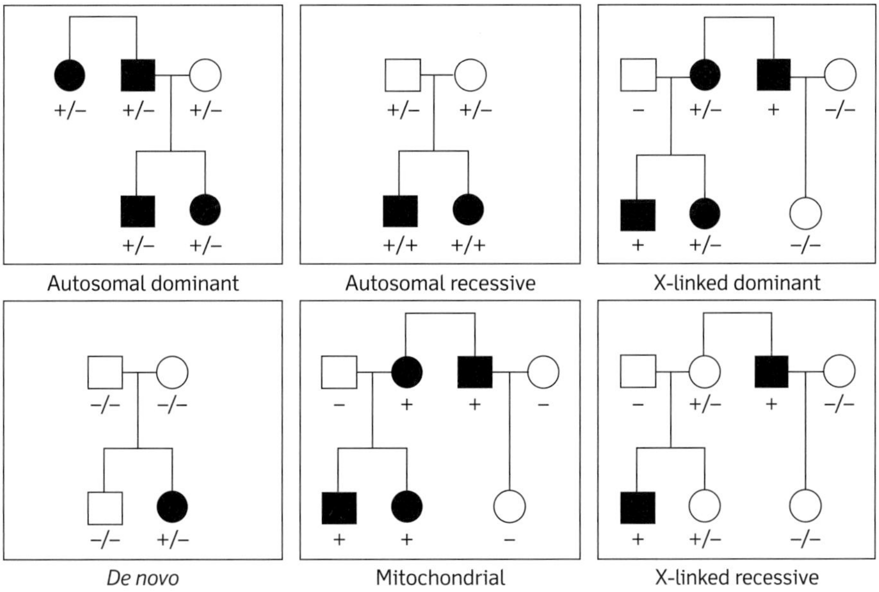

Fig. 9.1 Inheritance patterns that can be identified from the family history.

(homozygous) or different variants in the same gene (compound heterozygous). This often implies that both parents are carriers, that is, they have only one gene copy affected and no disease. In some cultures, where consanguinity is commonplace, genetic diseases due to homozygous gene variants should be suspected.

- X-linked: a gene on the X-chromosome is affected. Since males (XY) do not have another functional gene copy, they often have disease. Females (XX) are considered carriers, though in some cases can express disease. For dominant X-linked conditions, disease in the females can be severe. For many X-linked conditions, however, females are typically more mildly affected, if at all. Affected males cannot pass on the disease, and carrier females have a one in two risk of passing it on to their children.
- *De novo*: some variants arise at conception, meaning both parents are demonstrated to be gene negative in a setting where paternity is confirmed. *De novo* variants that cause disease often affect children, and reassuringly to families there is no recurrence risk to additional pregnancies or children. In rare cases, a *de novo* variant can appear to arise due to gonadal mosaicism, where some of the gonadal cells of a parent carry the genetic change. This situation is important to recognize as it means there is an inheritance risk to further children.
- Mitochondrial: genes that encode mitochondrial proteins can either be encoded by mitochondrial DNA or nuclear DNA. Nuclear DNA variants will follow inheritance patterns described previously. Mitochondrial DNA exists separate to nuclear DNA and is passed from the mother to offspring at conception. All children of an affected mother will inherit the affected mitochondrial DNA, though at varying levels (heteroplasmy). Importantly, males cannot pass on mitochondrial DNA variants.

Some common terms used in genetics are shown in ➤ **Table 9.1**.

Cardiac genetic testing

ICCs have a combined prevalence of up to 1 in 200–500 in the community. These encompass the inherited cardiomyopathies,[5] arrhythmia syndromes, and aortopathies,[6] among others, and are defined by their clinical and genetic heterogeneity. Most are autosomal dominantly inherited, meaning there is a one in two risk to first-degree relatives, and indeed a positive family history with multiple affected relatives is not an uncommon presentation. Historically, specialized centres drew in large kindreds with demonstrated familial disease that enabled their initial diagnoses. Indeed, these are the family descriptions that paved the way for our earliest understanding of the disease genes. Cardiac genetic testing is now a routine addition to management in many cases, largely driven by the evolution of next-generation sequencing technologies, making testing faster, more comprehensive, and widely available.

Genetic testing for ICCs has become widely available, and aims to identify the underlying genetic cause of the disease. In some cases, this can have benefit in clarifying the diagnosis in the affected individual, but for the most part, the true value lies in the ability to clarify disease risk for at-risk family members. Genetic testing for Mendelian genetic diseases is a two-step process. First, the disease-causing gene variant must be identified. Given many families have their own unique genetic cause of disease, this can be a challenge. Typically, a DNA sample is taken from the proband (i.e. the index case) and a large panel of genes associated with a specific phenotype are sequenced. In this setting, the potential outcomes can include (1) a genetic cause of disease is identified, (2) a genetic cause of disease is suspected but it cannot be reliably ascertained at this point in time, or (3) a genetic cause of disease is not identified (➤ **Table 9.2**).

If a variant is identified that is deemed to be causative, then cascade genetic testing can be offered to family members. This is a technically simpler test, evaluating the presence or absence of the causative variant in their DNA sample. If asymptomatic relatives are shown to be gene positive then they may at some point in future develop disease and should continue clinical screening with a cardiologist, and their own children have a one in two risk of disease. Those who are gene negative can be released from all future clinical screening, and likewise their children are no longer at risk. This is a powerful tool for use in families, and indeed the ability to release family members from lifetime periodic clinical surveillance is the basis for genetic testing being a very cost-effective addition to family management among those with hypertrophic cardiomyopathy (HCM)[7,8] and dilated cardiomyopathy (DCM).[9]

Cascade genetic testing can give at-risk family members options and greater certainty regarding their risk, but there can be additional considerations when children are concerned. Given many ICCs develop from teenage years and above, there is an argument that there is little urgency to determine a child's genetic status. In many cases, it may be prudent to offer cascade genetic testing

Table 9.1 Glossary of genetic terms

Variant	An alteration of the DNA sequence from the reference sequence
Gene	A part of the DNA sequence that encodes a specific protein
Protein	Proteins are comprised of amino acids and perform a multitude of tasks in our cells and body. These include structural, biochemical, transport, metabolic, cell signalling, and adhesion roles
Variant classification	Variants occur commonly. Some variants can be the underlying cause of genetic diseases. Distinguishing which are disease causing and which are not requires use of variant classification criteria. If there is robust evidence that the variant causes disease, it will be considered 'likely pathogenic' or 'pathogenic'. If there is enough evidence that it is not causative, then it will be considered 'likely benign' or 'benign'. Where there is insufficient or conflicting evidence, the variant will be termed a 'variant of uncertain significance' (VUS) and it should not be used for cascade screening in the family
Genetic testing	Genetic testing is the process of sequencing genes to determine if DNA variants exist. It is usually a two-step process (proband and cascade genetic testing)
Proband genetic testing	The first step in many cases requires finding the genetic variant causing disease in a member of the family who is definitely affected with disease
Cascade genetic testing	If a disease-causing variant is identified, at-risk relatives may be offered cascade genetic testing which tests for the presence or absence of the variant in the family
Phenotype	The clinical features due to a specific genetic variant. In many cases this is referring to a specific disease state
Disease penetrance	Whether or not the phenotype develops in those who have the genetic variant
Variable expression	The variability in clinical features present among those affected individuals who carry the same genetic variant

Source data from Ingles J, Macciocca I, Morales A, et al. Genetic Testing in Inherited Heart Diseases. Heart Lung Circ 2020; 29: 505–511.

once the child has reached an age where they can participate in the decision-making process. This is part of the pretest genetic counselling discussion when considering cascade genetic testing in children. However, ultimately, it will be the decision of the family, especially for risk of inherited arrhythmia syndromes where disease onset may be younger and where it is clinically challenging to diagnose.[10]

Currently the pick-up rate (diagnostic yield of cardiac genetic testing) can range from 10% to 70%, depending on the disease in question, the characteristics of the patient, and the gene panel sequenced.[11] Where genetic variants are not identified, it should be clarified to the family that it is believed that they may still have a familial disease, but that the current knowledge or available technologies are not sufficient to identify it. This can be frustrating for the patient, their family, and the treating clinician, and illustrates the critical role of research. With greater stringency in how gene variants are determined to be causative of disease, robust research methods that provide a high level of evidence for causation are needed.

Uncertain genetic results can be challenging in many ways. For the patient, comprehension of uncertain genetic findings can be difficult, causing confusion and being a barrier for further communication in the family.[12–14] For the clinician, it can be hard to know how to resolve whether the variant is the cause or not. In some cases, there can be further clarification of the role of the variant in disease. For example, in a family where there are multiple affected relatives, seeking permission to obtain DNA to determine if they do/do not carry the genetic variant. By segregating the variant to other affected relatives, we can increase the confidence that the variant is the cause of disease. For other families, research laboratories may choose to perform functional studies (e.g. using cells or animal models) to determine whether the variant causes disease.

Table 9.2 Outcomes of genetic testing in the proband (index case)

Meaning	Genetic result	Impact to the family
Pathogenic variant (class 5) Likely pathogenic variant (class 4)	Cause of disease is identified	Can be used for cascade genetic testing in the family
Variant of uncertain significance (class 3)	Cause of disease is suspected but cannot be reliably ascertained	Cannot be used in the family for cascade genetic testing, at-risk relatives should continue clinical surveillance
Likely benign variant (class 2) Benign variant (class 1) No variants identified	Only variants not considered to be causing disease, or no variants, are identified	Cascade genetic testing not available to the family, at-risk relatives should continue clinical surveillance

Genetics of sudden cardiac death in the young

Sudden cardiac death (SCD) is a tragic outcome of many ICCs, and in some cases, it is the presenting symptom of disease. Where a cause of death remains elusive, that is, sudden unexplained death or sudden arrhythmic death, an inherited cause is strongly suspected. For the surviving relatives, there are clinical, genetic, and psychological challenges, and thus distinct advantages to family-based approaches to care. Clarification regarding the cause of death is a key consideration, allowing clinicians to devise a more tailored clinical surveillance plan and family members to gain some closure. While clinical investigation of family members after a sudden unexplained death can reveal a diagnosis in 10–20% of families,[15] the molecular autopsy (i.e. genetic testing of postmortem DNA) can provide important insights. By identifying an underlying genetic cause, we can (1) provide a cause of death for the decedent, and (2) offer a useful tool to allow cascade genetic testing of asymptomatic family members.[16,17]

While the clinical and genetic aspects of care following a SCD have to date been a focus, the psychological care needs often garner less attention. There is a high risk of poor psychological outcomes, including post-traumatic stress symptoms and prolonged grief, with almost one in two first-degree relatives reporting clinically significant symptoms, on average 6 years after the death.[18,19] From a nursing perspective it is important that we recognize and advance our knowledge base in this area in order to optimize care to individuals and families.

Genetics of congenital heart diseases (CHD)

Genetic testing for CHDs has not been as widely adopted as other cardiac genetic testing. This is largely due to the complex inheritance of CHD, meaning very large numbers of genes need to be included on gene panels and often there can be a digenic inheritance pattern (i.e. multiple segregating variants). In large expert centres, genetic testing for CHD is performed in a research setting, often requiring multidisciplinary input to interpret the genetic findings. With the increasing availability of next-generation sequencing, however, there is a growing use of genetic testing in this setting. It is estimated that single-gene disorders can be identified in 3–5%, chromosomal abnormalities in 8–10%, and large structural variants in 3–25% of cases. The large majority, however, are considered multifactorial, due to a combination of environment and many genetic factors.

Nonetheless, genetic testing and counselling is recommended. Understanding the underlying genetic causes of CHD is important for the following reasons: to confirm diagnosis, to guide management, to prognosticate, to appraise the recurrence risk, and to assess the genetic risks in family members.[20] ➤ Fig. 9.2 gives a graphical illustration of the genetic counselling and testing process in CHD.

Challenges of cardiac genetic testing

While our understanding of the clinical and genetic aspects of these diseases has evolved in recent decades, challenges remain around clinical and genetic diagnosis. The phenotype may be subtle or difficult to detect using current cardiac investigations, while broad genetic testing will often implicate numerous rare variants with unknown impact. Rare variants are cumulatively common and at present there is little ability to determine their impact, with most being unlikely to cause disease. The dangers of misclassifying these as causative are well documented, often relating to issues with certain ethnicities being underrepresented in general population databases,[21] inconsistent variant classification,[22] and poorly defined

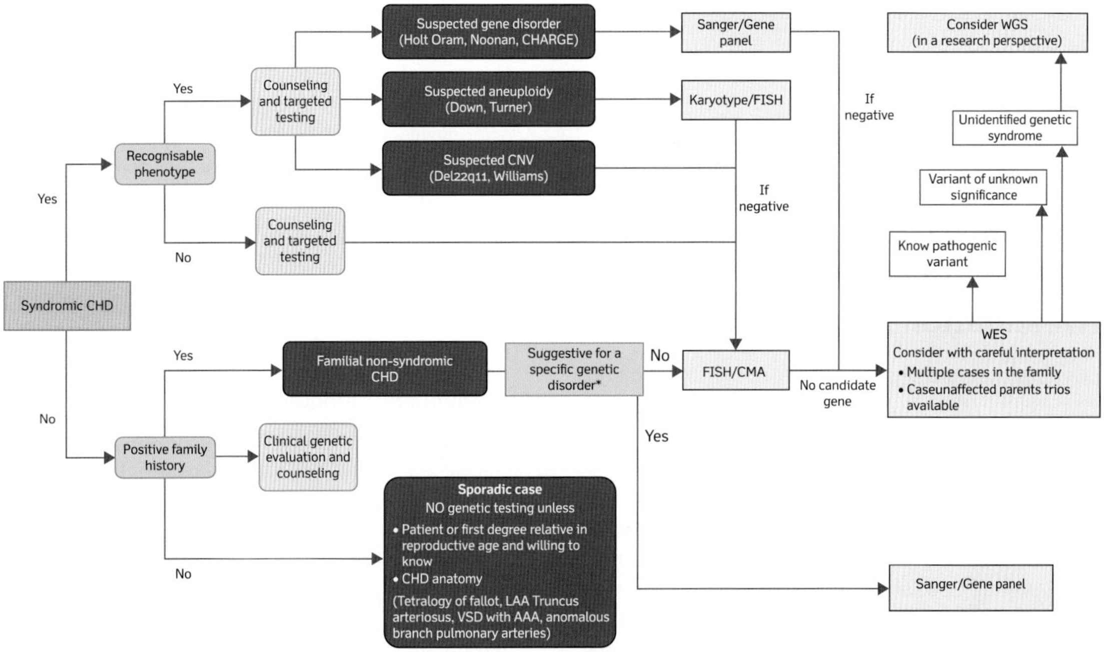

Fig. 9.2 Graphical illustration of the genetic counselling and testing process in congenital heart disease. AAA, ascending aortic aneurysm; AV, atrioventricular; CMA, chromosomal microarray; CNV, copy number variant; ELN, elastin; FISH, fluorescence *in situ* hybridisation; IAA, interrupted aortic arch; VSD, ventricular septal defect; WES, whole exome sequencing; WGS, whole genome sequencing; *e.g. *ELN* for familial supravalvular aortic stenosis; *TFAP2B* for familial patent ductus arteriosus, *NKX2.5* for familial atrial/ventricular septal defect with AV block.

De Backer J, Bondue A, Budts W, et al. Genetic counselling and testing in adults with congenital heart disease: A consensus document of the ESC Working Group of Grown-Up Congenital Heart Disease, the ESC Working Group on Aorta and Peripheral Vascular Disease and the European Society of Human Genetics. Eur J Prev Cardiol. 2020 Sep;27(13):1423–1435. doi: 10.1177/2047487319854552 with permission from SAGE.

association of a gene with a specific phenotype.[23,24] For the individual patient, putting together the pieces of the puzzle to understand the underlying genetic basis of disease is, therefore, difficult. In the setting of a positive family history, however, where the prior probability of a single gene causing disease is greater, the task may become easier and less prone to error. Likewise, interpretation of the phenotype in the context of a family means mild or incompletely penetrant traits, which may have been disregarded in isolation, can be more fully appreciated. The advantages of a well-constructed family history are far reaching in this setting, both for the management of patients and their relatives.

Role of genetic counselling

Genetic counselling is the process of providing information and emotional support to those with, or at risk of, genetic diseases.[25] It aims to assist patients and their families to understand and adapt to the medical, psychosocial, and familial aspects of genetic disease.[26] Genetic counselling, as a process, may be performed by appropriately trained health professionals, including genetic counsellors or genetic nurses.

Genetic counselling goes beyond provision of information, and an important focus is the psychosocial support offered, including empathic listening, crisis intervention, managing family dynamics, coping models, grief, and adjustment to disease diagnoses.[27] Awareness of the psychosocial considerations in the family, as well as a strong rapport with the patient, can help facilitate effective communication.[28] Additional support for some patients in communicating risk information to family members may be warranted. One recent study of patients with long QT syndrome (LQTS) showed that those with worse anxiety reported greater difficulty disseminating this information to relatives.[29] Consideration of the need for a clinical psychologist in the management of families with ICCs may also be warranted, and a referral pathway should be established. For families who have experienced a young SCD, this should be encouraged in all cases, given the known high prevalence of prolonged grief and post-traumatic stress symptoms.[18]

Inherited cardiovascular conditions (ICCs)—epidemiology, presentation, investigations, and management

ICCs is an overarching term for a range of conditions which affect the heart muscle (cardiomyopathies), electrical system (primary arrhythmia syndromes/channelopathies), and connective tissue disorders with major cardiovascular manifestations. Some of these conditions also have extracardiac manifestations, including abnormalities in the skeletal muscle, skin, and the neurological system. Specialized multidisciplinary teams integrate expertise to deal holistically with the complex needs of patients and families presenting with these conditions. These clinics provide individualized care with relevant members of staff covering the medical, genetic, psychological, and ethical issues.

Inherited cardiomyopathies

The cardiomyopathies are an important, heterogeneous group of heart muscle diseases that are associated with significant morbidity and mortality. Collectively, they are defined as a disorder of the myocardium where there is an abnormality in the structure and function of the heart muscle in the absence of coronary artery disease, hypertension, valvular disease, and CHD which could explain the observed myocardial abnormality.[30] ➤ Fig. 9.3 illustrates the classification of cardiomyopathies according to specific morphological and functional phenotypes which are then subclassified into familial and non-familial forms (➤ Table 9.3).

Hypertrophic cardiomyopathy

Epidemiology, pathology, and aetiology

HCM is a condition which affects approximately 1 in 500 of the general population. It is characterized by the development of a hypertrophied, non-dilated left ventricle (LV) in the absence of other predisposing conditions (such as aortic stenosis or hypertension). At a pathological level, the hallmark of the condition is myocardial disarray, or loss of the normal parallel alignment of the heart muscle cells.

The development of the hypertrophy is characteristically age related—in family settings, it is relatively uncommon for young children to manifest the disease before the age of 10 years and, while most genetically predisposed individuals develop hypertrophy during adolescence, there is increasing recognition of the development of late-onset disease. The hypertrophy is often asymmetrical, affecting the interventricular septum, but it is important to recognize that the hypertrophy can affect any part of the

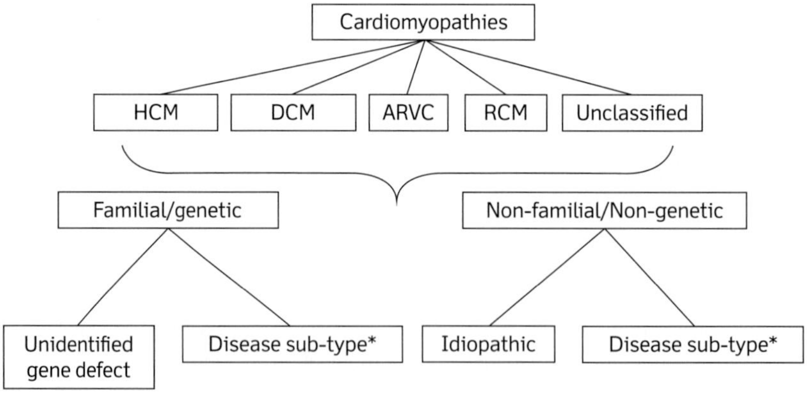

Fig. 9.3 Summary of proposed classification of cardiomyopathies. ARVC, arrhythmogenic right ventricular cardiomyopathy; DCM, dilated cardiomyopathy; HCM, hypertrophic cardiomyopathy; RCM, restrictive cardiomyopathy. (The asterisk refers to table 1 in reference[30].)

Elliott P, Andersson B, Arbustini E, et al. Classification of the cardiomyopathies: a position statement from the European Society Of Cardiology Working Group on Myocardial and Pericardial Diseases. Eur Heart J. 2008 Jan;29(2):270–6. doi: 10.1093/eurheartj/ehm342. Reprinted by permission of Oxford University Press on behalf of the European Society of Cardiology.

Table 9.3 Types of inherited cardiomyopathies

Condition and prevalence	Presentation	Investigations	Management
Hypertrophic cardiomyopathy (HCM) LV thickness ≥15 mm in one or more LV segment. 1:500 in general population	Often silent initially Dyspnoea Palpitations Syncope Chest pain	ECG Echocardiography (ECHO) Cardiac MRI HCM risk calculator Genetic testing	Reduction of proarrhythmic risk using: Drugs—beta-blockers, verapamil and disopyramide ICD Surgical techniques Exercise advice and avoidance of competitive sport Symptom management
Dilated cardiomyopathy (DCM) LV dilation and systolic dysfunction without CAD 1:250 general population Familial in 30%	Variable presentation Dyspnoea Palpitations Syncope/SCD Thromboembolism	ECG ECHO Chest X-ray Cardiac MRI Genetic testing	Symptom management and prevent complications—heart failure, SCD, and thromboembolism
Arrhythmogenic right ventricular cardiomyopathy (ARVC) 1:2500–5000 in general population	Usually presents in mid 30s Symptoms of heart failure or arrhythmia	ECG and signal-averaged ECG Cardiac MRI Angiography Genetic testing	Reduction of proarrhythmic risk using: Drugs—beta-blockers SCD risk stratification and ICD if indicated Tailored exercise advice
Restrictive cardiomyopathy (RCM) High ventricular pressure due to stiffness in myocardium Normal or reduced systolic and diastolic volume	Various causes: Idiopathic, familial, or associated with conditions such as amyloidosis, Fabry disease, and haemochromatosis Signs of heart failure or arrhythmia	ECG ECHO Cardiac MRI Angiography Endomyocardial biopsy	Treatment predicated by underlying cause Careful fluid management Drugs—diuretics, beta-blockers, calcium channel blockers Risk stratification and management—ICD and LV assist device where indicated
Left ventricular non-compaction (LVNC) Spongy myocardium usually restricted to LV apex	Idiopathic or associated with other congenital conditions, e.g. VSD or Ebstein anomaly	ECG ECHO Cardiac MRI	Prevention and treatment of heart failure, arrhythmia, and embolic events Genetic testing

myocardium. Up to one-third of patients have resting left ventricular outflow tract obstruction (LVOTO). However, in other patients without resting obstruction, it may be induced during exercise or if there are other haemodynamic strains, such as tachycardia, blood loss, or inadvertent use of inotropes. Atrial arrhythmias are common, and affected individuals have a high risk of thromboembolism. Progression to a 'burn-out' phase, which is characterized by progressive LV dilation, wall thinning, and systolic impairment, can occur in up to 15% of adults with HCM. More commonly, HCM is an autosomal dominant condition associated with pathogenic variants in sarcomere genes *MYBPC3*, *MYH7*, *TNNT2*, *TNNI3*, *TPM1*, *ACTC*, *MYL2*, and *MYL3*, which are implicated in 40% of cases.

It is important to recognize that there are many other conditions that can cause LV hypertrophy and appear to clinically mimic HCM, especially in the very young, as there are treatment implications, as well as implications for the risk of other family members. These include X-linked lysosomal disorders, such as Fabry disease caused by pathogenic variants in the alpha-galactosidase A (*GLA*) gene which typically presents in males over the age of 36 with concentric LV hypertrophy, and Danon disease where the dominant features include cardiomyopathy, skeletal myopathy, and developmental delay resulting from pathogenic variants in the lysosome-associated membrane protein-2 (*LAMP2*) gene. Other glycogen storage diseases which can include LV hypertrophy include Pompe disease (autosomal recessive) and a syndrome caused by pathogenic variants in the gamma-2 subunit adenosine monophosphate-activated protein kinase (*PRKAG2*) gene (autosomal dominant) which often includes conduction abnormalities and Wolff–Parkinson–White syndrome. LV hypertrophy is also a feature in primary mitochondrial disorders, Friedreich's ataxia, and syndromic conditions such as Noonan syndrome. The diagnosis of these conditions requires a high index of clinical suspicion and the use of appropriate diagnostic tools.

Furthermore, an important differential diagnosis in young healthy individuals is 'athlete's heart' which can show physiological hypertrophy. Various factors may be used to distinguish HCM from athlete's heart; these include extent of hypertrophy, LV cavity size, extent of left atrial enlargement, presence of LVOTO, changes in tissue Doppler parameters, peak VO_2 consumption, levels of N-terminal-pro-B-type natriuretic peptide, regression on cessation of exercise, and genetic testing.

Clinical presentation

An initial diagnosis of HCM is often made following an incidental finding of a heart murmur or an abnormal electrocardiogram (ECG) or in the context of family screening. Individuals with HCM generally have few or any symptoms. When present, these typically include dyspnoea, palpitations, and chest pain, which is commonly exertional but can also occur at rest following heavy meals. Syncope is a relatively common symptom which can be caused by multiple mechanisms such as LVOTO, abnormal vascular responses, and atrial and ventricular arrhythmias. Unexplained or exertional syncope is associated with increased risk of sudden death in the young. Extreme presentations include SCD and infants with symptoms of heart failure.

Investigations

Ninety-five per cent of individuals with HCM have an abnormal 12-lead ECG. Common features include a variable combination of pathological Q waves most often in the inferolateral leads, LV hypertrophy, and ST- and T-wave abnormalities. These should be interpreted in conjunction with findings on echocardiography and/or cardiac magnetic resonance imaging (MRI). In an adult, HCM is defined by a wall thickness of at least 15 mm in one or more LV myocardial segments—as measured by any imaging technique—that is not explained solely by loading conditions. In children, the diagnosis requires an LV wall thickness more than two standard deviations greater than the predicted mean. In first-degree relatives of patients with unequivocal disease, the presence of otherwise unexplained increased LV wall thickness greater than 13 mm in one or more LV myocardial segments, as measured by any cardiac imaging technique, will suffice. First-degree relatives of patients with HCM should be invited for cardiac screening commencing from the age of 10 years or even earlier and should continue at regular intervals due to the possibility of late-onset disease despite a normal initial screen. This also applies to genetic carriers, who remain phenotypically unaffected.

Management

Making an accurate diagnosis for HCM and the exclusion of conditions which mimic HCM ensures patients receive an appropriate management plan. Lifelong follow-up is required for monitoring disease progression, symptoms, and assessments for risk of SCD. Symptoms resulting from LVOTO may be initially managed with the addition of the antiarrhythmic, disopyramide, to beta-blockers or verapamil. Disopyramide is usually well tolerated but initiation at low doses is recommended, especially in the elderly. Prolongation of the QT interval may occur so patients will need regular ECG monitoring and other medications that prolong the QT interval should be avoided. Patients who are unable to tolerate medications or whose LVOTO-related symptoms do not respond to medical therapy may be offered septal reduction therapy. The traditional treatment is a septal myectomy which involves the removal of a portion of the heart muscle from the interventricular septum. A more recent option is alcohol septal ablation wherein 95% alcohol is injected to produce an area of localized necrosis within the basal septum. In patients without LVOTO, chest pain and dyspnoea are likely to be caused by LV diastolic impairment and microvascular ischaemia and these patients are, therefore, treated with beta-blockers or calcium antagonists. Other medications such as angiotensin-converting enzyme inhibitors or nitrates may be beneficial in selected patients with systolic dysfunction but should be avoided in patients who have inducible LVOTO as they can make symptoms worse. Patients who are in the end stage of the disease should receive standard heart failure therapy, including palliative care.

The overall risk for SCD in patients with HCM is around 1% per year. Nevertheless, high-risk patients should be identified and considered for a primary prevention ICD. The use of the HCM Risk-SCD calculator will facilitate this, considering age, cardiac imaging parameters, symptoms of syncope, and family history. Patients with HCM who present having survived an out-of-hospital cardiac arrest or have sustained ventricular tachycardia (VT) will typically have an ICD for secondary prevention. Advice against participation in competitive sport and intense physical activity should be given to high-risk patients for SCD and/or those with LVOTO.

Atrial fibrillation in HCM should be treated promptly as per European Society of Cardiology Guidelines as there is a high risk of thromboembolism in patients with HCM conveying a low threshold for commencing oral anticoagulants. The CHA_2DS_2-VASc score to calculate stroke risk is not recommended.

Dilated cardiomyopathy

Epidemiology, pathology, and aetiology

DCM is characterized by 'the presence of LV dilatation and systolic dysfunction in the absence of abnormal loading conditions or significant coronary artery disease'.[30] Right ventricular (RV) dilatation is often also present. The current data on the epidemiology of DCM estimates that it occurs in 1 out of 250 people in the population.[31] It is estimated that 25–35% of DCM cases are familial. Autosomal dominant, autosomal recessive, X-linked, and mitochondrial inheritance patterns have been reported, with a range of genes implicated, including cytoskeletal, sarcomere, and nuclear envelope proteins. Familial disease should also be suspected when there is a family history of sudden death, conduction system disease, or an associated skeletal myopathy. Acquired causes of DCM include autoimmune and systemic disorders, and inflammatory diseases, such as myocarditis; as well as past exposure to alcohol, drugs, or chemotherapeutic agents; metabolic/endocrine disorders; and other neuromuscular diseases.

Clinical presentation

Patients with DCM have signs and symptoms that are highly variable and depend on the degree of LV dysfunction. They may present with heart failure, arrhythmias, thromboembolic events, or SCD. Typical symptoms include reduced exercise tolerance, dyspnoea on exertion, palpitations, pre-syncope, and syncope.[32] Where family screening is being undertaken, several asymptomatic relatives may be identified to have isolated LV dilatation or asymptomatic LV dysfunction.

Investigations

The ECG in patients with DCM may be normal, but typically exhibits sinus tachycardia and non-specific ST-segment and T-wave changes. Evidence for atrial enlargement and ventricular hypertrophy is common as well as the presence of AF and ventricular arrhythmias. Atrioventricular (AV) block may also be present and raises the possibility for pathogenic variants in the lamin A/C gene (*LMNA*).[33] Chest X-ray is often abnormal in DCM reflecting LV and left atrial dilatation. Echocardiography is diagnostic for DCM in the presence of LV fractional shortening less than 25% and/or LV ejection fraction less than 45% with LV end-diastolic diameter greater than 117% of the predicted value corrected for age and body surface area. Cardiac MRI provides additional details beyond ventricular size and function, as it permits tissue characterization, including evidence of inflammatory processes and scarring. The absence of any other known cause of myocardial disease should be established and a diagnosis of idiopathic DCM is only assigned after all other possible explanations have been excluded.

Comprehensive or targeted genetic testing is recommended for patients with DCM, with truncating variants in *TTN* being the most common cause, but other genes including *RBM20*, *FLNC*, *DSP*, *BAG3*, and *PLN* also being potentially implicated. For patients with significant conduction disease, there should be a high level of suspicion of a causative variant in *LMNA*. Establishing a familial pattern of DCM helps confirm the diagnosis, thereby facilitating cascade screening within the family.[11] All first-degree relatives of a patient with familial or idiopathic DCM should have cardiac evaluation, including ECG and imaging.

Management

The management of DCM is targeted towards improvement of symptoms and the prevention of complications such as heart failure, SCD, and thromboembolism.[32] Treatment pathways are similar to those for established LV dysfunction/heart failure and include use of angiotensin-converting enzyme inhibitors (or angiotensin receptor antagonists), beta-blockers, mineralocorticoid antagonists, and I_f channel inhibitors. Device-based therapy, both pacemaker and ICD, may be indicated, according to established guidelines. Mechanical support with LV assist devices and heart transplantation may also be indicated in certain patients.

Arrhythmogenic right ventricular cardiomyopathy

Epidemiology, pathology, and aetiology

Arrhythmogenic right ventricular cardiomyopathy (ARVC) has an estimated prevalence of 1 in 2500–5000.[34] It is characterized by progressive fibro-fatty replacement of the myocardium, leading to both electrophysiological and contraction abnormalities. The pathological changes are found most commonly in the triangle of dysplasia (RV inflow, outflow, and apex) and are increasingly recognized in the LV. More recently, the triangle of dysplasia has been refined to include the RV basal inferior wall, the RV anterior wall, and the posterolateral LV wall.[35] Indeed, in the later stages, biventricular involvement resembling DCM is observed.

As greater understanding of the phenotype spectrum of the disease develops, the term arrhythmogenic cardiomyopathy has been suggested. This incorporates right-sided disease such as ARVC, and biventricular and left-sided disease which are known manifestations of these diseases.[36]

Autosomal dominant inheritance is the most common pattern of inheritance in ARVC, although autosomal recessive inheritance is also seen in the case of Naxos disease and Carvajal syndrome (often with hair and skin changes, such as woolly hair and palmoplantar keratoderma).[37] The genes involved mainly encode desmosomal genes *DSC2, DSG2, DSP, JUP, PKP2, PLN*, and *TMEM43*.

There is limited information on the natural history of the disease, although four stages are generally recognized:

- Concealed: early, generally asymptomatic phase; in very rare cases there may be ventricular arrhythmias preceding overt structural disease.
- Overt electrical disorder: unstable phase with symptomatic arrhythmias, generally left bundle branch block, and, thus, suggestive of RV origin.
- RV failure: phase of progressive deterioration in RV contractile function.
- Biventricular pump failure: phase of progressive biventricular dilatation.

Clinical presentation

It is rare for the condition to become manifest before the age of 12 years. Indeed, the median age of presentation is in the mid-thirties. Patients may present with a wide variety of symptoms related to arrhythmias and heart failure or as a sudden death. Affected asymptomatic relatives may be identified as part of family screening. There is some evidence to suggest that the rate of progression may be accelerated if patients participate in significant levels of exercise.

Investigations

Diagnosis of this condition is challenging and requires a detailed family history as well as multiple investigations, including imaging with echocardiography/cardiac MRI/angiography to define structure and function; 12-lead ECG, signal-averaged ECG, ambulatory ECG monitoring and exercise stress testing to look for resting T-wave abnormalities, delayed conduction on right-sided leads, and epsilon waves; late potentials on signal-averaged ECG; arrhythmias; and endomyocardial biopsies to detect histopathological changes. The original Task Force criteria for the diagnosis of ARVC were proposed in 1994 and modified in 2010; major and minor criteria are documented.[38,39] The main differential diagnoses include idiopathic right VT, myocarditis, sarcoidosis, RV infarction, and DCM.

Comprehensive or targeted genetic testing of desmosomal genes can be useful in patients with arrhythmogenic cardiomyopathy[36] and can help with cascade screening in family members.[11] The unpredictability of onset and symptoms complicates the evaluation of relatives and most will face lifelong comprehensive periodic cardiac screening in a specialist centre, particularly in the absence of a definitive pathogenic variant.

Management

The management of ARVC is focused on lifelong monitoring and treatment of symptoms, SCD risk stratification, and prevention of progression of the disease. Extreme physical exertion and participation in competitive sports or endurance training is not recommended due to the risk of disease progression and SCD. Beta-blockers are the mainstay for medical management. ICD implantation is considered according to risk for SCD[40]:

- High risk: patients who have experienced a cardiac arrest due to ventricular fibrillation or sustained VT and those with severe RV/LV dysfunction.

- Intermediate risk: includes those patients with unexplained syncope, non-sustained VT and/or moderate RV/LV dysfunction.
- Low risk: includes those with no risk factors and those who are gene carriers but do not currently show any phenotype.

Although an ICD may be lifesaving, it may also be associated with short-, medium-, and long-term complications that may require multidisciplinary involvement.[41]

Restrictive cardiomyopathy

Restrictive cardiomyopathy (RCM) is a less well-defined cardiomyopathy in which the pattern of ventricular filling caused by increased stiffness of the myocardium results in high ventricular pressures with small increases in volume in the presence of normal or reduced diastolic volumes, normal or reduced systolic volumes, and normal wall thickness. In many ways, it is a description of the pathophysiological state, which may represent various pathologies or cardiomyopathies rather than a distinct cardiomyopathy. This is the least common of all the cardiomyopathies.

RCM may be idiopathic, familial (related to pathogenic variants in the sarcomere genes), or associated with various systemic disorders, such as haemochromatosis, amyloidosis, Fabry disease, carcinoid syndrome, other metabolic disorders, hypereosinophilic syndromes, endomyocardial fibrosis, or previous radiation.

Clinical presentation

Adults with RCM have variable presentations but more commonly have signs and symptoms of heart failure and arrhythmias. There is usually an elevated jugular venous pressure. Disease progression is rapid in children with over 50% dying within 2 years of diagnosis.[41]

Investigations

In RCM, the ECG is typically abnormal with evidence of biatrial hypertrophy and non-specific ST-segment and T-wave changes. Cardiac imaging by echocardiography or cardiac MRI typically shows biatrial enlargement with evidence of diastolic dysfunction. Cardiac catherization may be required to distinguish it from constrictive pericarditis which has a similar presentation. Endomyocardial biopsy may be helpful in selected cases.

Management

Treatment of RCM should consider the underlying cause, if known, such as chemotherapy for those with amyloidosis.[42] Careful fluid management is an essential aspect in the treatment of patients with RCM. Diuretics are used to ameliorate symptoms and signs of pulmonary or venous congestion, but caution is required as they may reduce preload, thus decreasing blood pressure and cause dizziness. Beta-blockers and calcium channel blockers to increase filling time should be carefully introduced as patients may be intolerant, as is the case with angiotensin-converting enzyme inhibitors for which there is limited evidence of any benefit. Patients may have complex arrhythmias, including atrial fibrillation which will require anticoagulation, ICDs may be needed for the management of ventricular tachyarrhythmias. In severe cases, LV assist device therapy is now seen as a bridge to cardiac transplantation or as definitive therapy in RCM.[43] In familial RCM, screening and/or cascade testing of first-degree relatives should be advised accordingly, depending on the inheritance pattern associated with genetic aetiology.

Left ventricular non-compaction

Left ventricular non-compaction (LVNC) is characterized by the presence of spongy myocardium, thought to be as a result of an arrest in normal cardiac development, and predominantly involves the apical portion of the LV chamber (biventricular involvement has been described but is uncommon). The overall prevalence has been estimated as somewhere between 0.05% to 0.24% of the population and LVNC appears to be more common in males. LVNC can occur as an isolated condition or associated with other congenital heart anomalies (e.g. ventricular septal defect (VSD), Ebstein anomaly, bicuspid AV, alpha-dystrobrevin/ *NKX2.5* gene mutations). Inheritance patterns vary depending on the genes implicated, which include sarcomeric, mitochondrial, and X-linked genes (e.g. taffazin (*TAZ*)).

Clinical presentation

LVNC may be identified incidentally or when patients present with one or a combination of these clinical manifestations: heart failure, arrhythmias, or embolic events.

Investigations

Consensus on the diagnostic criteria for LVNC remains elusive. However, Jenni et al. (2001) proposed criteria based on an end-systolic ratio of non-compacted to compacted layers greater than 2 as seen on echocardiography.[44] Cardiac MRI has now been used more often as it allows for proper visualization of the apex in some cases.

Management

The management of LVNC is focused on the prevention and treatment of heart failure, arrhythmias, and embolic events.[45] The frequency of VT, risk for sudden death, and systemic embolism may warrant yearly ambulatory ECG monitoring. All first-degree relatives of patients with LVNC should be offered cardiac evaluation and cascade testing, where a causative pathogenic variant has been found in the proband.[11]

Inherited arrhythmias

Inherited arrhythmias are a group of disorders where there is an inherited susceptibility to heart rhythm defects due to pathogenic variants in genes mainly encoding the Na^+, and K^+ channels, and other arrhythmogenic mechanisms such as those linked to Ca^{2+} transport; typically in the context of a structurally normal heart.[46] This section will focus on the most common such as LQTS, Brugada syndrome (BS), and catecholaminergic polymorphic ventricular tachycardia (CPVT) (➤ **Table 9.4**), and the investigation of sudden arrhythmic death syndrome.

Long QT syndrome

Epidemiology, pathology, and aetiology

LQTS is a disease of myocardial ion channels causing delayed repolarization which can cause torsades de pointes and ventricular fibrillation and may lead to syncope and SCD. The exact prevalence of LQTS is uncertain; however, it is likely to be approximately 1:2000.[47]

While there are an increasing number of LQTS subtypes, the commonest are LQT1, LQT2, and LQT3. Of these LQT1 accounts for 30–35% of cases and is typically due to pathogenic variants in the *KCNQ1* gene. Patients with LQT1 present at a younger age with 86% experiencing a cardiac event by the age of 20 years, usually in the context of exercise, including swimming. Jervell and Lange Nielsen reported a rare, autosomal recessive form with deafness in the late 1950s. In the early 1960s, Romano and Ward reported autosomal dominant families without deafness. LQT2 and LQT3 are both autosomal dominant

Table 9.4 Types of inherited arrhythmias

Condition and prevalence	Presentation	Investigations	Management
Long QT syndrome (LQTS) Delayed repolarization caused by ion channel dysfunction	Variable from asymptomatic to syncope, epilepsy-type symptoms, or SCD	ECG History—precipitating factors, swimming, acoustic stimuli, stress Genetic testing to LQTS and CPVT Risk stratification Schwartz score, ICD where indicated Cascade screening	Beta-blockade Lifestyle modification—avoid competitive sports, swimming, and acoustic stimuli 'Drugs to Avoid' list to both LQTS and Brugada ICD in selected cases Left cardiac sympathetic denervation in selected cases
Brugada syndrome (BS) Complex genetic disorder	Variable from asymptomatic to syncope, epilepsy-type symptoms, SCD, nocturnal agonal breathing Arrhythmia more common at rest or sleeping	ECG Provocation test eg ajmaline Cascade screening	Avoidance of personal triggers Lifestyle modification ICD in selected cases
Catecholaminergic polymorphic ventricular tachycardia (CPVT) Bidirectional, polymorphic VT Prevalence 1:10,000	Palpitations or syncope during exercise in young, seizure-like symptoms, SCD	ECG Exercise stress testing Loop recorder Cascade screening	Avoidance of personal triggers Lifestyle modification Drug treatment ICD in selected cases left cardiac sympathetic denervation in selected cases

conditions and the onset of symptoms tends to be later in life compared to LQT1. LQT2 accounts for 25–30% of LQTS cases and is due to pathogenic variants in the *KCNH2* gene. Symptoms may be provoked by being startled by acoustic stimuli. In LQT3, cardiac events usually occur at rest or sleep and LQT3 is caused by pathogenic variants in *SCN5A*, which encodes the sodium ion channel. At least 12 genes have been implicated in LQTS encompassing the various subtypes.

Clinical presentation

Symptom patterns vary in LQTS, and patients can present asymptomatically with an incidental ECG finding, or epilepsy-type symptoms or indeed sudden death. Symptoms of transient loss of consciousness are typically caused by torsade de pointes and may be misdiagnosed as seizures.

It is important to note any precipitating situations, such as exercise and swimming, sudden acoustic stimuli or stress, and rest or sleep. A relevant family history of LQTS, SCD, recurrent syncope, epilepsy, and deafness should raise the suspicion of LQTS in individuals presenting with palpitations, dizziness, or syncope and an abnormal ECG.

Investigations

The QT interval reflects both depolarization and repolarization. As the QT interval varies with heart rate, several correction approaches have been advocated to ensure accurate measurement as this has important implications for diagnosis and management. The commonly used method is the Bazett formula. The Schwartz score has been used as a standard to diagnose LQTS based on ECG and clinical characteristics (➤ Table 9.5), and has now been incorporated in the updated consensus statement on the diagnosis and management of patients with inherited primary arrhythmia syndromes[6] (➤ Box 9.1).

Apart from the resting ECG, an exercise ECG is usually performed. In LQT1, the QTc interval on exercise does not shorten as much with increased heart rate compared to healthy individuals and this may be more pronounced in the immediate recovery phase (measurement should continue at least up to 4 minutes into recovery).

A 24-hour Holter recording can be helpful in recording T-wave changes not apparent at rest. Diurnal variation may be present, particularly in LQT3, with marked QTc prolongation seen overnight. Other arrhythmias such as ventricular ectopics, torsades de pointes, and non-sustained ventricular fibrillation may also be observed.

Management

Lifestyle modification is an important aspect of management in LQTS. Avoidance of competitive sport is advised, but an individualized approach should be undertaken. In LQT1, swimming should be avoided or under supervision as this is known to trigger an event in approximately 33% of patients. In LQT2, where triggers include

Table 9.5 Risk score for long QT syndrome (Schwartz score)

Criteria	Points
Electrocardiographic findinga	
A. QTc[b]	
≥480 ms	3
460–479 ms	2
450–459 ms (in males)	1
B. QTc[b] 4th minute of recovery from exercise stress test ≥480 ms	1
C. Torsade de pointes[c]	2
D. T wave alternans	1
E. Notched T wave in 3 leads	1
F. Low heart rate for age	0.5
Clinical history	
A. Syncope[c]	
With stress	2
Without stress	1
B. Congenital deafness	0.5
Family history	
A. Family members with definite LQTS[e]	1
B. Unexplained sudden cardiac death below age 30 among immediate family members[e]	0.5

[a] In the absence of medications or disorders known to affect these electrocardiographic features.
[b] QTc calculated by Bazett's formula where QTc = QT/√RR.
[c] Mutually exclusive.
[d] Resting heart rate below the 2nd percentile for age.
[e] The same family member cannot be counted in A and B.
SCORE: ≤1 point: low probability of LQTD.
1.5 to 3 points: intermediate probability of LQTS.
≥3.5 points high probability.
Reproduced from Schwartz PJ, Crotti L. QTc behavior during exercise and genetic testing for the long-QT syndrome. Circulation. 2011 Nov 15;124(20):2181–4. doi: 10.1161/CIRCULATIONAHA.111.062182 with permission from Wolters Kluwer.

Box 9.1 Diagnostic criteria for long QT syndrome

1. LQTS is diagnosed:
   a. In the presence of an LQTS risk score of 3.5 or higher in the absence of a secondary cause for QT prolongation *and/or*
   b. In the presence of an unequivocally pathogenic mutation in one of the LQTS genes *or*
   c. In the presence of a QT interval corrected for heart rate using Bazett's formula (QTc) of 500 ms or greater in repeated 12-lead ECG and in the absence of a secondary cause for QT prolongation.
2. LQTS can be diagnosed in the presence of a QTc between 480 and 499 ms in repeated 12-lead ECGs in a patient with unexplained syncope in the absence of a secondary cause for QT prolongation and in the absence of a pathogenic mutation.

Priori SG, Wilde AA, Horie M, et al; Heart Rhythm Society; European Heart Rhythm Association; Asia Pacific Heart Rhythm Society. Executive summary: HRS/EHRA/APHRS expert consensus statement on the diagnosis and management of patients with inherited primary arrhythmia syndromes. Europace. 2013 Oct;15(10):1389–406. doi: 10.1093/europace/eut272.

acoustic stimuli especially during sleep, telephones and alarm clocks should be removed from the bedroom. Drugs that prolong the QTc interval and those that deplete magnesium and potassium should be avoided (https://crediblemeds.org/).

Beta-blockers remain the mainstay of drug treatment with a very strong evidence base for LQT1 and LQT2. In some patients with LQT3, the sodium channel blocker mexiletine can be useful.

ICD implantation for secondary prevention is recommended for patients with LQTS who are survivors of cardiac arrest. A primary prevention ICD should be considered in the following patients:

- Patients with LQTS-related syncope while on beta-blockers.
- Patients with QTc greater than 500 ms and signs of electrical instability.
- Patients with high-risk genetic profiles (carriers of two variants, including Jervell and Lange–Nielsen syndrome).

In pregnancy, women with LQTS have an increased risk during the 9-month postpartum period (especially women with the LQT2 genotype) and should, therefore, have regular follow-up.

In patients who are unable to tolerate beta-blockers or remain high risk for sudden death with beta-blocker treatment, left cardiac sympathetic denervation is an option.[48] The procedure can be done surgically through a left supraclavicular incision or as a minimally invasive procedure in experienced centres. This procedure is frequently used in very-high-risk infants and children in whom ICD therapy may be relatively contraindicated due to the physical size of the patient.

All first-degree relatives of patients with LQTS should be offered cardiac screening. However, the exclusion of LQTS solely on clinical grounds has been difficult, and up to 6% of family members with normal QT intervals may ultimately have syncope or cardiac arrest.[49] If a causative gene defect has been found in the proband, it is recommended that family members are offered genetic counselling and predictive genetic testing. Nursing and psychosocial aspects of care are discussed on p. 274.

Brugada syndrome (BS)

Epidemiology, pathology, and aetiology

The prevalence of BS is uncertain but is reported to be 1:10,000 worldwide but can be as high as 0.5–1:1000 in Southeast Asia where it appears to be the most common cause of death in young men under the age of 50 years.[50] The syndrome typically presents in adulthood with a mean age of sudden death at 41 ± 15 years. BS is eight to ten times more prevalent in males than in females.

The genetic aspects of BS are complex and not yet fully understood, with some families demonstrating autosomal dominant inheritance of variants in *SCN5A*, and more recent evidence supporting a polygenic basis of disease.[51] BS leads to a reduction of Na^+ current and the ensuing conduction defects such as ventricular fibrillation in typically structurally normal hearts.

Clinical presentation

Patients with BS are frequently asymptomatic but they can present with palpitations, dizziness, syncope, chest discomfort, nocturnal agonal respiration, or cardiac arrest. Arrhythmias usually occur at rest or during sleep; or while in a febrile or vagotonic state but are rarely associated with exercise.

Investigations

The diagnosis of BS relies on the characteristic classical type 1 coved ST-segment elevation pattern (➤ **Fig. 9.4**)

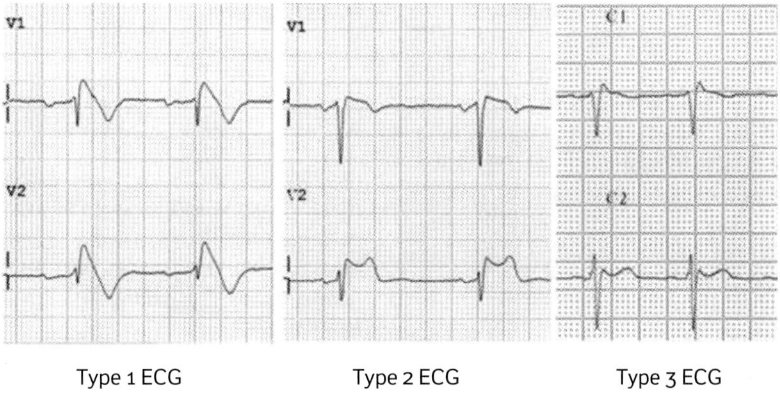

Fig. 9.4 Brugada ECG patterns.

present in the precordial ECG leads. The ECG should be performed with the right precordial leads (V1 and V2) positioned in the second and third intercostal spaces (high lead position) as well as the fourth intercostal space. The ECG changes may be present spontaneously or after administration of a sodium channel blocking drug, such as ajmaline or flecainide.

A diagnosis of BS is made in the presence of:

- ST-segment elevation with type 1 morphology of 2 mm or greater in one or among the right precordial leads V1, V2 in the standard or higher intercostal positions occurring either spontaneously *or* after drug provocation testing; *or*
- The induction of a type 1 ECG morphology after a drug provocation test in individuals with type 2 or type 3 ST-segment elevation in one or more leads among the right precordial leads V1, V2 in the standard or higher intercostal positions. Phenocopies that lead to Brugada-like ECG changes need to be ruled out. These include RV ischaemia, acute pulmonary embolism, pericarditis, myocardial infarction, and mechanical compression of the RV.

Management

Avoidance of triggers that lead to arrhythmias are key aspects of management in BS. This includes rapid treatment of fever and hypokalaemia, avoidance of high-carbohydrate meals close to bedtime, heavy drinking and very hot baths.[52] Patients should be advised against drugs that induce a type 1 ECG pattern—these include some antiarrhythmics, anaesthetic agents, cocaine, antidepressants, and antipsychotics (https://www.brugadadrugs.org/avoid/).

Risk stratification in BS is currently challenging but there is a consensus that those who survived a cardiac arrest should have an ICD implanted as recurrence remains high. The presence of a spontaneous type 1 ECG pattern or a history of syncope is considered high risk. Males tend to have a higher incidence of arrhythmias. There is still ongoing debate about the role of electrophysiological studies in risk stratification in BS.

Pharmacological therapy (isoproterenol or quinidine) may be of help in an arrhythmic storm situation, although there is currently no definitive evidence base for its use for prevention of SCD.

Genetic testing in BS makes little contribution to diagnosis, prognosis, and therapeutic management, in sharp contrast to LQTS and is, therefore, not routinely recommended. It is emerging that the familial pattern in BS may not be as simple as originally reported and that an oligogenic model may be more likely.[11] A clear exception is families where there is demonstrated familial inheritance of disease, and in these cases sequencing of *SCN5A* should be considered. Regardless of suspected inheritance risks, first-degree relatives should be offered clinical screening with a baseline ECG and drug provocation as appropriate.

Catecholaminergic polymorphic ventricular tachycardia (CPTV)

Epidemiology, pathology, and aetiology

CPVT is a rare condition characterized by bidirectional and polymorphic VT which is adrenergically mediated. The estimated prevalence of CPVT is approximately 1:10,000.[50]

Two types of CPVT have been noted which are linked to genes involved in calcium handling in the cells. CPVT1 is an autosomal dominant form which mainly involves pathogenic variants in the gene encoding the cardiac ryanodine receptor gene (*RYR2*). The rarer form, CPVT2, is the autosomal recessive form and is caused by pathogenic variants in the cardiac calsequestrin gene (*CASQ2*). Altogether, these account for 60% of the genetic causes of CPVT, suggesting that other genes are involved in this condition.

Clinical presentation

The first clinical manifestation in the form of palpitations or syncope usually presents in the first or second decade of life, typically occurring during exercise or heightened emotional stress. CPVT is a common cause of sudden unexplained cardiac death. Seizure-like activities may be seen during a syncopal episode which may be attributed to a neurological cause in the first instance, causing delays in the diagnosis of CPVT.

Investigations

The resting ECG is normal. However, ventricular arrhythmias generally occur during exercise stress testing. A classical pattern of monomorphic followed by polymorphic or bidirectional VT is noted with increasing arrhythmia burden as exercise progresses (➤ Fig. 9.5).[53] Holter monitors and implantable loop recorders can also be helpful investigations with regard to making a diagnosis. An echocardiogram will confirm a structurally normal heart. The diagnostic criteria for CPVT can be found in ➤ Box 9.2.[6]

A drug challenge with epinephrine or isoproterenol may be useful in eliciting arrhythmias in patients who cannot exercise.

Management

Avoidance of triggers is an important management aspect in CPVT and is focused on advice regarding exercise, particularly the limitation or avoidance of competitive

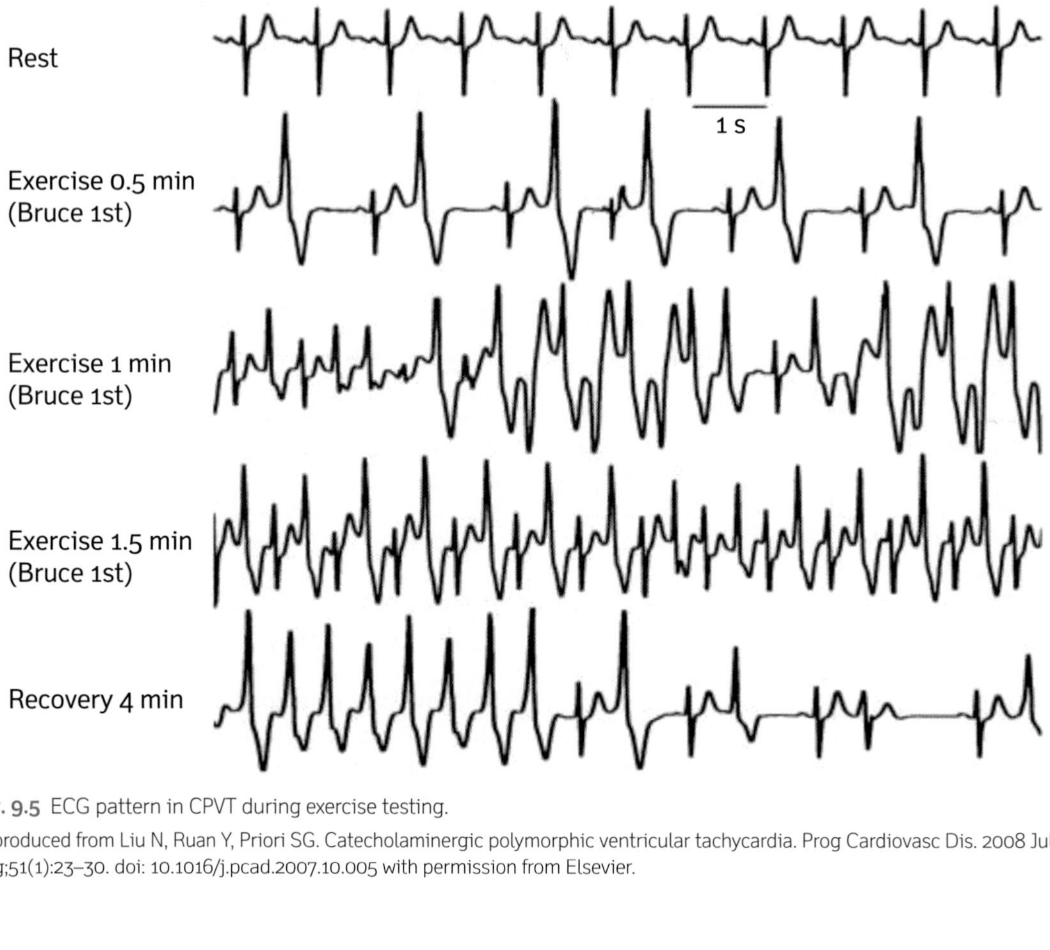

Fig. 9.5 ECG pattern in CPVT during exercise testing.

Reproduced from Liu N, Ruan Y, Priori SG. Catecholaminergic polymorphic ventricular tachycardia. Prog Cardiovasc Dis. 2008 Jul–Aug;51(1):23–30. doi: 10.1016/j.pcad.2007.10.005 with permission from Elsevier.

Box 9.2 Diagnostic criteria for catecholaminergic polymorphic ventricular tachycardia

1. CPVT *is diagnosed* in the presence of a structurally normal heart, normal ECG, and unexplained exercise or catecholamine-induced bidirectional VT or polymorphic ventricular premature beats or VT in an individual less than 40 years of age.
2. CPVT *is diagnosed* in patients (index case or family member) who have a pathogenic mutation.
3. CPVT *is diagnosed* in family members of a CPVT index case with a normal heart who manifest exercise-induced premature ventricular contractions or bidirectional/polymorphic VT.
4. CPVT *can be diagnosed* in the presence of a structurally normal heart and coronary arteries, normal ECG, and unexplained exercise or catecholamine-induced bidirectional VT or polymorphic ventricular premature beats or VT in an individual greater than 40 years of age.

Priori SG, Wilde AA, Horie M, et al; Heart Rhythm Society; European Heart Rhythm Association; Asia Pacific Heart Rhythm Society. Executive summary: HRS/EHRA/APHRS expert consensus statement on the diagnosis and management of patients with inherited primary arrhythmia syndromes. Europace. 2013 Oct;15(10):1389–406. doi: 10.1093/europace/eut272. © The European Society of Cardiology. Reprinted by permission of Oxford University Press.

sport and strenuous exercise, as well as stress-related environments.

Beta-blockers are used for patients who have a clinical diagnosis of CPVT and may be useful for asymptomatic gene carriers. Nadolol or propranolol are most widely prescribed and it is important to be aware that the maximal tolerated dose of beta-blockers should be prescribed to optimize control of arrhythmias. Exercise testing should be performed on a regular basis to monitor effectiveness of beta-blockers. Flecainide may be added to beta-blockers for further control of arrhythmias.

A diagnosis in childhood and the persistence of complex arrhythmias during the exercise stress test on a full dose of beta-blockers are independent predictors for arrhythmic events.[11] An ICD is recommended alongside beta-blockers for secondary prevention in patients who have survived a cardiac arrest and should be considered for primary prevention for those who have recurrent syncope or sustained VT despite beta-blocker therapy. The programming of the ICD should incorporate long delays before shock delivery, because painful shocks can increase the sympathetic tone and trigger further arrhythmias, leading to a malignant cycle of ICD shocks and even death.

Left cardiac sympathetic denervation may be recommended in the management of patients with CPVT intolerant to beta-blockers or those who continue to be symptomatic while on beta-blockers, as well as for those with recurrent VT storms.[48]

First-degree relatives are recommended to have clinical screening with an ECG, exercise stress test, and Holter monitor. They should also be offered genetic counselling and predictive genetic testing (if a causative gene has been identified) as there are lifestyle and treatment implications even for asymptomatic carriers.

Sudden cardiac death in the young (<40 years)

SCD is of major public health importance and prevention is key (REF) ESC 2016 Guidelines on Prevention of VA & SCD. However, most of these sudden deaths occur in older individuals and are secondary to coronary heart disease. The sudden, unexpected cardiac death of a young individual has profound effects not only for the family and friends but also for society in general. Accurate figures are not available but it has been estimated that the incidence of sudden death in young individuals is about 1–2:100,000 per year. Common causes include various types of cardiomyopathies and channelopathies, as well as atherosclerotic coronary artery disease, aortic dissection, and anomalous coronary arteries. However, in up to 40% of cases, no structural abnormality can be detected at autopsy and, where there is a negative toxicology result, this is termed sudden arrhythmic death syndrome.

In the event of SCD, it is very important to try to establish an accurate cause of death. Therefore, it is recommended that a thorough personal and family history and circumstance of the sudden death are collected. Expert cardiac pathology should be undertaken to rule out microscopic features of structural heart disease as well as collection of blood or suitable tissue for genetic evaluation/molecular autopsy. A molecular autopsy may be helpful in confirming a genetic cause of the SCD/make a diagnosis in up to 35% of cases. Establishing a pathogenic variant will enable cascade testing to the rest of the surviving family members.

Many conditions associated with SCD have a clear inherited basis, including many cases without a clear diagnosis established at postmortem. Therefore, clinical investigation, and, where indicated, genetic testing of surviving family members is warranted and should take place in a clinic with appropriately trained multidisciplinary staff. ➤ **Fig. 9.6** illustrates the clinical investigation pathway of surviving family members.[16]

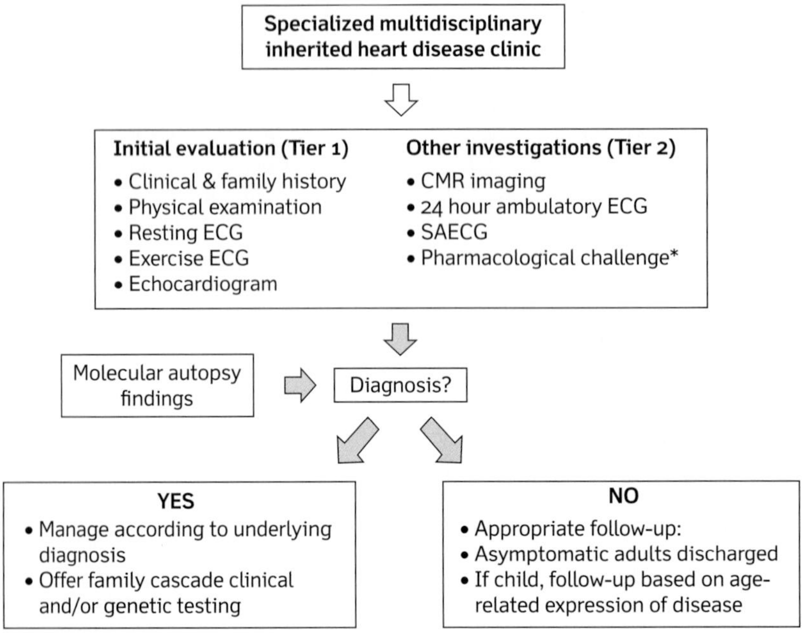

Fig. 9.6 Pathway for investigating SCD relatives.

Semsarian C, Ingles J, Wilde AA. Sudden cardiac death in the young: the molecular autopsy and a practical approach to surviving relatives. Eur Heart J. 2015 Jun 1;36(21):1290–6. doi: 10.1093/eurheartj/ehv063. Reprinted by permission of Oxford University Press on behalf of the European Society of Cardiology.

Inherited connective tissue disorders

The spectrum of signs and symptoms in inherited connective tissue disorders is extensive and may involve multiple body systems. Generally, patients will have progressive disease with mild to severe dermatological, joint, eye, and cardiovascular features. This section focuses on the cardiovascular manifestations and management in the most common inherited connective tissue disorders. Management of family members in inherited connective tissue disorders share a common approach where clinical screening of first-degree relatives is recommended and, in the presence of a pathogenic genetic variant in the proband, genetic counselling and cascade testing should be offered.

Marfan syndrome

Epidemiology, pathology, and aetiology

The minimal birth incidence of Marfan syndrome is 1:9800 with a prevalence of around 1:5000. Marfan syndrome is an autosomal dominant condition caused by pathogenic variants in the fibrillin-1 gene which has an important role in the stability of the extracellular matrix. These genetic defects bring about the characteristic features of Marfan syndrome found in the aorta, eye, and musculoskeletal system.

Loeys–Dietz syndrome appears to overlap with Marfan syndrome but has the additional features of arterial tortuosity and aneurysms, hypertelorism, and a bifid uvula. Genetic variants have been reported in the genes encoding the type 1 or type 2 transforming growth factor (TGF)-beta receptors.[54]

Diagnosis

The musculoskeletal features of Marfan syndrome are the most obvious on clinical examination, including long limbs, chest wall abnormalities, arachnodactyly (spider fingers), joint hypermobility, and stretch marks. Ophthalmic features include ectopia lentis, myopia, and retinal detachment. A diagnosis of Marfan syndrome is made if patients carry specific combinations of aortic, ophthalmic, skeletal, and genetic findings using the revised Ghent criteria[55] (https://www.marfan.org/dx/revised-ghent-nosology).

Due to multisystem involvement in Marfan syndrome, several diagnostic tools are needed and include cardiac and aortic imaging (transthoracic echocardiography and

MRI) to measure the aortic diameter at the sinuses of Valsalva and along the length of the aorta. Musculoskeletal evaluation may include pelvic X-ray and lumbar MRI scans.

Cardiovascular complications and management

Cardiovascular features of Marfan syndrome include mitral valve prolapse and regurgitation, LV dilatation and heart failure, and pulmonary artery dilatation, but the main cause of mortality and morbidity is aortic root dilatation leading to aortic dissection. Beta-blocker therapy should be considered at any age in those with a dilated aorta. However, prophylactic treatment may be more effective in those with an aortic diameter less than 4 cm.

Patients at high risk of aortic dissection include those with an aortic diameter greater than 5 cm, aortic dilatation extending beyond the sinus of Valsalva, a rapid rate of dilatation (>5%/year, or 1.5 mm/year in adults), and a family history of aortic dissection. Prophylactic aortic root surgery should be considered when the aortic diameter is greater than 5 cm at the sinus of Valsalva.

Pregnant women with Marfan syndrome are at an increased risk of aortic dissection if the aortic diameter is greater than 4 cm. Frequent cardiovascular monitoring is, therefore, warranted throughout pregnancy and the postpartum period.

Annual evaluation should be offered to patients with Marfan syndrome and will include a clinical history, examination, and cardiac and aortic imaging. Children should have more frequent surveillance with serial echocardiography every 6–12 months, depending on the aortic diameter and rate of increase.[56]

Vascular Ehlers–Danlos syndrome

Epidemiology, pathology, and aetiology

There are at least ten subtypes of Ehlers–Danlos syndrome (EDS) with overlapping features of skin laxity, easy bruising, delayed healing, joint hypermobility, and cardiovascular manifestations. The focus of this section is EDS IV which is associated with moderate to severe cardiovascular manifestations, including sudden death and stroke due to arterial rupture.

The pathology in EDS IV reveals vascular changes in the form of aneurysms, microscopic evidence of connective tissue changes, and abnormal type 3 collagen profile on biochemistry. EDS IV is caused by pathogenic variants in the collagen type 3 gene (*COL3A1*).

Cardiovascular complications and management

The clinical picture in EDS IV may be normal and skin thinning can be observed. Cardiovascular complications are a major concern in EDS IV and can be catastrophic and frequently fatal with arterial rupture and dissection commonly occurring. EDS IV may produce sudden arterial failure without evidence of gradual deterioration. Thus, the management of arterial complications in EDS IV is immediate and should not be delayed. Vascular surgery is potentially dangerous due to difficulty in establishing haemostasis in friable aneurysmal or dissected vessels.

Approaches in the event of a dissection include the conservative control of bleeding in smaller aneurysms and small arteries, coil embolization, the use of angiographic arteriography to aid in aneurysm resections, and grafting and endovascular repair.

Familial thoracic aortic aneurysm and dissection (FTAAD)

Epidemiology, pathology, and aetiology

Approximately 20% of thoracic aortic aneurysms and dissections relate to a genetic predisposition. Most are autosomal dominant with incomplete penetrance and variable clinical presentation. The genes involved in this group of conditions include *TGFBR1*, *TGFBR2*, *MYH11*, and *ACTA2*.

The mean age of presentation in familial thoracic aortic aneurysm and dissection (FTAAD) is younger than that of individuals with sporadic disease but older than those with Marfan syndrome.

Cardiovascular complications and management

The initial manifestations of FTAAD are either dilatation of the ascending aorta or dissection of the ascending aorta or both. Death usually results from aortic rupture. The onset and rate of progression of aortic dilatation is highly variable even within families but, tragically, the first presentation of FTAAD may be sudden unexplained death and a diagnosis is made at postmortem examination.[57]

Aortic dissection is rare in childhood but aortic dilatation may be present. In adults, the risk of aortic rupture is significant when the maximal aortic dimension reaches about 5.5 cm. Appropriate management with medical therapy and prophylactic repair of aneurysmal dilatation renders a similar life expectancy to that of the general population in those with FTAAD.

Family screening should improve the prognosis of those with a family history compared to those presenting with symptoms due to earlier surveillance. In at-risk family members, echocardiography should be performed at frequent intervals (every 1–3 years) from a young age (6–7 years) to monitor the status of the ascending aorta, with full imaging of the entire aorta every 4–5 years. Lifestyle advice should include avoidance of isometric exercises and competitive sport that has a risk for significant blows to the chest as this could accelerate aortic root dilatation. In pregnancy, serial monitoring of the aorta is warranted according to the prepregnancy assessment of the aorta.

Nursing care in inherited cardiac conditions

Psychological and emotional challenges of a diagnosis of an inherited cardiac condition

Patients diagnosed with an inherited condition have the dual challenge of dealing with their own health issues as well as the implications for the health of their family. It is common to experience a sense of guilt as the person 'who caused the condition'.[58] Furthermore, this stress and worry is compounded by the risk of sudden death at a young age.[59] In many cases, a diagnosis is brought about by a combination of a catastrophic family history of sudden death, significant morbidity, or a personal history of a cardiac arrest. These factors are known antecedents of significant psychological distress and, therefore, nursing care should be provided in the context of this background.[19,60] Patients with ICCs have varying signs and symptoms due to variable disease penetrance.[61] However, even if they are asymptomatic or have very few symptoms, they may be subjected to radical lifestyle changes to reduce the risk of sudden death.[62,63] The role of the nurse, alongside other clinicians, in supporting these adjustments can have a profound impact on the long-term coping of these patients and their families (see ➤ **Fig. 9.7** for a summary of some of these issues).

Specialized multidisciplinary clinics

International practice guidelines for the care of patients and families affected by inherited and congenital cardiac conditions have stipulated that clinical care for this population should be delivered within specialized multidisciplinary clinics due to the complex, long-term needs of these patient groups.[63–65] These clinics are typically comprised of a core team of cardiologists, clinical geneticists, specialist nurses, and genetic counsellors with experience and expertise in ICCs. The service has a full array of diagnostic capabilities in terms of cardiac imaging, arrhythmia interpretation, and genetic technologies. The core team works in collaboration with other disciplines, such as pathology, surgery, metabolic medicine, behavioural health, and many more, to bring about optimal outcomes for patients.[65] A nursing priority is, therefore, to facilitate early access to these specialized services and co-ordination of care.

The role of the cardiac genetics nurse

A cardiac genetics nurse is a core member of the ICC multidisciplinary team and is usually an experienced cardiovascular nurse with knowledge in heart failure, arrhythmias, and vascular disorders in both the inpatient and outpatient setting, who has undertaken additional academic and practical training in clinical genetics.[65–67] A main function of the role is to be the first point of care and contact for the patient and their families for access to the specialist service and also to coordinate the other associated specialties involved in their care.[67] Cardiac genetics nurses have the expertise to undertake a comprehensive family history, provide genetic and cardiac-related information and support, initiate tests and collate results for an multidisciplinary team evaluation, and facilitate family screening. They are responsible for addressing follow-up questions, providing health guidance, and ensuring timely and continued consultations long term. Where genetic services are mainstreamed, they also provide genetic counselling and facilitate diagnostic genetic testing.[66]

Principles of general nursing care in inherited cardiac conditions

While these specialist nursing roles exist, there are nursing responsibilities that every nurse in the cardiovascular specialty should be aware of and, at the centre of this, is the provision of holistic, person- and family-centred nursing care which aims to:

- In the acute, in-hospital phase, conduct a comprehensive assessment and the application of nursing interventions; and facilitate timely medical interventions to achieve homeostasis.
- Provide coordinated care within the multidisciplinary team for access to prompt expert consultations (i.e.

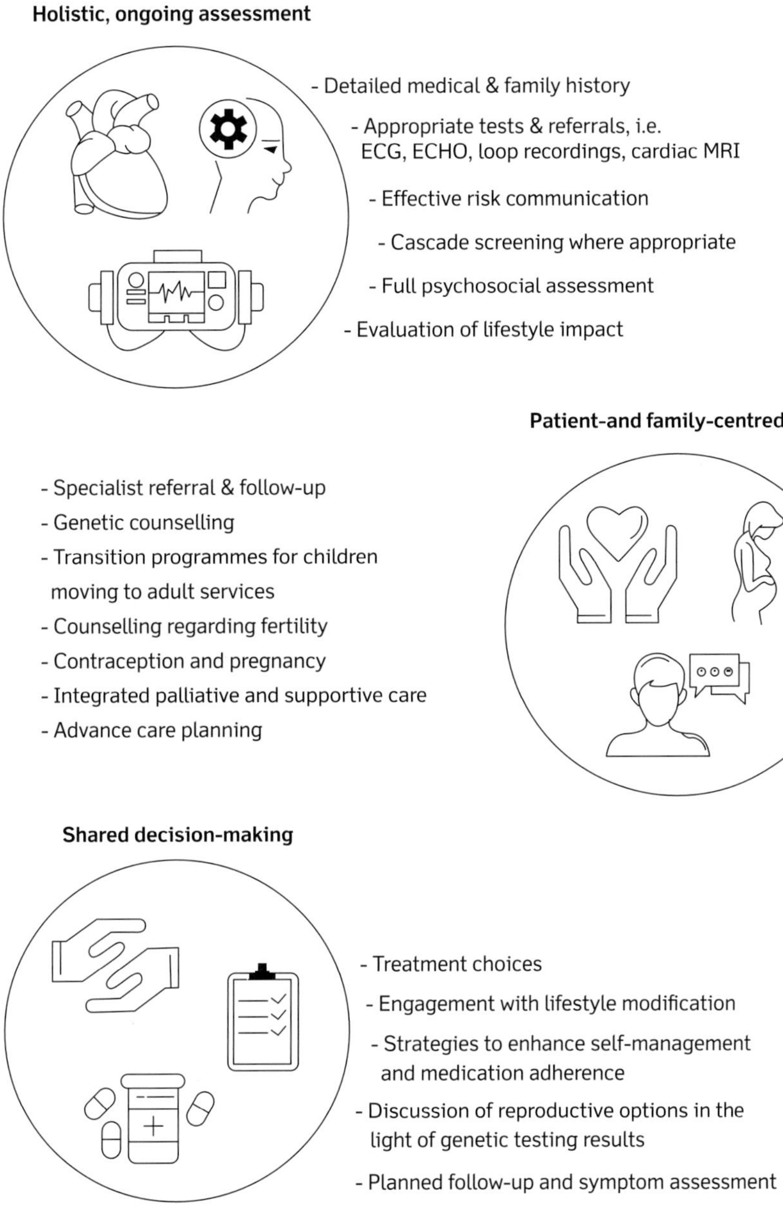

Holistic, ongoing assessment
- Detailed medical & family history
- Appropriate tests & referrals, i.e. ECG, ECHO, loop recordings, cardiac MRI
- Effective risk communication
- Cascade screening where appropriate
- Full psychosocial assessment
- Evaluation of lifestyle impact
Patient-and family-centred care
- Specialist referral & follow-up
- Genetic counselling
- Transition programmes for children moving to adult services
- Counselling regarding fertility
- Contraception and pregnancy
- Integrated palliative and supportive care
- Advance care planning
Shared decision-making
- Treatment choices
- Engagement with lifestyle modification
- Strategies to enhance self-management and medication adherence
- Discussion of reproductive options in the light of genetic testing results
- Planned follow-up and symptom assessment

Fig. 9.7 Issues surrounding the care of patients with inherited cardiac conditions.

cardiology, clinical genetics) and comprehensive diagnostic, genetic, and risk assessment work-up, as well as access to long-term follow-up.

- Ensure that patients and their families have comprehensive and clear health information to enable them to make balanced decisions about their clinical management, lifestyle, and genetic implications.
- Reinforce measures to prevent significant morbidity and SCD.
- Provide psychological support, tailored to the individual's needs and experience of the condition, personal coping skills, and family dynamics.
- Signpost to relevant patient support groups and resources.

- Ultimately, increase patient self-efficacy, harness their social and family networks, and develop their coping skills to enable adjustment, and optimal short- and long-term outcomes.

Nursing Assessment in inherited cardiac conditions

The diagnostic journey

An initial diagnosis or the beginning of the diagnostic work-up for an ICC may take place in the acute or out-patient setting. This period is usually marked by shock and disbelief as patients take in the events prior to the diagnosis, which could be as serious as a cardiac arrest.[68] It is important at this stage to establish an empathic therapeutic relationship with the patient and assess any additional psychological support needs signaling requirement for prompt referral.

Patients will undergo several diagnostic and risk stratification tests according to the guidance for each ICC. These can range from something as simple as an ECG or as invasive as cardiac catheterization. Preparing the patient by explaining the purpose of each test and ensuring prompt feedback of the results is essential to helping patients understand their diagnosis and provide reassurance when possible.[68] Uncertainty regarding signs and symptoms has been recognized as a source of emotional distress in this patient group[60] and can be ameliorated once the source is identified and a plan for treatment initiated.

Genetic studies will often be done as part of the diagnostic work-up and, therefore, access to genetic counselling will be crucial at this stage. The purpose and benefits of this were discussed at the start of this chapter (see 'Genetic principles and cardiac genetic testing' Pg 244).

Clinical management

Signs and symptoms

Many patients with ICCs may remain symptom free for most of their life. However, regular monitoring through serial investigations/regular follow-ups is essential to respond to any changes in their risk profile. Nursing responsibilities in this aspect include health education around signs and symptoms that herald the deterioration in cardiac function or dangerous ventricular arrhythmias summarized in ➤ Table 9.6.

Medications

When medications are initiated, a thorough discussion of the purpose, uptitration schedule, monitoring, and side effects, including possible effects on sexual performance, should be provided. Possible interactions should also be explored if patients have an existing medication regimen or are taking any supplements or herbal agents. Atrial fibrillation is also a common arrhythmia in HCM[69] and, therefore, requires the associated health education around the methods for cardioversion and anticoagulation which are discussed in detail in Chapter 7. Beta-blockers are the mainstay for patients with LQTS and CPVT to suppress ventricular arrhythmias and prevent SCD. Ensuring therapeutic levels through exercise testing should be facilitated.[6] Nursing input to support medication adherence is crucial, especially in the young, as it has been noted that this has been suboptimal in the LQT1 and LQT2 population despite a strong evidence base for its therapeutic benefits.[70]

A main aspect in the care of patients with inherited arrhythmias, particularly in LQTS and BS, is the avoidance of certain medications. In LQTS, these are medications that prolong the QTc interval and cause the depletion of potassium and magnesium.[71] In BS, the drugs to avoid are those associated with inducing a type 1 Brugada ECG pattern, such as antiarrhythmics, psychotropic drugs, certain anaesthetics, and other substances including cocaine, acetylcholine, ergonovine, and alcohol in excess.[72] Patients should, therefore, be advised regarding experimentation with recreational drugs and heavy drinking. They should also have access to the latest 'drugs to avoid' lists found online (for LQTS: https://crediblemeds.org/; for BS: https://www.brugadadrugs.org/).

Table 9.6 Potential health problem and associated signs and symptoms in inherited cardiac conditions

Potential health problem	Signs and symptoms
Decrease in myocardial function	Dyspnoea Easy fatigability Oedema/fluid retention Chest pain
Ventricular arrhythmias	Palpitations Dizzy spells Syncope or near-syncope Seizures or seizure-like episodes *Fever in Brugada syndrome may induce ventricular arrhythmias and requires rapid treatment

Devices

ICDs are used for primary prevention in high-risk groups and secondary prevention of SCD in ICCs and a decision should be made after a balanced discussion with the patient regarding the benefits and possible complications. Across cardiovascular diseases, ICDs are associated with depression and anxiety, particularly in the period post implantation and in those who received inappropriate or frequent shocks.[73] In an international study of patients with HCM, overall psychological well-being was not impacted by the ICD implantation. However, there was a heightened anxiety in anticipation of a future shock.[74] Furthermore, in a study focused on ICC patients with ICDs, the vulnerable groups for increased anxiety, depression, and post-traumatic stress were identified as those with a female sex, a history of syncopal episodes, other medical comorbidities, and complications with their ICD.[75] While the nursing care of patients undergoing ICD implantation should be delivered as per the guidance detailed in Chapter 7, it is worth noting that patients with ICCs may need extra support.

Lifestyle advice

Exercise and sport

Physical activity and exercise are essential for cardiovascular health and yet may be restricted in ICCs, as they are triggers for ventricular arrhythmias, particularly in LQT1 (unsupervised swimming should be avoided), CPVT, and HCM, and in the case of ARVC, lead to disease progression.[1] Studies have shown, particularly in ICC patients where participation in sport is part of their identity and main social group, that feelings of isolation, loneliness, and frustration are common when they are excluded for medical reasons.[76] Stricter guidelines exist for the participation of individuals with ICCs in competitive sport but, for general fitness and leisure, a person-centred approach is more appropriate as suited to the patient's risk profile for SCD.[62] An important nursing role is advocating for this tailored exercise advice and supporting patients as they adjust to these recommendations.

Other considerations

In patients with LQT2, acoustic stimuli, especially during sleep, should be avoided. Telephones and alarm clocks should not be present in sleeping areas.[69]

Sexual activity

Patients should be given the opportunity to discuss their concerns regarding sexual activity, not only because of the anxiety and depression they may experience due to the diagnosis, but also the physical activity itself which they may fear as precipitating symptoms.

Employment

Most patients diagnosed with an ICC can retain their usual employment. However, there will be cases where a decrease in physical functioning will make it impossible to carry on with heavy manual work, particularly in inherited cardiomyopathies.[63] Furthermore, certain occupations such as pilots, armed forces personnel, and heavy goods drivers have strict eligibility criteria which could exclude the patient depending on their physical status and clinical management. The loss of professional identity and role as a breadwinner can have a profound psychological impact on patients, not to mention the financial implications.[77] Input from social services, where relevant, should be considered as part of the initial nursing assessment.

Diet, weight, and smoking

Patients should be supported to maintain a healthy body mass index and diet. General advice on the health risks of smoking should be provided as well as referrals to a smoking cessation programme, as required. Patients with HCM and LVOTO should maintain hydration and may find smaller, more frequent meals more tolerable as large meals increase the propensity for chest pain.[63] Maintenance of good hydration to maintain electrolyte balance is also important in inherited arrhythmias. Therefore, there should be prompt treatment of diarrhoea and vomiting.[6]

Immunizations

In the absence of any contraindications, immunization schedules should be maintained. Patients should be encouraged to have yearly influenza vaccinations.[63]

Insurance

Patients diagnosed with ICCs may have difficulty getting life insurance and may see an increase in their travel insurance premiums, which can be a cause of anxiety and further limit their lifestyle choices.[78] Guidelines vary among different countries and local information should be shared with the patient.

Care of the family

The family at risk for inherited cardiac conditions

The inherited nature of these conditions automatically conveys a risk for first-degree relatives of the person first diagnosed with an ICC (the proband). Facilitation of screening and/or genetic testing for first-degree relatives is usually undertaken by members of the specialist ICC team. However, general nursing care should involve highlighting this risk to the patient and, if required, a referral to the specialist team should be made. Care should be taken to protect patient confidentiality, as in most countries the legal framework for conveying this risk information often stipulates that this risk information is communicated by the proband supported by the clinicians, and not communicated directly to relatives by the clinicians.[1] In most cases, patients and their families will work together to disseminate this information. However, not all will seek screening and/or pursue predictive genetic testing and this and/or a lack of communication can be a source of conflict within families.[60,79]

Engaging the family in the care of patients with long-term conditions is particularly helpful in supporting self-management and fostering increased social support.[80] However, the realization of their own risk may add further distress to family members already struggling with the proband's predicament.[1] Psychological support should, therefore, also be offered to the family members.

Psychological care in the context of sudden cardiac death

The psychological impact of ICCs in a relative is even more profound in the context of sudden death. The sudden, unexpected loss of an apparently healthy young relative is a major traumatic event for the bereaved.[81] Such situations are not uncommon in ICCs, as this group of conditions underlie at least half of SCDs in the under 45 age group.[82] This loss can interfere dramatically with established family routines and habits that have previously provided a sense of safety and purpose for the family unit.[83] Grief is a normal emotional response to the loss of a loved one. However, in sudden death in the context of ICCs, up to 44% of family members may experience prolonged grief and post-traumatic stress.[18] Mothers, in particular, are more likely to report symptoms of anxiety and depression.[19] Prompt assessment of needs and an appropriate referral to a clinical psychologist or other clinical professional skilled in psychological evaluation and treatment should be prioritized for bereaved relatives.

Strategies that have been known to help families include open lines of communication between patients and nurses and other clinicians over time as bereavement tends to continue despite a decrease of the acute shock, disbelief, and erratic emotional reactions which tends to occur early after the death of a family member. Health professionals can, and should, provide clear and accurate information about the cause of death and answer questions, while also recognizing that this information may need to be repeated several times.[83] Unanswered questions contribute to a lack of understanding related to causes and circumstances of a family member's death, which in turn appear to limit survivors' ability to make sense of their loss. Allowing family members to share stories of loss is also an important component of clinical care and peer support could be helpful in this respect.[84]

Support groups

There are patient support groups that are specific to ICCs. They aim to provide day-to-day experiential advice to patients with ICC and their families and patient-friendly health information. Support is provided in a variety of ways—via telephone, online, or group meetings and most have comprehensive websites. Support groups also focus on advocacy for the needs of patients and families in terms of clinical services and research priorities, and for increased awareness of ICCs.[85] Nurses should signpost patients and families to the appropriate support groups local to the patient.

Congenital heart diseases

CHD is a collection of gross structural abnormalities of the heart or intrathoracic great vessels that have actual or potential functional significance. CHD comprises a wide spectrum of simple, moderate, and complex severity lesions.[86] Globally, the birth prevalence of CHD is estimated to be 8.2:1000 newborns.[87] The highest birth prevalence is observed in Asia.[88] Since the first cardiosurgical operations on CHD 80 years ago, there have been spectacular medical, surgical, and technological evolutions, which yielded an increased life expectancy. To date, more than 90% of children born with CHD in Western countries can reach adulthood.[89,90] A slightly increasing birth prevalence over time, combined with improved survival rates, has resulted in a substantial growth of the population of people with CHD. In Western societies, adults with CHD have outnumbered the children with CHD. The number of adult patients with CHD in the population has been estimated to be about 3000 patients per million inhabitants.[91] There is even a growing group of older people with CHD, which is estimated to account for 11% of all adults with CHD by 2030.[92]

Irrespective of the surgical or medical treatment, these patients cannot be considered to be cured. Indeed, many patients have residual defects and they are vulnerable to developing complications over the course of life. In order to optimize longevity and long-term functioning, lifelong cardiac follow-up is indispensable. Therefore, a workforce of physicians, nurses, and allied professionals who are trained and equipped to provide such specialist care is required. Moreover, all cardiac care providers need to have a basic understanding of the particular features and unique needs of this growing population of people with CHD.[93]

Categorization of heart defects

Congenital heart defects can be categorized into simple, moderate, and complex severity lesions (➤ Box 9.3).[86] The birth prevalence of the respective heart defects is highly variable. Some defects are relatively common, whereas others can be considered as a rare disease. The treatment armamentarium and the prognosis vary for the different heart defects. Patients with a heart defect of great complexity are advised to have follow-up visits every 6–12 months at a specialist centre.[94] Patients with moderate-complexity lesions should receive check-ups every 1–2 years, preferably undertaken at specialist centres or in a shared care setting if the CHD course is uncomplicated.[95] In case of simple heart defects, patients need medical check-ups every 3–5 years, either in a non-specialized setting or at shared care facilities.[94,95] This indicates that almost all patients with CHD require lifelong surveillance. In the following sections, different types of important or common heart defects are discussed.

Congenital heart defects of great complexity

Single-ventricle physiology

The term single-ventricle physiology refers to a group of cardiac defects that share the common feature that only one of the two ventricles is of adequate functional size. Anomalies that are described as single-ventricle defects include tricuspid atresia (➤ **Fig. 9.8**a), mitral atresia, double-inlet LV, atrioventricular septal defect (AVSD)

Box 9.3 Categorization of heart defects according to the level of complexity

Mild

- Isolated congenital aortic valve disease.
- Isolated congenital mitral valve disease (except parachute valve, cleft leaflet).
- Mild isolated pulmonic stenosis.
- Isolated small (no relevant shunt) ASD, VSD, or PDA.
- Repaired secundum ASD, sinus venosus defect, VSD or PDA without residua, chamber enlargement, or elevated pulmonary artery pressure.

Moderate

(Repaired or unrepaired where not specified; alphabetic order.)

- Anomalous pulmonary venous connection (partial or total).
- Anomalous coronary artery arising from the pulmonary artery.
- Anomalous aortic origin of a coronary artery from the opposite sinus.
- Aortic stenosis—subvalvular or supravalvular.
- AVSD (partial or complete, including primum ASD).
- ASD (secundum), moderate or large unrepaired.
- Coarctation of the aorta.
- Double-chambered right ventricle.
- Ebstein anomaly.
- PDA, moderate or large unrepaired.
- Peripheral pulmonary stenosis.
- Pulmonic stenosis (infundibular, valvular, supravalvular), moderate or severe.
- Sinus of Valsalva aneurysm/fistula.
- Sinus venosus defect.
- Tetralogy of Fallot—repaired.
- VSD with associated abnormalities (excluding pulmonary vascular disease!) and/or moderate or greater shunt.

Complex

(Repaired or unrepaired where not specified.)

- Any congenital heart disease (repaired or unrepaired) associated with pulmonary vascular disease (including Eisenmenger).
- Any cyanotic congenital heart disease (unrepaired or palliated).
- Double-outlet ventricle.
- Fontan circulation.
- Interrupted aortic arch.
- Pulmonary atresia (all forms).
- Transposition of the great arteries (all forms).
- Univentricular heart (including double inlet left/right ventricle, tricuspid/mitral atresia, hypoplastic left heart, any other anatomic abnormality with a functionally single ventricle).
- Truncus arteriosus.
- Other complex abnormalities of atrioventricular and ventriculoarterial connection (i.e. crisscross heart, isomerism, heterotaxy syndromes, ventricular inversion).

Baumgartner H, De Backer J, Babu-Narayan SV, et al; ESC Scientific Document Group. 2020 ESC Guidelines for the management of adult congenital heart disease. Eur Heart J. 2021 Feb 11;42(6):563–645. doi: 10.1093/eurheartj/ehaa554.

<table>
<tr><td>Panel A: Tricuspid atresia</td><td>Panel B: Transposition of the great arteries</td><td>Panel C: Congenitally corrected transposition of the great arteries</td></tr>
<tr><td>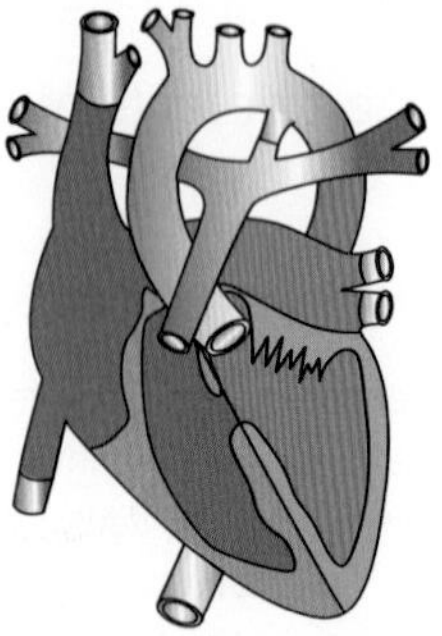</td><td>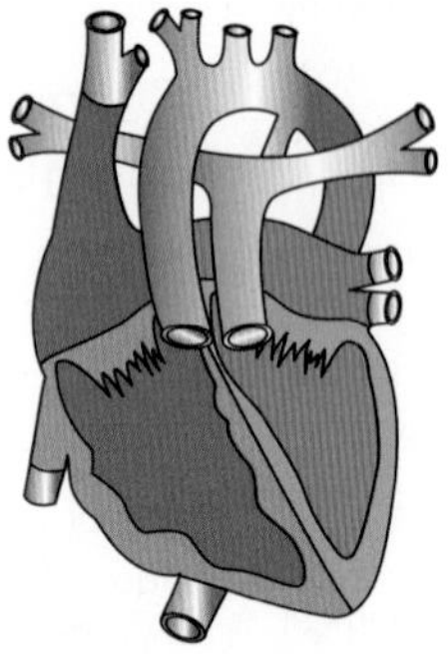</td><td>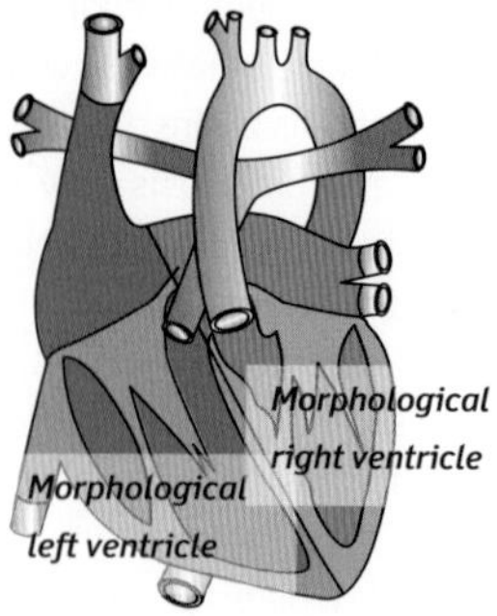</td></tr>
<tr><td>Panel D: Truncus arteriosus</td><td>Panel E: Tetralogy of Fallot</td><td>Panel F: Coarctation of the aorta</td></tr>
<tr><td>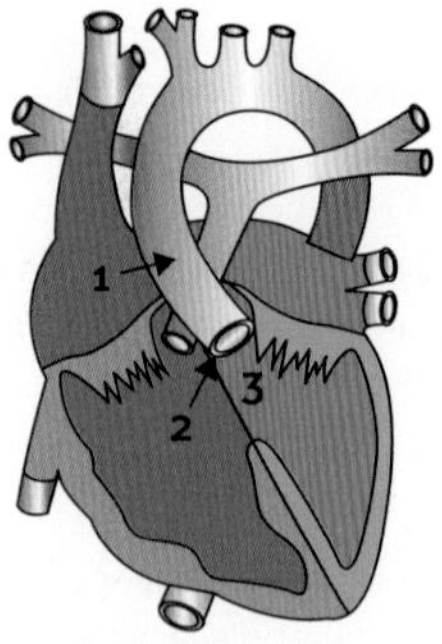
1: Common trunk; 2: Truncal valve; 3: VSD</td><td>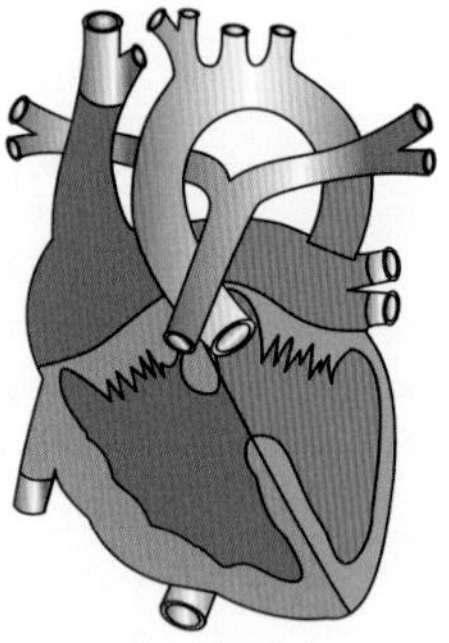</td><td>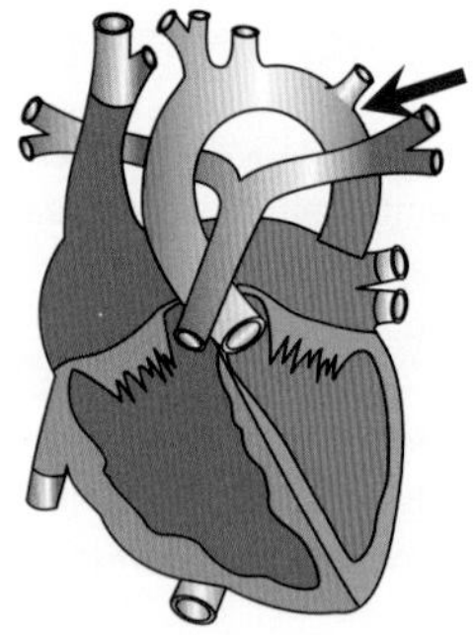</td></tr>
<tr><td>Panel G: Ebstein's anomaly</td><td>Panel H: Atrioventricular septal defect</td><td></td></tr>
<tr><td>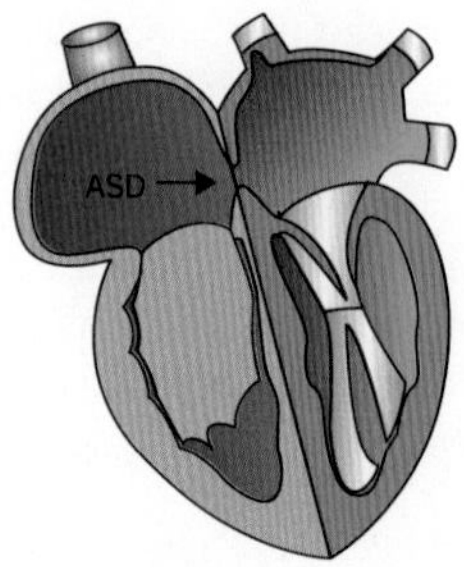</td><td>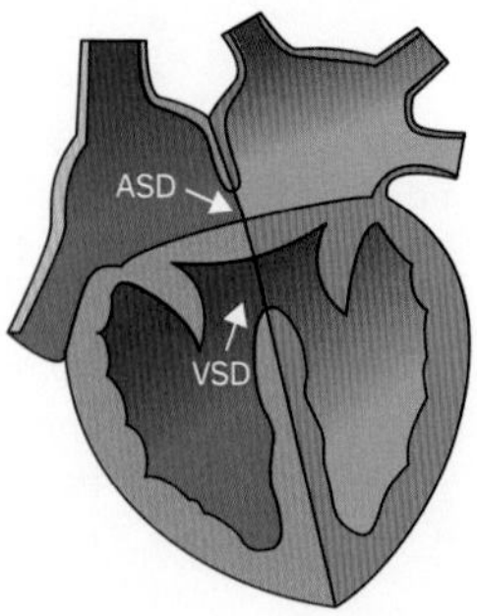</td><td></td></tr>
</table>

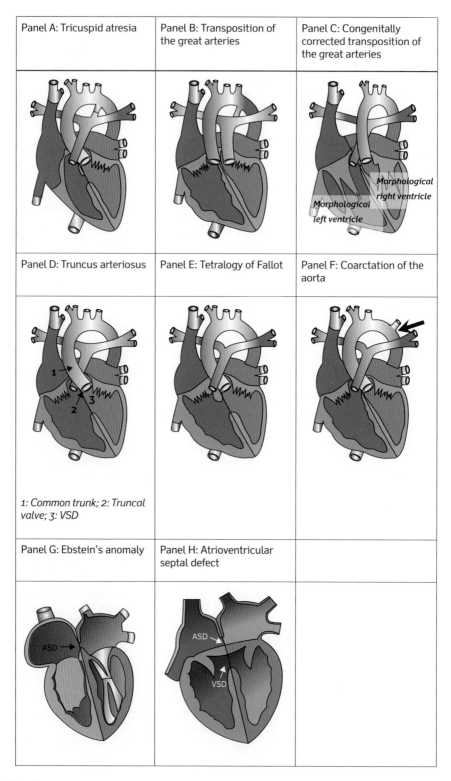

Fig. 9.8 Continued

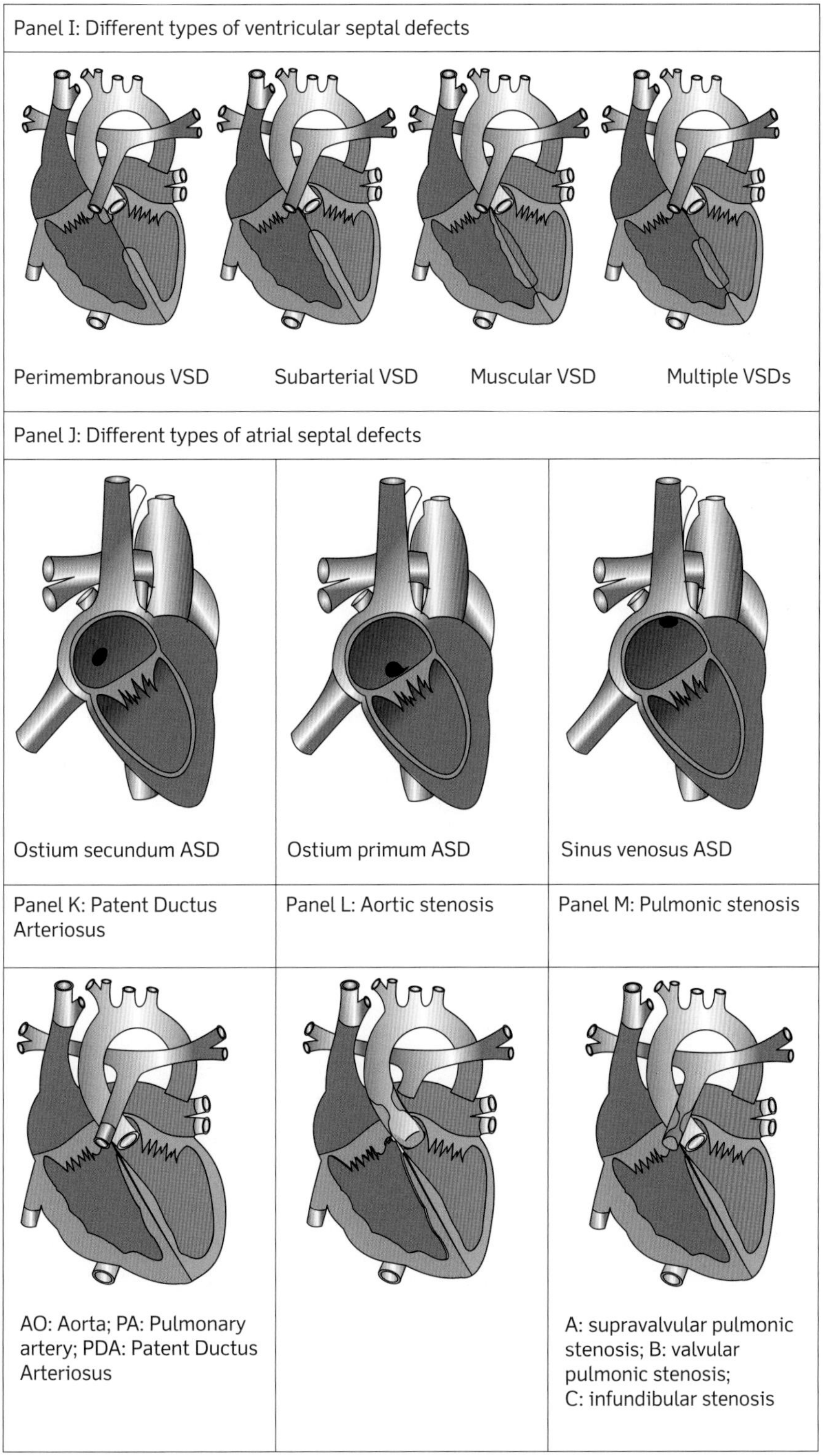

Fig. 9.8 Graphical representations of different congenital heart defects.

with a dominant LV or RV, hypoplastic left heart syndrome, and univentricular heart. Taken together, single-ventricle physiologies occur in about 6% of all congenital heart defects.[87] Hypoplastic left heart syndrome is the most common form, accounting for 2.5% of all CHD.[87]

Most patients with a single-ventricle physiology die in infancy or early childhood unless palliative surgery is performed. Biventricular repair is usually not possible. Today, all surgical approaches are either staged or palliative in nature. Norwood operations are performed in patients with hypoplastic left heart syndrome, and Fontan operations are performed on other types of single-ventricle physiology. These procedures can only be performed in well-selected patients.[96]

Life expectancy after palliation for single-ventricle physiology is considerably lower than that of other congenital heart defects. In historical cohorts, only 50% of patients with univentricular heart and 10% of patients with hypoplastic left heart survived into adulthood.[90] Due to the recent advances in surgical techniques, the survival rates will be better in contemporary patient groups.

Transposition of the great arteries

In transposition of the great arteries (TGA), also referred to as complete transposition of the great arteries or dextro-transposition of the great arteries (d-TGA), the aorta arises from the RV and is located anterior to the pulmonary artery; with the pulmonary artery arising from the LV (Fig. 9.8b). Blood returning to the heart from the systemic circulation is ejected from the RV into the aorta, sending unoxygenated blood back into the systemic circulation. This means that the systemic circulation and the pulmonic circulation form two parallel circuits, instead of one serial circuit. TGA occurs in about 4% of all CHDs.[87] There is a male preponderance in patients with TGA, with a sex ratio of 1.5.

Natural survival is extremely rare, and survival into adulthood is dependent on the early use of palliative shunting procedures (atrioseptectomy, atrioseptostomy), a pulmonary artery banding to regulate pulmonary flow, and later, the arterial switch procedure. In the arterial switch operation, the aorta and pulmonary artery are switched and the coronaries are reimplanted in the neo-aortic root. This operation has been performed since the late 1980s. Hence, the first patients who underwent this procedure are now in their third decade of life. Before the arterial switch operation, patients underwent an atrial rerouting procedure (e.g. the Mustard or Senning operation). Both of these procedures divert caval blood to the mitral valve and pulmonary venous blood to the tricuspid valve.

When directly compared, the outcomes of patients undergoing arterial switch operation is better than those of patients after atrial rerouting.[97] Indeed, 20-year transplant-free survival following atrial rerouting was 76% versus 82% after arterial switch operation.[97] Long-term follow-up studies have demonstrated that more than three-quarters of the patients who underwent a Mustard or Senning operation could survive into the fifth decade of life.[98] The long-term complications, such as arrhythmias, baffle obstruction, progressive failure of the systemic ventricle, and tricuspid regurgitation, are significant because of the demand placed on the RV to support the systemic circulation.

Congenitally corrected transposition of the great arteries

Congenitally corrected transposition of the great arteries (CCTGA), also known as levo-transposition of the great arteries (l-TGA), is a particular form of transposed great arteries. The aorta arises from the morphological RV and the pulmonary trunk from the morphological LV (Fig. 9.8c). However, the transposition is 'corrected' by the fact that the ventricles are inverted, with the morphological RV on the left and the morphological LV on the right. As a consequence, the circuit is physiologically correct, but the morphological RV serves as the systemic ventricle. Since the AV valves follow the ventricles, the left-sided AV valve is the anatomical tricuspid valve, whereas the right-sided valve is the anatomical mitral valve. Also, the coronary arteries are mirroring the normal situation. CCTGA occurs in less than 0.5% of all CHD.[99,100]

Most patients with CCTGA are managed conservatively. Indeed, surgical intervention is only indicated to repair associated anomalies such as VSD or pulmonary stenosis, which if left unrepaired can result in cyanosis or heart failure. Such operations are considered to be a 'physiological repair'. While patients are growing older, the function of the tricuspid valve may deteriorate and, consequently, dysfunction of the systemic ventricle emerges. To avoid or delay such complications, a selected group of patients may benefit from the double switch operation.[101] This is a combination of an atrial rerouting and an arterial switch operation, as described previously. A double switch operation is referred to as an 'anatomical repair' and makes the morphological LV the systemic ventricle.

Outcome data in CCTGA is limited. The largest cohort so far showed that there is a 20-year survival rate of 75% in patients with CCTGA.[101] Outcomes largely depend on the development of tricuspid regurgitation and systemic ventricular dysfunction.

Truncus arteriosus

Typical for a truncus arteriosus is that the primitive trunk failed to divide into two great arteries and, thus, a single great vessel emerges from the base of the heart through a single semilunar valve, straddling both ventricles over a large VSD (Fig. 9.8d). The truncus, which is the aorta, receives blood from both ventricles and gives rise to both pulmonary and systemic circulations, as well as coronary arteries. Hence, truncus arteriosus is a cyanotic heart defect with common mixing, and occurs in about 1% of all CHD.[87]

The Rastelli operation is the treatment of choice for truncus arteriosus. In this operation, the VSD is closed, the pulmonary arteries are disconnected from the common truncus, and a valved conduit is placed from the RV to the pulmonary arteries. Multiple reoperations to replace the conduit are common.

Before the availability of surgical corrections, 80% of children with truncus arteriosus died within the first year of life.[102] After corrective surgery, three-quarters of patients survive for 30 years.[103]

Congenital heart defects of moderate complexity

Tetralogy of Fallot

Tetralogy of Fallot (TOF) is a tetrad comprising a non-restrictive VSD, severe pulmonary stenosis causing obstruction to pulmonary blood flow, RV hypertrophy, and various degrees of overriding of the aorta (Fig. 9.8e). The degree of pulmonary obstruction is a primary determinant of clinical presentation. TOF accounts for approximately 5% of all CHD.[87] In about 15% of the patients with TOF, a deletion of chromosome 22q11 is observed.[96] TOF is treated surgically. Initially, the TOF correction was performed in two stages. In the first stage, a shunt is made between the subclavian artery and the pulmonary artery, in order to increase the pulmonary blood flow and reduce cyanosis while waiting for complete repair corrective surgery. In the second stage, the VSD is closed with a patch and the RV outflow tract is widened by removing some of the thickened muscle and/or by inserting a patch in the outflow tract. In this second stage, the shunt that was made in the first stage is closed. Nowadays, primary repair is performed in most patients.[104] Reoperations of the RV outflow tract for either regurgitation or restenosis are common. Mortality in patients with repaired TOF is low. Indeed, 25-year survival following repair is 94.5%.[105] However, mortality is increasing in the fourth and fifth decade of life and high morbidity is observed when patients are growing older.[106]

Coarctation of the aorta

Coarctation of the aorta is a deformity of the aortic isthmus, characterized by narrowing either proximal or distal to the left subclavian artery, where the ductus arteriosus joins the descending aorta (Fig. 9.8f). Occasionally, the coarctation occurs above the origin of the right subclavian. This narrowing results in obstruction of aortic blood flow within the lumen, resulting in upper extremity hypertension and decreased blood pressure in the lower extremities. Coarctation is strongly associated with other heart defects, such as bicuspid aortic valve, VSD, patent ductus arteriosus (PDA), and valve abnormalities. Coarctation of the aorta represents 3–5% of all congenital cardiac anomalies[87,100] and occurs with greater frequency in males than females.[99]

Surgical repair in infancy or childhood was the treatment of choice for many years. Such operations either resected the narrowed part or inserted a patch to widen the course of the aorta. Nowadays, the first treatment of choice in native coarctation of the aorta is also treated by balloon dilatation whether or not combined with stenting.[96] It is recommended that all patients with coarctation, regardless of absent clinical symptoms, undergo treatment, since untreated patients have a lower life expectancy due to congestive heart failure, cerebral haemorrhage, infective endocarditis, or dissection of the aorta.[107] Re-coarctation or aneurysms at the site of operation are common, and therefore require medical surveillance. Recoarctation is presumed when there is a difference in blood pressure of more than 30 mmHg between the upper and lower extremities. Contemporary survival rates in patients treated for coarctation of the aorta is 99% at 30 years and 88% at 50 years of age.[108]

Ebstein's anomaly

Ebstein's anomaly involves the tricuspid valve and is characterized by a downward displacement of portions of the tricuspid valve into the RV (Fig. 9.8g). The portion of the normal RV that underlies the tricuspid valve becomes mechanically a part of the right atrium (atrialized RV). As a result, the right atrium is exceptionally large, the RV is small, and the tricuspid valve is incompetent. In patients with Ebstein's anomaly, 80% have either an atrial septal defect (ASD) or patent foramen ovale, often resulting in a right-to-left shunt. Therefore, Ebstein's anomaly is typically considered to be a cyanotic heart defect. Ebstein's anomaly occurs in about 0.5% of all congenital heart defects. In general, the management of Ebstein's anomaly is conservative. Only when symptoms emerge, when ventricular function deteriorates and when cyanosis occurs (saturation less than 90%), is surgical intervention indicated. During such surgical procedures, the tricuspid valve is repaired, the interatrial communication is closed, and/or a pacemaker is placed. Tricuspid valve repair may include valvuloplasty, whether or not using an annuloplasty ring, or tricuspid valve replacement.

Ebstein's anomaly is compatible with a relatively long and active life.[109] Patients with Ebstein's anomaly may live beyond age 50 years. The largest current long-term outcome study showed that the mean age of initial operation was 24 years (range 8 days–79 years), and that the actuarial survival at 20 years post operation was 71.2%.[110]

Atrioventricular septal defect

AVSD, also called AV canal septal defects or endocardial cushion defects, are essentially a combination of both an ASD (ostium primum: see later) and a VSD (Fig. 9.8h). In patients with complete AVSDs, the endocardial cushions do not develop, resulting in a common AV valve, a primum ASD, and a VSD. Incomplete or partial AV canal defects typically consist of a primum ASD with a cleft mitral valve without VSD. Although AVSD can occur in those with normal chromosomes, it is much more frequently found in patients with Down syndrome. AVSD account for about 4% of all CHD.[87,100] Thirty-five per cent of patients with AVSD have Down syndrome.[96]

Patients with AVSD have invariably undergone some surgical intervention in infancy or childhood for incomplete or complete AVSD repair. Unrepaired complete AVSD results in Eisenmenger syndrome.[96] Incomplete repair includes an ASD patch closure and a mitral cleft suture. Complete repair includes not only ASD and VSD patch closure, but also mitral and tricuspid valve repair with valve reconstruction using available tissue from the common AV valve leaflets. Catheter closure of AVSD is not feasible.[96]

Long-term survival in patients who underwent surgery for AVSD is good, with 25-year survival rates of 88%.[111]

Congenital heart defects of mild complexity

Ventricular septal defect

VSDs are characterized by an abnormal opening between the LV and RV. There are three main categories of VSD: perimembranous (65%), muscular (30%), and malalignment/subarterial (5%) VSDs (Fig. 9.8i). In the perimembranous and muscular regions, spontaneous closure occurs in 50% of the patients. Furthermore, VSDs are categorized as restrictive or unrestrictive. Restrictive VSDs are small, resulting in a high gradient of pressure between RV and LV, and non-restrictive VSDs are large in which the pressure in the RV and LV is equal. Unrestricted defects are typically repaired in childhood, but restrictive VSDs can be newly found in the adult. VSDs are the most common heart defects, representing about 35% of all CHD.[87] Isolated small perimembranous VSDs do not require closure, as long as patients do not have problems with recurrent endocarditis. VSD closure can be done surgically or transcatheter with closing devices. Transcatheter closure is indicated in muscular VSDs that are located centrally in the interventricular septum, and in patients with increased risk for surgery, multiple previous cardiac surgical interventions, and VSDs that are poorly accessible for surgical closure.[96] Transcatheter procedures avoid arrhythmic and valvular complications from surgery.

The long-term survival of patients with isolated VSD is equal to that of the general population.[89] Nonetheless, when taking all VSDs together, the 30- and 40-year survival is 85% and 78%, respectively, which is lower than the general population.[112] Once patients survive the perioperative period, survival is similar to that of the general population again.[112] However, these patients are not free from complications and morbidity. Therefore, lifelong medical follow-up is also required for patients with this considerably mild heart defect.

Atrial septal defect

ASDs are abnormal communications between the left and right atria. There are different types of ASD, differentiated by their occurrence within the septum (Fig. 9.8j). *Ostium secundum* ASD, the most common type, occurs in the central region of the fossa ovalis. *Ostium primum* ASD, which occurs low in the atrial septum, has an associated cleft anterior mitral valve with varying degree of mitral insufficiency (see earlier: AVSD). *Sinus venosus* ASD occurs in the upper part of the atrial septum near the entry of the superior vena cava and may be associated with the partial anomalous right pulmonary venous connection. Owing to the trivial or absent physical signs, ASD may go undetected until the fourth or fifth decade. ASDs comprise 15% of all CHD,[87] and there is a female predominance.[99] In small ostium secundum ASDs (<6 mm), spontaneous closure occurs in one-third of the patients.[113] In patients with a persistent ASD, the defect is recommended to be closed if the pulmonary-to-systemic blood flow ratio (Qp/

Qs) is 1.5:1 or greater. Overall, closure is performed in about two-thirds of the patients with persistent ASD.[114] Transcatheter closure has become the first choice for ostium secundum ASD.[96]

Long-term survival in patients with ASD is very good and close to that of the general population. However, morbidity, even in small ASDs, is substantial. Patients who have undergone a surgical closure remain prone to developing arrhythmias, such as atrial fibrillation.[115] Long-term complications that occurred in patients following percutaneous closure of the ASD were device thrombosis, cardiac erosion, and atrial arrhythmias.[116] In small unrepaired ASDs, patients present with a higher prevalence of chronic comorbidities, particularly lung diseases.[114] The presence of long-term complications in this apparently mild condition stresses the need for lifelong follow-up, even in patients with small isolated ASDs.

Patent ductus arteriosus

The ductus arteriosus is a vascular connection, which during fetal life directs blood flow from the pulmonary artery to the aorta, bypassing the lungs. Functional closure of the ductus occurs within hours or days after birth. In some cases, it takes 6 months to several years to close. If the ductus remains patent, the direction of blood flow is reversed to left-to-right, because of high systemic pressure at the left side of the heart (Fig. 9.8k). A PDA, which can escape recognition until adulthood, accounts for about 10% of all cases of CHD[87] and predominates in females.[99] Initially, the treatment was surgical by ligating the PDA. Contemporary treatments entail a transcatheter closure, by using a plug. PDA is the only CHD that can be considered as 'cured' after closure.

Congenital aortic stenosis

A congenital stenosis of the aorta is characterized by an obstruction of the LV outflow (Fig. 9.8l). Three types of congenital aortic stenosis can be identified: valvular, subvalvular, and supravalvular. Valvular aortic stenosis represents 75% of all congenital aortic stenosis.[96] Supravalvular aortic stenosis is uncommon and refers to a stenosis of the ascending aorta. Three types of supravalvular stenosis have been described: hourglass, hypoplastic, and membranous. In about 20% of the patients, the valvular aortic stenosis is associated with other heart defects, mainly with coarctation of the aorta or PDA. Congenital aortic stenosis represents about 2.5% of all CHD.[87] When bicuspid valves are included, the prevalence is much higher, because bicuspid valves occur in 1–2% of the general population.[96]

Patients with non-calcified valves can be treated with balloon valvuloplasty. In patients with calcified valves, the treatment of choice is valve replacement.[96] Transcatheter aortic valve implantation currently has no place in the treatment of congenital aortic stenosis.[96] When patients develop symptoms, urgent surgery is required.[96] In supravalvular and subvalvular aortic stenosis, surgery is the primary treatment.[96] Long-term survival is good in patients who have undergone intervention in childhood or adolescence and in patients who are symptom free. The 25-year survival of patients treated for aortic stenosis is about 90%.[117] However, the 25-year freedom of intervention is only 40%.[117] Patients treated for supravalvular aortic stenosis had a 10-year survival of 80–95%.[118]

Pulmonary valve stenosis

Pulmonary valve stenosis can occur at the valvular, subvalvular (infundibular or subinfundibular), or supravalvular level (stenosis of the pulmonary artery and its branches) (Fig. 9.8m). In 90% of the cases, pulmonary stenosis is at valvular level. Supravalvular pulmonary stenosis results from the narrowing of the pulmonary trunk, its bifurcation, or its peripheral branches. Pulmonary stenosis may occur as an isolated defect or in combination with other congenital cardiac defects, including VSD, ASD, or as part of the TOF. Isolated pulmonary stenosis represents 6% of all CHD.[87] Balloon valvuloplasty is indicated in critical pulmonary stenosis, or if the RV systolic pressures are 50 mmHg or higher. If balloon valvuloplasty is not successful in critical stenosis, surgery with muscle resection or patch repair is required. Surgery is also recommended for patients with subinfundibular or infundibular stenosis.[96]

Life expectancy depends on the severity of the stenosis. Patients with mild pulmonary stenosis or patients who have undergone balloon valvuloplasty have an excellent survival, similar to that of the general population. They must, however, be periodically evaluated for mild residual pulmonary stenosis, or for pulmonary regurgitation which can occur as a result of the valvuloplasty. Patients following surgical correction for valvular pulmonary stenosis have a survival rate of 90% up to 40 years after the operation.[119]

From womb to tomb: continuity of care over the lifespan

It is obvious that patients with CHD cannot be considered as cured. Residua and sequelae indicate the need for lifelong follow-up by healthcare teams with expertise in CHD (➤ **Fig. 9.9**). During childhood, patients

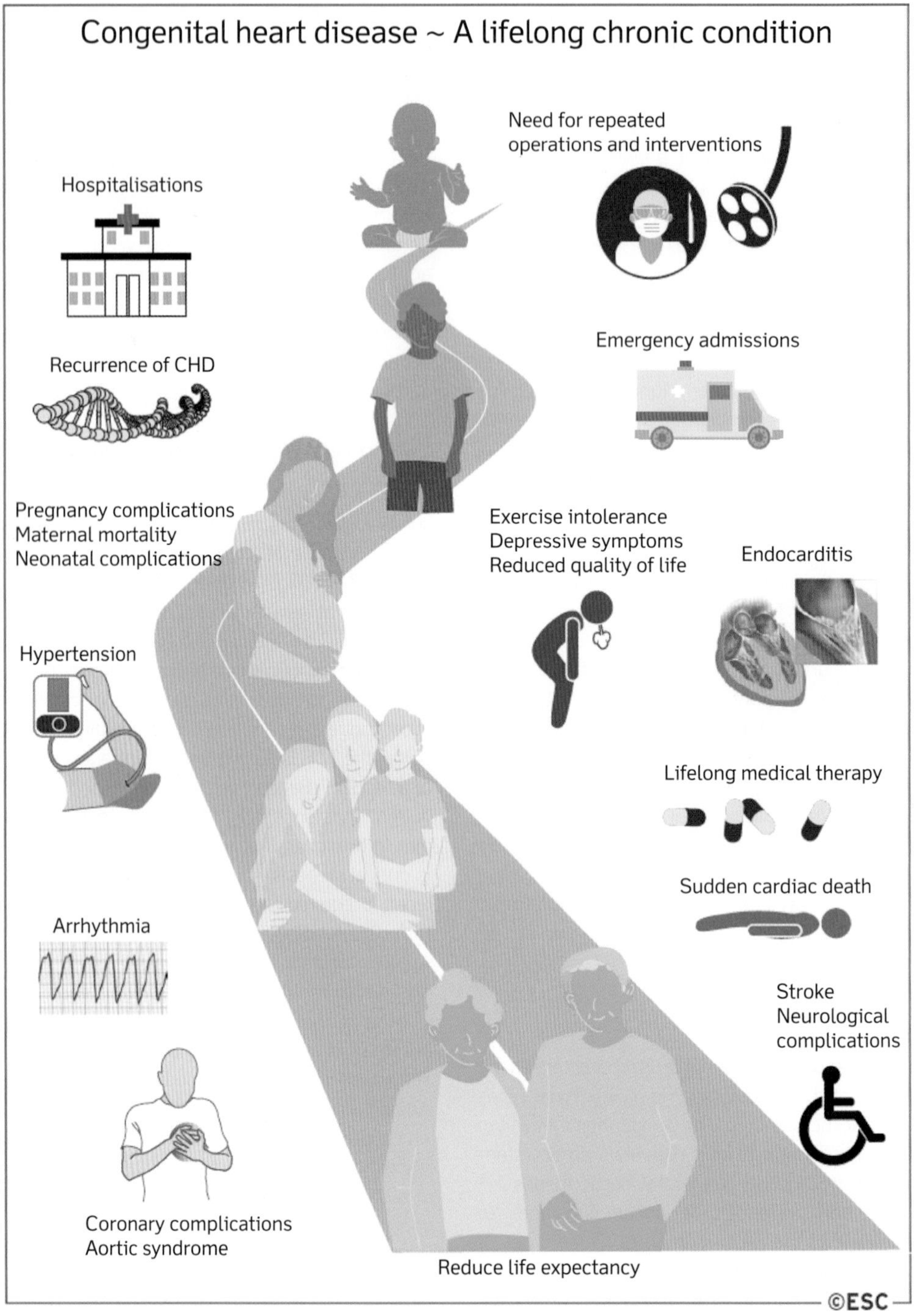

Fig. 9.9 Congenital heart disease (CHD) is a lifelong chronic condition. SCD, sudden cardiac death.

Baumgartner H, De Backer J, Babu-Narayan SV, et al; ESC Scientific Document Group. 2020 ESC Guidelines for the management of adult congenital heart disease. Eur Heart J. 2021 Feb 11;42(6):563–645. doi: 10.1093/eurheartj/ehaa554. © The European Society of Cardiology. Reprinted by permission of Oxford University Press.

are typically followed up at paediatric cardiology. When they are growing up, patients ought to be seamlessly transferred from paediatrics to adult-oriented healthcare. Nonetheless, empirical evidence showed that a substantial number of patients have gaps in their care. Care gaps rates range from 7% to 76%,[120] with a median proportion of 42%. The phase of adolescence seems to be a very vulnerable period for care gaps. However, care gaps occur throughout the entire life spectrum.[121] Clinicians should identify patients at risk for discontinuity of care and need to implement intervention plans that keep patients in care.[120]

The growing number of patients is an impetus for the increasing number of specialized centres for adults with CHD.[122] Minimal requirements for such centres have been proposed.[64] However, only a limited number of centres fulfil the proposed criteria.[122] The professions that are lacking most are allied professions, such as masters-prepared nurses, psychologists, and social workers. Given the complexity of CHD and the high prevalence of psychosocial problems, such professionals are indispensable in the interdisciplinary teams.

Although survival has improved dramatically over the past decades, premature death is still prevalent in patients with CHD. In line with this, increasing attention is given to end of life issues. It was found that the last year of life of patients with CHD is more expensive and more burdensome than that of patients with cancer.[123] Furthermore, 53% of patients indicated that they would like to die at home; 1% stated that their healthcare providers talked to them about end of life planning, although 62% of the patients preferred an early end of life discussion.[124] Current clinical practice is mismatched with the preferences of the patients. Therefore, more attention has to be given to end of life discussions and care for patients with CHD.

Nursing care in congenital heart diseases

Psychological, physical, and social impact

There must be careful consideration of the unique care needs of patients with CHD. Patients may experience a psychological, physical, and social impact of the condition, which requires dedicated nursing care. Historically, the 'feeling of being different' is a recurrent theme in the studies of the lived experience of patients with CHD, particularly in those with the most severe forms.[125–127] They not only perceive themselves as different but also feel that they are perceived as different by others. This tends to emerge in the adolescent phase where differences due to visible signs and symptoms and physical activity restrictions become a focus. These often persist through young adulthood, where this 'difference' relates more to limitations in career choices or personal relationships.[128] Coping with this sense of being different is highly individualized and is influenced by the patient's personality and attitudes. For example, those who feel that they are able to affect their environment (internal locus of control) will often use active strategies to cope with their situation. Parental overprotection also appears to be a factor in creating difficulties in integration of the illness in daily life. Parents who offer a realistic view on living with the heart defect early on may ultimately facilitate better coping. Healthcare providers can also impact this 'feeling of difference' as lack of information, particularly in the perioperative period, leads to feelings of insecurity, fear of the unknown, and disappointments regarding the patients' outcomes.[128]

Patients with CHD may have residual problems and sequelae from conservative medical management, as well as the initial surgical or interventional procedures.[96] These include risks for complications such as bacterial endocarditis, arrhythmias, and heart failure. Therefore, they require regular medical follow-up and are often instructed to adhere to lifelong health behaviours, such as adherence to preventive measures for endocarditis, medications, and the avoidance of heavy physical activity.

A topic that is particularly of concern for people with CHD are reproductive issues.[96] Patients need to be counselled about the most appropriate contraceptive methods for them, the risk for complications in case of pregnancy, the need for follow-up during pregnancy, and the recurrence risk. Also advanced care planning needs to be discussed in this counselling. For instance, the couple need to discuss if the partner is able and wants to raise the children alone, in case of severe adverse events in the patient.

A significant proportion of patients with CHD also experience difficulties with employability and gaining life insurance which is a further source of insecurity and could result in declined social integration.[129]

Specialized facilities and healthcare professionals

To meet the specific needs of the growing CHD patient population and to minimize the negative impacts of the condition, specialized clinics providing lifelong care to adult patients with CHD are now established internationally.[96] These specialized clinics consist of a team of health professionals—CHD cardiologists, cardiac surgeons, obstetricians, specialist nurses, psychologists, and cardiac physiologists—who are trained and educated in this field.[122]

The nurse specialist tends to have a pivotal role in the collaborative care needed to deliver the best outcomes for the patient and has a key role in transition from paediatric to adult cardiology, identifying patient needs, educating patients and their families, initial screening for psychological problems, and onward referral to a social worker, psychologist, legal adviser, or other professionals.[130]

Specific attention ought to be given to transitional care. When patients are transitioning from a child towards an adult, they need to develop the skills to become the manager of their condition. Comprehensive transitional care is recommended. Therefore, the CHD team needs to include staff with expertise in adolescent health.

Key elements in the care for adults with congenital heart disease

Recommendations relevant for nurses to provide holistic care for patients with CHD include[93]:

1. A formal transition programme should be instituted when patients with CHD are moving on from paediatric to adult cardiology. This ensures that patients will have a seamless follow-up in a specialist clinic, with adequate support in all aspects of their care.
2. Individualized patient education regarding a patient's diagnosis and specific health behaviours must be provided to maximize good outcomes. This should include education around their specific lesion, procedures or interventions planned or already undertaken, medications, exercise modifications, signs and symptoms of deterioration, need for regular clinic follow-up, and reproductive risk and contraception.
3. Tools for screening of psychosocial problems should be available for rapid identification of concerns and referral to the appropriate health professional. Psychosocial concerns that have been identified in this population include anxiety, depressive symptoms, lack of self-esteem, issues with family functioning, and social integration.
4. Specific issues have been identified which require prompt and appropriate counselling input in patients with CHD. Vocational counselling and advice regarding employability and insurance difficulties should be provided, which are timed at key periods to tie in when making choices regarding education and training.
5. Women will require careful and timely counselling regarding pregnancy and choice of contraception. While CHD is not always genetic, it is important to discuss the recurrence risk in an offspring prospectively with all patients and, therefore, adequate genetic counselling should be provided.

References

1. Kumar D, Elliott P. Principles and Practice of Clinical Cardiovascular Genetics. Oxford: Oxford University Press; 2010.
2. Inouye M, Abraham G, Nelson CP, Wood AM, Sweeting MJ, Dudbridge F, et al. Genomic risk prediction of coronary artery disease in 480,000 adults: implications for primary prevention. J Am Coll Cardiol. 2018;72(16):1883–93.
3. Choi SH, Jurgens SJ, Weng LC, Pirruccello JP, Roselli C, Chaffin M, et al. Monogenic and polygenic contributions to atrial fibrillation risk: results from a national biobank. Circ Res. 2020;126(2):200–209.
4. Ingles J, Macciocca I, Morales A, Thomson K. Genetic testing in inherited heart diseases. Heart Lung Circ. 2020;29(4):505–11.
5. Watkins H, Ashrafian H, Redwood C. Inherited cardiomyopathies. N Engl J Med. 2011;364(17):1643–56.
6. Priori SG, Wilde AA, Horie M, Cho Y, Behr ER, Berul C, et al. Executive summary: HRS/EHRA/APHRS expert consensus statement on the diagnosis and management of patients with inherited primary arrhythmia syndromes. Europace. 2013;15(10):1389–406.
7. Ingles J, McGaughran J, Scuffham PA, Atherton J, Semsarian C. A cost-effectiveness model of genetic testing for the evaluation of families with hypertrophic cardiomyopathy. Heart. 2012;98(8):625–30.
8. Wordsworth S, Leal J, Blair E, Legood R, Thomson K, Seller A, et al. DNA testing for hypertrophic cardiomyopathy: a cost-effectiveness model. Eur Heart J. 2010;31(8):926–35.
9. Catchpool M, Ramchand J, Martyn M, Hare DL, James PA, Trainer AH, et al. A cost-effectiveness model of genetic testing and periodical clinical screening for the evaluation of families with dilated cardiomyopathy. Genet Med. 2019;21(12):2815–22.
10. Christian S, Somerville M, Taylor S, Atallah J. When to offer predictive genetic testing to children at risk of an

inherited arrhythmia or cardiomyopathy. Circ Genom Precis Med. 2018;11(8):e002300.

11. Ackerman MJ, Priori SG, Willems S, Berul C, Brugada R, Calkins H, et al. HRS/EHRA expert consensus statement on the state of genetic testing for the channelopathies and cardiomyopathies this document was developed as a partnership between the Heart Rhythm Society (HRS) and the European Heart Rhythm Association (EHRA). Heart Rhythm. 2011;8(8):1308–39.
12. Fanos JH. New 'first families': the psychosocial impact of new genetic technologies. Genet Med. 2012;14(2):189–90.
13. Ormondroyd E, Oates S, Parker M, Blair E, Watkins H. Pre-symptomatic genetic testing for inherited cardiac conditions: a qualitative exploration of psychosocial and ethical implications. Eur J Hum Genet. 2014;22(1):88–93.
14. Burns C, Yeates L, Spinks C, Semsarian C, Ingles J. Attitudes, knowledge and consequences of uncertain genetic findings in hypertrophic cardiomyopathy. Eur J Hum Genet. 2017;25(7):809–15.
15. Bagnall RD, Weintraub RG, Ingles J, Duflou J, Yeates L, Lam L, et al. A prospective study of sudden cardiac death among children and young adults. N Engl J Med. 2016;374(25):2441–52.
16. Semsarian C, Ingles J, Wilde AAM. Sudden cardiac death in the young: the molecular autopsy and a practical approach to surviving relatives. Eur Heart J. 2015;36(21):1290–96.
17. Ingles J, Bagnall RD, Semsarian C. Genetic testing for cardiomyopathies in clinical practice. Heart Fail Clin. 2018;14(2):129–37.
18. Ingles J, Spinks C, Yeates L, McGeechan K, Kasparian N, Semsarian C. Posttraumatic stress and prolonged grief after the sudden cardiac death of a young relative. JAMA Intern Med. 2016;176(3):402–405.
19. Yeates L, Hunt L, Saleh M, Semsarian C, Ingles J. Poor psychological wellbeing particularly in mothers following sudden cardiac death in the young. Eur J Cardiovasc Nurs. 2013;12(5):484–91.
20. De Backer J, Bondue A, Budts W, Evangelista A, Gallego P, Jondeau G, et al. Genetic counselling and testing in adults with congenital heart disease: a consensus document of the ESC Working Group of Grown-Up Congenital Heart Disease, the ESC Working Group on aorta and Peripheral Vascular Disease and the European Society of Human Genetics. Eur J Prev Cardiol. 2020;27(13):1423–35.
21. Manrai AK, Funke BH, Rehm HL, Olesen MS, Maron BA, Szolovits P, et al. Genetic misdiagnoses and the potential for health disparities. N Engl J Med. 2016;375(7):655–65.
22. Harrison SM, Dolinsky JS, Knight Johnson AE, Pesaran T, Azzariti DR, Bale S, et al. Clinical laboratories collaborate to resolve differences in variant interpretations submitted to ClinVar. Genet Med. 2017;19(10):1096–104.
23. Walsh R, Buchan R, Wilk A, John S, Felkin LE, Thomson KL, et al. Defining the genetic architecture of hypertrophic cardiomyopathy: re-evaluating the role of non-sarcomeric genes. Eur Heart J. 2017;38(46):3461–68.
24. Walsh R, Thomson KL, Ware JS, Funke BH, Woodley J, McGuire KJ, et al. Reassessment of Mendelian gene pathogenicity using 7,855 cardiomyopathy cases and 60,706 reference samples. Genet Med. 2017;19(2):192–203.
25. Biesecker BB. Goals of genetic counseling. Clin Genet. 2001;60(5):323–30.
26. National Society of Genetic Counselors' Definition Task Force, Resta R, Biesecker BB, Bennett RL, Blum S, et al. A new definition of genetic counseling: National Society of Genetic Counselors' Task Force report. J Genet Couns. 2006;15(2):77–83.
27. Austin J, Semaka A, Hadjipavlou G. Conceptualizing genetic counseling as psychotherapy in the era of genomic medicine. J Genet Couns. 2014;23(6):903–909.
28. Burns C, James C, Ingles J. Communication of genetic information to families with inherited rhythm disorders. Heart Rhythm. 2018;15(5):780–86.
29. Burns C, McGaughran J, Davis A, Semsarian C, Ingles J. Factors influencing uptake of familial long QT syndrome genetic testing. Am J Med Genet A. 2016;170A(2):418–25.
30. Elliott P, Andersson B, Arbustini E, Bilinska Z, Cecchi F, Charron P, et al. Classification of the cardiomyopathies: a position statement from the European Society of Cardiology working group on myocardial and pericardial diseases. Eur Heart J. 2008;29(2):270–76.
31. Hershberger RE, Hedges DJ, Morales A. Dilated cardiomyopathy: the complexity of a diverse genetic architecture. Nat Rev Cardiol. 2013;10(9):531–47.
32. Elliott P. Cardiomyopathy. Diagnosis and management of dilated cardiomyopathy. Heart. 2000;84(1):106–12.
33. Sweet M, Taylor MRG, Mestroni L. Diagnosis, prevalence, and screening of familial dilated cardiomyopathy. Expert Opin Orphan Drugs. 2015;3(8):869–76.
34. Haugaa KH, Haland TF, Leren IS, Saberniak J, Edvardsen T. Arrhythmogenic right ventricular cardiomyopathy, clinical manifestations, and diagnosis. Europace. 2016;18(7):965–72.
35. Goff ZD, Calkins H. Sudden death related cardiomyopathies—arrhythmogenic right ventricular cardiomyopathy, arrhythmogenic cardiomyopathy, and exercise-induced cardiomyopathy. Prog Cardiovasc Dis. 2019;62(3):217–26.
36. Towbin JA, McKenna WJ, Abrams DJ, Ackerman MJ, Calkins H, Darrieux FCC, et al. 2019 HRS expert consensus statement on evaluation, risk stratification,

and management of arrhythmogenic cardiomyopathy. Heart Rhythm. 2019;16(11):e301–72.

37. Awad MM, Calkins H, Judge DP. Mechanisms of disease: molecular genetics of arrhythmogenic right ventricular dysplasia/cardiomyopathy. Nat Clin Pract Cardiovasc Med. 2008;5(5):258–67.
38. McKenna WJ, Thiene G, Nava A, Fontaliran F, Blomstrom-Lundqvist C, Fontaine G, Camerini F. Diagnosis of arrhythmogenic right ventricular dysplasia/cardiomyopathy. Task force of the working Group myocardial and pericardial Disease of the European Society of Cardiology and of the Scientific Council on cardiomyopathies of the International Society and Federation of Cardiology. Br Heart J. 1994;71(3):215–18.
39. Marcus FI, McKenna WJ, Sherrill D, Basso C, Bauce B, Bluemke DA, et al. Diagnosis of arrhythmogenic right ventricular cardiomyopathy/dysplasia: proposed modification of the Task Force Criteria. Eur Heart J. 2010;31(7):806–14.
40. Corrado D, Wichter T, Link MS, Hauer RN, Marchlinski FE, Anastasakis A, et al. Treatment of arrhythmogenic right ventricular cardiomyopathy/dysplasia: an international task force consensus statement. Circulation. 2015;132(5):441–53.
41. Norekval T, Kirchhof P, Fitzsimons D. Patient centred care of patients with ventricular arrhthymia at risk of sudden cardiac death: What do the ESC 2015 Guidelines add? *Eur Jour Cardiovascular Nursing* 2017;16;7,58–564.
42. Nugent AW, Daubeney PEF, Chondros P, Carlin JB, Cheung M, Wilkinson LC, et al. The epidemiology of childhood cardiomyopathy in Australia. N Engl J Med. 2003;348(17):1639–46.
42. Muchtar E, Blauwet LA, Gertz MA. Restrictive cardiomyopathy: Genetics, pathogenesis, clinical manifestations, diagnosis, and therapy. Circ Res. 2017;121(7):819–37.
44. Sajgalik P, Grupper A, Edwards BS, Kushwaha SS, Stulak JM, Joyce DL, et al. Current status of left ventricular assist device therapy. Mayo Clin Proc. 2016;91(7):927–40.
45. Jenni R, Oechslin E, Schneider J, Attenhofer Jost C, Kaufmann PA. Echocardiographic and pathoanatomical characteristics of isolated left ventricular non-compaction: a step towards classification as a distinct cardiomyopathy. Heart. 2001;86(6):666–71.
46. Oechslin E, Jenni R. Left ventricular non-compaction revisited: a distinct phenotype with genetic heterogeneity? Eur Heart J. 2011;32(12):1446–56.
47. Leenhardt A, Denjoy I, Guicheney P. Catecholaminergic polymorphic ventricular tachycardia. Circ Arrhythm Electrophysiol. 2012;5(5):1044–52.
48. Schwartz PJ, Stramba-Badiale M, Crotti L, Pedrazzini M, Besana A, Bosi G, et al. Prevalence of the congenital long-QT syndrome. Circulation. 2009;120(18):1761–67.
49. Cho Y. Left cardiac sympathetic denervation: an important treatment option for patients with hereditary ventricular arrhythmias. J Arrhythm. 2016;32(5):340–43.
50. Perez MV, Kumarasamy NA, Owens DK, Wang PJ, Hlatky MA. Cost-effectiveness of genetic testing in family members of patients with long-QT Syndrome. Circ Cardiovasc Qual Outcomes. 2011;4(1):76–84.
51. Skinner JR, Winbo A, Abrams D, Vohra J, Wilde AA. Channelopathies that lead to sudden cardiac death: clinical and genetic aspects. Heart Lung Circ. 2019;28(1):22–30.
52. Bezzina CR, Barc J, Mizusawa Y, Remme CA, Gourraud JB, Simonet F, et al. Common variants at SCN5A-SCN10A and HEY2 are associated with Brugada syndrome, a rare disease with high risk of sudden cardiac death. Nat Genet. 2013;45(9):1044–49.
53. Vohra J, Rajagopalan S, CSANZ Genetics Council Writing Group. Update on the diagnosis and management of Brugada syndrome. Heart Lung Circ. 2015;24(12):1141–48.
54. Liu N, Ruan Y, Priori SG. Catecholaminergic polymorphic ventricular tachycardia. Prog Cardiovasc Dis. 2008;51(1):23–30.
55. Loeys BL, Chen J, Neptune ER, Judge DP, Podowski M, Holm T, et al. A syndrome of altered cardiovascular, craniofacial, neurocognitive and skeletal development caused by mutations in TGFBR1 or TGFBR2. Nat Genet. 2005;37(3):275–81.
56. Loeys BL, Dietz HC, Braverman AC, Callewaert BL, De Backer J, Devereux RB, et al. The revised Ghent nosology for the Marfan syndrome. J Med Genet. 2010;47(7):476–85.
57. Dean JCS. Marfan syndrome: clinical diagnosis and management. Eur J Hum Genet. 2007;15(7):724–33.
58. Guo DC, Regalado ES, Minn C, Tran-Fadulu V, Coney J, Cao J, et al. Familial thoracic aortic aneurysms and dissections: identification of a novel locus for stable aneurysms with a low risk for progression to aortic dissection. Circ Cardiovasc Genet. 2011;4(1):36–42.
59. McAllister M, Davies L, Payne K, Nicholls S, Donnai D, MacLeod R. The emotional effects of genetic diseases: implications for clinical genetics. Am J Med Genet A. 2007;143A(22):2651–61.
60. Christiaans I, van Langen IM, Birnie E, Bonsel GJ, Wilde AA, Smets EM. Quality of life and psychological distress in hypertrophic cardiomyopathy mutation carriers: a cross-sectional cohort study. Am J Med Genet A. 2009;149A(4):602–12.
61. Hamang A, Eide GE, Rokne B, Nordin K, Bjorvatn C, Øyen N. Predictors of heart-focused anxiety in patients undergoing genetic investigation and counseling of long QT syndrome or hypertrophic cardiomyopathy: a one year follow-up. J Genet Couns. 2012;21(1):72–84.
62. Lobo I. Same genetic mutation, different genetic disease phenotype. Nat Educ. 2008;1(7):64.

63. Hammond-Haley M, Patel RS, Providência R, Lambiase PD. Exercise restrictions for patients with inherited cardiac conditions: current guidelines, challenges and limitations. Int J Cardiol. 2016;209:234–41.
64. Elliott PM, Anastasakis A, Borger MA, Borggrefe M, Cecchi F, Charron P, et al. ESC Guidelines on diagnosis and management of hypertrophic cardiomyopathy. Kardiol Pol. 2014;72(11):1054–26.
64. Baumgartner H, Budts W, Chessa M, Deanfield J, Eicken A, Holm J, et al. Recommendations for organization of care for adults with congenital heart disease and for training in the subspecialty of 'Grown-up Congenital Heart Disease' in Europe: a position paper of the Working Group on Grown-up Congenital Heart Disease of the European Society of Cardiology. Eur Heart J. 2014;35(11):686–90.
66. Ahmad F, McNally EM, Ackerman MJ, Baty LC, Day SM, Kullo IJ, et al. Establishment of specialized clinical cardiovascular genetics programs: recognizing the need and meeting standards: a scientific statement from the American Heart Association. Circ Genom Precis Med. 2019;12(6):e000054.
67. Kirk M, Simpson A, Llewellyn M, Tonkin E, Cohen D, Longley M. Evaluating the role of cardiac genetics nurses in inherited cardiac conditions services using a Maturity Matrix. Eur J Cardiovasc Nurs. 2014;13(5):418–28.
68. Burton H, Alberg C, Hall A, Sagoo GS, Stewart A, Inherited cardiovascular conditions services. Inherited cardiovascular conditions: the challenges of genomic medicine. Heart. 2010;96(6):474–76.
69. Andersen J, Øyen N, Bjorvatn C, Gjengedal E. Living with long QT syndrome: a qualitative study of coping with increased risk of sudden cardiac death. J Genet Couns. 2008;17(5):489–98.
70. Elliott P, Lambiase P, Kumar D. Inherited Cardiac Disease. Oxford: Oxford University Press; 2011.
71. Waddell-Smith KE, Li J, Smith W, Crawford J, Skinner JR, Cardiac Inherited Disease Group New Zealand. β-blocker adherence in familial long QT syndrome. Circ Arrhythm Electrophysiol. 2016;9(8):e003591.
72. Postema PG, Neville J, de Jong JSSG, Romero K, Wilde AA, Woosley RL. Safe drug use in long QT syndrome and Brugada syndrome: comparison of website statistics. Europace. 2013;15(7):1042–49.
73. Postema PG, Wolpert C, Amin AS, Probst V, Borggrefe M, Roden DM, et al. Drugs and Brugada syndrome patients: review of the literature, recommendations, and an up-to-date website (www.brugadadrugs.org). Heart Rhythm. 2009;6(9):1335–41.
74. Shiga T, Suzuki T, Nishimura K. Psychological distress in patients with an implantable cardioverter defibrillator. J Arrhythm. 2013;29(6):310–13.
75. Maron BJ, Casey SA, Olivotto I, Sherrid MV, Semsarian C, Autore C, et al. Clinical course and quality of life in high-risk patients with hypertrophic cardiomyopathy and implantable cardioverter-defibrillators. Circ Arrhythm Electrophysiol. 2018;11(4):e005820.
76. Ingles J, Sarina T, Yeates L, Semsarian C. Psychosocial impact of implantable cardioverter-defibrillator therapy in genetic heart disease patients: a prospective study. Eur J Cardiovasc Nurs. 2014;13:S69–70.
77. Bratt EL, Sparud-Lundin C, Östman-Smith I, Axelsson AB. The experience of being diagnosed with hypertrophic cardiomyopathy through family screening in childhood and adolescence. Cardiol Young. 2012;22(5):528–35.
78. Etchegary H, Enright G, Audas R, Pullman D, Young TL, Hodgkinson K. Perceived economic burden associated with an inherited cardiac condition: a qualitative inquiry with families affected by arrhythmogenic right ventricular cardiomyopathy. Genet Med. 2016;18(6):584–92.
79. Aatre RD, Day SM. Psychological issues in genetic testing for inherited cardiovascular diseases. Circ Cardiovasc Genet. 2011;4(1):81–90.
80. Geelen E, Van Hoyweghen I, Doevendans PA, Marcelis CL, Horstman K. Constructing 'best interests': genetic testing of children in families with hypertrophic cardiomyopathy. Am J Med Genet A. 2011;155A(8):1930–38.
81. Buck HG, Harkness K, Wion R, Carroll SL, Cosman T, Kaasalainen S, et al. Caregivers' contributions to heart failure self-care: a systematic review. Eur J Cardiovasc Nurs. 2015;14(1):79–89.
82. Wisten A, Zingmark K. Supportive needs of parents confronted with sudden cardiac death—a qualitative study. Resuscitation. 2007;74(1):68–74.
83. Miles CJ, Behr ER. The role of genetic testing in unexplained sudden death. Transl Res. 2016;168:59–73.
84. Mayer DD, Rosenfeld AG, Gilbert K. Lives forever changed: family bereavement experiences after sudden cardiac death. Appl Nurs Res. 2013;26(4):168–73.
85. Neimeyer RA, Sands DC. Meaning reconstruction in bereavement: from principles to practice. In: Neimeyer RA, Harris DL, Winokuer HR, Thornton GF (Eds), Grief and Bereavement in Contemporary Society: Bridging Research and Practice. New York: Routledge/Taylor & Francis Group; 2011:9–22.
86. Hayes H, Buckland S, Tarpey M. Briefing notes for researchers: public involvement in NHS, public health and social care research. National Institute for Health Research; 2012. http://www.invo.org.uk/wp-content/uploads/2012/04/INVOLVEBriefingNotesApr2012.pdf.
87. Stout KK, Daniels CJ, Aboulhosn JA, Bozkurt B, Broberg CS, Colman JM, et al. 2018 AHA/ACC guideline for

the management of adults with congenital heart disease: executive summary: a report of the American College of Cardiology/American Heart Association Task Force on Clinical Practice guidelines. Circulation. 2019;139(14):e637–97.

88. Liu Y, Chen S, Zühlke L, Black GC, Choy MK, Li N, Keavney BD. Global birth prevalence of congenital heart defects 1970–2017: updated systematic review and meta-analysis of 260 studies. Int J Epidemiol. 2019;48(2):455–63.
89. van der Linde D, Konings EEM, Slager MA, Witsenburg M, Helbing WA, Takkenberg JJ, et al. Birth prevalence of congenital heart disease worldwide: a systematic review and meta-analysis. J Am Coll Cardiol. 2011;58(21):2241–47.
90. Mandalenakis Z, Rosengren A, Skoglund K, Lappas G, Eriksson P, Dellborg M. Survivorship in children and young adults with congenital heart disease in Sweden. JAMA Intern Med. 2017;177(2):224–30.
91. Moons P, Bovijn L, Budts W, Belmans A, Gewillig M. Temporal trends in survival to adulthood among patients born with congenital heart disease from 1970 to 1992 in Belgium. Circulation. 2010;122(22):2264–72.
92. Mulder BJM. Epidemiology of adult congenital heart disease: demographic variations worldwide. Neth Heart J. 2012;20(12):505–508.
93. Baumgartner H. Geriatric congenital heart disease: a new challenge in the care of adults with congenital heart disease? Eur Heart J. 2014;35(11):683–85.
94. Moons P, De Geest S, Budts W. Comprehensive care for adults with congenital heart disease: expanding roles for nurses. Eur J Cardiovasc Nurs. 2002;1(1):23–28.
95. Landzberg MJ, Murphy DJ, Davidson WR, Jarcho JA, Krumholz HM, Mayer JE, et al. Task force 4: organization of delivery systems for adults with congenital heart disease. J Am Coll Cardiol. 2001;37(5):1187–93.
96. Deanfield J, Thaulow E, Warnes C, Webb G, Kolbel F, Hoffman A, et al. Management of grown up congenital heart disease. Eur Heart J. 2003;24(11):1035–84.
97. Baumgartner H, Bonhoeffer P, De Groot NMS, de Haan F, Deanfield JE, Galie N, et al. ESC Guidelines for the management of grown-up congenital heart disease (new version 2010). Eur Heart J. 2010;31(23):2915–57.
98. Kiener A, Kelleman M, McCracken C, Kochilas L, St Louis JD, Oster ME. Long-term survival after arterial versus atrial switch in d-transposition of the great arteries. Ann Thorac Surg. 2018;106(6):1827–33.
99. Couperus LE, Vliegen HW, Zandstra TE, Kiès P, Jongbloed MRM, Holman ER, et al. Long-term outcome after atrial correction for transposition of the great arteries. Heart. 2019;105(10):790–96.
100. Moons P, Sluysmans T, De Wolf D, Massin M, Suys B, Benatar A, et al. Congenital heart disease in 111 225 births in Belgium: birth prevalence, treatment and survival in the 21st century. Acta Paediatr. 2009;98(3):472–77.
101. Bjornard K, Riehle-Colarusso T, Gilboa SM, Correa A. Patterns in the prevalence of congenital heart defects, metropolitan Atlanta, 1978 to 2005. Birth Defects Res A Clin Mol Teratol. 2013;97(2):87–94.
102. Rutledge JM, Nihill MR, Fraser CD, Smith OE, McMahon CJ, Bezold LI. Outcome of 121 patients with congenitally corrected transposition of the great arteries. Pediatr Cardiol. 2002;23(2):137–45.
103. Marcelletti C, McGoon DC, Mair DD. The natural history of truncus arteriosus. Circulation. 1976;54(1):108–11.
104. Naimo PS, Fricke TA, Yong MS, d'Udekem Y, Kelly A, Radford DJ, et al. Outcomes of truncus arteriosus repair in children: 35 years of experience from a single institution. Semin Thorac Cardiovasc Surg. 2016;28(2):500–11.
105. Hussain S, Al-Radi O, Yun TJ, Hua Z, Rahmat B, Rao S, et al. Survey of multinational surgical management practices in tetralogy of Fallot. Cardiol Young. 2019;29(1):67–70.
106. Smith CA, McCracken C, Thomas AS, Spector LG, St Louis JD, Oster ME, et al. Long-term outcomes of tetralogy of Fallot: a study from the pediatric cardiac care consortium. JAMA Cardiol. 2019;4(1):34–41.
107. Dennis M, Moore B, Kotchetkova I, Pressley L, Cordina R, Celermajer DS. Adults with repaired tetralogy: low mortality but high morbidity up to middle age. Open Hear. 2017;4(1):e000564.
108. Brown ML, Burkhart HM, Connolly HM, Dearani JA, Cetta F, Li Z, et al. Coarctation of the aorta: lifelong surveillance is mandatory following surgical repair. J Am Coll Cardiol. 2013;62(11):1020–25.
109. Lee MGY, Babu-Narayan SV, Kempny A, Uebing A, Montanaro C, Shore DF, et al. Long-term mortality and cardiovascular burden for adult survivors of coarctation of the aorta. Heart. 2019;105(15):1190–96.
110. Brown ML, Dearani JA, Danielson GK, Cetta F, Connolly HM, Warnes CA, et al. Functional status after operation for Ebstein anomaly: the Mayo Clinic experience. J Am Coll Cardiol. 2008;52(6):460–66.
111. Brown ML, Dearani JA, Danielson GK, et al. The outcomes of operations for 539 patients with Ebstein anomaly. J Thorac Cardiovasc Surg. 2008;135(5):1120–36.
112. Schleiger A, Miera O, Peters B, Schmitt KRL, Kramer P, Buracionok J, et al. Long-term results after surgical repair of atrioventricular septal defect. Interact Cardiovasc Thorac Surg. 2019;28(5):789–96.

113. Menting ME, Cuypers JAAE, Opić P, Utens EM, Witsenburg M, van den Bosch AE, et al. The unnatural history of the ventricular septal defect: outcome up to 40 years after surgical closure. J Am Coll Cardiol. 2015;65(18):1941–51.
114. Hanslik A, Pospisil U, Salzer-Muhar U, Greber-Platzer S, Male C. Predictors of spontaneous closure of isolated secundum atrial septal defect in children: a longitudinal study. Pediatrics. 2006;118(4):1560–65.
115. Udholm S, Nyboe C, Karunanithi Z, Christensen AI, Redington A, Nielsen-Kudsk JE, et al. Lifelong burden of small unrepaired atrial septal defect: results from the Danish National Patient Registry. Int J Cardiol. 2019;283:101–106.
116. Piechowiak M, Banach M, Ruta J, Barylski M, Rysz J, Bartczak K, et al. Risk factors for atrial fibrillation in adult patients in long-term observation following surgical closure of atrial septal defect type II. Thorac Cardiovasc Surg. 2006;54(4):259–63.
117. Jalal Z, Hascoet S, Baruteau AE, Iriart X, Kreitmann B, Boudjemline Y, et al. Long-term complications after transcatheter atrial septal defect closure: a review of the medical literature. Can J Cardiol. 2016;32(11):1315.e11–18.
118. Hochstrasser L, Ruchat P, Sekarski N, Hurni M, von Segesser LK. Long-term outcome of congenital aortic valve stenosis: predictors of reintervention. Cardiol Young. 2015;25(5):893–902.
119. Liu H, Gao B, Sun Q, Du X, Pan Y, Zhu Z, et al. Surgical strategies and outcomes of congenital supravalvular aortic stenosis. J Card Surg. 2017;32(10):652–58.
120. Cuypers JAAE, Menting ME, Opić P, Utens EM, Helbing WA, Witsenburg M, et al. The unnatural history of pulmonary stenosis up to 40 years after surgical repair. Heart. 2017;103(4):273–79.
121. Goossens E, Bovijn L, Gewillig M, Budts W, Moons P. Predictors of care gaps in adolescents with complex chronic condition transitioning to adulthood. Pediatrics. 2016;137(4):e20152413.
122. Mackie AS, Ionescu-Ittu R, Therrien J, Pilote L, Abrahamowicz M, Marelli AJ. Children and adults with congenital heart disease lost to follow-up: who and when? Circulation. 2009;120(4):302–309.
123. Thomet C, Moons P, Budts W, De Backer J, Chessa M, Diller G, et al. Staffing, activities, and infrastructure in 96 specialised adult congenital heart disease clinics in Europe. Int J Cardiol. 2019;292:100–105.
124. Steiner JM, Kirkpatrick JN, Heckbert SR, Sibley J, Fausto JA, Engelberg RA, et al. Hospital resource utilization and presence of advance directives at the end of life for adults with congenital heart disease. Congenit Heart Dis. 2018;13(5):721–27.
125. Tobler D, Greutmann M, Colman JM, Greutmann-Yantiri M, Librach LS, Kovacs AH. End-of-life in adults with congenital heart disease: a call for early communication. Int J Cardiol. 2012;155(3):383–87.
126. Gantt LT. Growing up heartsick: the experiences of young women with congenital heart disease. Health Care Women Int. 1992;13(3):241–48.
127. McMurray R, Kendall L, Parsons JM, Quirk J, Veldtman GR, Lewin RJP, et al. A life less ordinary: growing up and coping with congenital heart disease. Coron Health Care. 2001;5(1):51–7.
128. Tong EM, Sparacino PSA, Messias DKH, Foote D, Chesla CA, Gilliss CL. Growing up with congenital heart disease: the dilemmas of adolescents and young adults. Cardiol Young. 1998;8(3):303–9.
129. Claessens P, Moons P, de Casterlé BD, Cannaerts N, Budts W, Gewillig M. What does it mean to live with a congenital heart disease? A qualitative study on the lived experiences of adult patients. Eur J Cardiovasc Nurs. 2005;4(1):3–10.
130. Sluman MA, Apers S, Sluiter JK, Nieuwenhuijsen K, Moons P, Luyckx K, et al. Education as important predictor for successful employment in adults with congenital heart disease worldwide. Congenit Heart Dis. 2019;14(3):362–71.
131. Vernon S, Finch M, Lyon J. Adult congenital heart disease: the nurse specialist's role. Br J Card Nurs. 2011;6(2):88–91.

10 Care of the patient with heart failure

TINY JAARSMA, ANNA STROMBERG, EKATERINI LAMBRINOU, ANDREAS PROTOPAPAS, LOREENA HILL, ANA LJUBAS, AND DAVID R. THOMPSON

CHAPTER CONTENTS

This chapter covers the care of patients with heart failure. It looks at heart failure management programmes and the importance of self-care in this patient population.

KEY MESSAGES

- Heart failure is a major and growing health problem that imposes a significant human and economic burden on individuals, families, and society.
- This condition is associated with high mortality, morbidity, and hospital readmission rates.
- It impairs health-related quality of life and well-being of patients, families, and carers.
- Management depends on a detailed, systematic clinical assessment.
- Treatments include both pharmacological agents and devices.
- Patients with heart failure and their families need education and support to help them understand and cope with treatments and their complications and have an active role in the care plan design based on their needs and preferences, make adjustments to their lifestyle, adhere to the therapy, and take responsibility for their self-care management.

Introduction

Heart failure (HF) is a progressive and complex syndrome as a consequence of structural or functional cardiac diseases, including coronary heart disease, high blood pressure, valvular disease, and cardiomyopathies.[1] It progresses rapidly with an escalating ageing population and causes considerable morbidity, mortality, and rehospitalization, resulting in a tremendous burden on the global healthcare system but also at personal, family and societal levels.[2] Health professionals need to determine the best therapy by integrating the patient's and family's characteristics and needs, clinical signs, and diagnostic tests.[1]

Nurses, including nurse specialists, are important in HF care,[3] and nurse-led HF management programmes reduce HF-related and all-cause readmissions.[4] The aim of this chapter is to present an overview of HF, including its pathophysiology, epidemiology, clinical presentations, clinical features, management, including self-care, complications, and devices, and describe the important role of nurses throughout the trajectory of HF.

Pathophysiology and epidemiology

HF is a complex and fatal clinical condition characterized by a prototype of symptoms (dyspnoea, orthopnoea, lower limb swelling) and signs (elevated jugular venous pressure, pulmonary congestion) often caused by a structural and/or functional cardiac abnormality resulting in reduced cardiac output and/or elevated intracardiac pressures. It encompasses patients with normal left ventricular ejection fraction (LVEF), typically considered as HF with a preserved ejection fraction (HFpEF) of 50% or greater; an LVEF in the mid-range of 40–49% is considered as HFmrEF; and an LVEF less than 40% as HF with a reduced ejection fraction (HFrEF)[1] (➤ Table 10.1).

Approximately 1–2% of the population in high- and middle-income countries have HF although this depends on what definitions are applied. Prevalence increases with age to 10% or higher among people more than 70 years of age. In the population over 65 years old presenting to their general practitioner with breathlessness on exertion, a significant minority will have undiagnosed HFpEF.[5] Patients with HFpEF are generally older, female, and are more likely to have a history of hypertension and atrial fibrillation than a previous myocardial infarction. However, in all patients with HF, there will often be a history of many pathologies which can include myocardial infarction, both inherited and acquired cardiomyopathies, valvular heart disease, alcohol abuse, and some infectious diseases (e.g. Chagas disease and rheumatic fever). Aetiology varies widely according to geographic region,[6] although coronary heart disease and hypertension are the most common primary causes of HF globally. Improvements in treatment over the last few decades have improved survival and reduced hospitalization, in particular, for HFrEF. Between 17% and 45% of deaths from HF occur within 1 year of diagnosis,[6] mainly due to cardiovascular causes. Deaths from non-cardiovascular causes occur more in patients with HFpEF.[1] Most of our understanding of HF comes from studies conducted in high-income countries, although most HF, like cardiovascular disease in general, occurs in low- and middle-income countries.

Advances in health sciences have increased the life expectancy of individuals with HF, changing at the same time the demographic and clinical characteristics contributing to an increase in the proportion of patients diagnosed with HF.[7,8] A strong correlation has been found between advanced age and increased incidence of HF, of which hypertension appears to be a major precursor.[9] Consequently, the combination of advanced age, elderly patients, and coronary heart disease is expected to increase the prevalence of HFrEF in patients across European countries[10] (see also Chapter 14).

Approximately half of HF patients were reported as experiencing all-cause hospitalization at 1-year follow-up, with non-cardiovascular disease hospitalizations associated with a risk of subsequent mortality similar to cardiovascular disease hospitalizations.[11] Often acute events and rehospitalizations are due to non-cardiac reasons such as complications of other diseases or polypharmacy, behavioural reasons such as non-adherence to the therapy, and

Table 10.1 Classifications of heart failure (see the ESC HF Guidelines[1] for more information)

HF with a preserved ejection fraction (HFpEF)	Symptoms ± signs, normal LVEF ≥50%, elevated natriuretic peptides, evidence of structural, and/or functional abnormality
HF with a mid-range ejection fraction (HFmrEF)	Symptoms ± signs, LVEF in the mid-range 40–49%, elevated natriuretic peptides evidence of structural, and/or functional abnormality
HF with a reduced ejection fraction (HFrEF)	Symptoms ± signs, LVEF <40%

socioeconomic determinants, with many people with HF reporting a variety of emotional and physical symptoms that substantially impair their health-related quality of life, mobility, and daily living.[8,12] The incidence and prevalence of HF increase significantly with age and HF is the most common reason for hospitalization in older adults.[7,13] As the HF profile changes towards a more elderly cohort, there is a subsequent rise in the number of comorbidities (see also Chapter 14) and need for multiple medications (polypharmacy) (see also Chapter 14) along with the challenge of diagnostic difficulty and complex management.[5,7,13] Furthermore, older people with HF have additional symptoms and needs: cognitive impairment, dementia, anorexia, muscle wasting, cachexia (see definition later in this chapter), frailty (described in Chapter 8), and depression (described in Chapter 11). Respiratory disorders, depression, obesity, and arthritis in older people can present with similar symptoms as those with HF (e.g. dyspnoea and fatigue).

Clinical presentations

Aetiology

Risk factors for HF are likely to vary depending on the quality of healthcare and the geographical area.[1] Other causes of HF are shown in ➤ Table 10.2.

The decreased cardiac output activates compensatory mechanisms such as increased activation of the sympathetic nervous system, the renin–angiotensin–aldosterone system (RAAS), and other neurohormonal mechanisms, in an attempt to maintain cardiovascular homeostasis and increased cardiac output.[14] In clinical practice, pharmacological treatment of HF is targeted at neurohormonal activation based on pathophysiological mechanisms.[15]

The Frank–Starling mechanism

In the early stages of HF, the Frank–Starling mechanism plays an important role in increasing cardiac output. In HF, for the same preload, the heart muscle is unable to increase the stroke volume and cardiac output (➤ Fig. 10.1). Thus, HF treatment aims to decrease preload and afterload using diuretics and vasodilators[15] (see also Chapter 4).

Neurohormonal activation

Sympathetic nervous system

Increased sympathetic tone by baroreceptors leads to increased heart rate in order to maintain cardiac output. Stimulation of the sympathetic nervous system causes peripheral vasoconstriction and increased afterload due to release of catecholamines in the circulation. As a negative effect, tachycardia causes increased myocardial oxygen demand and shortens ventricular filling time.

Table 10.2 Aetiologies of heart failure

Heart diseases	Coronary artery disease • Myocardial infarction • Ischaemia
	Hypertension
	Valvular heart disease/ rheumatic
	Cardiomyopathy
	Arrhythmia
	Congenital
	Pericardial diseases
Toxic damage	Alcohol, cocaine
	Heavy metals (e.g. iron, cobalt)
	Medications (e.g. immunomodulating, antidepressant, antiarrhythmics, non-steroidal anti-inflammatory, anaesthetic agents, and chemotherapeutic)
Immune -infections and metabolic diseases	Autoimmune diseases
	Chagas disease, viruses, fungi, bacteria
	Amyloidosis, haemochromatosis
	Thyroid diseases, thyrotoxicosis
	Nutritional deficiencies
Other	Iatrogenic fluid overload, renal failure
	Sepsis
	Severe anaemia

Source data from Ponikowski P, Voors AA, Anker SD, Bueno H, Cleland JGF, Coats AJS, et al. 2016 ESC Guidelines for the diagnosis and treatment of acute and chronic heart failure: The Task Force for the diagnosis and treatment of acute and chronic heart failure of the European Society of Cardiology (ESC). Developed with the special contribution. Eur J Heart Fail. 2016;37(27):2129–200.

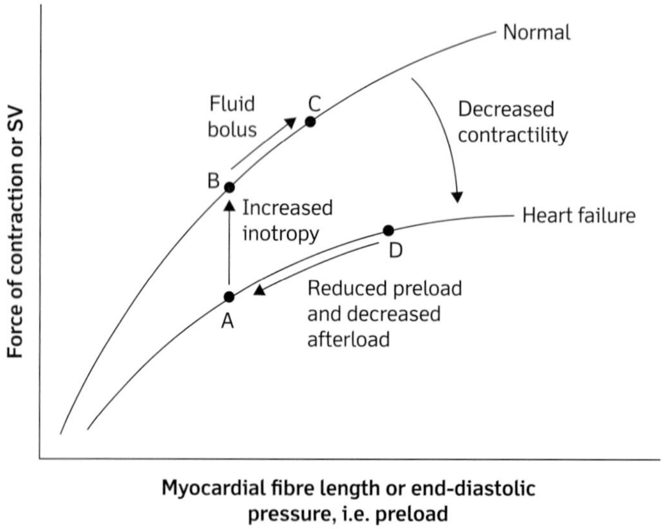

Fig. 10.1 Starling curves effect of filling and increased inotropy. Y-axis: force of contraction can be represented by cardiac output, stroke volume (SV), or stroke work. X-axis: myocardial fibre length can be represented by end-diastolic volume or end-diastolic pressure. A→B represents increased contractility from inotropic therapy. B→C represents a fluid bolus. D→A represents preload or afterload reduction by vasodilators and/or diuretics.

Reproduced from Barry P, Morris K, Ali T. Applied physiology and bedside assessment. In: Paediatric Intensive Care. Oxford UK: Oxford University Press, 2010 with permission from Oxford University Press.

Renin–angiotensin–aldosterone system

Activation of the RAAS aims to increase the intravascular volume and preload of the left ventricle via the Frank–Starling mechanism in order to improve cardiac output and maintain blood pressure and renal flow at a normal level. Renin converts angiotensinogen, which is produced in the liver, into angiotensin I. Angiotensin I is then converted, by the angiotensin converting enzyme, to angiotensin II. Angiotensin II is an active factor of the RAAS and causes vasoconstriction, activation of the sympathetic nervous system, myocyte hypertrophy, and aldosterone release. In addition, the RAAS is also responsible for releasing other neurohormones. Consequently, aldosterone release causes sodium and water retention and potassium excretion (➤ Fig. 10.2).

Ventricular remodelling

Ventricular remodelling is the response of the myocardium to insult in conditions such as ischaemia, inflammation, and mechanical pressure (changes in haemodynamic load), with changes in the geometry (volume and mass) and the structure of the left ventricle (mass and shape).[16] Changing the shape of the left ventricle contributes to increased wall stress and dilation of the mitral valve ring causing functional or ischaemic mitral valve failure. The process of ventricular remodelling is characterized by a neurohormonal response and activation of RAAS secretion of catecholamines, cortisol, and oxidative stress.[17] Ventricular remodelling can lead to electrical and mechanical complications, such as ventricular arrhythmia and ventricular dyssynchrony, and further reduced cardiac output.[16]

Other hormonal responses

Release of natriuretic peptides

As a compensatory mechanism, the main action of natriuretic peptides is to promote diuresis, natriuresis, and vasodilation in order to reduce the extracellular volume and control of cardiovascular homeostasis. Release of these peptides is due to increased mechanical tension in the walls of the atria and ventricles.[18]

Release of antidiuretic hormone.

Vasopressin regulates osmotic pressure and circulating blood volume. Baroreceptors detect a decrease in mean arterial pressure due to the failing heart and this leads to elevated vasopressin release. As a result, vasoconstriction and water retention occur in an effort to increase mean arterial pressure.

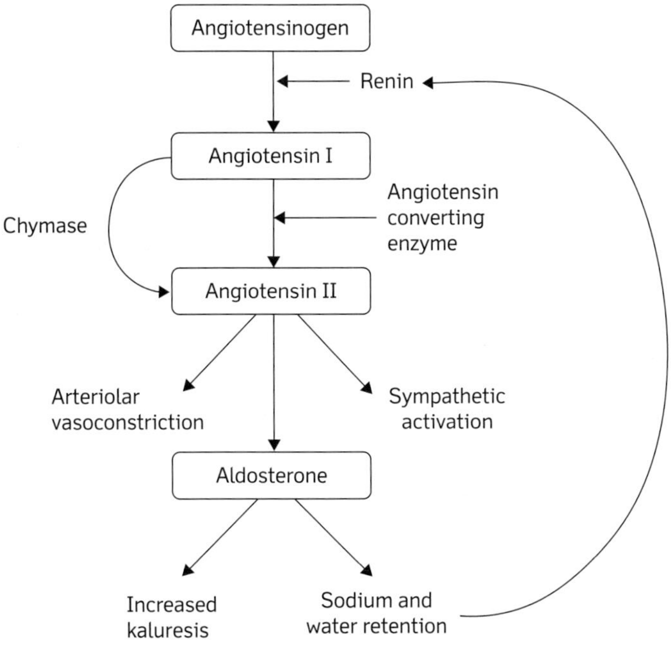

Fig. 10.2 The renin–angiotensin–aldosterone system.

Reproduced from Gardner R, McDonagh T, Walker, N. Definition of heart failure, basic epidemiology, and pathophysiology. In: Heart Failure. Oxford, UK: Oxford University Press, 2014 with permission from Oxford University Press.

Symptoms and signs

The symptoms and signs of HF (➤ **Table 10.3**) are determined by a careful, systematic, detailed clinical assessment that requires skill, experience, and time.[19]

Symptom classification

The New York Heart Association (NYHA) functional classification (➤ **Table 10.4**) is used to determine the severity of HF which has been particularly useful in clinical practice and is used in most clinical studies, describing patient functionality in four stages based on symptoms and ability to exercise.[20]

Medical investigations for heart failure diagnosis

Assessment pathway

Essential initial investigations include natriuretic peptides, electrocardiogram (ECG), and echocardiogram. Patients with normal plasma concentrations are unlikely to have HF. An ECG is useful in ruling out HF as it is unlikely for patients with HF to have a completely normal ECG. However, the most useful test to confirm the presence of HF is an echocardiogram.

Algorithms for the diagnosis of HF in both acute and non-acute settings are presented in ➤ **Fig. 10.3** and ➤ **Fig. 10.4**. These are as described in the European Society of Cardiology (ESC) Guidelines for the management of HF.[1] More information on cardiogenic shock is available in Chapter 5 where track and trigger systems to identify and monitor deterioration are covered.

Nursing assessment

History

Taking a detailed history is essential for further nursing care plans. History should include information about previous medical history and any other comorbidities, NYHA classification, implanted devices, sexual and exercise activity, and sleep disorders. Nurses need to consider the common factors that cause hospitalization as a consequence of decompensated HF, for example compliance with evidence-based medications, diet, fluid and sodium restriction, self-care strategies such as daily weighting,

Table 10.3 Symptoms and signs of heart failure

Symptoms	Signs
Typical	**More specific**
Breathlessness Orthopnoea Paroxysmal nocturnal dyspnoea Fatigue, tiredness, increased time to recover after exercise Reduced exercise tolerance Ankle swelling	Elevated jugular venous pressure Hepatojugular reflux Third heart sound (gallop rhythm) Laterally displaced apex
Less typical	**Less specific**
Nocturnal cough Wheezing Bloated feeling Loss of appetite Confusion (especially in the elderly) Depression Palpitations Dizziness Syncope Bendopnoea	Weight gain (>2 kg/week) Weight loss (in advanced HF) Tissue wasting (cachexia) Cardiac murmur Peripheral oedema (ankle, sacral, scrotal) Pulmonary crepitations Pleural effusion Tachycardia Irregular pulse Tachypnoea Cheyne–Stokes respiration Hepatomegaly Ascites Cold extremities Oliguria Narrow pulse pressure

McDonagh TA, Metra M, Adamo M, Gardner RS, Baumbach A, Böhm M, et al. 2021 ESC Guidelines for the diagnosis and treatment of acute and chronic heart failure: Developed by the Task Force for the diagnosis and treatment of acute and chronic heart failure of the European Society of Cardiology (ESC) With the special contribution of the Heart Failure Association (HFA) of the ESC. Eur Heart J. 2021, ehab368 © The European Society of Cardiology. Reprinted by permission of Oxford University Press.

'over the counter' medication, and social and psychological aspects.

Physical examination

Inspection, palpation, percussion, and auscultation are the four basic methods of physical examination with which nurses should be familiar (see Chapter 5 for more detail). Despite advances in technology, performing a physical examination is an important skill not only for the diagnosis of HF, but also the optimization and follow-up strategies and therapeutic plans.[19] Specifically, a physical examination reveals valuable information about the patient's clinical status such as volume overload, congestion, perfusion, and adherence to the therapy.[20,21]

Table 10.4 NYHA functional classification of heart failure

Class I	No limitation of physical activity. Ordinary physical activity does not cause undue breathlessness, fatigue, or palpitations
Class II	Slight limitation of physical activity. Comfortable at rest, but ordinary physical activity results in undue breathlessness, fatigue, or palpitations
Class III	Marked limitation of physical activity. Comfortable at rest, but less than ordinary activity results in undue breathlessness, fatigue, or palpitations
Class IV	Unable to carry on any physical activity without discomfort. Symptoms at rest can be present. If any physical activity is undertaken, discomfort is increased

McDonagh TA, Metra M, Adamo M, Gardner RS, Baumbach A, Böhm M, et al. 2021 ESC Guidelines for the diagnosis and treatment of acute and chronic heart failure: Developed by the Task Force for the diagnosis and treatment of acute and chronic heart failure of the European Society of Cardiology (ESC) With the special contribution of the Heart Failure Association (HFA) of the ESC. Eur Heart J. 2021, ehab368 © The European Society of Cardiology. Reprinted by permission of Oxford University Press.

Respiratory manifestations

Common symptoms in HF are breathlessness, orthopnoea, paroxysmal nocturnal dyspnoea and reduced exercise tolerance. Less typical symptoms are nocturnal cough, wheezing, bloated feeling. Dyspnoea or breathlessness is associated with high pressures in the left ventricle and in the pulmonary capillary. Depending on the severity of the patient's condition, dyspnoea occurs in three clinical forms:

Exertional dyspnoea

During physical activity, the patient complains of shortness of breath and is forced to stop the activity and rest. For example, dyspnoea can occur when climbing stairs or while running. In advanced stages of HF, dyspnoea may appear with minimal effort such as in speech.

Orthopnoea and paroxysmal nocturnal dyspnoea

Orthopnoea is defined as dyspnoea appearing in the supine position and relieved when the patient adds more

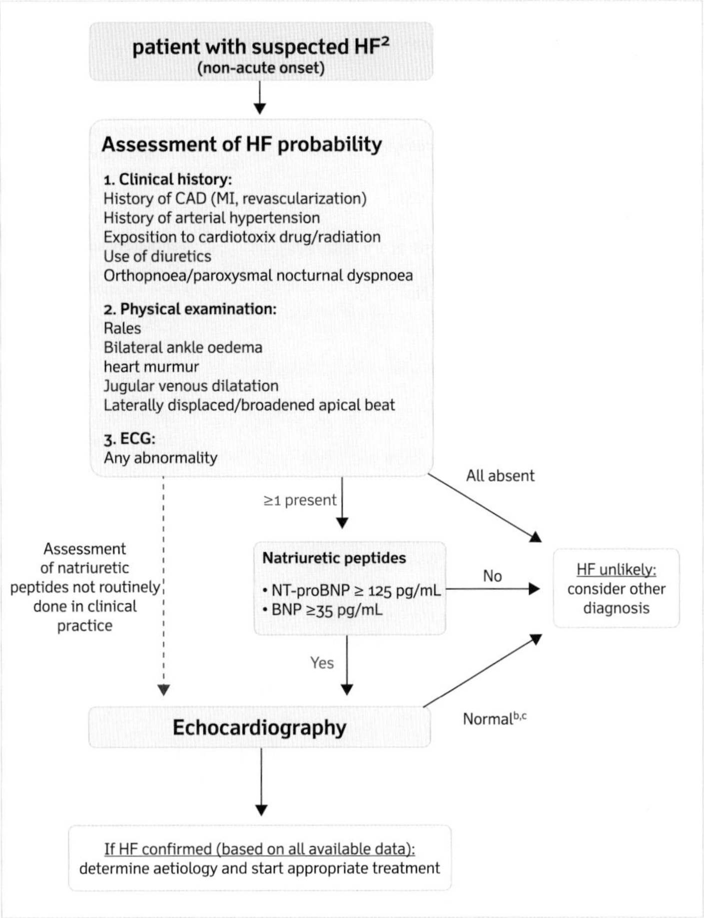

Fig. 10.3 The diagnostic algorithm for heart failure. BNP = B-type natriuretic peptide; ECG = electrocardiogram; HFmrEF = heart failure with mildly reduced ejection fraction; HFpEF= heart failure with preserved ejection fraction; HFrEF= heart failure with reduced ejection fraction; LVEF = left ventricular ejection fraction; NT-proBNP = N-terminal pro-B type natriuretic peptide. McDonagh TA, Metra M, Adamo M, et al; Authors/Task Force Members; Document Reviewers. 2021 ESC Guidelines for the diagnosis and treatment of acute and chronic heart failure: The Task Force for the diagnosis and treatment of acute and chronic heart failure of the European Society of Cardiology (ESC). Developed with the special contribution of the Heart Failure Association (HFA) of the ESC. Eur Heart J. 2021 Aug 27; 00, 1_128. doi:10.1093/eurheartj/ehab368. © The European Society of Cardiology. Reprinted by permission of Oxford University Press.

pillows or sits up, whereas paroxysmal nocturnal dyspnoea occurs at night. The patient wakes up suddenly after a few hours of bedtime and is frightened, anxious, and has shortness of breath, being forced to sit or stand in order to relieve his/her symptoms. This kind of dyspnoea is caused by congestion of the lungs due to redistribution of blood volume.

Pulmonary oedema

Pulmonary oedema constitutes the most dramatic clinical feature of HF and may occur suddenly or progressively. It is a life-threatening situation and the patient can develop severe respiratory distress with use of accessory muscles, orthopnoea, tachypnoea, cough, low oxygen saturation (hypoxaemia), and signs of pulmonary congestion. In severe situations, the cough may be accompanied by frothy bloody sputum, excessive sweating, anxiety, and pale skin. On pulmonary auscultation, initially crackles are heard over the lung bases at the end of inspiration but soon these occupy all the pulmonary fields. This is caused by an increase in pulmonary capillary hydrostatic pressure which forces fluid into the alveoli.

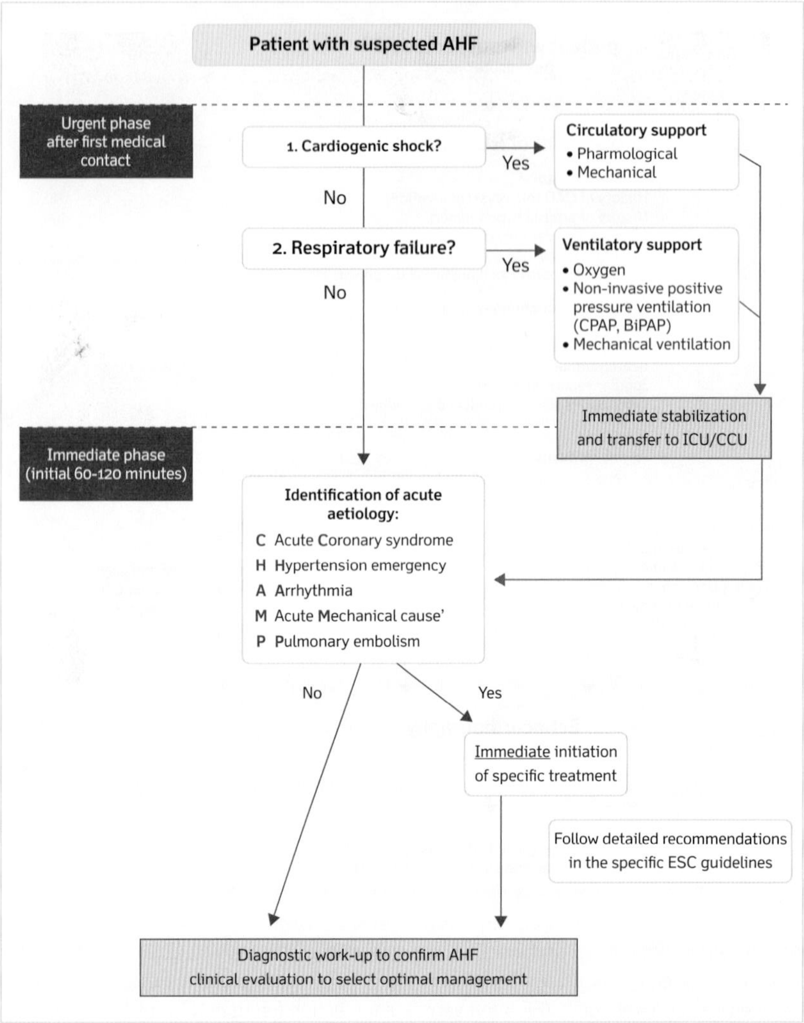

Fig. 10.4 Diagnosing heart failure of acute onset. AHF, acute heart failure; BiPAP, bilevel positive airway pressure; CCU, coronary care unit; CPAP, continuous positive airway pressure; ESC, European Society of Cardiology; ICU, intensive care unit. [a] Acute mechanical cause: myocardial rupture complicating acute coronary syndrome (free wall rupture, ventricular septal defect, acute mitral regurgitation), chest trauma or cardiac intervention, acute native or prosthetic valve incompetence secondary to endocarditis, aortic dissection, or thrombosis.

Ponikowski P, Voors AA, Anker SD, et al; Authors/Task Force Members; Document Reviewers. 2016 ESC Guidelines for the diagnosis and treatment of acute and chronic heart failure: The Task Force for the diagnosis and treatment of acute and chronic heart failure of the European Society of Cardiology (ESC). Developed with the special contribution of the Heart Failure Association (HFA) of the ESC. Eur J Heart Fail. 2016 Aug;18(8):891–975. doi: 10.1002/ejhf.592. © The European Society of Cardiology. Reprinted by permission of Oxford University Press.

Volume status

Symptoms and signs of HF vary widely, with some signs resulting from fluid retention and volume overload, while common symptoms include dyspnoea and fatigue. The volume status can be assessed by estimating the jugular venous pressure, testing the hepatojugular reflux, auscultation of the lungs and heart, evaluating the presence of oedema (➤ **Fig. 10.5**a), and measuring weight.

Jugular venous distention is a sign of volume overload and is common in decompensated HF. In order to examine

(a) (b)

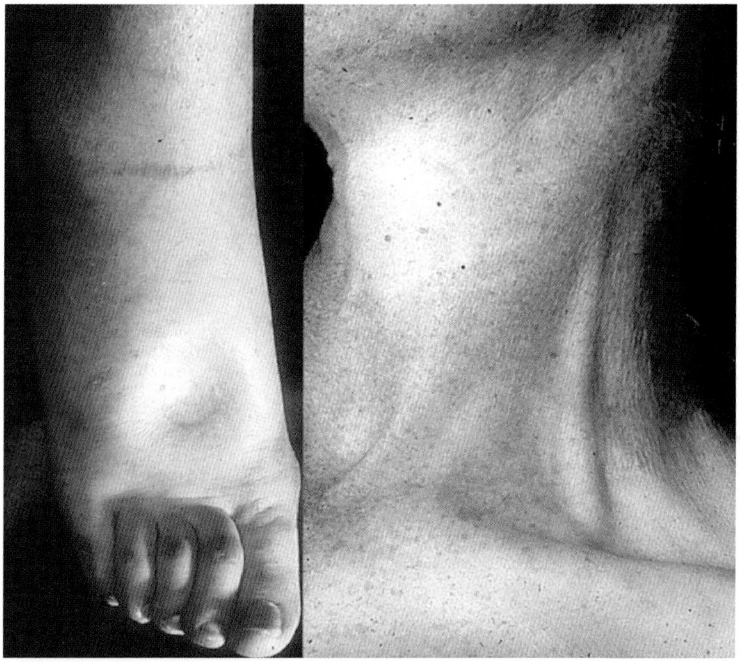

Fig. 10.5 Signs of congestion in heart failure: (a) peripheral oedema; (b) raised jugular venous pressure.

Reproduced from Dargie HJ, McDonagh TA. Diagnosing heart failure. In: Oxford Textbook of Heart Failure. Oxford, UK, Oxford University Press, 2011 with permission from Oxford University Press.

it, the patient should be placed at 45 degrees from the supine position and the right internal jugular vein evaluated. It indicates increased pressure in the right atrium, elevated pulmonary capillary wedge pressure, and left atrial pressure (➤ **Fig. 10.5**b). Jugular pressure may be normal at rest but increased when steadily compressing the patient's abdomen for 10 seconds. This test is called the hepatojugular reflux and is positive when the jugular venous pressure is raised more than 3 cmH_2O and maintained for a few seconds (10–15 seconds) after removal of the pressure. A positive hepatojugular reflux reflects elevated ventricular filling pressures. Hepatomegaly is also a common sign in right HF.

Another finding which commonly occurs in patients with HF is oedema. Oedema can be present as a pitting oedema of the lower extremities (➤ **Fig. 10.5**a); oedema in the abdomen is called ascites. Due to the oedema, the patient's body weight may increase. A daily record of the patient's body weight, at the same time every day, is necessary in order to detect early decompensated HF. For example, unexpected weight gain of more than 2 kg in 3 days is a sign of alarm. Daily measurement of fluid intake and output helps determine efficacy of diuretic therapy and volume status.

Sometimes, a pleural effusion can be present, typically indicated by dullness on percussion of the lung and no sounds heard during auscultation. Cardiac auscultation is useful for evaluating volume status. As a sign of left ventricular failure, the third heard sound can be heard and is associated with increased left ventricular end-diastolic pressure.

Vital signs

Examining vital signs is crucial to determine abnormalities (see Chapter 5). Increased sympathetic activity results in decreased peripheral perfusion due to vasoconstriction with cold extremities, increased capillary refill time, and even high blood pressure. On the other hand, hypotension (systolic blood pressure <90 mmHg) can be caused as a side effect of medication such as angiotensin-converting enzyme (ACE) inhibitors (or angiotensin II receptor blockers), beta-blockers, and diuretics due to hypovolaemia. Hypotension is also a sign of hypoperfusion. However, it is important to measure blood pressure in a supine and standing position in order to assess volume status and to exclude hypotension that is not caused by a reduced preload possibly due to aggressive diuretic or ACE inhibitor treatment.

The pulse pressure (the difference between systolic blood pressure and diastolic blood pressure) reflects stroke volume and vascular stiffness. Patients with HF who have a narrow pulse pressure have worse prognosis.

Examining the pulse rate provides information on efficacy of treatment or indicates a worsening situation. For example, a rapid rhythmic pulse (such as sinus tachycardia) in a patient with HF may be due to fever, anaemia, or hyperthyroidism. It is also a sign of decompensated HF due to increased sympathetic activity. Conversely, bradycardia can be caused by side effects of medicines such as beta-blockers, digoxin, and antiarrhythmics. However, a slow heart rate can also occur due to other causes such as heart block. Palpation of the pulse will identify if it is rhythmic or arrhythmic, supported and evidenced by an ECG. The latter (e.g. atrial fibrillation, see Chapter 7) may be caused by infection, valvular disease (see Chapter 8), thyroid disease, or decompensated HF. In the case of atrial fibrillation, precordial auscultation is recommended instead of measuring peripheral pulse by palpation.[1]

Left-sided HF is characterized by the symptoms and signs of pulmonary congestion due to ineffective pumping of the left ventricle, whereas right-sided HF is characterized by those of systemic venous congestion (➤ Table 10.5).

Table 10.5 Summary of symptoms and signs of congestion

Left sided	Right sided
Orthopnoea	Jugular venous dilation
Paroxysmal nocturnal dyspnoea	Bilateral peripheral oedema
Bilateral pulmonary crackles, wheezing	Hepatomegaly
Bilateral peripheral oedema	Hepatojugular reflux
Hypoxia	Ascites
Cough	Symptoms of gut congestion (e.g. abdominal pain, nausea, vomiting, reduced appetite)

Laboratory tests

Laboratory tests also provide significant clinical information for the diagnosis and treatment of HF. Due to the pathophysiology and medications, electrolyte imbalance (e.g. hyponatraemia, hypo/hyperkalaemia, and hypomagnesaemia) and renal failure are common in HF.[21] See the ESC Guidelines on HF for more information on laboratory tests.[1]

Comprehensive management and nursing care

Heart failure management programmes

Clinical guidelines recommend that patients with HF, especially after hospitalization, are enrolled in multidisciplinary HF management programmes to reduce the risk of HF hospitalization and mortality and improve quality of life.[22,23] Different organizational forms can be used to include a combination of components that guarantee optimal HF care. HF management programmes can vary in their components and apply different service models, such as a clinic-based approach (in primary, secondary, or tertiary care), a home-based programme, case management, or a hybrid-based model.[24]

However, it is not a matter of who provides the best care for the HF patient, but rather how we can provide patients with integrated interdisciplinary care where healthcare professionals collaborate with each other in providing person-centred care that fits the individual patient's situation as well as each local healthcare system (see Chapter 14). The following characteristics and components are recommended:

Characteristics

- Use a patient/person-centred approach.
- Employ a multidisciplinary/interdisciplinary approach (e.g. nurse, cardiologist, primary care physician, pharmacist, physiotherapist, dietician, psychologist, social worker, and surgeon) (see also Chapter 3).
- Target high-risk symptomatic patients and have a proactive approach for prevention.
- Have competent and professionally educated staff.
- Encourage patient/carer engagement in the condition and its management.

Components

- Optimized medical and device treatment.
- Adequate patient education, with special emphasis on self-care including patient involvement in symptom monitoring.
- Provision of psychosocial support to patients and family caregivers with respect to sociocultural characteristics and needs.

- Follow-up after discharge (regular clinic and/or home-based visits; possibly telephone support or telemonitoring).
- Easy access to healthcare (through in-person follow-up and by telephone contact) and facilitated access to care during episodes of decompensation.
- Assessment of (and appropriate intervention in response to) an unexplained change in weight, nutritional status, functional status, quality of life, sleep problems, psychosocial problems, or other findings (e.g. laboratory values).
- Access to advanced treatment options, supportive care, and palliative care.

As with any complex intervention, HF management programmes should be tailored to individual patient (and partner, family, caregiver) needs, choices, and preferences. The nurse will need to discuss through communication with the patient, family, and other members of the team the most desirable and appropriate outcomes for the patient along the HF trajectory. These are likely to be related to health-related quality of life and well-being, but also to issues such as satisfaction with and experiences of their care.[25,26]

Self-care

Self-care is essential in the long-term management of chronic illnesses such as HF. Self-care is defined as the process of maintaining health through health-promoting practices and managing illness and can be performed in both healthy and ill states.[27] Self-care can be seen as an overarching concept built from the three key concepts: self-care maintenance (e.g. taking medication as prescribed), self-care monitoring (e.g. regular weighing), and self-care management (e.g. changing diuretic dose). For patients with HF, it might be necessary to regulate and adapt self-care during the course of the disease, for example, in times of deterioration, if comorbidities occur, or in case of specific advanced treatment.[27–30] Self-care has proven to be very important to influence both medical and person-centred outcomes in patients with HF. Those who report more effective self-care have better quality of life, lower mortality, and lower readmission rates than those who report poor self-care.[24,31,32] However, despite the obvious relationship of good self-care with positive health outcomes, many patients find it difficult to adhere to self-care advice. This lack of adherence might be related to the complexity of self-care, lack of perceived need for self-care, the long-term character of the behavioural changes needed, or a lack of motivation, to mention a few (see also Chapter 11).

A challenge faced by healthcare professionals (nurses) is in understanding the complex process of self-care and to develop appropriate, theory-driven interventions that support patients and their caregivers to maintain their health and manage their chronic illness. The middle-range theory of self-care of chronic illness[27] and the situation-specific theory of HF self-care[31] can assist healthcare professionals (nurses) in their assessment of patients with HF and identify individual factors that hinder their engagement in self-care.

Self-care behaviour in heart failure patients

Self-care maintenance

Self-care maintenance refers to those behaviours performed to improve well-being, preserve health, or maintain physical and emotional stability. These behaviours can be related to lifestyle or the medical regimen, and they may be imposed by healthcare professionals or chosen by the patients in order to meet their own goals. Important self-care maintenance behaviours for HF patients are listed here[1] (see also Chapter 11 and Chapter 12):

- Taking medication (including careful use of non-prescription medication).
- Being physically active.
- Cessation of smoking (and drug use).
- Eating a healthy diet.
- Updating immunization.
- Restricting alcohol.
- Balancing activity and rest (sleep and rest).
- Adapting leisure and travel (if relevant).

Self-care monitoring

Self-care monitoring is the process of observing oneself for changes in symptoms and signs (when they occur). In HF patients, this includes monitoring weight changes, or changes in symptoms. Active monitoring for symptoms is needed for awareness and interpretation of bodily changes as symptoms.[30,33]

Important self-care monitoring behaviours for HF patients are:

- Fluid accumulation (weight gain, leg/ankle oedema, shortness of breath, impendence).
- Activity.

- Increasing fatigue.
- Sleep problems.
- Appetite.
- Other symptoms (dizziness, nausea).

Self-care management

Self-care management is defined as the response to symptoms and signs. It is important that patients and their caregivers receive individualized advice on what the most optimal self-care management is for them.[30]

Important self-care management behaviours for HF patients can include:

- Adapting diet or fluid prescription in accordance with their symptoms.
- Adapting their exercise levels in case of fatigue.
- Taking extra diuretics if there are symptoms of fluid retention, such as sudden weight gain and dyspnoea.
- Consulting a healthcare provider.

Case studies

➤ Table 10.6 includes two case studies in HF care which demonstrate the principles of care outlined in this chapter.

Complications

As HF progresses, complications are likely to occur (➤ Box 10.1). The most common are muscle atrophy, anaemia, arrhythmias, valvular heart disease, and kidney, liver, and lung damage. Complications may result from adverse reactions to medications (e.g. headache, hypotension, nausea, and vomiting); however, the most serious complication is sudden cardiac death.

Arrhythmias

Atrial fibrillation is the most common arrhythmia in HF (see also Chapter 7). Atrial and ventricular contractions are not synchronized and that causes blood stasis which can lead to thrombus formation and thromboembolism. Symptoms of atrial fibrillation include dyspnoea in minimal physical activity, fatigue, palpitations, anxiety caused by irregular heart rhythm, and episodes of lightheadedness and syncope caused by brain hypoperfusion. Furthermore, patients can feel frustrated and anxious by a lack of knowledge and understanding of the disease, complications, and therapy. The main goals of treatment are rhythm or rate control and the patient's comfort and feelings of trust and staying calm. Sudden cardiac death is a major cause of mortality in a growing population of HF patients.[34] Malignant heart disorders such as ventricular tachycardia and ventricular fibrillation are the most common cause of sudden cardiac death. The incidence of malignant arrhythmias is higher in patients with HF than in the general population, therefore implantable cardioverter defibrillators (ICDs) are an option in such patients for prevention of sudden cardiac death. No test can predict sudden cardiac death, but timely assessment of a high-risk patient, optimal drug therapy, and preventive implantation of ICDs can surely help prevent a lethal outcome.

Valvular heart disease

Valvar heart disease in HF is the result of heart enlargement and morphological changes in valve structure (see also Chapter 8). All valves can be affected. The result of valve disease is a worsening in haemodynamics. Fluid accumulates in the lungs and affects gas exchange. It can also result in acute pulmonary oedema. The main symptoms are dyspnoea and orthopnoea.

Thromboembolism

Embolic events are also a complication of HF. When the heart isn't working effectively, blood clots are more likely to form in the blood vessels or in the heart (especially in case of atrial fibrillation). A stroke occurs when a clot(s) lodges in a blood vessel in the brain and cuts off the necessary blood flow and tissue perfusion. Ischaemic stroke symptoms include numbness on one side of the body, confusion, trouble speaking, and loss of balance or coordination. If the patient does not receive medical care in a timely manner, there can be permanent neurological damage. A pulmonary embolism is a blockade of a blood vessel in the lungs. Symptoms include shortness of breath, chest pain on breathing, and tachycardia. Depending on the size of the blocked vessel, it can be an acute or chronic complication.

Organ damage

HF affects other organs too, predominantly the liver and kidneys.[21] As heart function declines, kidney blood flow and glomerular filtration decreases. Sodium filtration also decreases which results in fluid retention. With reduced

Table 10.6 Case studies: heart failure

	Heart failure (1)	Heart failure (2)
1. Patient population and medical history	Elizabeth is an independent 64-year-old lady. She lives alone and has good family and friend support. She enjoyed an alcoholic drink on social occasions, but over the last 12 months her intake has increased to 4–6 units every night. Her medical history included chronic obstructive pulmonary disease, compliant with inhalers, and ex-smoker. Over the past 3 weeks Elizabeth felt more breathless when carrying out her household chores. She also noticed swelling in her ankles and lower legs	John is a 49-year-old gentleman who presented with anterolateral myocardial infarction, treated with primary percutaneous coronary intervention and stenting 5 years ago. He has a manual job, smokes 40 cigarettes per day, and has a positive family history of coronary artery disease. Echocardiogram post myocardial infarction demonstrated moderate left ventricular dysfunction. He was initiated on guideline-directed medications, and provided with information and support to make necessary lifestyle changes, including smoking cessation. He was followed up by the HF nurses in secondary care
2. Clinical presentation	Elizabeth became concerned when she could not lie comfortably in bed. Instead, she would awaken three or four times during the night, feeling so breathless she had to sit on the side of the bed. Her inhaler for chronic obstructive pulmonary disease helped slightly. She decided to attend the accident and emergency (A&E) department. A B-type natriuretic peptide was markedly elevated at 4800 ng/L and an urgent echocardiogram demonstrated a severely impaired left ventricle	Over the past year, John has noted a deterioration in his exercise tolerance. He now would become breathless on walking upstairs or when feeling anxious. He denied any chest pain, dizziness, or palpitations. His general practitioner performed N-terminal pro-B-type natriuretic peptide blood test which was elevated at 510 ng/L. A cardiac magnetic resonance imaging scan was arranged which showed severe left ventricular impairment (ejection fraction 30%)
3. Evaluation pathway	Elizabeth was reviewed by the cardiology team in A&E and admitted directly to the ward for close monitoring. An ECG showed sinus rhythm with broad QRS duration (152 ms). A cardiac magnetic resonance imaging scan demonstrated severely dilated and impaired left ventricle in keeping with non-ischemic cardiomyopathy	The HF team reviewed John and discussed referral to an electrophysiologist for device implantation. As John's ECG was sinus rhythm with no prolongation of QRS, the option was an ICD. Medications were also amended, with perindopril changed to sacubitril/valsartan. Six months later John was reviewed by the electrophysiologist. An echocardiogram showed an improvement in left ventricular impairment; however, ICD implantation remained warranted

(continued)

Table 10.6 Continued

	Heart failure (1)	Heart failure (2)
4. Treatment	Elizabeth was fluid restricted to 1200 mL and strict recording of her urinary output. Intravenous diuretic therapy was commenced, which Elizabeth found difficult as she became embarrassed due to occasional incontinence. A SRC was inserted, at her request for the first 4 days. Elizabeth was weighed every morning and over the course of the initial days lost 2 kg. She became less breathless and subsequently more mobile around the ward. When her condition stabilized, Elizabeth was commenced on an ACE inhibitor and beta-blocker, both guideline-directed medications. Her kidney function was checked daily. After 10 days she was ready for discharge. Elizabeth was feeling much better, but decided a close friend would stay with her at home to assist with daily household chores, such as shopping. On discharge, the treatment plan was for further titration of EB medication and consideration of device therapy	John is admitted for primary prevention ICD implantation. The device was implanted using local anesthetic into the pectoral muscle in the left upper chest region. Steristrips were applied and the wound covered with a dressing
5. In-hospital nursing care and priorities	During her hospital stay Elizabeth was reviewed by the HF nurse. Information on her condition as well as the subsequent need for lifestyle changes (including cessation of alcohol) was provided. Her medication regimen was discussed and the need for adherence. This verbal advise was supplemented with a booklet which had a table to record daily weights as well as the contact details of the HF nurse, should Elizabeth notice her signs or symptoms deteriorate. Contact details of her local cardiac patient support organization were also provided	John is transferred back to the ward after his procedure. An ECG and chest X-ray are carried out. John is monitored in the cardiac ward overnight to ensure no arrhythmia or bleeding from the wound site. He is reviewed by the electrophysiologist and the cardiac scientist in the morning. The cardiac scientist checks his device and provides important lifestyle advice, as required following device implantation. This information is reinforced by the HF nurse and an important review date at the ICD clinic arranged. Contact details of the local support group for cardiac device patients are also given, which will provide John and his wife with ongoing psychoeducational support. John is discharged following receipt of this information and device checks
6. Discharge planning and follow-up	Elizabeth was reviewed by the HF nurse 2 weeks later. Her blood pressure and pulse were recorded and kidney function checked. Elizabeth was making good progress, describing breathless only when she exerted such as climbing stairs (NYHA II) and had no dizziness. Weight was stable and she had not taken any alcohol. Her medications were therefore increased and a date confirmed to be reviewed by the electrophysiologist for consideration of CRT-D implantation	John lives with his wife. He returned home with the plan to be reviewed by the ICD clinic in 1 month. He also has the contact details of the ICD clinic and the HF nurse should he experience any problems. He is aware of the driving and travel restrictions, which have an impact on his work. He was reviewed by his general practitioner 1 week after discharge and reviewed at the ICD clinic after 1 month. No arrhythmias were noted and he has had a phased return to less manual work

SRC, self retaining catheter; EB, evidence based.

Box 10.1 Complications of heart failure

- Arrhythmias:
  - Atrial fibrillation.
  - Ventricular arrhythmias (ventricular tachycardia, ventricular fibrillation).
  - Bradyarrhythmias.
  - Sudden cardiac death.
- Thromboembolism:
  - Stroke.
  - Peripheral embolism.
  - Deep venous thrombosis.
  - Pulmonary embolism.
- Gastrointestinal:
  - Hepatic congestion and hepatic dysfunction.
  - Malabsorption.
- Musculoskeletal:
  - Cardiac cachexia.
- Respiratory:
  - Pulmonary congestion.
  - Respiratory muscle weakness.
  - Pulmonary hypertension.
- Renal:
  - Fluid retention.
  - Kidney failure.
- Haematological:
  - Anaemia.
- Electrolyte disbalance:
  - Hypokalaemia.
  - Hyperkalaemia.
  - Hyponatraemia.
- Drugs side effects:
  - Hypotension.
  - Electrolyte disbalance.
- Anxiety and depression.
- Impaired health-related quality of life.

function of the right ventricle, the liver can become congested affecting its function and leading to ascites. Furthermore, congestion in the intestines can cause malabsorption. In monitoring patients with liver and kidney complications, it is important to provide education on diet and nutrition (see also Chapter 11 and Chapter 13).

It is essential that patients adhere to a low-sodium diet.

Pulmonary complications

Patients with HF who have prolonged or severe pulmonary congestion can develop lung complications, especially pneumonia and pulmonary embolus. Because their breathing is already compromised by the HF itself, these pulmonary complications can be particularly dangerous in a patient with HF. In addition, patients who have repeated episodes of acute pulmonary oedema may simply reach the point where an acute episode causes death before they can get medical care.

Cardiac cachexia

Cardiac cachexia is a condition in which a patient loses a significant amount of body fat, muscle, and bone. It is common in advanced HF patients. Once it begins, it cannot be reversed simply by eating more. Weight loss is the main symptom of cardiac cachexia; however, it is associated with increased fatigue and generalized weakness.[35] It is possibly caused by fluid retention in the intestines which prevents absorption of nutrients, liver failure which causes hypoalbuminemia, and chronic inflammation which can cause muscle breakdown.

Drug side effects

Diuretics are often use in the management of HF. Diuretics can cause hypotension, hypokalaemia, and dehydration. Hyperkalaemia can be a side effect of ACE inhibitors and angiotensin II receptor blockers. More information on drug treatments used in HF can be found in the ESC Guidelines on HF.[1]

Anxiety and depression

Suffering from chronic illness is a risk factor for depression or anxiety (see also Chapter 11). The rate of depression in the general population with HF is 25%, and in a population with advanced HF is higher than 50%.[36] Patients need to successively adapt to changing physical and psychosocial situations, and not adapting well enough leads to depression or anxiety. Symptoms of depression in HF are not specific and include persistent sadness, hopelessness, and lack of affect. Nurses and clinicians should offer emotional support, and education about HF and its symptoms and signs.

Impaired health-related quality of life

HF and its related complications and possible comorbidities present a condition which implies many unpleasant symptoms for the patient. The quality of life in HF patients is more significantly impaired than is the case with some other chronic diseases.[37] Dyspnoea, sleep disorders, oedema, nausea, and fatigue are some of the symptoms which affect not only the physical aspect of a person's life, but its psychosocial and economic dimensions as well.

Lifestyle changes caused by the illness, physical limitations in daily activities, losing a job, increased costs, reversed social roles in the family, or uncertainty regarding the course of illness, all present a burden to the patient and their caregivers. All of the above-mentioned aspects impair the patient's quality of life. Such a state, as well as social isolation and depression, reduce the patient's cooperation in the disease treatment, which has a direct influence on their chances of survival. The early introduction of palliative care may help in relieving the symptoms and reducing suffering. A multidisciplinary approach, the development of self-care programmes, patient education, and social support all have a positive impact on the quality of life and they reduce the frequency of rehospitalization.

Care of patients with devices

Device therapy is a cornerstone in the management of HF patient[1] (see also Chapter 7). Nevertheless, over one-quarter of patients with an implanted cardiac device feel insufficiently informed of potential complications and future implications of living with the device.[38] Patients and families should receive tailored information and psychological support to understand the risks and benefits, therefore ensuring informed consent, promotion of self-care, and enabling future control in daily life[39,40] (see also Chapter 13).

Many of the implanted devices used in HF management are solely appropriate for patients with HFrEF, for example, ICDs, cardiac resynchronization therapy (CRT), and ventricular assist devices (VADs).[1,41]

Types of devices

Implantable cardioverter defibrillator

An ICD is a small electromagnetic device inserted into the pectoral muscle to pace the heart if it beats too slow, to pace if it beats too quickly (known as antitachycardia pacing), and discharge a shock when a life-threatening arrhythmia occurs. HF patients may be given the option of a subcutaneous ICD, which just discharges a 'shock'. For symptomatic patients with HFrEF (ejection fraction ≤35%), an ICD is implanted for primary prevention. For patients with HFpEF, there are no data to support the use of an ICD.[1,42] The decision to implant a device should be taken carefully, with involvement of the family for patients of advanced age or debilitating comorbidities.[42,43]

Many patients with an ICD experience psychological distress following the receipt of shock therapy and the realization of the device's impact on daily living (i.e. driving restrictions, work, and leisure activities). Younger age, depression, and type D personality have been found to be associated with an increased vulnerability for post-traumatic stress and anxiety symptoms.[44] To date, there is limited evidence on the effectiveness of non-pharmacological therapies, therefore most patients receive the prescription of an antidepressant.

Combined with biventricular pacing, an ICD can reduce hospitalization rates, decrease mortality,[45,46] and improve HF symptoms and quality of life.[47]

Cardiac resynchronization therapy

The CRT device works by pacing the two ventricles in a synchronized motion to improve the contractibility of the heart, thus improving cardiac output. The device can include an ICD (CRT-D) or be a pacemaker only (CRT-P). For a CRT-D to be implanted, the patients must fulfil criteria for both a CRT device and the ICD device.[1]

Clear communication and information regarding the prognostic benefit of an implanted device is vital to enable informed choice. Despite its proven effectiveness, the 'non-response' rate remains approximately 30%[48] (see also Chapter 14).

Ventricular assist device

The VAD, developed as a mechanical circulatory support for haemodynamically unstable HF patients awaiting cardiac transplantation, is surgically implanted, acting as an artificial pump to assist the dysfunctional ventricle.[49] It comprises a blood pump, system monitor, system controller, and a driveline wire which protrudes out of the body and connects to the battery power source.

Most VADs implanted are left ventricular assist devices (LVADs), the type of device depends on the ventricle that is failing to function efficiently, for example, the right ventricle (RVAD) or both ventricles (biventricular assist device: BiVAD). Since the decline in heart donors for transplantation, VADs are being used more as 'destination therapy', with improved patient survival rates (80%) and quality of life.[50,51] However, VADs are not without complications, such as infection, bleeding and pump thrombosis, and mechanical pump failure.[52]

Successful outcome of the implantation procedure relies on thorough patient and family education before hospital discharge, including regular monitoring, VAD maintenance, and the safe performance of activities of daily living.[53] Patient safety is a priority; therefore, the patient and family must learn techniques including redressing the driveline site, monitoring and management of anticoagulation therapy, and care of the batteries in current use and 'on charge' for future use.

Following discharge, patients will be regularly reviewed by their HF multidisciplinary team with input from the VAD centre regarding drug therapy, blood profiles, and lifestyle, with referral to cardiac rehabilitation to assess and improve exercise tolerance and potentially reduce the risk of hospitalization and mortality.[54]

Long-term management

All patients with an ICD are regularly reviewed, face to face or via telemonitoring,[55] usually at the hospital where the device was implanted. During a face-to-face meeting, the device can be reprogrammed to prevent, for example, unnecessary shocks, optimization of resynchronized pacing, or alteration of the threshold for antitachycardia pacing, in order to improve outcomes. The patient and family must be informed of the importance to attend routine reviews, what to do in 'emergency' or out-of-hours' situations, and given a contact number for advice and support. In services where remote monitoring is available, nurses must inform, educate, and introduce patients and family to the facility.

References

1. Ponikowski P, Voors AA, Anker SD, Bueno H, Cleland JGF, Coats AJS, et al. 2016 ESC Guidelines for the diagnosis and treatment of acute and chronic heart failure: The Task Force for the diagnosis and treatment of acute and chronic heart failure of the European Society of Cardiology (ESC). Developed with the special contribution. Eur J Heart Fail. 2016;37(27):2129–200.
2. Lambrinou E, Kalogirou F, Lamnisos D, Sourtzi P. Effectiveness of heart failure management programmes with nurse-led discharge planning in reducing re-admissions: a systematic review and meta-analysis. Int J Nurs Stud. 2012;49(5):610–24.
3. McDonagh TA, Blue L, Clark AL, Dahlström U, Ekman I, Lainscak M, et al. European Society of Cardiology Heart Failure Association Standards for delivering heart failure care. Eur J Heart Fail. 2011;13(3):235–41.
4. Oyanguren J, Latorre García PM, Torcal Laguna J, Lekuona Goya I, Rubio Martín S, Maull Lafuente E, et al. Effectiveness and factors determining the success of management programs for patients with heart failure: a systematic review and meta-analysis. Rev Esp Cardiol. 2016;69(10):900–14.
5. Kalogirou F, Forsyth F, Kyriakou M, Mantle R, Deaton C. Heart failure disease management: a systematic review of effectiveness in heart failure with preserved ejection fraction. ESC Heart Fail. 2020;7(1):194–214.
6. Ferreira JP, Kraus S, Mitchell S, Perel P, Piñeiro D, Chioncel O, et al. World Heart Federation roadmap for heart failure. Glob Heart. 2019;14(3):197–214.
7. Coats A. Ageing, demographics, and heart failure. Eur Heart J. 2019;21(Suppl L):L4–7.
8. Tromp J, Ferreira JP, Janwanishstaporn S, Shah M, Greenberg B, Zannad F, et al. Heart failure around the world. Eur J Heart Fail. 2019;21(10):1187–96.
9. Mahmood SS, Wang TJ. The epidemiology of congestive heart failure: the Framingham Heart Study perspective. Glob Heart. 2013;8(1):77–82.
10. Guha K, McDonagh T. Heart failure epidemiology: European perspective. Curr Cardiol Rev. 2013;9(2):123–27.
11. Bello NA, Claggett B, Desai AS, McMurray JJV, Granger CB, Yusuf S, et al. Influence of previous heart failure hospitalization on cardiovascular events in patients with reduced and preserved ejection fraction. Circ Heart Fail. 2014;7(4):590–95.
12. Lambrinou E, Protopapas A, Kalogirou F. Heart failure: a challenging syndrome for health care professionals. Cardiovasc Disord Med. 2018;3(3):1–5.
13. Dharmarajan K, Rich MW. Epidemiology, pathophysiology, and prognosis of heart failure in older adults. Heart Fail Clin. 2017;13(3):417–26.
14. Arrigo M, Parissis JT, Akiyama E, Mebazaa A. Understanding acute heart failure: pathophysiology and diagnosis. Eur Heart J. 2016;18(Suppl G):G11–18.
15. Yancy CW, Jessup M, Bozkurt B, Butler J, Casey DE, Colvin MM, et al. 2017 ACC/AHA/HFSA focused update of the 2013 ACCF/AHA guideline for the management of heart failure: a report of the American College of Cardiology/American Heart Association Task Force on Clinical Practice Guidelines and the Heart Failure Society of America. J Card Fail. 2017;23(8):628–51.
16. Cohn JN, Ferrari R, Sharpe N. Cardiac remodeling-concepts and clinical implications: a consensus paper from an International Forum on Cardiac Remodeling. J Am Coll Cardiol. 2000;35(3):569–82.
17. Lymperopoulos A, Rengo G, Koch WJ. Adrenergic nervous system in heart failure: pathophysiology and therapy. Circ Res. 2013;113(6):739–53.
18. Ghosh N, Haddad H. Atrial natriuretic peptides in heart failure: pathophysiological significance, diagnostic and prognostic value. Can J Physiol Pharmacol. 2011;89(8):587–91.
19. Thibodeau JT, Drazner MH. The role of the clinical examination in patients with heart failure. JACC Heart Fail. 2018;6(7):543–51.
20. Harinstein ME, Flaherty JD, Fonarow GC, Mehra MR, Lang RM, Kim RJ, et al. Clinical assessment of acute heart failure syndromes: emergency department through the early post-discharge period. Heart. 2011;97(19):1607–18.

21. Harjola VP, Mullens W, Banaszewski M, Bauersachs J, Brunner-La Rocca HP, Chioncel O, et al. Organ dysfunction, injury and failure in acute heart failure: from pathophysiology to diagnosis and management. A review on behalf of the Acute Heart Failure Committee of the Heart Failure Association (HFA) of the European Society of Cardiology (ESC). Eur J Heart Fail. 2018;19(7):821–36.
22. Krumholz HM, Currie PM, Riegel B, Phillips CO, Peterson ED, Smith R, et al. A taxonomy for disease management: a scientific statement from the American Heart Association Disease Management Taxonomy Writing Group. Circulation. 2006;114(13):1432–45.
23. Jonkman NH, Westland H, Groenwold RHH, Ågren S, Atienza F, Blue L, et al. Do self-management interventions work in patients with heart failure? An individual patient data meta-analysis. Circulation. 2016;133(12):1189–98.
24. Van Spall HGC, Rahman T, Mytton O, Ramasundarahettige C, Ibrahim Q, Kabali C, et al. Comparative effectiveness of transitional care services in patients discharged from the hospital with heart failure: a systematic review and network meta-analysis. Eur J Heart Fail. 2017;19(11):1427–43.
25. Thompson DR, Clark AM. Heart failure disease management interventions: time for a reappraisal. Eur J Heart Fail. 2020;22(4):578–80.
26. Kyriakou M, Middleton N, Ktisti S, Philippou K, Lambrinou E. Supportive care interventions to promote health-related quality of life in patients living with heart failure: a systematic review and meta-analysis. Heart Lung Circ. 2020;29(11):1633–47.
27. Riegel B, Jaarsma T, Strömberg A. A middle-range theory of self-care of chronic illness. Adv Nurs Sci. 2012;35(3):194–204.
28. Kato N, Jaarsma T, Ben Gal T. Learning self-care after left ventricular assist device implantation. Curr Heart Fail Rep. 2014;11(3):290–98.
29. Jaarsma T, Cameron J, Riegel B, Stromberg A. Factors related to self-care in heart failure patients according to the middle-range theory of self-care of chronic illness: a literature update. Curr Heart Fail Rep. 2017;14(2):71–77.
30. Jaarsma T, Hill L, Bayes-Genis A, La Rocca HPB, Castiello T, Čelutkienė J, et al. Self-care of heart failure patients: practical management recommendations from the Heart Failure Association of the European Society of Cardiology. Eur J Heart Fail. 2020;23(1):157–74.
31. Van Der Wal MHL, Van Veldhuisen DJ, Veeger NJGM, Rutten FH, Jaarsma T. Compliance with non-pharmacological recommendations and outcome in heart failure patients. Eur Heart J. 2010;31(12):1486–93.
32. Lee KS, Lennie TA, Dunbar SB, Pressler SJ, Heo S, Song EK, et al. The association between regular symptom monitoring and self-care management in patients with heart failure. J Cardiovasc Nurs. 2015;30(2):145–51.
33. Riegel B, Jaarsma T, Lee CS, Strömberg A. Integrating symptoms into the middle-range theory of self-care of chronic illness. ANS Adv Nurs Sci. 2019;42(3):206–15.
34. Lane RE, Cowie MR, Chow AWC. Prediction and prevention of sudden cardiac death in heart failure. Heart. 2005;91(5):674–80.
35. Jaarsma T, Beattie JM, Ryder M, Rutten FH, McDonagh T, Mohacsi P, et al. Palliative care in heart failure: a position statement from the palliative care workshop of the Heart Failure Association of the European Society of Cardiology. Eur J Heart Fail. 2009;11(5):433–43.
36. Pintor L. Heart failure and depression, an often neglected combination. Rev Esp Cardiol. 2006;59(8):761–65.
37. Zambroski CH, Moser DK, Bhat G, Ziegler C. Impact of symptom prevalence and symptom burden on quality of life in patients with heart failure. Eur J Cardiovasc Nurs. 2005;4(3):198–206.
38. Haugaa KH, Potpara TS, Boveda S, Deharo JC, Chen J, Dobreanu D, et al. Patients' knowledge and attitudes regarding living with implantable electronic devices: results of a multicentre, multinational patient survey conducted by the European Heart Rhythm Association. Europace. 2018;20(2):386–91.
39. Ezzat VA, Lee V, Ahsan S, Chow AW, Segal O, Rowland E, et al. A systematic review of ICD complications in randomised controlled trials versus registries: is our 'real-world' data an underestimation? Open Heart. 2015;2(1):e000198.
40. Groarke J, Beirne A, Buckley U, O'Dwyer E, Sugrue D, Keelan T, et al. Deficiencies in patients' comprehension of implantable cardioverter defibrillator therapy. Pacing Clin Electrophysiol. 2012;35(9):1097–102.
41. Yancy CW, Jessup M, Bozkurt B, Butler J, Casey DE, Drazner MH, et al. 2013 ACCF/AHA guideline for the management of heart failure: a report of the American College of Cardiology Foundation/American Heart Association Task Force on Practice Guidelines. J Am Coll Cardiol. 2013;62(16):e147–239.
42. Lee MC, Sulmasy DP, Gallo J, Kub J, Hughes MT, Russell S, et al. Decision-making of patients with implantable cardioverter-defibrillators at end of life: family members' experiences. Am J Hosp Palliat Med. 2017;34(6):518–23.
43. Hill L, McIlfatrick S, Taylor BJ, Jaarsma T, Moser D, Slater P, et al. Patient and professional factors that impact the perceived likelihood and confidence of healthcare professionals to discuss implantable cardioverter defibrillator deactivation in advanced heart failure. J Cardiovasc Nurs. 2018;33(6):527–35.
44. Habibović M, Denollet J, Pedersen SS. Posttraumatic stress and anxiety in patients with an implantable cardioverter defibrillator: trajectories and vulnerability factors. Pacing Clin Electrophysiol. 2017;40(7):817–23.
45. Cleland JGF, Daubert JC, Erdmann E, Freemantle N, Gras D, Kappenberger L, et al. The CARE-HF study

(CArdiac REsynchronisation in Heart Failure study): rationale, design and end-points. Eur J Heart Fail. 2001;3(4):481–89.

46. Bristow MR, Feldman AM, Saxon LA. Heart failure management using implantable devices for ventricular resynchronization: Comparison of Medical Therapy, Pacing, and Defibrillation in Chronic Heart Failure (COMPANION) trial. J Card Fail. 2000;6(3):276–85.
47. Young JB, Abraham WT, Smith AL, Leon AR, Lieberman R, Wilkoff B, et al. Combined cardiac resynchronization and implantable cardioversion defibrillation in advanced chronic heart failure: the MIRACLE ICD trial. JAMA. 2003;289(20):2685–94.
48. Naqvi SY, Jawaid A, Goldenberg I, Kutyifa V. Non-response to cardiac resynchronization therapy. Curr Heart Fail Rep. 2018;15(5):315–21.
49. Parameshwar J, Hogg R, Rushton S, Taylor R, Shaw S, Mehew J, et al. Patient survival and therapeutic outcome in the UK bridge to transplant left ventricular assist device population. Heart. 2019;105(4):291–96.
50. Modica M, Ferratini M, Torri A, Oliva F, Martinelli L, De Maria R, et al. Quality of life and emotional distress early after left ventricular assist device implant: a mixed-method study. Artif Organs. 2015;39(3):220–27.
51. Kirklin JK, Naftel DC, Pagani FD, Kormos RL, Stevenson LW, Blume ED, et al. Sixth INTERMACS annual report: a 10,000-patient database. J Heart Lung Transplant. 2014;33(6):555–64.
52. Dang G, Epperla N, Muppidi V, Sahr N, Pan A, Simpson P, et al. Medical management of pump-related thrombosis in patients with continuous-flow left ventricular assist devices: a systematic review and meta-analysis. ASAIO J. 2017;63(4):373–85.
53. Casida JM, Marcuccilli L, Peters RM, Wright S. Lifestyle adjustments of adults with long-term implantable left ventricular assist devices: a phenomenologic inquiry. Heart Lung J Acute Crit Care. 2011;40(6):511–20.
54. Adamopoulos S, Corrà U, Laoutaris ID, Pistono M, Agostoni PG, Coats AJS, et al. Exercise training in patients with ventricular assist devices: a review of the evidence and practical advice. A position paper from the Committee on Exercise Physiology and Training and the Committee of Advanced Heart Failure of the Heart Failure Association. Eur J Heart Fail. 2019;21(1):3–13.
55. Hernández-Madrid A, Lewalter T, Proclemer A, Pison L, Lip GYH, Blomstrom-Lundqvist C. Remote monitoring of cardiac implantable electronic devices in Europe: results of the European Heart Rhythm Association survey. Europace. 2014;16(1):129–32.

11 Cardiovascular prevention and rehabilitation

CATRIONA JENNINGS, KATHY BERRA, LAURA L. HAYMAN, IRENE GIBSON, JENNIFER JONES, ALISON ATREY, DAVID R. THOMPSON, CHANTAL F. SKI, MARY KERINS, TARA CONBOY, LIS NEUBECK, ROBYN GALLAGHER, AND SUE KOOB

CHAPTER CONTENTS

KEY MESSAGES

- There is a global imperative for the prevention of cardiovascular disease which includes primordial, primary, and secondary prevention.
- Prevention requires a multifactor risk reduction approach because of the multifaceted aetiology of cardiovascular disease.
- Components of cardiovascular disease prevention include behavioural strategies to encourage the

adoption of healthy lifestyle habits, the use of medications to manage biological risk factors, and strategies to manage psychological conditions such as anxiety and depression.
- Risk estimation allows the detection of those at highest risk, so they can be identified for management as a priority.
- Nurses have an important role to play in the implementation of prevention programmes which, when led by this professional group working in interdisciplinary models with physicians and allied health professionals, have been shown to be successful in reducing total mortality.
- Integrating digital technology can address barriers to participation in programmes and improve adherence. Healthcare providers need to be familiar with these modes of delivery and equipped on what to recommend.
- Professional societies, associations, and heart foundations play an important role in supporting healthcare professionals, patients, and caregivers to maximize the effectiveness of prevention initiatives.

Introduction

In this chapter we will look at the priorities for cardiovascular prevention and rehabilitation (CVPR). This perspective reflects an integrated approach to prevention and rehabilitation. In 1993, the World Health Organization (WHO) provided a definition for cardiac rehabilitation as follows[1]:

> **The sum of activities required to influence favourably the underlying cause of the disease, as well as to provide the best possible physical, mental and social conditions, so that the patients may, by their own efforts, preserve or resume when lost as normal a place as possible in the community.**

This definition alludes to the need for efforts to manage risk factors, that is, underlying causes of cardiovascular disease (CVD) which have an impact on preventing the development of CVD. More recently, calls to action have been published, firstly in 2011 under the auspices of the Preventive Cardiovascular Nurses' Association (PCNA) and the Council on Cardiovascular Nursing and Allied Professions (now known as the Association of Cardiovascular Nursing and Allied Professions (ACNAP)).[2] This supplement was directed specifically at nurses working in cardiovascular care. Secondly, an international charter was published[3] under the auspices of the Canadian Institutes for Health Research which calls for the harmonization of efforts to promote CVPR and to provide an international consensus on its core components.

The global imperative: why nurses need to be involved in cardiovascular prevention and rehabilitation

Cardiovascular prevention and rehabilitation

CVPR programmes, a common setting for secondary prevention (➤ Table 11.1), demonstrate that providing multifactor risk reduction (MFRR) for patients with atherosclerotic heart disease reduces both morbidity and mortality from vascular diseases including stroke and myocardial infarction and some cancers.[4] Following cancer prevention guidelines reduces the risk of cancer, CVD, and all-cause mortality.

CVPR programmes achieve this through managing well-known cardiovascular risk factors such as blood pressure, lipids, diabetes, obesity, poor diet, physical inactivity, tobacco use, depression, and numerous other health-related conditions.[5] As part of the emphasis on cardiovascular risk reduction, these programmes have been successful in developing healthcare professionals as primary and secondary prevention specialists. Although these programmes have proven to be successful, data show that they only reach a minority of all eligible patients. The fifth EUROASPIRE survey of preventive care in coronary patients reported that only one-third of patients post cardiac event attended a CVPR programme. In fact, less than half (46%) were advised, but if advised, two-thirds (69%) attended.[6] Numerous barriers exist that prevent individuals from participating in cardiovascular risk reduction programmes (➤ Table 11.2). Thus, there is much to be done in order to improve access these programmes.

Table 11.1 Definitions of terms used in prevention

Primordial prevention	Prevention of the development of cardiovascular risk factors in the first place
Primary prevention	Modifying adverse health behaviours and cardiovascular risk factors to reduce the risk of incident CVD
Secondary prevention	Managing cardiovascular risk factors to prevent recurrence of CVD events

Table 11.2 Barriers to participation in cardiovascular risk reduction programmes

Cost	Programmes are not reimbursed sufficiently in many countries and do not cover all groups who should be eligible
Availability	In many countries, programmes are not available
Lack of transportation	Programmes may be located far from where people who need it live and transport is not reimbursed
Complex comorbidities	For example, depression and other mental illnesses, arthritis, and chronic pulmonary disease (see also Chapter 14)
Lack of referral from physicians and other healthcare providers	Programmes are often not seen as an integral part of cardiovascular care and physicians, among others, may not refer their patients or emphasize the importance of attending
Literacy	Ability to understand verbal communication and written information particularly about health and illness management (see also Chapter 13)
Cultural beliefs	Values and perceptions that may be represented in health behaviours and practices (see also Chapter 14)

Wagner's Chronic Care Model (➤ **Fig. 11.1**)[7] captures key components for delivering a successful cardiovascular risk reduction programme. Wagner defines the importance of healthcare systems interfacing with communities to provide self-management and decision-making support[8] (https://www.kingsfund.org.uk/audio-video/edward-wagner-chronic-care-model-and-integrated-care). This outreach is augmented by clinical information systems and healthcare delivery systems. The interface of community with healthcare systems must be patient centred (see also Chapter 2), timely and efficient, and supported by evidence-based guidelines. Careful cooperation

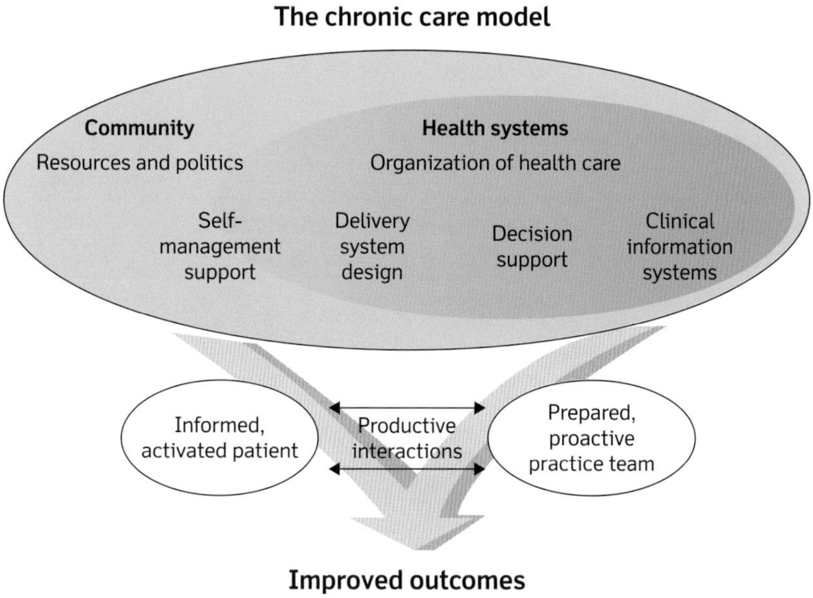

Fig. 11.1 Wagner's Chronic Care Model.

between the community and healthcare systems supports the development of informed and activated patients and families and creates a proactive healthcare team of physicians, nurses, and allied health professionals.

The evidence for multifactor risk reduction

The INTERSTROKE and INTERHEART studies clearly demonstrated that patients suffering from a stroke or an acute myocardial infarction share common cardiovascular risk factors. For stroke risk, these include hypertension, smoking, waist-to-hip ratio (abdominal obesity), physical inactivity, and the ratio of apolipoprotein B to A1. For acute myocardial infarction, similar shared risk factors such as hypertension, smoking, waist-to-hip ratio, and the ratio of apolipoprotein B to A1 were also found. Other important risk cardiovascular factors such as poor diet, diabetes, alcohol intake, psychosocial stress, and depression were predictive of stroke and acute myocardial infarction.[9,10]

Two systematic reviews and meta-analyses of prevention and rehabilitation trials, published in 2016,[11,12] the first reviewing trials of exercise-based cardiac rehabilitation programmes and the second reviewing trials of CVPR programmes, both showed no effect on total mortality (➤ **Table 11.3**). However, a significant effect was seen on cardiovascular mortality in both reviews. Importantly, van Halewijn's et al's review[9] showed in two subanalyses—the first comparing programmes that addressed six or more cardiovascular risk factors with those addressing less, and the second comparing programmes which included medication prescription and monitoring with those that did not—a significant effect on total mortality, demonstrating that a MFRR approach is an effective strategy for prevention and rehabilitation. Focusing on exercise alone is less effective.

➤ **Table 11.4**[13–23] and ➤ **Table 11.5**[14,17,18,20,24–28] show the evolution of the research into MFRR since the 1990s and implementation of this research into clinical practice. Our challenge is to build on this important clinical research and develop similar programmes to offer integrated primary and secondary CVD risk reduction across all ages, ethnicities, and both sexes. Salisbury nicely described how CVPR programmes are an excellent place to create healthy communities.[29] Cardiac rehabilitation programmes are directed by well-educated healthcare professionals and also have resources such as psychosocial counselling, nutrition, and physical activity expertise. Their knowledge regarding the promotion of self-management including shared decision-making and patient-centred care (see also Chapter 2) creates an environment conducive to successful behaviour change. They wisely pointed out that patients want convenience when accessing MFRR programmes. Patients look for individualized care plans, they need the support of healthcare providers including continuity of relationships, and seek healthcare providers

Table 11.3 Systematic reviews of prevention and rehabilitation trials

Randomized controlled trials (RCTs)	Year trials conducted	N of trials	*N* of patient	Effect on total mortality	Effect on cardiovascular mortality
RCTs of exercise-based cardiac rehabilitation[11]	1975–2013	47	12,455	RR 0.96, 95% CI 0.88–1.04	
RCTs of exercise-based cardiac rehabilitation[11]	1975–2013	27	7469		RR 0.74, 95% CI 0.64–0.86
RCTs of prevention and rehabilitation[12]	2010–2015	18	7691	RR 1.00, 95% CI 0.88–1.14	
RCTs of prevention and rehabilitation[12]	2010–2015	4	1046		RR 0.42, 95% CI 0.21–0.88
RCTs of prevention and rehabilitation—subanalysis of programmes addressing 6 or more risk factors[12]	2010–2015	6	2470	0.63, 95% CI 0.43–0.93	
RCTs of prevention and rehabilitation—subanalysis of programmes including medication prescription and monitoring[12]	2010–2015	3	1035	0.35, 95% CI 0.18–0.70	

CI, confidence interval; RR, relative risk.

Table 11.4 Evolution of the research into delivery of multifactor risk reduction programmes

Study name, design (year) and country	Patient population and number	Intervention	Follow-up	Important results
SCRIP RCT[13] (1994) US	Known coronary heart disease 300	Intensive nurse-led case management of multiple cardiovascular risk factors	4 years	1. Reduction in acute myocardial infarction and total cardiac events—rate ratio 0.61 (CI 0.03–0.9) 2. Significant reduction in need for PCI and coronary artery bypass grafting 3. Angiographic evidence of improved atherosclerotic plaque burden compared to usual care
MULTIFIT RCT[14] (1994) US	Post acute myocardial infarction 585	Nurse-led case management of multiple risk factors	1 year	1. Smoking cessation rates: 70% vs 53% ($P = 0.03$) 2. LDL-C 2.77 ± 0.69 mmol/L vs 3.41 ± 0.90 mmol/L (107 ± 30 mg/dL vs 132 ± 30 mg/dL) ($P = 0.001$) 3. Functional capacity 9.3 ± 2.4 METS vs 8.4 ± 2.5 METS ($P = 0.001$)
Grampian RCT[15] (1998) UK	Known coronary heart disease 1343	Nurse-led lifestyle and risk factor consultations in general practice with regular follow-up over 1 year	1, 4, and 10 years	1. At 4 years, cumulative death rates: 14.5% and 18.9%, respectively ($P = 0.038$). 2. At 10 years, survival analysis: proportional hazard ratios were 0.88 (0.74–1.04) for total mortality and 0.96 (0.79–1.18) for coronary death or non-fatal myocardial infarction
CHAMP Quasi experimental design[16] (2001) US	Post acute myocardial infarction 558	Multidisciplinary team approach to ensure hospitalized patients with known coronary disease are discharged with guideline-based therapies	1 year	Significant reduction in total mortality between pre (7%) and post (3.3%) CHAMP groups
COACH RCT[17,18] (2003, 2004) Australia	Known coronary heart disease 792	4 coaching sessions (total 2 hours) from dietitians and nurses to achieve lifestyle and risk factor goals over 6 months	4 years	Despite superior lifestyle and risk factor management in COACH patients, no difference seen in survival but significantly reduced number of hospital admissions (16% any cause) and bed days (15% cardiac; 20% any cause)
COURAGE RCT[19] (2007) US and Canada	Known coronary heart disease 2287	Comparison of optimal medical therapy + PCI with optimal medical therapy alone	Mean 4.7 years	No difference in primary composite death rates between the groups—demonstrated importance of adhering to practice guidelines on medical therapy and deferring PCI in stable coronary heart disease

Continued

Table 11.4 *Continued*

EUROACTION[20] (2008) Europe	Incident coronary heart disease in hospital, and high multifactorial risk in general practice 5396	Intensive nurse-led, family-centred, interdisciplinary programme to manage multiple lifestyle (smoking, diet, and physical activity) and risk factors (weight, blood pressure, lipids, and diabetes) in hospital for coronary heart disease patients and in general practice for high multifactorial risk patients	1 year	In incident coronary heart disease patients in hospital: 1. Fruit and vegetables intake (≥400 g per day) 72% vs 35% $P = 0.004$ 2. Moderate intensity physical activity (≥30 min, ≥4 times per week) 54% vs 20% $P = 0.002$ 3. Blood pressure (<140/90 mmHg; <130/85 mmHg in patients with diabetes) 65% vs 55% $P = 0.04$
COACH—community outreach and cardiovascular health RCT[21] (2011) US	Known coronary heart disease, hypercholesterolaemia, hypertension, diabetes type 2 (African American or Caucasian) 525	Nurse practitioners and community health workers led aggressive pharmacological management and tailored educational and behavioural counselling for lifestyle modification and problem-solving to address barriers to adherence and control	1 year	Significant improvements in: 1. LDL-C (difference, 15.9 mg/dL) 2. Triglycerides (difference, 16.3 mg/dL) 3. Systolic blood pressure (difference, 6.2 mmHg) 4. HbA1c (difference, 0.5%) 5. Perceptions of the quality of their care (difference, 1.2 points)
RESPONSE[22,23] (2013, 2017) The Netherlands	Post acute myocardial infarction	Nurse-led consultations for 6 months to manage lifestyle and risk factors in hospital and community setting	1 year	1. 17.4% reduction in estimated 10-year cardiovascular mortality 2. 7–9 risk factors at goal in 35% vs 24.7% $P = 0.003$

Table 11.5 Translating MFRR evidence into working models of care

The model of care	Country and health system where implemented	Evidence supporting model of care
The Stanford Chronic Care Management System: home care for patients with chronic conditions (e.g. heart failure, coronary heart disease) The Stanford Cardiac Rehabilitation Programme—MULTIFIT—care management programme for chronic diseases	US Stanford University and the Kaiser Permanente Health Care System 2015: Moving Analytics, Inc. given an exclusive licence to use MULTIFIT—includes remote care management programmes for coronary heart disease, heart failure, diabetes, hypertension, and acute coronary syndrome. http://www.stanfordchroniccaresystem.com/about.html	14
MyAction for Our Hearts (see also 'Integrated models of community-based cardiovascular disease care')	UK National Health Service and CROI Heart Charity in Galway in collaboration with Ireland Health Service Executive MyAction Pilot, Bromley, Southeast London, UK NHS Cardiovascular Health and Rehabilitation Service, Imperial College Healthcare NHS Trust, London UK Our Hearts Our Minds, Western Health and Social Care Trust, Eniskillen, Northern Ireland CROI Heart and Stroke Centre, Galway, Western Ireland	20,24–27
Heart to Heart Project	The Stanford and San Mateo County Heart to Heart Project, US http://med.stanford.edu/ppop/heart.html	28
COACH Program https://www.thecoachprogram.com/telemedicine/	Throughout the public health system in Australia	17,18

with skills in behavioural change techniques, medical therapies, and communication skills.

The important role of nurses

Nurses have an important role to play in the implementation of MFRR programmes. Many of the studies mentioned previously included programmes that were coordinated and led by nurses. A systematic review and meta-analysis from 2016[30] of 12 trials of secondary prevention of CVD conducted between 1994 and 2008 including 4886 patients showed significant reductions in total mortality (0.78, 95% confidence interval (CI) 0.65–0.95) and improvements in both adherence to lipid-lowering therapy (1.57, 95% CI 1.14–2.17) and antiplatelet therapy (1.42, 95% CI 1.01–1.98).

Nurses are equipped to lead these programmes for a number of reasons. They are accustomed to working closely with the medical profession and to implementing medical decisions about care. They follow professional recommendations and protocols well and are trained to understand symptoms and monitor patients' signs, such as blood pressure. They are also trained to safely administer medicines and are familiar with medications, doses, potential medication interactions, and side effects. In some countries, legislation now permits nurses and other health professionals, for example, nurse practitioners and pharmacists, to have prescribing rights. While this has been driven by economic circumstances, diminishing numbers of physicians and unavailability of health services in rural areas has been challenging. Enabling nurse practitioners and pharmacists has proven to be safe and successful with patients, physicians, and nurses who report a higher quality of care and greater flexibility and convenience for patients and their families (see also Chapter 12).

However, as importantly, nurses bring a holistic and health-promoting approach to care. Nurse training and bachelor degree programmes incorporate the medical, biological, social, and behavioural sciences as well as health psychology. In addition, nurses are taught to use counselling and teaching skills. This prepares them for a holistic approach to care as opposed to the disease-oriented approach. Rather, they see their patients in the context of their physical, psychological, and spiritual needs, their family, and their social environment. The promotion of health, nurture, and caring are central to the profession of nursing and an integral part of their expertise. It is this model of care which they adopt rather than the medical model.

Nurses are formally taught management theory, because, in their professional role, they are required to coordinate interdisciplinary care delivered by nursing teams and other disciplines. This includes physiotherapists, pharmacists, and occupational therapists, who provide important care for their patients. They learn to become managers from an early stage in their career when they are put in charge of overseeing groups of hospitalized patients. They learn to cope with patients' emotional and medical problems because they are the professional who spend the most time with patients. They have time to listen, perhaps during the administration of basic care. They have to cope with patients' anger, their fears, and their denial. They have to deal with death and dying and loss. They are the frontline to deal with families, relatives, and friends.

Having the knowledge, skills, and experience equips nurses with skills which they can apply to the management of preventive and rehabilitative care. Nurses must know their capabilities, access adequate training for extended roles, accept their limitations, and know when it is appropriate to refer to other disciplines or to seek the advice of physicians. For example, in the UK, nurses are governed by the Nursing and Midwifery Council and its code of professional conduct (https://www.nmc.org.uk/standards/code/), and they have access to university modules and in-service training to further their knowledge and give them extra skills. Provision of this kind varies between countries.

In taking on this management role, nurses work closely with physicians who provide the medical leadership to ensure that prevention and rehabilitation programmes are an integral part of the care plan. Nursing responsibilities in hospitals and clinical practice settings includes the management of cardiovascular patients. Physicians are responsible for encouraging patients to participate in prevention and rehabilitation programmes. Close collaboration between nurses and physicians is required to ensure that risk factor management and medications therapies are optimal. With physician support, patients are more likely to participate in programmes and achieve their healthcare goals. Both nursing and medical professionals are important to successful healthcare. As nurses assume more responsibility for medical decision-making and achieve advanced skills (physical assessment, nurse prescribing), implementation of medical decisions becomes much more collaborative (see also Chapter 3). Nurse-coordinated care is applied differently based on individual country health cultures. It is dependent upon the professional standing and provision for expanding roles (see also Chapter 3) and physician/nurse ratios by country.

Nurses do not work in isolation from other professionals. Working in collaboration, not only with physicians but with an interdisciplinary approach, is essential. A transdisciplinary approach may be preferable to a multidisciplinary approach where single disciplines work in silos with no reference to each other to coordinate preventive care which requires a broad spectrum of expertise. The transdisciplinary team recommended to deliver a CVPR service ideally includes a specialist nurse, dietician, physiotherapist or exercise specialist, psychologist, pharmacist, occupational therapist, vocational counsellor, social worker, and supported by a cardiologist.[31]

Examples of research evaluations of practice models which were subsequently implemented in clinical practice can be seen in ➤ **Table 11.5**. Further on in this chapter we describe the components of prevention and rehabilitation and the settings in which they can be delivered.

Family

In order to be successful with implementing primary and secondary prevention of CVD, we need to focus on barriers that prevent patients from achieving MFRR. A key component of this is the family, including both younger and older generations. Lloyd-Jones and others found a strong association between a family history of premature heart disease and adult-onset coronary artery disease.[32] The association is strong when there is a parent and a sibling with premature disease. Also, children whose parents develop early CVD tend to be more obese, have worse lipid profiles, are more likely to be hypertensive, have glucose abnormalities, and other physiological measurements associated with cardiac and other vascular diseases.[33] Children in high-risk families have a higher risk of developing CVD risk factors and CVD due to genetic susceptibility, lifestyle behaviours, and commonly shared environmental factors. Importantly, they also showed that family history does not necessarily predict improved CVD reduction behaviours.

The Multi Ethnic Study of Atherosclerosis (MESA), showed that for Caucasians, African Americans, Hispanics, and American Chinese, the prevalence of a family history of CVD predicted a higher Framingham Risk Score for those under 10% and for those between 10% and 20% measured risk.[34] A history of CVD in the family indicates a higher risk for family members. Results of a very recent study designed to examine the association between parental cardiovascular health (CVH) and time to onset of CVD in offspring found that maternal CVH was a more robust predictor of an offspring's CVD-free survival than paternal CVH.[35] In this analysis of data generated from the Framingham Heart Study, offspring of mothers with ideal cardiovascular health (ICVH) lived 9 more years free of CVD than offspring of mothers with poor cardiovascular health (P<0.001). Maternal poor CVH was associated with a twice as high hazard rate of early-onset CVD compared with maternal ICVH (adj. hazard rate = 2.09, 95% CI 1.50–2.92). Collectively, results underscore the importance of family in CVD prevention and suggest the need for clinical and policy interventions that break the intergenerational cycle of CVD-related morbidity and mortality. It has also been shown that parental lifestyle influences childhood behaviours. Steinberger and colleagues[33] evaluated television watching plus an overweight parent in children. They found that the children with more than 1 hour of TV watching per day or an overweight parent had a higher likelihood of developing CVD risk factors during their lives. They also found that families who consumed a Mediterranean diet, one high in fruits, vegetables, wholegrains, and fish plus healthy oils, had a beneficial effect on the cardiovascular risk factors in adults and their children. Families are critically important for successful primary and secondary CVD prevention programmes.

Ageing

The world's population is ageing and data show clearly that older adults benefit from CVD prevention programmes. The global median age, as reported by 'Our World in Data', was 21.5 years in 1970 and 30 years in 2019 (https://ourworldindata.org/age-structure). This report showed that 8% are older than 65 years, with half of the world's population working between 25 and 65 years of age. Focusing preventive measures across all ages is a clear direction for prevention programmes and research.

It is known that chronic diseases in males and females increase by age. Uijen and colleagues studied men and women across the age span of 24 to 75 years of age.[36] They identified the presence of one or more chronic diseases (hypertension, diabetes mellitus, ischaemic heart disease, chronic obstructive pulmonary disease, osteoarthritis of the knee or hip) by age groups. The presence of three or more risk factors for those over 75 years of age was approximately 85%, between the ages of 65 to 74 years was approximately 70%, and between the ages of 45 and 64 years was approximately 42%. Thus, comprehensive MFRR is necessary across the lifespan.

Technology

Innovation and technology have been shown to benefit both primary and secondary prevention services and are becoming essential in clinical care. The Internet provides access to important health information and is the most commonly used source for health-related topics. In addition, increasingly more people are using their smartphones and other technology to access healthcare information. In 2016, Google processed greater than 1 trillion searches per year or about 90 billion searches per month regarding healthcare. The Internet has been shown to be successful in delivering behaviourally guided weight loss programmes and programmes for heart failure management and cardiovascular risk factor modification.[37–39] Burke and colleagues looked at consumer use of mobile health for CVD prevention and provided an overview in a scientific statement from the American Heart Association (AHA).[40] They encouraged embracing the challenge to produce new evidence on the effectiveness of technology and how this evidence can be adopted into clinical practice and help support primary and secondary CVD prevention. Later on in this chapter, examples of innovation in technology for delivering prevention and rehabilitation interventions are described and discussed.

Primordial and primary prevention of cardiovascular disease: supporting evidence, challenges, and opportunities for nurses and nursing

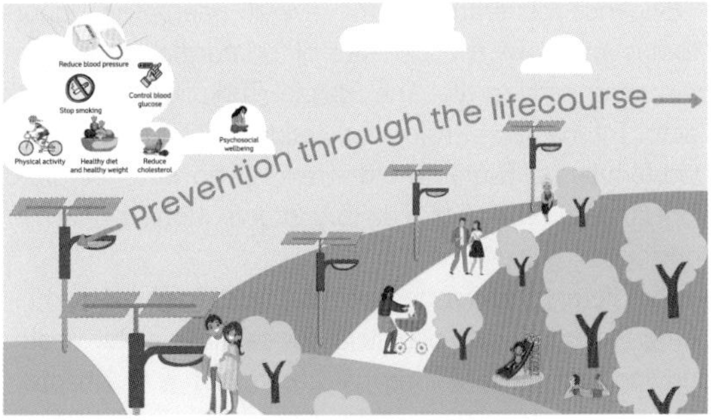

What is primordial and primary prevention?

While there is substantial evidence for the effectiveness of nurse case-managed secondary CVD prevention programmes globally in both clinical and community-based settings, there is considerably less research focused on the important role of nurses and nursing in primordial prevention. Primary prevention focuses on modifying adverse health behaviours and risk factors to reduce the risk of incident CVD (➤ **Table 11.1**). The global prevalence and trends in the intra-individual clustering of risk factors (obesity, hypertension, dyslipidaemia) and adverse health behaviours points to the importance of primary prevention efforts.[41] Primordial prevention, prevention of the development of risk factors in the first place, includes both individual/clinical approaches while emphasizing macrolevel strategies such as environmental and policy initiatives that enable development and maintenance of healthy behaviours.[42] The AHA has prompted considerable global attention on primordial and primary prevention and the promotion of ICVH across the lifespan.[43]

Addressing lifestyle and risk factors early in life

Most children are born with ICVH as operationalized by AHA metrics that include four health behaviours (smoking status, body-mass index (BMI), physical activity, and healthy diet score) and three health factors (total cholesterol, blood pressure, and fasting plasma glucose). Substantial data generated from clinical and epidemiological studies indicate that atherosclerotic processes begin early in life and are influenced over time by potentially modifiable behaviours, health factors, and environmental exposures.[44,45] Data also indicate that individuals who maintain optimal levels of established risk factors for CVD through adult life have dramatically lower lifetime CVD risk and longer survival than their adult counterparts who developed one or more risk factors earlier in life.[46]

Evidence generated from several paediatric cohort studies highlight the benefits of primordial prevention beginning early in life. The Special Turku Coronary Risk Factor Intervention Project for Children (STRIP), randomized families of 6-month-old infants (who were recruited from clinics in Turku) to a dietary intervention ($n = 540$) or control ($n = 522$).[47]

The dietary intervention was designed to guide participants towards a diet beneficial for cardiovascular health and focused on replacing saturated fats with unsaturated fats. Individualized dietary counselling transitioned from parent to child at approximately 7 years of age, continued at least biannually until 20 years of age, and also focused on reduction of salt intake and increase in wholegrain products, fruit, and vegetables. At follow-up in adolescence, those in the control group who received usual paediatric primary care had increased risk of low ICVH (≤ 3 metrics) compared with intervention adolescents; the number of ICVH metrics was inversely associated with aortic intima–media thickness ($P < 0.0001$) while the risk of high intima–media thickness (>85th percentile) was substantially higher in adolescents with a low number of ICVH metrics compared with those with a higher score (risk ratio = 1.78, 95% CI 1.31–2.43). In another analyses of STRIP data, conducted when participants were 20 years of age, the long-term relative risk of metabolic syndrome was significantly lower in the intervention group (relative risk 0.59, 95% CI, 0.40–0.88; $P < 0.009$).[48] Taken together, the results from this landmark study support the importance of clinical, individual, and family-focused life course approaches to primordial prevention of CVD and provided evidence to inform guidelines for promoting cardiovascular health early in life.[49]

The importance of psychosocial factors and health inequalities

Adding to the evidence supporting life course approaches to primordial prevention are findings from the Cardiovascular Risk in Young Finns Study, a multicentre study that included participants ($n = 1089$) who were 3–18 years of age at baseline.[50] A major aim was to examine the cumulative effect of psychosocial exposures and factors (socioeconomic and emotional environments, life events, self-regulation, health behaviours, social adjustment) in youth on AHA-defined ICVH in adulthood. Results indicated that a favourable socioeconomic environment and participants' self-regulatory behaviour were the strongest predictors of ICVH 27 years later in adulthood. Of note, individuals exhibiting favourable levels in all psychosocial factors in youth had the healthiest profiles in adulthood. In contrast, highlighting the association of adverse environmental exposures and experiences in early life and cardiometabolic health in adulthood are results from several studies summarized in a statement from the AHA. This statement supported the need for both individual and population-based primordial prevention.[51] Central to population-based prevention and to reducing disparities in cardiovascular health are macrolevel strategies targeting contexts in which healthy lifestyles develop and are maintained.

Relevant contexts include family, schools, worksites, and communities (including the built environment and quality and quantity of available foods). As suggested in socioecological models of health and behaviour, local, national, and global policies that influence these contexts are of critical importance. For example, local and national school policies impact the food and physical activity environments of schools, recognized venues for population-based primordial and primary prevention for children and youth.[52] The MESA study provides evidence reaffirming associations between neighbourhood characteristics (socioeconomic status, availability of healthy foods, and outlets for physical activity) and level of cardiovascular health.[53] Harper and colleagues[54] suggest that the interactions among early-life socioeconomic environments/contexts and risk factor trajectories influence both the development and maintenance of health behaviours and their 'cumulative biologic' sequelae as part of a major life course process linking socioeconomic position in early life to CVD in adulthood.

Which public health measures are the most important?

Collectively, the accumulated evidence supports life-course clinical and population-based approaches and strategies in order to realize optimal cardiovascular health for diverse populations. A 2019 global impact assessment analysis argues convincingly for three public health interventions that have potential to save approximately 100 million lives globally within 25 years.[55] Specifically, the high-impact interventions targeted are improving treatment of high blood pressure to 70%, reducing sodium intake by 30%, and eliminating the intake of artificial trans fatty acids. Of note, programmes and policies targeting these interventions have been shown to be effective but will require multipronged approaches with tailoring to region/country-specific needs and resources. Increasing coverage for the identification of hypertension and treatment will require availability of and access to medications, blood pressure monitors, dose-specific treatment protocols, expansion of primary healthcare coverage, and healthcare information systems that facilitate tracking and monitoring of rates of treatment and control. Policies that target primary sources of sodium in each country will be required to reduce sodium intake by 30%. Since it is well established that packaged food and food eaten away from the home are major contributors to sodium intake worldwide, evidence-based policy options focused on industry targets, front-of-pack labelling, and institutional food standards in schools, government offices, and other institutions are recommended. In low- and middle-income countries, homemade food is the major source of sodium intake indicating a need for public education and media campaigns to reduce intake. Similarly, policies and regulatory mechanisms will facilitate the elimination of trans fat worldwide. Of note, approximately 23 countries have such regulations (as of 2018) and the WHO has offered specific recommendations including promoting replacement with healthier oils, and creating awareness among industry, policymakers, and consumers.[56]

How can nurses help?

The potential for primordial prevention to promote optimal cardiovascular health on a global level has been demonstrated. While multilevel efforts will be essential in realizing the World Heart Federation and AHA goals for cardiovascular health, nurses are the largest healthcare discipline managing CVD risk factors globally and are well positioned in healthcare and community settings to implement evidence-based, country/region-specific prevention guidelines.

Recognizing the importance of policies necessary to create healthy food and physical environments, access to affordable, quality healthcare, and as advocates for the health of the public worldwide, nurses must participate in targeted activities designed to allocate resources and increase capacity for promoting primordial as well as primary prevention.

Conclusion

In summary, it is time to embrace the multifactor, multilevel challenges and opportunities for improved CVD prevention. Focusing on guideline-based multifactor care management for multiple comorbidities, along with the emerging importance of technology, will help us to better manage community-based patients living at home with CVD, stroke, and for those with high-risk comorbidities. Medical therapies and interventions must be easily available, accessible, affordable, and financially supported to improve utilization. Optimizing prevention across the life course includes primordial, primary, and secondary interventions. As such, prevention begins early in life, extends beyond the individual level, and includes contexts/environments where healthy behaviours and lifestyles are developed and the policies that impact those environments. Successful prevention is also family focused and addresses the unique needs of the family across the lifespan. Telemedicine, computers, handheld devices, and wearable and other technologies are important advancements for home and community-based care. Computer-based support is essential including social media, email, Internet, text messaging, and the use of iPhone reminders. By expanding our reach, developing our tools for prevention, and coordinating care across all ages and communities, we can provide the much-needed services of primordial, primary, and secondary prevention around the world.

Concept of total cardiovascular risk and total risk management

In the previous section, we defined primordial, primary, and secondary prevention of CVD. While primordial prevention of CVD is very important, this chapter focuses principally on primary and secondary prevention. In order to define the patient population eligible for primary and secondary prevention, the European Society of Cardiology (ESC) has categorized risk into four levels[57] and described methods to assess the level of risk in individuals (➤ Table. 11.6). This allows us to focus efforts on the right people (see also Chapter 1).

Risk assessment plays a central role in CVPR and is a key component of CVD prevention guidelines in most countries across the globe. Yet, despite the use of this risk estimation in clinical practice across Europe, implementation of MFRR is suboptimal.[58] A large majority of individuals at high CVD risk are not achieving the recommended blood pressure, lipid, diabetes, and lifestyle goals.[59] This calls for wider utilization of risk assessment tools, which are specific to different patient groups, are efficient to use, accurate, and support a more personalized approach to communicating risk.[60] Adding a MFRR score into the electronic medical record can support clinicians in identifying and initiating MFRR counselling and treatment.[17,61] Assessment of total cardiovascular risk in individuals should be multifactorial, which represents a paradigm shift from the traditional approach of treating single risk factors in isolation. This is because the total risk of developing CVD (the probability of having an event over a given period of time) is determined by the combined effect of cardiovascular risk factors present, including age, sex/gender, smoking status, blood pressure, and total cholesterol[62] or body mass index (BMI). For example, an individual with several mildly raised risk factors may be at a higher total risk of CVD than someone with just one elevated risk factor; this is demonstrated in ➤ Table 11.7.[57] Evidence from randomized controlled trials shows that assessment based on total risk leads to more optimal prevention with a strong association between the level of the patient's pre-intervention total CVD risk and the degree of treatment benefit.[61]

Risk estimation tools are useful for clinicians in identifying individuals at high multifactorial risk for CVD and directing the intensity of the prevention intervention accordingly. Estimating CVD risk forms the basis for initiating a conversation with the patient about risk reduction strategies, leading to shared decision-making regarding lifestyle goals, medical risk factor management, and the initiation and adjustment of preventive

Table 11.6 Risk categories

Very high-risk	Subjects with any of the following. • Documented CVD, clinical or unequivocal on imaging. Documented clinical CVD includes previous AMI, ACS, coronary revascularization and other arterial revascularization procedures, stroke and TIA, aortic aneurysm and PAD, Unequivocally documented CVD on imaging includes significant plaque on coronary angiography or carotid ultrasound. It does NOT include some increase in continuous imaging parameters such as intima-media thickness of the carotid artery. • DM with target organ damage such as proteinuria or with a major risk factor such as smoking or marked hypercholesterolaemia or marked hypertension. • Severe CKD (GFR <30 mL/min/1.73 m2). • A calculated SCORE ≥10%.
High-risk	Subjects with: • Markedly elevated single risk factors, in particular cholesterol >8 mmol/L (>310 mg/dL) (e.g. in familial hypercholesterolaemia) or BP ≥180/110 mmHg. • Most other people with DM (with the exception of young people with type I DM and without major risk factors that may be at low or moderate risk). • Moderate CKD (GFR 30–59 mL/min/1.73 m²). • A calculated SCORE ≥5% and <10%.
Moderate risk	SCORE is ≥1% and <5% at 10 years. Many middle aged subjects belong to this category.
Low-risk	SCORE <1%

ACS = acute coronary syndrome; AMI = acute myocardial infarction; BP = blood pressure; CKD = chronic kidney disease; DM = diabetes mellitus; GFR = Glomerular filtration rate; PAD = peripheral artery disease; SCORE = systematic coronary risk estimation; TIA = transient ischaemic attack.

Table 11.7 Impact of combinations of risk factors on SCORE 10-year risk of fatal cardiovascular disease

Sex	Age (years)	Cholesterol (mmol/L)	SBP (mmHg)	Smoker	Risk (10-year risk of fatal CVD)
F	60	7	120	No	2%
F	60	7	140	Yes	5%
M	60	6	160	No	9%
M	60	5	180	Yes	21%

SBP, systolic blood pressure.

medication (avoiding undertreatment of high-risk patients and overtreatment of low-risk patients) as appropriate.

How to estimate total cardiovascular disease risk

Adopting a total risk approach to CVD prevention ensures that individuals at highest CVD risk gain the most from preventive measures. There are several tools that can be used to estimate cardiovascular risk and all have their own unique features which should be considered prior to use.[60] European guidelines recommend estimating risk in apparently healthy individuals using the Systematic Coronary Risk Evaluation (SCORE) tool.[57] SCORE predicts the likelihood of fatal CVD events, with the threshold for very high risk being defined as a risk of death of 10% or greater. The level of 10-year CVD risk whether low (<1%), moderate (≥1% to 5%), high (≥5% to <10%), or very high (≥10%) should guide the intensity of the preventive action. To learn more about utilizing the SCORE risk estimation tool in clinical practice and the various categories of risk, please visit the ESC website (https://www.escardio.org).[63] Risk can also be estimated using charts where access to the electronic tool is unavailable (https://www.escardio.org/Education/Practice-Tools/CVD-prevention-toolbox/SCORE-Risk-Charts). While SCORE has many advantages in terms of its intuitive nature and objective assessment of risk, it is only suitable for apparently healthy individuals between 40 and 65 years of age. It is not suitable for patients over 65 years of age as it will overestimate risk and is not intended for use in patients with established CVD as these patients are automatically considered high risk. The use of SCORE in young people with multiple risk factors poses a challenge as a low absolute risk may conceal a high relative risk, which would require intensive lifestyle modification. To overcome this, the relative risk chart is recommended for use,[57] demonstrating to young people that through making the recommended lifestyle changes, risk can be significantly reduced. Risk age is another effective tool for communicating with young people with a low absolute risk. The risk age of a person with multiple CVD risk factors is the age of a person with the same level of risk, but with risk factors within recommended levels.[57]

To address CVD risk across all patient categories, ensuring optimization of patient outcomes, there are increasing calls for different risk algorithms for different population groups.[60] For example the Second Manifestation of Arterial Disease (SMART) risk score (https://www.escardio.org/Education/ESC-Prevention-of-CVD-Programme/Risk-assessment/SMART-Risk-Score) is suitable for estimating risk in patients with previous CVD. It recognizes that not all CVD patients are alike and that there can be variation in 10-year risk. In addition, given the very high-risk status of these patients, tools such as SMART can provide ongoing motivation regarding adherence to a healthy lifestyle and medication adherence.

Risk estimation tools provide objective estimates of CVD risk and their use should be complementary to clinical decision-making, while promoting patient empowerment and self-management. The utilization of health behaviour change techniques is an essential component to communicating CVD risk effectively and engaging the patient in the shared decision-making process. With many high-risk patients remaining undiagnosed and untreated,[59] all opportunities whether systematic or opportunistic to identify patients at increased CVD risk must be promoted.

Components of prevention and rehabilitation in clinical practice

Lifestyle and risk factor management

As described earlier in this chapter, nurses play an important role in an interdisciplinary approach in preventive and rehabilitation programmes. They have the important clinical skills for monitoring and managing lifestyle and risk factors across the age span. The ESC Guidelines in collaboration with experts from the disciplines of dietetics, physical activity, exercise, medicine, psychology, and social care provide nurses with knowledge and tools to become effective CVD prevention specialists. In this section, we will cover the principles of this practice and cross-reference to other resources as appropriate. The settings in which this care can be delivered will be covered in 'Settings and delivery modes for cardiovascular prevention and rehabilitation'.

Adverse lifestyle habits—smoking, poor diet, and sedentary behaviour—are associated with obesity, raised blood pressure, abnormal lipid profiles, and glucose dysregulation. All of these factors are linked to premature mortality from CVD (see also Chapter 1). Therefore, priorities for intervention should include support to stop smoking, to adopt a healthy diet, to increase physical activity and exercise, and to manage body weight using behavioural approaches and taking psychosocial factors into account. In addition, medication will be required in most cases to manage blood pressure, lipids, and diabetes. Nurses are well positioned within the healthcare system to support patients with adherence to these therapies.

All of these risk factors should be managed to the goals outlined in the evidence-based guidelines. The ESC has multiple resources to facilitate this management. Health professionals can access evidence-based clinical practice guidelines on the ESC website (https://www.escardio.org/Guidelines/Clinical-Practice-Guidelines). The following guidelines are relevant to preventive care:

- 2021 ESC Guidelines on cardiovascular disease prevention in clinical practice. Developed by the Task Force for CVD prevention in clinical practice with representatives of the European Society of Cardiology and 12 medical societies. With the special contribution of the European Association of Preventive Cardiology (EAPC).[57]
- '2018 ESC/ESH Guidelines for the management of arterial hypertension: the Task Force for the management of arterial hypertension of the European Society of Cardiology (ESC) and the European Society of Hypertension (ESH).'[64]
- '2019 ESC/EAS Guidelines for the management of dyslipidaemias: lipid modification to reduce cardiovascular risk: the Task Force for the management of dyslipidaemias of the European Society of Cardiology (ESC) and European Atherosclerosis Society (EAS).'[65]
- '2019 ESC Guidelines on diabetes, pre-diabetes, and cardiovascular diseases developed in collaboration with the EASD: the Task Force for diabetes, pre-diabetes, and cardiovascular diseases of the European Society of Cardiology (ESC) and the European Association for the Study of Diabetes (EASD).'[66]

The ESC Guidelines webpage also includes a number of tools to facilitate implementation of guidelines in clinical practice, including summary cards and pocket guidelines. There is also a pocket guidelines app (https://www.escardio.org/Guidelines/Clinical-Practice-Guidelines/Guidelines-derivative-products/ESC-Mobile-Pocket-Guidelines) which can be downloaded to a smart device. ACNAP has a toolkit (https://www.escardio.org/Sub-specialty-communities/Association-of-Cardiovascular-Nursing-&-Allied-Professions/Education/be-guidelines-smart) which provides materials to empower nurses to participate in guidelines implementation. The ESC Association of Preventive Cardiology website (https://www.escardio.org/Sub-specialty-communities/European-Association-of-Preventive-Cardiology-(EAPC)/Education) has an education section and prevention toolbox.

Supporting patients and families to make healthy lifestyle changes

In order to successfully support healthy lifestyle changes in our patients, there are a number of factors to take into account. These include the different ways in which people define and view their health,[67] beliefs and perceptions patients may have about their condition, the social and environmental context in which people are living, psychological comorbidities, and the level of support from family, carers, friends, and colleagues. Health behaviours are influenced by all of these factors. For example, cultural beliefs and habits in relation to food, legislation pertaining to tobacco and unhealthy foods, the cost of healthy foods, provision of exercise facilities in the built environment, social support, stressful work environments, and psychological factors such as anxiety and depression. Nurses and other health professionals need to have an understanding of these complexities in order to prepare themselves for supporting

Box 11.1 The environmental context and behavioural change

Example: people make lifestyle choices in the context of their environment. An understanding of the environmental context allows more empathy when addressing behavioural change, for example, quitting smoking. This context may include the following:

1. Social pressure—the rest of the family smokes; friends, carer(s), and others in the leisure environment smoke.
2. Social isolation—there is no one to reinforce the messages the patient receives from the nurse, no 'buddy' to accompany them in this task, no one to encourage them and give them confidence.
3. Psychological need—smoking may be perceived as being one of the only comforts the patient has in life, a way of coping with stress at work and in general.
4. Social conditioning—smoking may be seen as the social norm. Anecdotal accounts of longevity associated with smoking may be recounted.
5. Socioeconomic status—smoking is more prevalent in manual compared to non-manual workers and those with a lower educational attainment.
6. The government receives substantial revenue from cigarette taxes and is therefore reluctant to take drastic measures such as banning cigarette advertising to reduce the prevalence of smoking.

individuals and families to change their lifestyle. ➤ Box 11.1 demonstrates how the environment may influence people in relation to making behavioural changes.

Other influencing factors for healthy change include the balance of power between professionals and patients. Patients and family members should feel empowered to make healthy choices and not coerced to do so. A helping partnership empowers patients to take control of their illness, set their own priorities for change, and to engage in self-care and self-management. Sharing information, sharing agenda setting, and planning jointly, all encourage patients to participate in shared decision-making. Motivation and intention to initiate behaviour changes requires professional follow-up and support. Effective communication and counselling skills are essential to encourage the initiation of these changes.

Theories and approaches to health behaviour change

Over the years, several empirical theories have been described in the literature to explain health behaviour change such as the Health Belief model,[68] the theory of self-efficacy,[69] and the transtheoretical model.[70] More recently, Michie and colleagues have developed a taxonomy of behaviour change strategies used in clinical practice[71] and elaborated the COM-B model (➤ **Fig. 11.2**) for behaviour change[71] which categorizes the ability for individuals to make changes according to their capability (available knowledge, skills, and capacity to engage in desired behaviour), opportunity (factors external to an individual that allow or prompt them to engage in a behaviour), and their motivation (all brain processes that lead an individual to decide to behave in a certain way). ➤ Fig. 11.3[72] outlines the complexity of the change process and characterizes interventions and how they relate to policy and behaviour.

A pragmatic approach to helping people change behaviours, which was first used for addiction treatment, is motivational interviewing.[73] This strategy is based on a number of principles:

- Encouraging patients to take an active role in therapy.
- Enhancing internal motivation.
- Encouraging patients to explore and resolve ambivalence.
- Exchanging information rather than 'telling' to find solutions.
- Developing a collaborative relationship between professional and patient.
- Drawing on patient's resources and motivation.
- Allowing autonomy and avoiding being authoritative.
- Resisting the 'righting' reflex.
- Supporting self-efficacy.

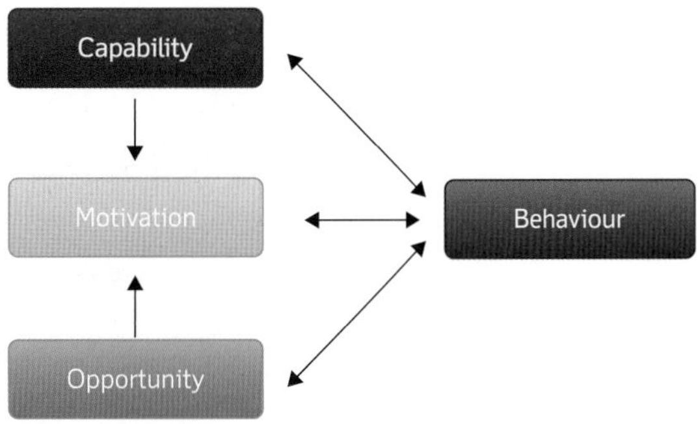

Fig. 11.2 The COM-B Model.
http://www.behaviourchangewheel.com/about-wheel.

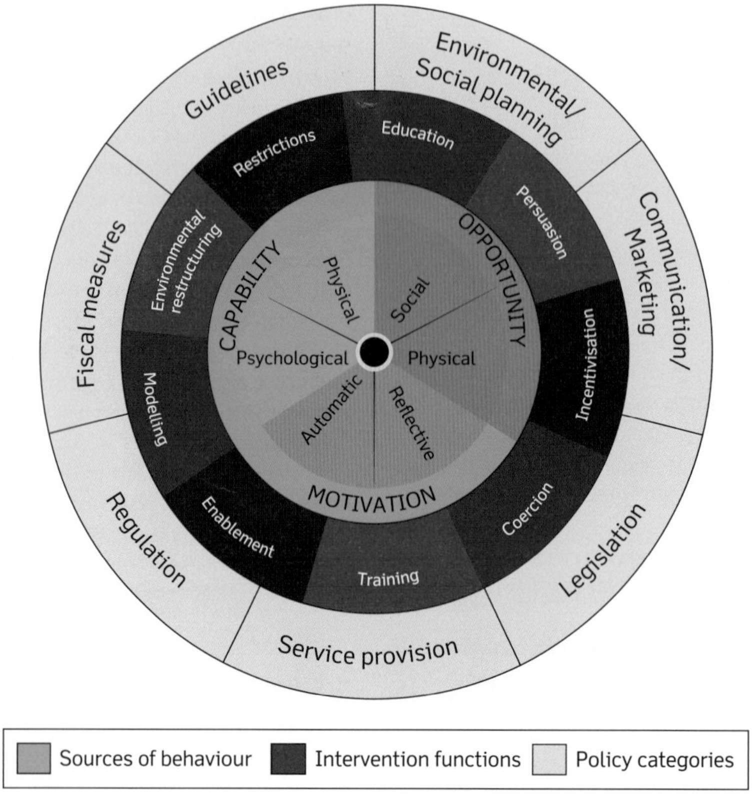

Fig. 11.3 The Behaviour Change Wheel.

- Using a counselling approach which includes expressing empathy and active listening techniques (➤ Box 11.2).

The important contribution of family members and other caregivers should also be stressed in relation to making behaviour change more successful.

Box 11.2 Using OARS principles when counselling patients

Open-ended questions: 'Since you had your heart attack there are a number of things that are concerning you. What would you like to talk about first?'

Affirmation: 'It takes a lot of strength and determination to stay away from smoking like you have done over the last week.'

Reflective listening: 'I can see that you are quite concerned you may have another heart attack.'

Summarizing: 'So we have talked about ... and you have decided that you would like to ...'

Use of behavioural approaches includes the negotiation of realistic goals using 'SMART' principles. Goals should be specific, measurable, achievable, realistic, and timely and graded so that they represent what will be achieved in both the longer and shorter ('1 day at a time' goals) terms. Follow-up and progress monitoring towards reaching goals, managing lapses and problems, and developing a contingency plan to prevent relapse is essential.

Tobacco and smoking cessation management

All patients and families should be supported to become tobacco free. The risks associated with continued tobacco use and the benefits of quitting are clear.[74–76] The best way to achieve and maintain abstinence in cardiac patients and their families is to integrate tobacco cessation support into CVPR programmes. In order to do this, nurses and other members of the interdisciplinary team require training in skills to support patients and families in a quit attempt. In the UK, there is a national centre for smoking cessation and training which provides online training internationally

Box 11.3 The 5As

- *Always* ask your patients about smoking.
- *Advise* those who are smoking to quit.
- *Assess* nicotine dependence in smokers and motivation to quit.
- *Agree* on a treatment plan which encompasses counselling and pharmacology in those motivated to quit.
- *Arrange* follow-up.

(https://elearning.ncsct.co.uk/). The '5As' (➤ **Box 11.3**) provide a reminder of the steps to be taken by all health professionals practising in any setting preparing themselves to provide tobacco cessation support.

The basis for a successful quit attempt is a comprehensive assessment which incorporates the following:

- Smoking status and biomarker validation.
- Measurement of nicotine dependence.
- Readiness to quit and when (e.g. in a month or in 6 months).
- Motivation—importance and confidence. Identify ambivalence.
- Past quit attempts.
- Psychological comorbidities (e.g. depression).
- Others in the household who smoke.

Assessing smoking status

Smoking status can be assessed using the following questions:

1. Have you ever smoked?
2. How many years have you smoked?
3. How long ago did you stop smoking?
4. Do you smoke now?

Self-reported smoking status is more reliable if validated with a biomarker. An expired breath carbon monoxide monitor provides a pragmatic way to measure this in a clinical setting because it is inexpensive, provides an immediate result, and has the benefit of visual demonstration of the harms of tobacco to patients.

Assessing dependence on tobacco

The nicotine contained in tobacco is extremely addictive, which is why the early stage of a quit attempt is challenging. Once dependent on tobacco, being deprived of a cigarette induces 'nicotine hunger' in a smoker which manifests in several symptoms of withdrawal including irritability, aggression, depression, restlessness, anxiety, poor concentration, light-headedness, insomnia, and urges to smoke. Most of these symptoms will disappear within 1 month of quitting, although urges to smoke can persist or re-emerge some time after a quit attempt has been made. However, it is reassuring to be able to tell patients that they are not likely to feel the discomfort of physical withdrawal a month beyond their quit date.

Smokers with a high dependency on nicotine will benefit most from pharmacological and counselling support during their quit attempt. Many cardiac and high CVD risk patients who are smokers will fall into this category as they have been smoking several cigarettes per day for many years. Validated available measures of nicotine dependence include the Heavy Smoking Index[77] (➤ **Table 11.8**) and the Fagerström Test for Nicotine Dependence.[78] The most important indicators of dependence are time of the first cigarette of the day and number of cigarettes smoked per day. A higher score on both measures is an indicator of higher dependence.

Table 11.8 Heavy Smoking Index to measure dependence on nicotine

Heavy Smoking Index		
How many cigarettes do you smoke each day?		
• 31 plus	(1.5 pack plus)	= 3 points
• 21 – 30	(1 – 1 and half packs)	= 2 points
• 11 – 20	(half – 1 pack)	= 1 point
• 1 – 10	(half pack or less)	= 0 points
How soon after waking do you smoke your first cigarette?		
• Within 5 minutes		= 3 points
• From 6 – 30 minutes		= 2 points
• From 30 minutes – 1 hour		= 1 point
• More than one (1) hour		= 0 points
Heavy Smoking Index Score (add points from 1 & 2 above)		
0 - 1 = Light Smoker	2 - 3 = Moderate Smoker	4 - 6 = Heavy Smoker

Box 11.4 Using scaling questions to measure motivation and build self-efficacy

Build self-efficacy:

- 'On a scale of 1–10, how important is it for you to quit?'
- 'Using the same scale, how confident are you that you can quit?'
- 'So why are you a ... on the scale and not 10?'
- 'What would it take to move you from ... to 10?'

Assessing readiness to quit and motivation

Many smokers want to quit but are often ambivalent and lacking confidence and about how and when they will stop. An important role for the professionals is to build self-efficacy by providing information on pharmacotherapy and exploring the pros and cons of quitting with their patients. ➤ Box 11.4 shows one of the tools you can use to do this.

Assessing past quit attempts

Many patients believe that a failed attempt in the past to stop smoking means they cannot succeed in a future attempt. It is important to explore these past attempts in order to understand possible reasons which may include, for example, suboptimal use of pharmacotherapy. This exploration also provides an opportunity to reframe perceptions. A past quit attempt which lasted for a few years can be seen as a success to build on rather than a failure which cannot be redeemed.

Assessing psychological comorbidities

Dependence on nicotine may be a way for some smokers to lift their mood given the antidepressant properties of nicotine. However, in the long term, mental health is improved with smoking cessation.[79] Therefore, it is important not to deter quit attempts due to this concern.

Assessing smoking in the family

Smokers attempting to quit will be facing significant barriers if there are other members of the household, close friends, or carers who smoke. It is important to assess the level of available social support and engage spouses, partners, and others in supporting patients attempting to quit. Quitting smoking at the workplace where smoking is permitted makes quitting difficult. Public policies and workplace policies prohibiting smoking are essential. Quit attempts can be all the more successful if they are embarked on with others. Quitting smoking with a spouse or significant other who smokes contributes greatly to success.

Key components of behavioural support

Some patients may have quit at the time of their cardiovascular event but will need support to sustain their quit attempt in the form of pharmacotherapy and counselling, and others will be embarking on a quit attempt when they join a CVPR programme. This setting has the opportunity of providing smoking cessation support over the duration of the programme where a quit attempt can be initiated, monitored, and followed up in participants. Support delivered at this important time has the advantage of preventing relapse so often associated with the early stages of a quit attempt. While this should include support from all members of the interdisciplinary programme team, it should be coordinated by a particular member of the team. Nurses are ideal to take on this task.

Behavioural support should be provided alongside pharmacotherapy. The key components of this support[80] are outlined as follows and can be carried out using a group based or individual one-to-one approach:

1. Ask patients to identify and record their personal reasons for quitting—they will be able to revisit these in moments of weakness and reinvigorate their quit attempt.
2. Ensure that patients are realistic about the challenges they face in making the quit attempt, the importance of using pharmacotherapy, and identify ways of coping with withdrawal.
3. Set a quit date and reinforce the importance of not having one puff of a cigarette. Encourage patients to prepare for the attempt by disposing of ashtrays, cigarettes, letting friends and family know that they are quitting and asking for their support, and so on.
4. Remind patients of the seriousness of their decision to quit and how important it is to remain abstinent especially during the challenging first week.
5. Record the baseline breath carbon monoxide reading and chart the decline to normal after the quit date. Record a carbon monoxide reading each time the patient visits the programme to check adherence. This will provide an opportunity to discuss lapses and avoid long-term relapse.
6. Ask patients to identify 'triggers' for lapsing and discuss ways to manage them.

Box 11.5 How to manage lapses and get back on track

- Where the patient fails to stick to their quit date—set a new date or a reduction plan (see 'Medication to support quit attempts').
- Reinforce the need to stay in contact even if a lapse occurs.
- Remind the patient to look at their original reasons for quitting to rejuvenate commitment.

7. Remind patients that withdrawal from nicotine is unlikely to last more than a month.
8. Discuss medication choices and explain how to take it. Monitor tolerance and adherence.
9. Use remote support strategies like texting, telephone helpline, and emailing if urgent support with lapses is required. See ➤ **Box 11.5** for how to help with lapses.

Medication to support quit attempts

In this section, the most effective medications to support stop smoking attempts will be covered, that is, varenicline (Champix®) and nicotine replacement therapy (NRT). More details and information on other medications used in smoking cessation can be found in *The ESC Textbook of Preventive Cardiology*[81] and *The ESC Handbook of Preventive Cardiology*.[82] Using medication to support a quit attempt is essential and especially in cardiovascular patients. Medications are mostly prescribed to support abrupt quit attempts, that is, where a patient quits completely on a set quit date. However, medication can also be used to help a patient to reduce tobacco in the run up to a quit date. In addition, medication has been shown to be useful in supporting temporary abstinence (e.g. on long-haul flights and in other settings where abstinence is required for a temporary period), and to provide harm reduction in those who are unable to quit completely.

Varenicline (Champix®)

What is it?

This medication comes in tablet form and contains a partial receptor agonist, which provides relief from withdrawal and reduces the desire to smoke.

How is it prescribed and taken?

Varenicline is taken over a 12-week course. Initially it is uptitrated over a 1-week period from a dose of 0.5 mg daily (days 1–3), followed by a dose of 0.5 mg twice daily (days 4–7), to a maintenance dose of 1 mg twice daily from day 8 onwards.

Does it have any side effects?

It can cause nausea in around one-third of patients; however, this is usually mild and often tolerated. Some patients report vivid dreams. None of these side effects are dangerous.

Is it safe for patients with heart disease or risk factors?

This medication has been shown to be safe in both the general and cardiac populations.[83–85] Despite early reports of neuropsychiatric and other adverse events, subsequently research has confirmed its safety in both acute and chronic cardiovascular settings.[86]

What is the best way to use it?

Varenicline is effective when used on its own as described previously. In addition, it can be used in combination with nicotine products. Some success has been reported and some studies are still ongoing.[87]

How effective is it?

This medication has been demonstrated to have the most efficacy for smoking cessation.[83] The minimum treatment period is 12 weeks but this can be extended depending on how long after starting treatment the patient quits.[88]

Nicotine replacement therapy

What is it?

This medication comes in various forms including transdermal patches, gum, inhalators, lozenges, and nasal spray. While it contains nicotine, it does not contain all the other harmful constituents present in cigarettes. The nicotine is absorbed through the skin and oral, buccal, or nasal mucosa. It replaces some of the nicotine which a smoker would normally get through their cigarettes and thus provides relief from withdrawal and reduces the urge to smoke.

How is it prescribed and taken?

NRT is most commonly used over a 12-week course. It is most effective when the long-acting patch is used in combination with a short-acting product such as the gum or inhalator.

Does it have any side effects?

Some skin irritation can be experienced with the patch although this is less likely to occur when the site is rotated. This is also true of the mouth and nose.

Is it safe for patients with heart disease or risk factors?

This medication has been shown to be safe in both the general and cardiac populations.[86]

What is the best way to use it?

As described previously, long- and short-acting NRT are best used together. In addition, NRT can be used in combination with varenicline. Some success has been reported and some studies are still ongoing.[87]

How effective is it?

When long- and short-acting NRT are used in combination, they are about as effective as varenicline.[83] The minimum treatment period is 12 weeks but this can be extended up to 9 months and beyond if necessary.

Using varenicline and nicotine replacement therapy to reduce smoking with a view to an eventual quit attempt

There is evidence to show that using NRT and varenicline to reduce smoking with an eventual quit in mind is effective. The UK charity Action on Smoking and Health (ASH) describes a 'Cut down to stop' (https://ash.org.uk/home/) programme which spreads reduction and quitting over a duration of up to 6 months or more.[89]

Issues with weight gain and smoking cessation

Weight gain is common after a successful stop-smoking attempt with an average of 4–5 kg body weight gain over a year.[90] Patients who start off their quit attempt overweight or obese gain the most weight; however, while weight gain has an adverse effect on the cardiovascular risk profile, smoking cessation should be prioritized over weight loss as excess weight carries less risk. In addition, weight management can be delayed until a quit attempt has been sustained in the long term. During a programme of CVPR, patients should be offered a tailored programme of healthy diet advice and support to safely increase physical activity and this may mitigate against weight gain.[91]

Suggested resources

- *The ESC Handbook of Preventive Cardiology* (chapter 10).[82]
- *The ESC Textbook Preventive Cardiology* (chapter 10).[81]

Adopting healthy eating habits and achieving and maintaining optimal weight and shape

In order to reduce cardiovascular risk, all patients and families require advice and support to adopt a cardioprotective diet and to achieve and maintain a healthy weight and shape. CVD has multiple modifiable risk factors many of which can be improved by adapting a healthier diet and shape. Patients often have more than one comorbidity so understanding how dietary advice can be integrated with the overall care given within a CVPR programme is essential. Support to achieve dietary and body weight goals should be an integral part of a programme. The whole interdisciplinary team therefore requires extended dietary knowledge and understanding. Ideally the team should include a dietitian; however, other team members can play an important role in dietary and weight management supported with the necessary education and training in the required skills.

A healthy diet associated with the lowest risk for cardiovascular disease

There is extensive evidence that diet influences CVD. This is either directly or through its beneficial effect on CVD risk factors. This evidence is available from both population-based studies and RCTs. However, there is often conflicting information due to methodological problems including small sample sizes, short study durations, and the difficulties in identifying the effect of a single dietary factor independent of other changes. As diet is made up of whole foods and not individual nutrients, it is hard to attribute the health effects of a food when it has many nutrient components. This is especially so if reducing one component results in the increase of another. The observed effect would be dependent on the quality of the replacement.

In more recent years, nutritional research has placed greater focus on dietary patterns and foods rather than nutrients. The most commonly referenced dietary patterns are the Dietary Approaches to Stop Hypertension (DASH)[92] diet and the Mediterranean diet from the Prevención con Dieta Mediterránea (PREDIMED) trial.[93] The essential difference between these two diets is the additional focus on extra virgin olive oil or nuts in the latter study. The two trials diets in PREDIMED showed a 30% reduction in incidence of major cardiovascular events compared to those on a low-fat diet.

The Mediterranean diet has a focus on unprocessed, plentiful wholegrain products, vegetables, fruit, fish, and unsaturated fats but is also low in saturated fat. It also advises on a pattern of eating a large variety of whole foods that are fresh and local when possible. This is more important than promoting a single nutrient intake.

Within a CVPR programme, there are the additional challenges of comorbidities and often multiple risk factors which are concurrently being addressed. Working as a team, with the patient and their carers, is essential to establish realistic short- and long-term goals.

Assessing dietary intake

To provide a tailored dietary and/or weight management programme requires a detailed dietary assessment in combination with all other aspects of a CVD assessment.

The two principal methods of assessing dietary intake include what patients recall eating and what they record they have eaten. A quick and useful tool to collect recall information from patients is to use the interview-led validated 9- or 14-point Mediterranean diet score tool.[94] The 14-item version, known as the Mediterranean Diet Adherence Screener (MEDAS-14), was originally validated for use in the Spanish PREDIMED study[95] but has since been validated in many other European countries including UK, Germany, and Italy.[96–99] ➤ **Table 11.9** shows the components of the diet that are assessed when using this tool and how it is scored. An increase of 2 points in this score has been shown to be associated with a 9% reduction in cardiovascular risk.[100] In addition to using this tool, patients can be asked to record what they have eaten in a 3- or 7-day food diary. Keeping a food diary helps patients to become more aware of the content, quantity, and pattern of their eating (➤ **Table 11.10**). The following hints can make the process of keeping a diary easier:

- Record everything that you eat, however small.
- Take the diary everywhere you go.
- Record what you have eaten immediately after eating it so you don't forget.
- Record how you feel when you eat something.
- Record any physical activity you do.

Assessing dietary intake using recall and recording will generate discussion with the patient on how diet can be modified and improved. More information on dietary assessment methods can be found in *The ESC Handbook of Preventive Cardiology*.[82]

Behavioural strategies to improve dietary patterns

Professionals can use counselling and motivational interviewing techniques (e.g. 'OARS'— Open-ended questions, Affirmation, Reflective listening, Summarizing) to support patients to make healthy dietary changes, including negotiating 'SMART' goals, monitoring

Table 11.9 The 14-point Mediterranean diet score

Mediterranean diet score tool question	Yes/no
Is olive oil the main culinary fat used?	
Are 4 tbs olive oil used each day?	
Are 2 servings (of 200g each) of vegetables eaten each day?	
Are 3 servings (of 80g each) of fruit eaten each day?	
Is <1 serving (100–150 g) red meat, hamburgers, other meat products eaten each day?	
Is <1 serving (12g) of butter, margarine, cream eaten each day?	
Is <1 serving (330 mL) of sweet or sugar sweetened carbonated beverages consumed each day?	
Are 3 glasses (of 125 mL) of wine consumed each week?	
Are 3 servings (of 150 g) of legumes consumed each week?	
Are 3 servings (of 100–150 g) of fish or (200 g) of seafood eaten each week?	
Are <3 servings of commercial sweets/pastries eaten each week?	
Is 1 serving (50 g) of nuts consumed each week?	
Is chicken, turkey or rabbit routinely eaten instead of veal, pork, hamburger, or sausages?	
Are pasta, vegetable or rice dishes flavoured with garlic, tomato, leek, or onion eaten 2 times per week?	
TOTAL SCORE (total number of 'yes' answers)	

Table 11.10 An example of a food diary

DAY:
DATE:

Time of day	What you ate	How much you ate	Thoughts, Feelings & Physical Activity
Early Morning:	Coffee with Skimmed milk	1 cup 1 tbsp	
Breakfast:	Wholemeal bread (large loaf) Salted butter Hard Cheese Egg -boiled	2 medium slices 2 tsp 2 matchbox size pieces 1 medium egg	
During Morning:	Coffee with skimmed milk Apple (eaten with skin)	1 mug 1 tbsp 1 medium	Used stairs rather than lift when shopping
Midday:	Sandwiches: wholemeal bread (brand) large loaf, sliced Butter Ham (no fat) Tomato Banana Diet Cola	4 slices 4 level tsp 2 thin slices 1 large 1 large 1 can (330ml)	Sunny day, felt happy
During Afternoon:	Water Roasted salted peanuts	1 glass 25g packet	Craved something salty
Evening Meal:	Chicken & mushroom casserole (home-made with skimmed milk in the sauce) Rice (steamed) Broccoli, boiled Plain yoghurt with honey Medium orange Half mineral water/half natural orange juice Coffee with skimmed milk	4 heaped tbsp 1 apple sized 3 tbsp 3 tablespoons and 2 teaspoons 1 medium 1 glass 1 cup 1 tbsp	
During Evening:			
Bedtime Snack:	Milk Chocolate.	8 squares	

progress, and exploring strategies to overcome challenges and barriers (see also 'Supporting patients and families to make healthy lifestyle changes'). Some useful educational topics are included in ➤ Box 11.6.

Regarding behavioural changes, creating a supportive network is very important. Professionals can help by providing advice and contact to existing support groups. They can also ensure the involvement of family, friends, and carers. Technology in the form of websites and smartphone apps may also be useful (see 'Technology to support prevention and rehabilitation initiatives').

Box 11.6 Educational topics to support dietary change

- Healthy cooking tips.
- Making healthy choices when shopping and when eating away from home.
- Understanding how to read food labels.
- How to budget when buying healthy foods.
- Understanding portion sizes and how a healthy plate of food looks to ensure a balanced diet (Fig. 11.7).
- Buying local fruit and vegetables in season.

Translating ESC dietary guidelines into understandable messages for patients and families

When advising on the adoption of a healthy diet, professionals should be aware of ways to translate the evidence-based guidelines into language that is meaningful to the lay public. Guidelines are often written is a way that is hard for untrained personnel to interpret. ➤ **Table 11.11** shows the ESC prevention guidelines in the left column with some practical advice in the right column.

Table 11.11 Translating guidelines into messages for patients and families to use for patients. An example of this is the table shown below. (REF)

ESC guideline	Practical advice example
• Adopt a more plant and less animal based food pattern	Try to have 1-2 vegetarian meals in a week to support environmental sustainability as well as CV health.
• Saturated fat should account for less than 10% of total energy intake, through replacement by polyunsaturated fatty acids, monounsaturated fatty acids and carbohydrates from wholegrains	Foods including saturated fat include butter, full fat milk, cream, meaty pies and fatty meat for example. Mono-unsaturated fat includes olive oil, rapeseed oil, groundnut oil. Polyunsaturated fat includes sunflower oil or corn oil. Be careful to monitor overall fat intake, especially if attempting to lose weight
• Red meat should be reduced to a maximum of 350-500g a week, in particular processed meat should be minimized.	Replace red meat options with white meat or fish. Choose fresh or frozen cuts of meats that are not processed (e.g. burgers, sausages, cured, breaded, battered). Try to have meat free days
• Limit trans-unsaturated fatty acids as much as possible with preferably none from processed foods,.	Trans fatty acids include margarine, shop bought cakes, biscuits and other convenience foods.
• 30–45 g of fibre per day, preferably from wholegrain products	Increasing intake of dietary fibre can be achieved by eating more fruit and vegetables, porridge oats, pulses (lentils, kidney beans, chickpeas, baked beans, peanuts), wholemeal bread, wholemeal breakfast cereals (shredded wheat) and potato skins.
• ≥ 200 g of fruit per day (2–3 servings)	A portion equals for example: 4 heaped tablespoons of French beans or cooked greens, a 5 cm piece of cucumber, two whole canned plum tomatoes, two dried figs, an orange or apple, two handfuls of raspberries, a heaped tablespoon of sultanas, two small tangerines. Be realistic about increasing targets gradually (see figure [ ] for more information on portion size)
• ≥ 200 g of vegetables per day (2–3 servings)	
• Fish is recommended once or twice a week, in particular fatty fish.	Examples of fatty fish are sardines, pilchards, mackerel, tuna, salmon or trout.
• 30g unsalted nuts per day	Choose raw nuts with no added flavouring. Monitor amount eaten.
• Consumption of alcoholic beverages should be limited to a maximum of 100g per week.	A glass or unit (approx. 10g of alcohol) of alcohol is equal to 25 mls of spirits, a 125 mls glass of 9% wine and 250 mls of standard beer.
• Less than 5 g of salt per day	Use other flavourings instead, such as herbs, spices, lemon juice, garlic, pepper, vinegar and chilli. Avoid convenience meals, stock cubes and salty snacks because they contain a lot of salt and sugar.
• Sugar-sweetened beverages such as soft drinks and fruit juices must be discouraged	Replace with water, water flavoured with a squeeze of lime, coffee/tea without sweeteners. Fruit juices are high in sugar as the fibre has been broken down and many portions are required to produce one glass.

Representing guidelines as real foods will make them easier to use for patients.

Encouraging patients to eat from the major food groups is important to ensure a balanced diet. The advice outlined in ➤ **Table 11.11** breaks the guidelines into practical foods groups with examples of foods and recommended intake frequency. More detail on food groups is available in *The ESC Handbook of Preventive Cardiology*.[82]

When giving dietary advice, it is also important for the healthcare provider to be respectful to any cultural, religious, or socioeconomical restrictions. In addition, it is important to incorporate the environmental issues related to food and food manufacturing. As the Mediterranean diet has such a high focus on diverse plant foods, it not only addresses environmental drive to help the planet, but it also will help to improve the gut biome.

There is currently no evidence to support the use of supplements or fortified foods unless deficiencies are identified or if the patient's diet is severally restricted. If this is the case, they would need an individual session with a dietician for additional assessments.

Food choices to lower low-density lipoprotein cholesterol and improve the overall lipoprotein profile

See ➤ **Table 11.12**.

Achieving and maintaining optimal weight and shape

Overweight and obesity are associated with increases in cardiovascular death and all-cause mortality. All-cause mortality is lowest in those with a BMI of 20–25

Table 11.12 Food choices to modify the blood lipid profile

	To be preferred	To be used in moderation	To be chosen occasionally in limited amounts
Cereals	Wholegrains	Refined bread, rice, and pasta, biscuits, corn flakes	Pastries, muffins, pies, croissants
Vegetables	Raw and cooked vegetables	Potatoes	Vegetables prepared in butter or cream
Legumes	Lentils, beans, fava beans, peas, chickpeas, soybean		
Fruit	Fresh or frozen fruit	Dried fruit, jelly, jam, canned fruit, sorbets, ice lollies/popsicles, fruit juice	
Sweets and sweeteners	Non-caloric sweeteners	Sucrose, honey, chocolate, sweets/candies	Cakes, ice creams, fructose, soft drinks
Meat and fish	Lean and oily fish, poultry without skin	Lean cuts of beef, lamb, pork, and veal, seafood, shellfish	Sausages, salami, bacon, spare ribs, hot dogs, organ meats
Dairy food and eggs	Skimmed milk and yoghurt	Low-fat milk, low-fat cheese and other milk products, eggs	Regular cheese, cream, whole milk, and yoghurt
Cooking fat and dressings	Vinegar, mustard, fat-free dressings	Olive oil, non-tropical vegetable oils, soft margarines, salad dressing, mayonnaise, ketchup	Trans fats and hard margarines (better to avoid them), palm and coconut oils, butter, lard, bacon fat
Nuts/seeds		All, unsalted (except coconut)	Coconut
Cooking procedures	Grilling, boiling, steaming	Stir-frying, roasting	Frying

kg/m².[101] While this is true in those less than 60 years of age, it may not be so in the elderly, where a higher body weight is healthier. Having a healthy weight and shape is also associated with superior cardiovascular risk factor control.

Obesity is the result of an imbalance in energy intake and expenditure; however, this occurs because of complex behavioural and societal factors. Effective weight management requires a three-pronged approach encompassing dietary management, physical activity, and behavioural strategies. Even losing as little as 10% of body weight can be of benefit to an obese person. Calorie reduction depends on eating less, replacing unhealthy with healthy food options, and changing the balance of food eaten throughout the day (➤ Fig. 11.4).

The European prevention guidelines[57] recommend that people with healthy weight, that is, a BMI between 20–25 kg/m², maintain their weight and that overweight and obese people achieve a healthy weight (or aim for a reduction in weight) in order to reduce cardiovascular risk. The WHO has further refined this goal taking ethnicity into account (➤ Table 11.13).[102]

Anthropometric measurements used in assessment of overweight and obesity

Measuring obesity is an important part of a cardiovascular assessment. Body fat can be measured in different ways, each with pros and cons. The most common is the BMI which classifies weight according to height. It is calculated

Traditional meal	Healthy 'balanced' meal	Weight reducing meal
Unhealthy meal proportions	Changing the proportions of food in this way leads to a healthier meal.	Changing the proportions in this way will reduce energy intake, help you lose weight, but allow you to eat the same amount of food.

Tips:

- Cook more vegetables than you would normally prepare.
- Put vegetables on your plate first so that they take up half the plate.
- Followed by starch, such as potatoes/rice.
- Followed by fish/meat/cheese portion last, therefore reducing your intake of these products.

Fig. 11.4 Balancing nutrition: food plates.

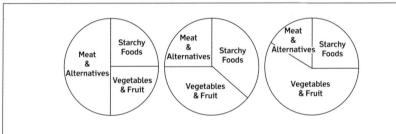

Table 11.13 WHO BMI recommendations

White European population (kg/m²)	Asian population (kg/m²)	Description
<18.5	<18.5	Underweight
18.5–24.9	18.5–23	Increasing but acceptable risk
25–29.9	23–27.5	Increased risk
≥30	>27.5	High risk

using the following formula: weight (kg)/(height (m))². It is inexpensive, simple to calculate, and strongly correlates with body fat levels as measured by the most accurate methods. It is also supported by many studies showing a correlation between increased BMI and higher risk of chronic disease. Other methods that are common in clinical practice for measuring body fat are waist circumference (see following subsection), waist-to-hip ratio, skinfold thicknesses, and bioelectrical impedance. Other methods such as magnetic resonance imaging or dual-energy X-ray absorptiometry are expensive and more complex to measure and so are not suitable for everyday community practice.

Measuring body weight and height

- Shoes should be removed along with heavy overclothes and any heavy items from the patient's pockets like keys or loose change.
- Height should be measured without shoes and with the heels together, with the so-called Frankfurt plane of the head in a horizontal position.
- The patient should breathe in deeply and reach up to their maximum height.
- The feet should be flat on the ground.

Waist circumference provides a measure of central obesity which is important in assessing cardiovascular risk. Although waist circumference and waist-to-hip ratio provide the same information, the latter requires two measurements so the risk of error is increased resulting in the former being used more frequently. Body fat stored in the abdomen carries a higher risk than subcutaneous fat. For every 5 cm increase in waist circumference over 4 years, there is an increased risk of total and cardiovascular mortality.[103] The European thresholds for advising on weight reduction are a waist circumference of at least 102 cm in men and at least 88 cm in women. In addition, a waist circumference of at least 94 cm in men and at least 80 cm in women represents the threshold at which no further weight should be gained. The International Diabetes Federation (IDF) has refined these thresholds by ethnicity (➤ **Table 11.14**).[104]

Table 11.14 International Diabetes Federation guidance on waist circumference

European	Men >94 cm (37 inches) Women ≥80 cm (31.5 cm)
South Asian	Men >90 cm (35 inches) Women ≥80 cm (31.5 cm)
Chinese	Men >90 cm (35 inches) Women ≥80 cm (31.5 cm)
Japanese	Men >90 cm (35 inches) Women ≥80 cm (31.5 cm)
Ethnic South and Central America	Use European data until more specific ones are available
Sub-Saharan Africa	Use European data until more specific ones are available
Easter Mediterranean, Middle East, and Arab populations	Use European data until more specific ones are available

Measuring waist circumference

- Sit in front of the patient and ensure they are standing straight with both feet together, arms relaxed down by their side (supporting themselves on a piece of furniture if they cannot balance) and looking straight ahead.
- Measure next to the skin or over one piece of light clothing.
- Palpate the lowest rib and iliac crest (➤ **Fig. 11.5**) and measure the midpoint between the two points.
- Pass the tape around the patient ensuring it is horizontal and not twisted from the midpoint.
- The tape must be taut but not tight. Encourage the patient to breathe normally, taking the measurement at the end of expiration.

Interventions to support weight loss

Achieving the BMI goal of 20–25 kg/m² is often unrealistic. Even a 10% reduction of total body weight has been shown to have health benefits relating to total mortality,[101] diabetes-related deaths/morbidity, reduction of blood pressure, and reduction of cholesterol.

It is important to identify the root causes of weight gain as well as physical, mental, and psychosocial barriers when working with patients who have identified weight loss as a goal during their time on the CVPR programme. Reducing weight is a long-term process. When planning an individual's interventions, the patient's longer-term support should be identified early. Nutrition and exercise are the cornerstone to any weight loss intervention but adjunctive therapies outside the scope of the CVPR team maybe appropriate (additional psychological behavioural, pharmacotherapy, and surgical interventions).

Negative energy balance is required to lose weight, achieving this can be done in multiple ways. One way is by working with patients and their families to reduce portion sizes of foods or change the proportion of food groups in their diet alongside increasing their lifestyle activity levels (➤ Fig. 11.4 and ➤ Table 11.15).

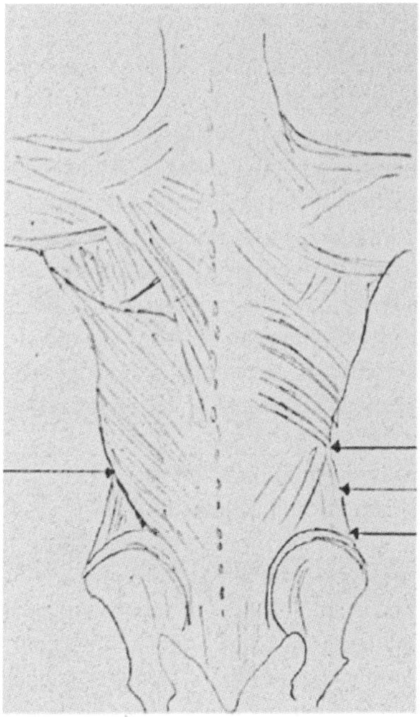

Fig. 11.5 Where to measure waist circumference.

As many patients with CVD have comorbidities, having the support from nutritionally qualified healthcare providers (preferably a dietician) is essential to do this effectively and safely. While a Mediterranean diet has been shown to reduce CVD risk, if an alternative pattern is more suitable to enable particular patients to achieve the necessary weight loss and would be of benefit in improving CVD risk factors, it should be considered. There is increasing evidence of the effectiveness of low-carbohydrate diets[105,106] and very low-calorie diets.[107] This is particularly so in patients with type 2 and pre-diabetes. In these groups, successful weight loss can even result in a reversal of the diabetes. These diets must be carefully planned and monitored closely to ensure they remain nutritious. Without this planning, these diets can be very poor quality. Incorporating this type of intervention within a CVPR programme would only be sensible if the team had access to a qualified dietician.

Measuring servings of food

See ➤ Table 11.15.

Suggested resources

- *The ESC Handbook of Preventive Cardiology* (chapter 11).[82]
- *The ESC Textbook of Preventive Cardiology* (chapters 11 and 13).[81]

Physical activity and exercise

It is important for nurses working in cardiovascular care and particularly in prevention and rehabilitation services to have an understanding of the cardiovascular risks associated with a sedentary lifestyle and the benefits of supporting patients to become physically active for their health and recovery.

Physical inactivity is the fourth leading risk factor for global mortality and accounts for 12.2% of the global burden of acute myocardial infarction and 6% of deaths that occur worldwide (➤ Fig. 11.6).[108] In the WHO European region, it accounts for 1 million deaths per year, which is around 10% of total deaths. It also accounts for 8.3 million disability-adjusted life years which is around 5% of the total. More than half of this WHO region's population is not active enough to meet health recommendations. This translates into enormous costs for the region. For a population of 10 million people, where half the population is insufficiently active, the overall cost is estimated to be €910 million annually.

Since the turn of the century, evidence has been mounting to show that more active adults, including older adults,

Table 11.15 Measuring portion size

Food groups	Standard serving	Visual equivalent
Bread, cereal, rice, pasta, and potato	One cup of pasta 30 g cereal 1 medium potato	Tennis ball A fist A computer mouse
Fruits	1 medium apple or orange 1 tablespoon raisins ½ avocado	Tennis ball ½ cupped hand
Vegetables	2 spears of broccoli 8 Brussel sprouts 3 tbsp frozen mixed veg	1 cupped hand
Milk, yogurt, and cheese	200 mL semi-skimmed milk 30 g of hard cheese 125 g of yogurt	Average glass 1 matchbox Average pot
Meat, poultry, and fish	100 g meat/chicken or fish	Deck of cards
Dry beans, eggs, and nuts	3 heaped tsps cooked beans 28 g nuts Large teaspoon peanut butter 2 whole eggs	Light bulb Cupped hand Ping pong ball
Fats, oils, and sweets	1 tsp of salad dressing 1 tsp of butter /margarine or oil ½ cup ice cream	½ thumb ½ forefinger Tennis ball

consistently have a lower risk for cardiovascular and all-cause mortality compared to inactive adults. These studies include evidence from across Europe and the US including the Framingham Heart Study, the Canada Health Survey, the Swedish Annual Level of Living Survey, the Puerto Rico Heart Health Program, and the Nordic Research Project on Aging, among several others.[109–115] The benefits[116] include not only all-cause and cardiovascular mortality, but also improved cardiovascular risk factor profiles (blood pressure, lipids, and blood glucose), reduction of some cancers, improved cognition, less dementia, improved physical function, less frailty and risk of falls, improved bone health, and improved psychological health.

Identifying people who are sedentary and working with them to increase physical activity levels and meet evidence-based guidelines can lead to reduced mortality. Estimates have shown that even if one in five people who are physically inactive become active this could translate into more than 100,000 deaths averted, equal to one life saved every 5 minutes[117] (➤ **Table 11.16**).

Looking in more depth at the benefits of increasing activity for the cardiovascular risk profile, it has become clear that while physical inactivity is an independent risk factor for CVD, it also interacts with several other risk factors, including poor lipid profiles, high blood pressure, diabetes, obesity, and mental health. Thus, in addressing physical inactivity, there are important benefits for the cardiovascular risk profile as a whole. In this way, increasing physical activity becomes a powerful cardioprotective therapy. In ➤ **Fig. 11.7**, the cardioprotective effects of aerobic endurance training can be seen in relation to atherosclerosis, thrombosis, ischaemia, and arrythmias as well as the psychological benefits which are important for cardiovascular health.[118]

Specifically, in relation to weight loss and lowering low-density lipoprotein cholesterol (LDL-C), the minimum guideline of 150 minutes of moderate intensity exercise per week is beneficial to numerous other risk factors. As an example, physical activity supports weight loss in conjunction with low-density lipoprotein (LDL) lowering. For many risk factors, evidence suggests more is better and as such, achieving levels between 250 and 300 minutes per week of moderate aerobic physical activity intensity exercise is encouraged where possible.

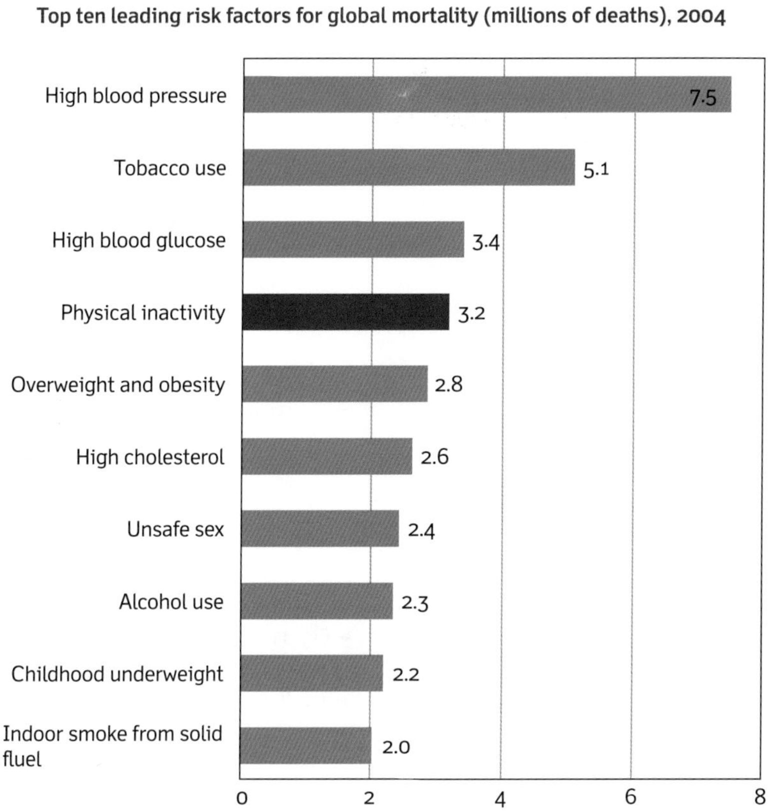

Fig. 11.6 Physical inactivity as a leading global risk factor.

Table 11.16 Reducing deaths by reducing inactivity.

Estimated reductions in European disorder prevalence and deaths associated with given declines in inactivity, 2012			
Percentage decline in physical inactivity	5%	10%	20%
Potential decline in breast cancer cases	8,200	16,300	32,600
Potential decline in colorectal cancer cases	5,600	11,200	22,400
Potential decline in type II diabetes cases	115,000	231,000	462,000
Potential decline in CHD cases	8,400	16,700	33,400
Potential deaths averted	25,600	51,100	102,200

Data Source; Lee et al., (2012), WHO, OECD, Eurostat, IDA, EUCAN, Cebr analysis Infographics Source; Inactivity Time Bomb – Now We Move Report https://inactivity-time-bomb.nowwemove.com/

Anti atherosclerotic	Psychological	Anti thrombotic	Anti ischaemic	Anti arrhythmic
Improved lipids	↓ Depression	↓ Platelet adhesiveness	↓ Myo cardial O_2 demand	↑ Vagal tone
↓ Blood pressure	↓ Stress	↑ Fibinolysis	↑ Coronary blood flow	↑ Heart rate variability
↓ Adiposity	↑ Social support	↓ Fibrinogen	↓ Endothelial dysfunction	↓ Adrenergic activity
↑ Insulin sensitivity		↓ Blood viscosity	↑ Endothelial progenitor cells (EPCS)	
↓ Inflammation			↑ Circulating angiogenic cells	
			↑ Nitric oxide	

Fig. 11.7 Cardioprotective effects of exercise training.

Regular aerobic exercise can increase high-density lipoprotein cholesterol (HDL-C) by 3–10% (up to 0.16 mmol/L), especially at a more vigorous intensity. It can also reduce triglycerides by around 11% (up to 0.34 mmol/L). In conjunction with a reduction in saturated fat intake, it can slow down the reduction in protective HDL-C.[119–122]

A recent systematic review and meta-analysis[123] of RCTs investigating the effects of different types of exercise training on blood pressure lowering found that both aerobic and resistance (endurance, dynamic resistance, and isometric resistance training) all help to lower both systolic and diastolic blood pressure. As far back as 1995, the insulin resistance atherosclerosis prospective observational study[124] of 1467 patients with glucose tolerance ranging between normal and mild non-insulin-dependent diabetes mellitus showed that regular exercise can improve insulin sensitivity and lower fasting insulin levels (➤ Fig. 11.8).

This multifactorial effect that physical activity has on the cardiovascular risk profile has been likened to that of the polypill[125] and strengthens the case for including it as an important part of a CVD prevention intervention.

Threshold for benefit

Importantly, most recent evidence shows that there is no lowest threshold for benefit with the most benefit being in those who are the most sedentary becoming a little more active (➤ Fig. 11.9). Reducing sedentary behaviour is now as important as getting people to become active. In such cases, the health benefits can be immediate. In individuals who exercise regularly but are otherwise sedentary, cardiovascular risk is much higher than in regular

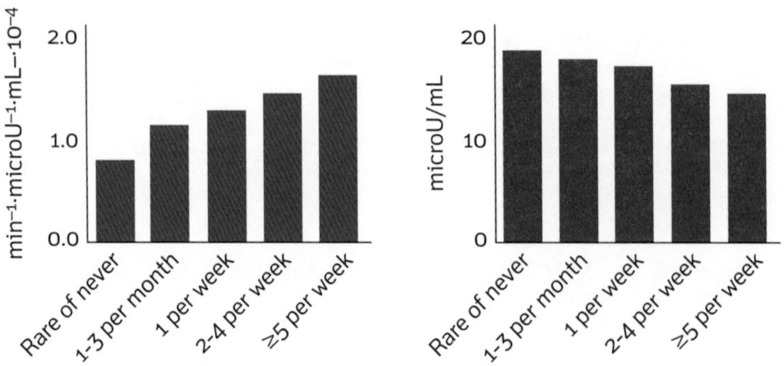

Fig. 11.8 Effects of exercise on insulin.

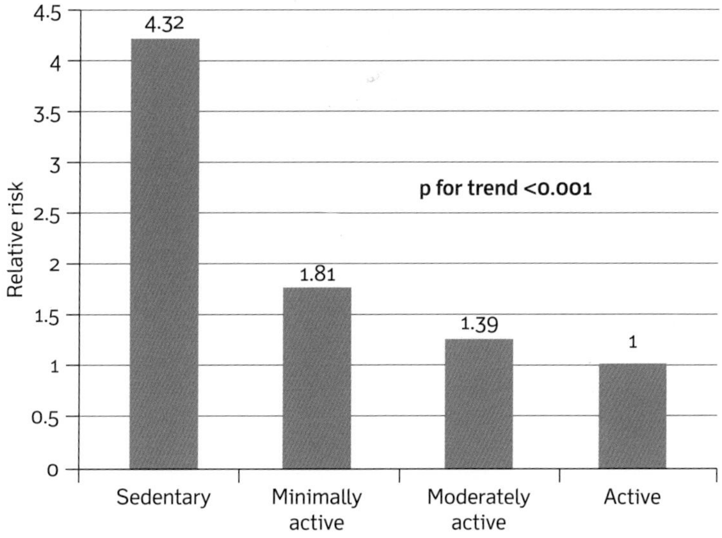

Fig. 11.9 Relative risks for classification of activity at the time of a treadmill test among veterans.

exercisers who limit the amount of time they are sedentary.[127,128] These studies demonstrated that any amount of activity helps. However, most benefits are associated with 150–300 minutes of moderate physical activity per week[57] (➤ Box 11.7).

The amount of time in the day spent sitting is related to survival. Katzmarzyk and colleagues, in a 14-year follow-up of 17,013 individuals,[128] showed that compared with those who were sedentary almost none of the time, in those who were sedentary almost all of the time, survival was lower (➤ Fig. 11.10).

Box 11.7 Recommendations for your patients

150 minutes of moderate intensity activity (or 75 minutes of vigorous) (or equivalent combination) per week.

Example: in the last week a patient reports they have walked briskly (moderate intensity) for 30 minutes, twice. They also went jogging (vigorous intensity) for 25 minutes, twice?

Is this patient achieving the guidelines?

The answer is YES!

30 minutes × 2 of moderate intensity activity = 60 minutes.

25 minutes × 2 of vigorous activity translates into 100 minutes of moderate intensity activity.

Total = 160 minutes of moderate intensity activity.

For every 2 hours of sitting time per day replaced with standing time there will be an 11% lower triglyceride level, 6% lower total to HDL-C ratio, and 0.06 mmol/L higher HDL. Replacing sitting time with stepping had even more significant benefits. More than 4 hours of screen time per day significantly lowers HDL-C levels. Those in the highest screen time category also had significantly higher triglyceride levels.[129,130]

Making every contact count

When interacting with patients, health professionals have the opportunity to make every contact count. In doing so they need to draw on behavioural approaches to assess activity levels, identify barriers and intervene (see more about behavioural approaches elsewhere in this chapter). According to a recent 'call to action', the first recommendation to all health professionals is to treat physical activity as a 'vital sign' and assess it at every meeting with patients.[131] Two questions are proposed (➤ **Table 11.17**). A score can be calculated from the responses to these questions which informs the health professional of how many minutes per week the respondent says they are active. In addition, this call to action includes an adaptation of the 5As model used in smoking cessation brief interventions (see ➤ **Box 11.3** earlier in this chapter) and for providing support to increase physical activity (➤ **Fig. 11.11**). This builds on asking about physical activity at every visit and prompts the professional to give advice, assess motivation, negotiate a treatment plan, and organize follow-up.

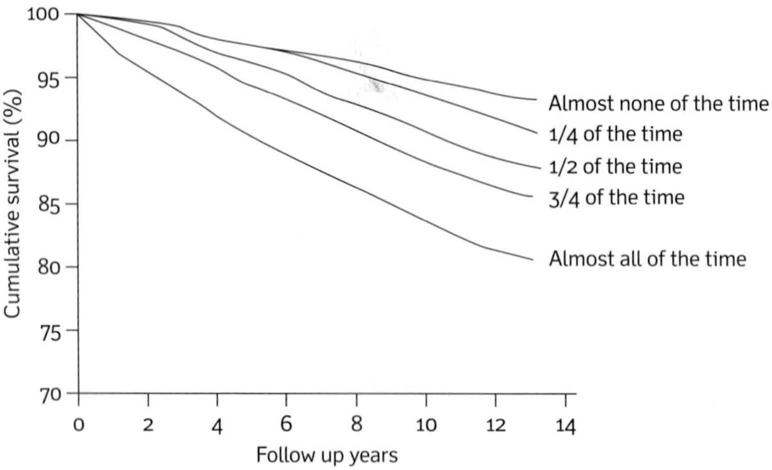

Fig. 11.10 Differences in survival according to proportion of the day spent sitting.

The treatment plan includes providing an exercise prescription as part of the intervention which works towards accumulating 150 minutes of activity per week. It also encourages patients to measure and record their physical activity on paper, using a wearable device or their smartphone,[132] referring to a specialist as appropriate who may be a physician or nurse with expertise, a physiotherapist, an exercise physiologist, or a certified fitness instructor. Follow-up allows both professional and patient to chart progress, set goals, solve problems, and identify and draw on social support.

In summary, physical activity prescription is effective. Healthcare providers have an important opportunity to make physical activity an integral component of the prevention and treatment of chronic disease. All healthcare providers should include physical activity assessment and prescription as part of routine care for patients. Recommendations from physicians influence patient engagement and improve the likelihood of adoption. Any amount of physical activity has benefit and importantly, a strong emphasis should be placed on reducing sedentary time.

Table 11.17 Measuring and calculating physical activity and exercise participation as a vital sign.

The Physical Activity Vital Sign 1. On average, how many days per week do you engage in moderate to strenuous exercise (like a brisk walk)?	_ days
2. On average, how many minutes do you engage in exercise at this Level?	_ minutes
Total minutes per week of physical activity (multiply #1 by #2)	_ minutes per week

Finally, if health professionals are going to be effective in helping their patients to become more active, they need to consider their own behaviour and lead by example, remembering that even the smallest increases in activity levels can have benefit.

Suggested resources

- *The ESC Handbook of Preventive Cardiology* (chapter 12).[82]
- *The ESC Textbook of Preventive Cardiology* (chapters 12 and 13).[81]

Biological risk factor management

Biological risk factors include raised blood pressure, abnormal lipid profile and dysglycaemia, and diabetes mellitus. As outlined already in this chapter, a multiple risk factor management approach is required to manage CVD prevention because the total risk of developing CVD or its recurrence is determined by the combined effect of cardiovascular risk factors present, including age, sex/gender, smoking status, blood pressure, and total cholesterol or BMI.

Nurses play an important role in the management of cardiovascular risk factors in collaboration with physicians and other allied professional colleagues. In addition

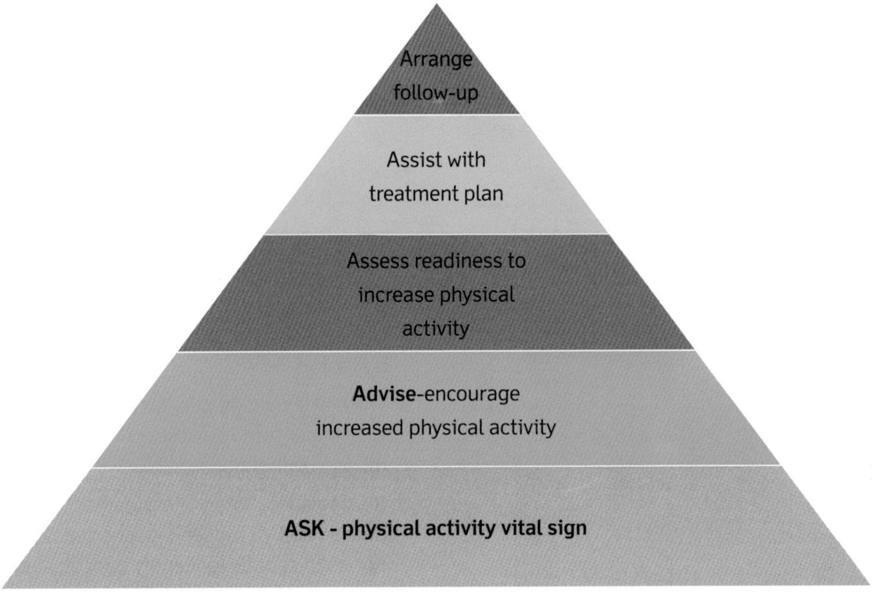

Fig. 11.11 5As used to guide physical activity brief intervention.

to providing education for self-management and using behavioural strategies to achieve lifestyle goals, they are ideally placed to monitor treatment and progress. Increasingly, with the advent of non-medical prescribing (see more in Chapter 12), they play a role in initiating and titrating treatment. Importantly, they work with allied professional experts to evaluate and manage adherence to both lifestyle and medical treatments.

Blood pressure

Classification of blood pressure

Blood pressure should be classified as either optimal, normal, high normal, or grade 1, 2, or 3 hypertension when measured in the clinical setting (office measurement). The most recent ESC Guidelines[64] defines this as shown in ➤ Table 11.18. Diagnosis of hypertension should be based

Table 11.18 Classification of office blood pressure based on office measurements

Category	Systolic (mmHg)		Diastolic (mmHg)
Optimal	<120	and	<80
Normal	120–129	and/or	80–84
High normal	130–139	and/or	85–89
Grade 1 hypertension	140–159	and/or	90–99
Grade 2 hypertension	160–179	and/or	100–109
Grade 3 hypertension	≥180	and/or	≥110
Isolated systolic hypertension[a]	≥140	and	<90

BP, blood pressure; SBP, systolic blood pressure.
BP category is defined according to seated clinic BP and by the highest level of BP, whether systolic or diastolic.
[a] Isolated systolic hypertension is graded 1, 2, or 3 according to SBP values in the ranges indicated.
The same classification is used for all ages from 16 years.

Table 11.19 Definitions of hypertension according to office, ambulatory, and home blood pressure levels

Category	SBP (mmHg)		DBP (mmHg)
Office BP[a]	≥140	and/or	≥90
Ambulatory BP			
Daytime (or awake) mean	≥135	and/or	≥85
Night-time (or asleep) mean	≥120	and/or	≥70
24 h mean	≥130	and/or	≥80
Home BP mean	≥135	and/or	≥85

BP, blood pressure; DBP, diastolic blood pressure; SBP, systolic blood pressure.
[a] Refers to conventional office BP rather than unattended office BP.

on repeated office measurements conducted during more than one clinic visit. Alternatively, diagnosis should be based on ambulatory blood pressure monitoring (ABPM) or on home blood pressure monitoring (HBPM) where this is feasible. In particular, ABPM and HBPM, especially HBPM, provide opportunities to confirm a diagnosis of hypertension, detect white-coat and masked hypertension, and to monitor blood pressure control.

Where measurements are taken outside the clinical environment (ABPM and HBPM), the definition of hypertension should be based on different parameters (➤ **Table 11.19**).

Measuring blood pressure

As blood pressure varies enormously depending on the day and time it is measured, it is necessary to take several measurements in each individual on separate occasions. The decision to start treatment with medication should be based on two measurements taken on two to three separate occasions.

In order to take and record an accurate and reliable blood pressure reading in the clinic setting, technique is important (➤ **Fig. 11.12**). The following guidelines should be followed:

1. The patient should be seated quietly for 5 minutes before measurement.
2. Three readings should be recorded 1–2 minutes apart. The measurements should be repeated if there is a difference of greater than 10 mmHg between the first two readings. The blood pressure recorded should be an average of the last two readings.
3. Additional measurements may be required in patients with unstable values due to arrhythmias (e.g. patients with atrial fibrillation). In these patients, it is preferable to use auscultatory methods rather than an automated device.
4. Use a standard size bladder cuff, 22–42 cm, for most patients.
5. The cuff should be positioned at the level of the heart with the arm and back supported so as to avoid muscle contraction.
6. If using auscultatory measurement methods, use phase I and V (sudden reduction/disappearance) Korotkoff sounds to identify systolic and diastolic blood pressure respectively.
7. Take measurements on both arms for the first visit to detect between arm differences. Use the measurement from the arm with the higher value as reference.
8. Take a measurement 1 and 3 minutes after standing up from a seated position in all patients for the first visit measurement in order to exclude orthostatic hypertension. Lying and standing measurements should also be considered in the following patients: older patients, patients with diabetes, and patients with other conditions where orthostatic hypertension may frequently occur.
9. Record heart rate and use palpation where arrhythmia is likely to be present.

Measurements taken in a home (HBPM) or ambulatory (ABPM) setting will likely vary from those taken in a clinic setting. While both HBPM and ABPM can be useful in diagnosing whitecoat hypertension, they have their advantages and disadvantages (➤ **Table 11.20**).

Interventions to lower blood pressure

Blood pressure treatment goals can be seen in ➤ **Table 11.21**. Interventions to lower blood pressure include those based on providing support with healthy lifestyle changes (➤ **Box 11.8**) and those based on drug therapy. More information on providing support for healthy lifestyle habits can be found elsewhere in this chapter. More information on drugs used in the management of blood pressure can be found in Chapter 12.

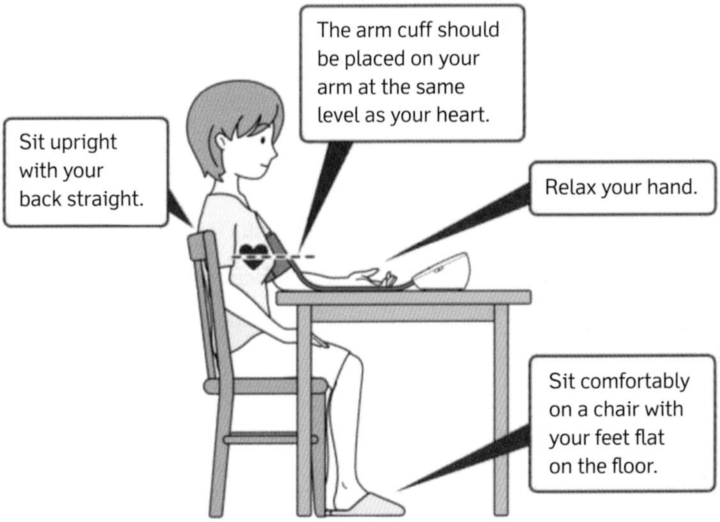

Fig. 11.12 Maintaining the correct posture for measurement: upper arm blood pressure monitor (regular cuff wrapping type). https://www.healthcare.omron.co.jp/zeroevents/english/bloodpressuremonitor/howtouse.html.

Initiating drug therapy in patients who are not already at high or very high risk due to established CVD, renal disease, or diabetes, a markedly elevated single risk factor (e.g. cholesterol), or hypertensive left ventricular hypertrophy should be based not only according to blood pressure classification, but also on a total cardiovascular risk assessment using the ESC SCORE risk estimation tool (https://www.heartscore.org/). Classification of cardiovascular risk and risk estimation is explained elsewhere in this chapter (see 'Concept of total cardiovascular risk and total risk management'). Drug treatment may be considered for high normal blood pressure (i.e. 130–139 mmHg systolic blood pressure/ 85–89 mmHg diastolic blood pressure) when cardiovascular risk is high due to established heart disease.

Table 11.20 Comparison of ambulatory blood pressure monitoring and home blood pressure monitoring

ABPM	HBPM
Advantages	**Advantages**
• Can identify white-coat and masked hypertension • Stronger prognostic evidence • Night-time readings • Measurement in real-life settings • Additional prognostic BP phenotypes • Abundant information from a single measurement session, including short-term BP variability	• Can identify white-coat and masked hypertension • Cheap and widely available • Measurement in a home setting, which may be more relaxed than the doctor's office • Patient engagement in BP measurement • Easily repeated and used over longer periods to assess day-to-day BP variability
Disadvantages	**Disadvantages**
• Expensive and sometimes limited availability • Can be uncomfortable	• Only static BP is available • Potential for measurement error • No nocturnal readings[a]

ABPM, ambulatory blood pressure monitoring; BP, blood pressure; HBPM, home blood pressure monitoring.
[a] Techniques are being developed to enable nocturnal BP measurement with home BP devices.

Table 11.21 Blood pressure treatment goals (based on office measurements)

Blood pressure targets	
<140/80 mmHg	In all patients
<130/80 mmHg	In most patients if treatment is tolerated
SBP <120–129 mmHg	In most patients <65 years receiving drug treatment
SBP 130–139 mmHg	In patients ≥65 years receiving drug treatment

SBP, systolic blood pressure.

When considering treatment of older patients, the biological rather than the chronological age should be taken into account with consideration being given to frailty, independence, and tolerability of treatment. Grade 1 hypertension (140–159 mmHg) can be treated with blood pressure-lowering drugs and lifestyle interventions in patients older than 65 years if fit and provided they are well tolerated, but not in patients over the age of 80 years.

Medication to manage blood pressure

Most patients requiring medication can be considered for a single-pill treatment strategy, that is, a drug that contains two or more different treatments in one tablet. A two-drug combination can be used to initiate treatment. Simplified treatment algorithms include the use of an angiotensin-converting enzyme inhibitor or angiotensin receptor blocker combined with a calcium channel blocker or a thiazide/thiazide-like diuretic as core treatment strategy with beta-blockers used for specific indications. More information about drug regimens and combinations for the treatment of hypertension can be found in the ESC Guidelines[57,64] (see also Chapter 12).

Box 11.8 Lifestyle interventions to lower blood pressure

- Restrict salt to less than 5 g per day.
- Restrict alcohol:
  - Less than 14 units per week for men.
  - Less than 8 units per week for women.
- Increase consumption of fruit and vegetable, fish, nuts, unsaturated fatty acids (olive oil), and low-fat dairy and reduce consumption of red meat.
- Control body weight to avoid obesity and aim for healthy weight and shape (see section 'Adopting healthy eating habits and achieving and maintaining optimal weight and shape').
- Take regular aerobic exercise (see 'Physical activity and exercise').
- No tobacco exposure.

Blood lipids

Classification

Management of the lipid profile should be guided by the level of total cardiovascular risk (see 'Concept of total cardiovascular risk and total risk management'). ➤ Table 11.22 shows the goals for LDL-C according to the level of risk.

Measuring lipids

In patients who are found to be at high cardiovascular risk, a full lipid profile should be measured to guide management. The lipid profile is expressed using a number of different parameters including total cholesterol, LDL-C, HDL-C, and triglycerides (TG). LDL-C is not directly measured from the blood, but is usually calculated according to the Friedewald formula:

$$\text{LDL-C} = \text{total cholesterol} - \text{HDL-C} - (\text{TG}/2.2)$$

This calculation should be based on a fasting lipid profile (after 12 hours). If fasting triglycerides are more than 4 mmol/L, the calculation will not be valid. Following an acute coronary syndrome, lipid levels should be assessed within the first 24 hours as after this, during the following 6–8 weeks, they will lower and reduce the accuracy of the baseline reading. Alcohol can raise triglyceride levels and, over a longer period can raise HDL-C levels.

Interventions to manage the lipid profile

Lipid treatment goals can be seen in ➤ Table 11.22. Interventions to manage lipids include those based on providing support with healthy lifestyle changes and those based on drug therapy.

Lifestyle interventions to achieve lipid goals include making healthy food choices (see 'Adopting healthy eating habits and achieving and maintaining optimal weight and shape' and ➤ Table 11.12). In addition, quitting smoking has a small effect on raising HDL-C. Increasing habitual physical activity has a large effect on raising HDL-C, a small effect on reducing total cholesterol and LDL-C, and a moderate effect on reducing triglycerides. Reducing excessive body weight has a moderate effect on reducing total cholesterol and LDL-C, a small effect on reducing triglycerides,

Table 11.22 Lipid goals

LDL-C targets	
At very high cardiovascular risk[a]	An LDL-C reduction of ≥50% from baseline and LDL-C goal of <1.4 mmol/L (<55 mg/dL)[b]
At high cardiovascular risk[a] LDL-C <1.8 mmol/L (<70 mg/dL)	An LDL-C reduction of ≥50% from baseline and LDL-C goal of <1.8 mmol/L (<70 mg/dL)
At moderate cardiovascular risk[a]	LDL-C <2.6 mmol/L (<100 mg/dL)
At low cardiovascular risk[a]	LDL-C <3 mmol/L (<116 mg/dL)

LDL-C, low-density lipoprotein cholesterol.
[a] See text for definitions of level of risk.
[b] In patients with CVD who experience a second event within 2 years and LDL-C goal of <1 mmol/L (40 mg/dL) may be considered

and a moderate effect on increasing HDL-C. A summary of this evidence is provided in the ESC Guidelines on lipid.[57,65]

The main drugs used in the management of lipids include statins, a combination of statins and ezetimibe and PCSK9 inhibitors. (see also Chapter 12). ➤ Table 11.23 summarizes the indications for use of these drugs.

The decision to start lipid-lowering medication depends not only on the lipid levels but also on total CVD risk. In all cases, it is important to look at and manage all risk factors. Risk estimation (see 'Concept of total cardiovascular risk and total risk management') should be used to guide the treatment of asymptomatic adults aged over 40 years without CVD, diabetes mellitus, chronic kidney disease, familial hypercholesterolaemia, or LDL-C greater than 4.9 mmol/L (>190 mg/dL).

Table 11.23 Drug therapies used to treat lipids

Statins	High intensity up to highest tolerated dose to achieve goal appropriate for level of risk
Ezetimibe + statin	If above does not achieve goal
PCSK9 inhibitors	For secondary prevention patients and familial hypercholesterolaemia patients at very high risk, add in PCSK9 inhibitors

Blood glucose and diabetes

Classification and diagnosis

Like blood pressure and lipids, glucose has a continuous relationship with cardiovascular risk. This risk is worsened by the presence of other lifestyle risk factors such as smoking, poor diet, and physical inactivity. People with diabetes are classified either at very high risk or high risk of developing CVD depending on the presence of other cardiovascular risk factors (see 'Concept of total cardiovascular risk and total risk management')[66] and in those with coronary disease, around two-thirds will have either frank diabetes or dysglycaemia (impaired glucose tolerance or impaired fasting glucose).[133]

It is therefore very important to screen for diabetes in these patients. Type 2 diabetes is much more common than type 1 although the risk of developing CVD is elevated in both. The ESC Guidelines[57,66] recommend using either fasting plasma glucose or haemoglobin A1c (HbA1c) for diagnosis, and an oral glucose tolerance test (OGTT) for the diagnosis of impaired glucose tolerance. While these guidelines recommend the use of an OGTT for diagnosis in individuals with established CVD only if fasting plasma glucose and HbA1c are inconclusive, ideally, and where possible, screening should include both an OGTT and fasting HbA1c levels. An OGTT was found in the EUROASPIRE IV survey of patients with coronary artery disease to identify the largest number of patients with undetected diabetes.[133]

An OGTT requires that the patient has fasted for 8–12 hours. A fasting glucose sample is then performed followed by the administration of an oral glucose load with 75 g of anhydrous glucose. A second blood sample should be analysed for glucose 2 hours later. During this time, the patient should not eat or drink anything else. This test allows classification of blood glucose as either impaired fasting glycaemia, impaired glucose tolerance, or diabetes mellitus. The WHO criteria for the diagnosis of dysglycaemia based on the OGTT can be seen in ➤ Table 11.24.[134]

HbA1c has been recognized by the WHO as a diagnostic test for diabetes since 2011.[135] Prior to this, HbA1c was used more to monitor the control of existing diabetes. It reflects the average level of glucose to which the red blood cells have been exposed over a period of between 4 weeks to 6 months. A diagnosis is made if the HbA1c is greater than 48 mmol/mol or 6.5% on two occasions. However, if a diagnosis had already been made using other tests like the OGTT, a value of less than this would not exclude diabetes.

Table 11.24 WHO criteria for the diagnosis of dysglycaemia based on the OGTT

Diabetes	Fasting plasma glucose ≥7 mmol/L OR 2-hour plasma glucose ≥11.1 mmol/L
Impaired glucose tolerance (IGT)	Fasting plasma glucose <7 mmol/L AND 2-hour plasma glucose* ≥7.8 and < 11.1 mmol/L
Impaired fasting glucose (IFG)	Fasting plasma glucose 6.1 to 6.9 mmol/L AND (if measured) 2-hour plasma glucose* <7.8 mmol/L

*The 2-hour plasma glucose is measured after the ingestion of 75 g of oral anhydrous glucose.

OGTT which includes post-prandial glucose testing, should definitely be recommended for patients who have a fasting glucose value at target but an HbA1c above target because post-prandial glucose values (impaired glucose tolerance) are associated with greater cardiovascular risk, independent of fasting plasma glucose.[66]

Interventions to manage dysglycaemia and diabetes

Interventions to manage dysglycaemia and diabetes include those based on providing support with healthy lifestyle changes and those based on drug therapy. ➤ Table 11.25 shows the most recent ESC recommended targets for risk factor control in patients with diabetes. Control of blood pressure and lipids to target is as important as the control of glycaemia and in these patients will lead to a substantial impact on cardiovascular risk. Combined reduction in HbA1c, systolic blood pressure, and lipids decreases cardiovascular events by 75%.[66] Multifactorial treatment is still underused. Therefore, in the context of CVPR, it is important first to look for and

Table 11.25 Risk factor goals for patients with diabetes

Glycaemic targets	
HbA1c <7% (<53 mmol/mol), i.e. near normal	To reduce risk of microvascular complications
Tighter glucose control to be initiated early on in the course of DM	Leads to reduction in cardiovascular outcomes in younger people over 20-year timescale
Individualized targets according to duration of DM, comorbidities and age: HbA1c <8% (64 mmol/mol) for the elderly	
Blood pressure	
SBP 130 mmHg for most SBP <120 mmHg if tolerated SBP 130–139 mmHg older patients	
Lipids[a] (see also 'Concept of total cardiovascular risk and total risk management')	
• At very high cardiovascular risk[a] LDL-C <1.4 mmol/L (<55 mg/dL)	And at least 50% reduction
• At high cardiovascular risk[a] LDL-C <1.8 mmol/L (<70 mg/dL)	And at least 50% reduction
• At moderate cardiovascular risk[a] LDL-C <2.6 mmol/L (<100 mg/dL)	

DM, diabetes mellitus; HbA1c, glycated haemoglobin; SBP, systolic blood pressure; LDL-C, low-density lipoprotein cholesterol.
[a] <Footnote to be confirmed>

Box 11.9 Lifestyle goals

- No exposure to tobacco, support for quit smoking attempts (see 'Tobacco and smoking cessation management').
- A Mediterranean diet supplemented with olive oil and/or nuts reduces the incidence of major cardiovascular events (see 'Adopting healthy eating habits and achieving and maintaining optimal weight and shape').
- Lower excessive body weight (see 'Adopting healthy eating habits and achieving and maintaining optimal weight and shape').
- Moderate to vigorous physical activity of at least 150 minutes/week is recommended for the prevention and control of diabetes mellitus (see 'Physical activity and exercise').

confirm dysglycaemia and diabetes and to provide expert lifestyle management, providing smoking cessation support where appropriate, dietary advice, weight management, and safe access to physical activity and exercise (➤ Box 11.9). In addition, screening for microalbuminuria is recommended to identify renal dysfunction.

The principal drug therapies used to manage diabetes are listed here (more information about these therapies can be found in Chapter 12):

- Sodium–glucose co-transporter 2 (SGLT2) inhibitors.
- Glucagon-like peptide-1 receptor agonists (GLP-1RAs).
- Angiotensin-converting enzyme inhibitor or angiotensin receptor blocker for blood pressure control and renal protection.
- Statins plus added ezetimibe (if necessary) to manage lipids.
- PCSK9 inhibitors if above mentioned drugs not tolerated or ineffective.

Lifestyle goals are listed in ➤ Box 11.9.

Addressing psychosocial aspects, illness perceptions, and health-related quality of life

In most CVPR programmes, efforts are focused primarily on encouraging people to take more exercise, lose weight, stop smoking, and eat a healthy diet. While these are important, issues such as mood changes, lack of social support, illness misconceptions, and health-related quality of life are often relegated as secondary considerations.[136,137] Yet addressing psychosocial issues often impacts directly on how well people manage their health and initiate behaviour changes and adhere to them and their medications.[138–140] These are vital considerations not only for patients but for their partners, carers, and families as demonstrated by a large and growing body of empirical research identifying that psychosocial risk factors such as low socioeconomic status, social isolation, stress, depression, and anxiety increase the risk of CVD and stroke and also contribute to poorer health-related quality of life and prognosis in patients with established heart disease.[57,141] For example, depression and anxiety are common in people with CVD, with over 30% of women and 20% of men reporting symptoms of depression and 39% of women and 22% of men reporting symptoms of anxiety.[142] Depression and anxiety are associated with female gender, lower educational level, more sedentary lifestyle, lower quality of life, poorer somatic symptoms, higher mortality, and higher healthcare costs.[142,143] Moreover, as CVD and depression are the two most common causes of disability in high-income countries, and are expected to become so globally by 2030,[144] the challenges they pose in CVD prevention and rehabilitation are great.

Lower socioeconomic status, loneliness, and social isolation are significant risk factors and commonly found among people with CVD and associated with depression, both as a cause and sequela,[145–147] and are compounded by factors such as unemployment, occupational stress, job strain, financial insecurity, loss of independence, and low self-esteem.[141] Thus, social and environmental factors are important. For example, living alone, particularly among men in middle and lower socioeconomic positions, is associated with all-cause and cardiovascular mortality.[148] Furthermore, social support provides protection from depression.[149]

Perceptions of illness are also important. Illness perceptions are cognitive frameworks which patients construct to make sense of their illness, and which subsequently, guide their behaviour directed at managing the illness.[150] These perceptions include beliefs about the cause, expected symptoms, cure/control, timeline, and consequences. They vary widely among patients including both positive and negative perceptions that influence an individual's ability to cope with disease and to perceive it as manageable or threatening. Hence, poorer illness perceptions are related to outcomes such as depressive symptoms and treatment adherence.[150]

All of these factors have potential to impact adversely on a patient's health-related quality of life: their physical, mental, emotional, social, and spiritual functioning, including activity limitations and personal perceptions.[151]

The challenge is to try to address these issues, some more difficult than others, with the choice of intervention guided by an individual assessment of need, patient choice and preference, and taking account of considerations such as health and social care referral systems, resources, personnel, location, and surveillance. Thus, for example, interventions may be delivered in the home or community setting, depending on ease of access, monitoring, follow-up, continuity of care and use of technologies such as telehealth or eHealth. For example, psychosocial well-being and quality of life among other factors have been shown to improve, at least in the shorter term, among mobile app users.[152] Counselling, education, and feedback will be informed by factors such as culture, race, ethnicity, language, and health literacy. The goal is to offer appropriate, holistic, and patient-centred care that will enhance a patient's experience and health outcome.

Effective communication is fundamental to patient assessment and determining if and what intervention is required (see also Chapter 13). This involves establishing a mutually respectful active partnership with the patient and their partner, family, or social support network. This requires communication skills such as active listening, summarizing, reflecting, and chunking information.[141] By using counselling skills and OARS principles, a rapport can be established with the patient and an assessment made of their readiness, willingness, and ability to make any necessary changes.[141] The person is likely to feel anxious, fearful, and uncertain and should be reassured that such reactions are normal and given ample time to discuss their feelings and concerns with family members.

Assessment

Patients should be assessed for the risk factors outlined using appropriate, brief, valid, and reliable measures. A routine structured clinical diagnostic interview is often impractical and the use of self-screening tools in the cardiac rehabilitation centre, outpatient clinic, or patient's home is a realistic alternative.

Suitable measures for mood include the Patient Health Questionnaire-9 for depressive symptoms,[153] the Generalized Anxiety Disorder Scale-7 for anxiety symptoms,[154] or the Hospital Anxiety and Depression Scale (HADS) for both depression and anxiety.[155] Measures for social support include the Multidimensional Scale of Perceived Social Support,[156] and for illness perceptions the Brief Illness Perception Questionnaire.[157] If it is deemed that patients have developed inaccurate or unrealistic illness perceptions, referral to a mental health professional may be warranted. Alternatively, brief psychoeducational interventions aimed at modifying such illness perceptions have been shown to improve quality of life and treatment adherence and reduce anxiety and depression.[158]

In people with CVD, health-related quality of life is usually measured by a combination of generic and disease-specific measures.[159] Generic measures are designed to address multiple aspects of health-related quality of life across a range of different patient or disease groups. Thus, they focus on general issues of health (or ill health, such as functional capacity, disability, and distress), rather than specific features of a particular disease. Examples of generic measures include the Short-Form 36-item (SF-36) health survey[160] and the EuroQoL 5D (EQ-5D).[161] Disease-specific measures are designed to examine those aspects of health-related quality of life that are relevant to a specific disease group and are, overall, more clinically sensitive and potentially more responsive in detecting change. Examples of disease-specific measures include the Seattle Angina Questionnaire (SAQ),[162] the Myocardial Infarction Dimensional Assessment Scale (MIDAS),[163] and the Minnesota Living with Heart Failure (MLHF) questionnaire.[164] In addition to psychometric properties such as reliability, validity, and responsiveness, the choice of measure will depend on factors such as the patient/clinician burden its use may impose, resources, costs, and intellectual property and copyright issues (see also Chapter 2).

Interventions

In order to be effective, interventions require a friendly and positive interaction to enhance a patient's ability to cope and adhere to recommended lifestyle changes and treatments. Such empowerment means gauging the patient's experiences, thoughts, attitudes, beliefs, worries, knowledge and understanding, and their motivation and commitment. This is likely to be enhanced by including the patient's partner or family member who can reinforce information, correct misconceptions, dispel myths, and allay fears. Behavioural interventions such as motivational interviewing are designed to increase motivation and self-efficacy by helping set realistic, incremental goals in combination with self-monitoring to reduce targeted risk factors. The focus of such interventions should be on coping and empowerment strategies and include measurable and feasible goal setting and pacing (see also

'Supporting patients and families to make healthy lifestyle changes').

The choice of intervention will depend on the issue to be addressed. However, many people will respond to brief advice (5 minutes) using the 5As (Ask, Advise, Assess, Assist, Arrange). Some may require brief behaviour counselling (15–20 minutes) or more specialized counselling such as motivational interviewing, mindfulness, cognitive behaviour therapy, or behavioural activation. Goals can be negotiated using 'SMART' principles and graded in terms of priority and duration. For successful behaviour change to occur, three conditions (COM-B) are necessary: capability, opportunity, and motivation[72] (see also section 'Supporting patients and families to make healthy lifestyle changes').

Specialized psychological interventions have additional beneficial effects in terms of distress, depression, and anxiety.[165] These interventions include individual or group counselling regarding psychosocial risk factors and coping with illness, stress management programmes, meditation, autogenic training, biofeedback, breathing, yoga, and/or muscular relaxation. Multimodal behavioural interventions, integrating health education, physical exercise, and psychological therapy, for psychosocial risk factors and coping with illness are recommended in patients with established CVD and mental health symptoms in order to improve their mental health.

Whatever approach is adopted, consideration should be given to a person's preferences, personal circumstances, and technical skills. Tailoring and adapting the content and delivery of interventions to the capacity of the individual has the potential to exert the most impact. For instance, for some, text-based materials may be seen as too strenuous or time-consuming to read, and telephone calls may be offered as an alternative to written feedback.

It is important that healthcare professionals recognize issues such as financial worries, cultural, racial, ethnic, and linguistic backgrounds, rural and remote locations, family circumstances, social networks, sleep difficulties, and travel restrictions as barriers for patients. For example, CVD can result in loss of workability and early retirement and return to work is associated with better psychosocial well-being and health-related quality of life.[166]

Gender and culturally sensitive interventions may be needed, as notions of masculine/feminine social roles and sexual orientation can determine social norms and traditions to support self-care and self-management, which vary by race and ethnicity.

Many patients, particularly those who are young, are heavy users of technology for connecting with friends and finding information and support. The challenge for online health services is to design interventions specifically suitable for them that are action based and focus on changing short- and long-term behaviours, rather than just increasing knowledge. In considering the use of new technologies, app characteristics such as brevity of interactions, minimal on-screen text, and a solutions-oriented approach are deemed essential.

Depression and anxiety

Psychological interventions are likely to improve a person's function, quality of life, and general health,[160] although it is recognized that psychological problems are underreported and undertreated. Patients who are screened at 'moderate to high' risk of depression have higher levels of depression and anxiety, and lower levels of well-being and social support at follow-up, than those at 'no to low' risk of depression. Importantly, screening and referral alone is insufficient to achieve optimal disease management: a collaborative care approach with integrated pathways to primary care is necessary.[167] A promising approach is one that takes a patient preference, stepped-care approach in which depressed patients participate in decision-making on whether to initiate medications and/or psychotherapy and receive frequent follow-up assessments with decisions as to whether to intensify, switch, or maintain therapies.[168,169]

eHealth services such as guided Internet-based cognitive behaviour therapy may improve access to acceptable, effective, and cost-effective interventions to reduce symptoms of anxiety and depression.[170] Given that mood disorders are common and impose a considerable burden on quality of life,[171] attention should be focused on alleviating these. Apart from pharmacotherapy, cognitive behaviour therapy is a frontline option, with novel approaches such as Panic Attack Treatment in Comorbid Heart Diseases (PATCHD) showing promise.[172] Another promising and less intensive and costly approach, for depression at least, is the use of behavioural activation, a simpler psychological treatment than cognitive behaviour therapy.[173]

Psychological interventions can improve psychological symptoms and reduce mortality in people with CVD, but there remains considerable uncertainty regarding the magnitude of these effects and the specific techniques most likely to benefit people with different presentations of CVD.[165]

Partners

Partners may have more distress than the patient, although they can share the emotional burden and provide social support. They can also bolster confidence, instil hope, and encourage the patient to seek healthcare, attend CVPR, and adhere to lifestyle and medications.[141] While family and friends are often the preferred source of support for many, there is a fear of placing undue worry on loved ones. The role of partners in caring for patients and serving as their primary source of support has the potential to place an undue burden on them. Hence, they need support themselves.

Cardiovascular prevention and rehabilitation

Encouraging patients to attend a CVPR programme that integrates counselling for psychosocial risk factors and exercise is effective in reducing anxiety, distress, and stress, and may be home or community based.[138–140] Indeed, all eligible patients with CVD should be automatically referred to such a programme as it is a useful vehicle for not only addressing psychosocial issues but also for encouraging adherence to secondary prevention measures. It also provides an ideal opportunity for addressing through vocational counselling particular concerns such as return to work or early retirement. Whatever interventions are deemed appropriate will depend on an individual consultation and assessment of capability, motivation, and opportunity for behaviour change and realistic goal setting and support including self-help information, teaching techniques that support understanding and knowledge, and peer support.

Conclusion

Psychosocial factors, illness perceptions, and quality of life are important factors in the cause of, coping with, and outcome of CVD and need to be considered on an individual basis. A successful experience and outcome for patients will depend on an assessment of their risk factors, characteristics, and expectations, their engagement in shared decision-making, and ongoing outcome monitoring to evaluate their responsiveness to any intervention.

Settings and delivery modes for cardiovascular prevention and rehabilitation

The aim of CVPR is to promote secondary prevention in patients with coronary heart disease by promoting lifestyle changes, with a multifactorial interdisciplinary approach. It is a comprehensive programme which includes exercise, education, lifestyle and risk factor assessment and management, and motivational and psychological support for cardiac patients.[174,175] The benefits and efficacy have been well documented and the core components have been standardized; however, the length and structure of programmes varies greatly across Europe depending on national guidelines and government policy.[176]

Hospital setting

Historical perspective

For many years now, CVPR has been recognized as making an important contribution in the protection of physical and psychological health of patients with heart disease. It has evolved over time and the use of exercise in the treatment of heart disease is not a new concept. As far back as 1768, Herberden observed that his patient with angina pectoris was 'nearly cured' by sawing wood for half an hour every day. This valuable information was forgotten and overlooked. By the early twentieth century, heart disease was recognized as a grave problem. When a diagnosis of myocardial infarction was made, prolonged bedrest was thought to be the cure if the patient's life was to be saved and improved. The treatment was strict bedrest, which inevitably led to deconditioning of patients and subsequently to them becoming 'cardiac cripples'.[177] Nonetheless, it was around this time that the treatment began to change. Levine and Lown[178] established that getting out of bed and sitting in a chair for 7 days after the onset of acute coronary symptoms was safe and had physical and psychological benefits. Additionally, the use of physical training to aid post-infarction recovery began, following findings in the 1950s that coronary patients have responses to exercise that are similar to normal, but modified by deconditioning. Research suggested that many patients led miserable unproductive lives after their cardiac event. They were frightened to return to work and needlessly, became cardiac invalids. Coexisting with gradual changes from sedentary convalescence to early mobilization, the importance of lifestyle and risk factors was realized and the concept of 'cardiac rehabilitation' was born.

Hospital-based programmes

Many programmes include exercise for the patients while still in hospital in phase 1 of rehabilitation. Education was introduced in phase 1 by Johnson et al. in 1976,[179] when they included advice on smoking, diet, and activities post discharge. In order to supervise early activity, Harrington et al. devised a programme with electrocardiogram telemetry monitoring in 1981.[180] This was to detect arrhythmias while carrying out activities of daily living and light exercise.

Gottheiner pioneered the first outpatient programme in Israel in 1955 and by 1968 had experience of over 1000 patients.[181] The exercise programme started with several months of build-up exercises, which graduated to endurance training such as running, cycling, or swimming. When enrolled, the patients were expected to stay in the programme for life. The early cardiac rehabilitation programmes developed in the 1950s and 1960s were mainly exercise based. Following Gottheiner in Israel, other researchers such as Kellerman and Brunner developed programmes of exercise twice or three times a week for 3 months. Brunner reported the reduction of angina in his study group.[182] In addition, his subjects were fitter after the programme than before and were even fitter than non-trained healthy individuals of the same age. The first controlled trial of exercise was conducted by Naughton et al.[183] in 24 post myocardial patients. After 8 months of exercise, the exercise group had lower heart rates and blood pressure at rest and at exercise than the sedentary groups. Subsequently, comprehensive guidelines for exercise in cardiac rehabilitation were established.

In America in 1975, Hellerstein and Ford[184] were the first to develop a more comprehensive programme for post-myocardial infarction patients. This included education, vocational advice, and a listing of the different energy expenditure of different daily activities at work and at leisure. They introduced exercise testing before and after the exercise programme with the aim of exercising patients to approximately 60–70% of their aerobic capacity. This led to the belief that a more comprehensive programme was more beneficial to cardiac patients than exercise alone.

From this early development, CVPR has advanced worldwide and the programmes are now integral to the comprehensive care of patients with coronary heart disease and are coordinated multifactorial interventions.

CVPR differs in delivery from country to country. In Ireland and the UK, the duration of programmes varies from 6 to 12 weeks. Whereas in the US and Canada, programmes can last up to 6 months or a year.

The Carinex study[185] reported duration, content of programmes, staffing, and organizational activities across Western Europe. It is evident from the study that programmes are varied but well organized. The most notable difference is the length of the programme, which varied from 3 weeks in France to 20 weeks in parts of Belgium. CVPR in Eastern Europe and parts of Germany and Switzerland, is organized differently and is mostly on an inpatient basis in residential clinics. These clinics are usually run by a cardiologist with a follow-on maintenance programme. In western Europe, many programmes are still based in hospital outpatient services; however, there are now several examples of community-based services. Most programmes are now set up on a rolling basis where patients start and finish at different times, thus allowing for flexibility. CVPR programmes amalgamate an exercise programme with education and counselling, which includes aggressive risk factor management, psychosocial and vocational counselling, and the use of cardioprotective medicines which has been shown to be efficient in secondary prevention of CVD.[186]

The mode of delivery of programmes varies throughout Europe and the rest of the world, as local resources and population needs dictate what can be done.[185,186] However, most programmes incorporate the goals of CVPR into their delivery, which can be identified specifically as medical, psychological, behavioural, social, and health services goals.[186] To achieve these goals, an interdisciplinary team is recommended to deliver a CVPR service. The team may include cardiologists, nurses, physiotherapists, psychologists, dieticians, pharmacists, occupational therapists, vocational counsellors, social workers, and others. The programme carried out by the team should be flexible and individualized since patients' medical problems and needs, educational level, and social and vocational situations vary. Consequently, it may not be necessary for all patients to attend every component of the programme and such flexibility within programmes could increase attendance.[187]

Patients should be assessed on an individual basis and risk stratified prior to commencing a structured programme. Hospital programmes may include high-risk stratified patients monitoring with telemetry and easy access to a cardiology department (Irish Association of Cardiac Rehabilitation guidelines, American Heart Association guidelines). Exercise capacity assessment should be conducted using recommended methods such as exercise stress testing, which is the gold standard, or the incremental shuttle walk test.

More recently, a European survey[188] found that CVPR was available in 40/44 (90.9%) of European countries. Programme availability was greatest in western European countries, but overall were higher than in other high-income countries (P <0.001). Typically, throughout Europe, there was only one CVPR slot per seven cardiac patients, with a vital need of 3,449,460 slots annually. Guidelines were used in 70% or more of programmes with no regional variation. Programmes had a multidisciplinary team of 6.5 ± 3.0 staff number with a variation in type of staff regionally. Notably, European programmes had more staff than other high-income countries, offering 8.5 ± 1.5/10 core components over 24.8 ± 26.0 hours (regional differences, $P < 0.05$).

Guidelines, standards, and core components for CVPR have been developed and updated by various expert associations across the world. The Scottish Intercollegiate Guideline network, Working Group on Cardiac Rehabilitation and Exercise Physiology, American Association of Cardiovascular and Pulmonary Rehabilitation, and many European countries offer guidance on the most effective method of CCPR to be provided.

Regarding exercise, eminent societies recommend that patients progress from moderate to vigorous intensity aerobic exercise over the timeframe of the programme, with resistance training introduced in the latter half of the programme as an important extra. This mode of delivery has been deemed safe and provides for a better outcome for the cardiac patient.[176]

The British Association for Cardiovascular Prevention and Rehabilitation (BACPR) published the third edition of its standards and core components for CVPR in 2017.[189] The aim of this publication was to further emphasize to commissioners, clinicians, politicians, and the public the significance of robust, quality indicators of CVPR service delivery. The 2017 revision has six standards and six core components (➤ **Fig. 11.13**), with greater emphasis on quantifiable clinical and health outcomes, audit, and certification. The standards are outlined as follows:

1. The delivery of six core components by a qualified and competent multidisciplinary team, led by a clinical coordinator.
2. Prompt identification, referral, and recruitment of eligible patient populations.
3. Early initial assessment of individual patient needs which informs the agreed personalized goals that are reviewed regularly.
4. Early provision of a structured CVPR programme, with a defined pathway of care, which meets the individual's goals and is aligned with patient preference and choice.
5. Upon programme completion, a final assessment of individual patient needs and demonstration of sustainable health outcomes.
6. Registration and submission of data to the National Audit for Cardiac Rehabilitation and participation in the National Certification Programme.

A six-step clinical pathway has been developed from inpatient stay to discharge following a CVPR programme which can be used in most countries depending on local logistics[190] (➤ **Fig. 11.14**).

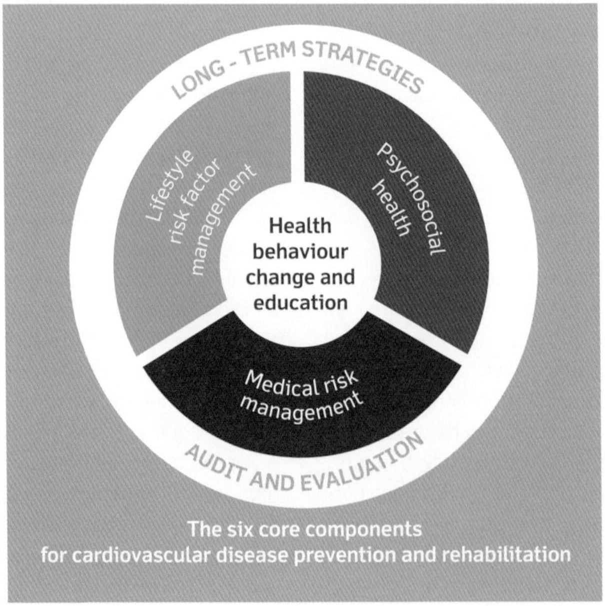

Fig. 11.13 The British Association for Cardiovascular Prevention and Rehabilitation (BACPR) six core components.

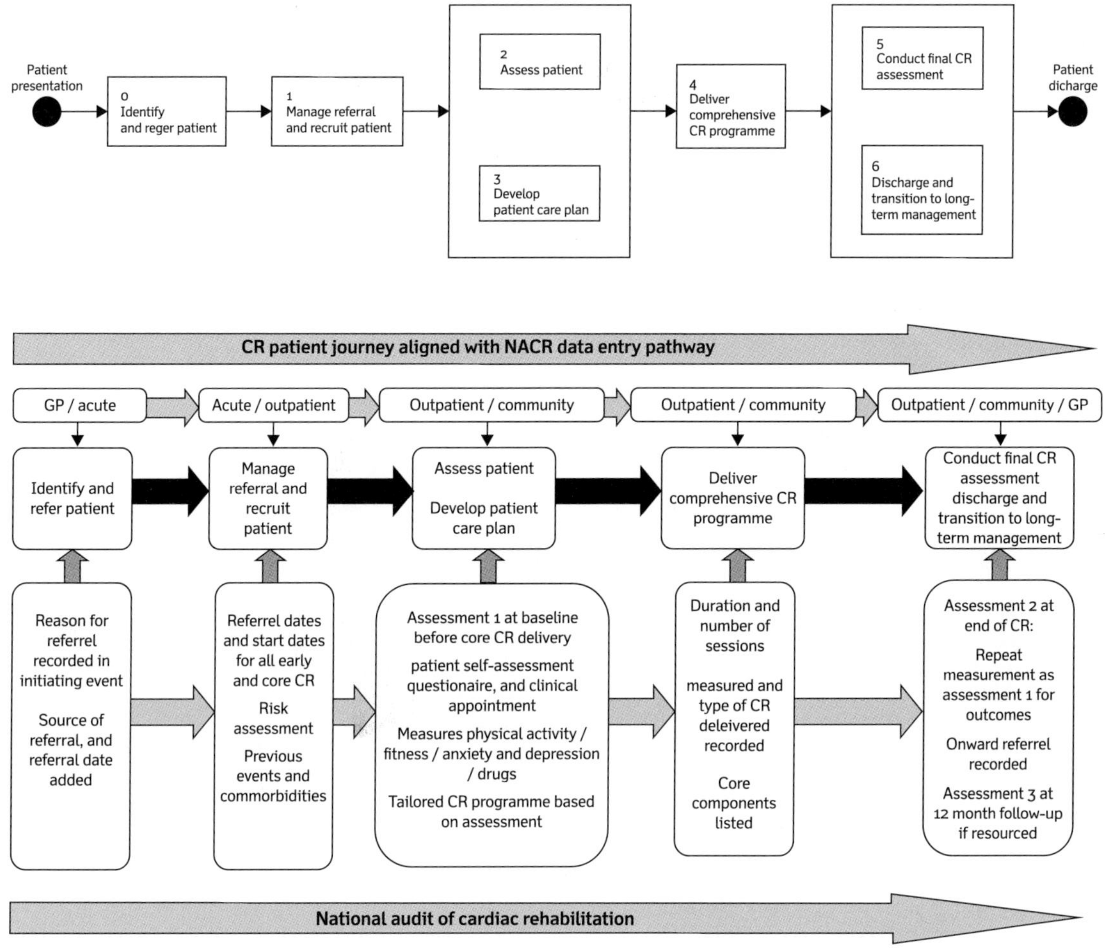

Fig. 11.14 Cardiac rehabilitation patient pathway aligned with National Audit of Cardiac Rehabilitation (NACR) data entry pathway. CR, cardiac rehabilitation; GP, general practitioner.

In a consensus document,[175] strategies are outlined to implement prevention programmes in post-myocardial infarction patients (➤ **Fig. 11.15**). The main thrust of the strategy is that CVPR should begin in hospital during the admission for the acute event or intervention procedure. At this stage, all professionals involved in patient care should encourage and promote lifestyle changes with prevention as a priority. Lifestyle changes and preventive medications should be pivotal to discharge planning. This early intervention along with automatic referral to structured, ambulatory programmes post discharge is designed to promote uptake. Maintenance will be promoted by family involvement and integrated care process with healthcare providers outside secondary care settings.[175]

The European Cardiac Rehabilitation Inventory Survey[191] assessed topics including national guidelines, legislation and funding mechanisms, types of CVPR provided, and characteristics of included patients. It found that less than half of eligible cardiovascular patients benefit from CVPR in most European countries.

The results yielded responses from 28 of 39 (72%) countries; 61% had national CVPR associations and 57% had national professional guidelines. Most countries (86%) provided early CVPR during the acute inpatient phase, although service provision varied; 29% reported delivery to over 80% patients. Support in the early post-discharge period was available; however, 15 countries reported provision in less than 30%. Almost half (46%) had national legislation for this kind of support. Three-quarters had

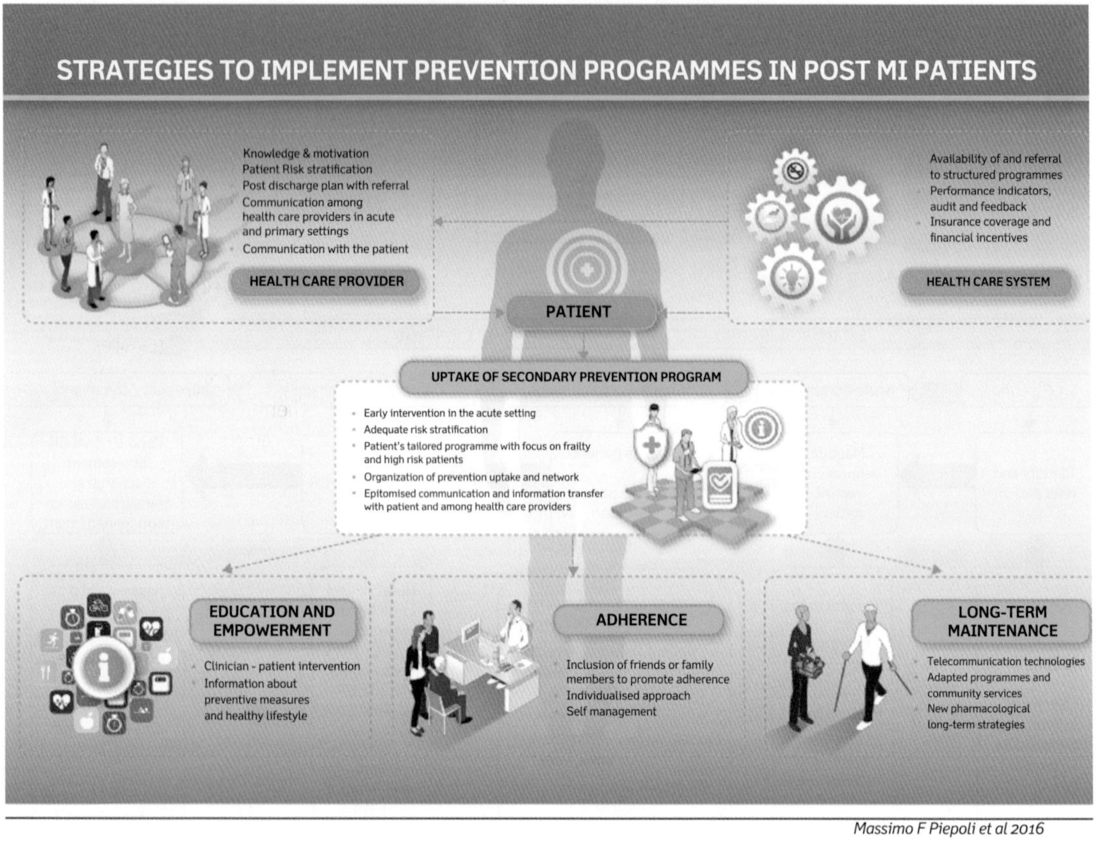

Fig. 11.15 Strategies to implement prevention programmes in post-myocardial infarction patients.

government funding and an associated tariff. Structured ambulatory programmes to follow early support were less supported. Although they were available in most countries, 11 could not provide estimates of numbers participating. Thirteen reported that all costs were met by patients.

Primary care setting

The World Health Organization

The WHO defines primary care as a place of first contact for healthcare, but more than just 'gate keeping', for example, in deciding where patients should be referred for specialist care (https://www.euro.who.int/en/health-topics/Health-systems/primary-health-care/main-terminology). Primary care should provide continued, comprehensive, and coordinated care in the long term.

An ageing population, adverse trends in cardiovascular risk factors, and the burden of chronic non-communicable disease has intensified the demand for high-quality primary care services.[57,192] As cardiovascular risk is predominantly driven by poor lifestyle habits learned early in life, preventive efforts should begin in childhood (see also 'The global imperative'). Embracing this concept, primary care addresses health over the life course providing an optimal environment to deliver health promotion and integrated primary and secondary prevention. Its wide reach into the population (via routine check-ups, episodic visits, and chronic disease support), unrivalled knowledge of patients' social situation, and access to continuous care and coordination highlight its suitability.[193]

While combining all healthcare professionals' diverse knowledge and skills into multimodal interventions can optimize preventive efforts, nurses working in primary care are integral members of the primary care team, which also can include general practitioners and other professionals such as community or district nurses, midwives, feldshers, dentists, physiotherapists, social workers, psychiatrists, speech therapists, dietitians, pharmacists, and administrative staff and managers. Their holistic approach and frequent patient contact provide unlimited opportunities to address the needs of patients and families including screening, healthy lifestyle promotion, and planned evidence-based interventions. Given the compelling data demonstrating the impact of nurse-led prevention programmes,[30,196] there is a critical need to expand nurses' roles in primary care as this could increase access to these services, alleviating general practitioner shortages while enhancing care at a lower cost. However, various constraints including time and educational preparation prevent them from practising to their full potential.[195]

Although preparing and maintaining a well-educated workforce is fundamental, nurse training programmes routinely focus on acute care settings with less emphasis on primary care, leading to a weakness in training for nurses working in primary care. Existing undergraduate programmes need to revise curricula to reflect emerging healthcare needs with a clear focus on prevention and primary care health delivery. It is equally important that nurses maintain their competence to practise, after basic training, through ongoing education. This gap has been acknowledged within the European context through the development by ACNAP of a core curriculum intended to guide the continuing education of nurses working in cardiovascular care (see also Chapter 3).[196] In addition, highly beneficial postgraduate masters' programmes are available, although currently are not a prerequisite for employment.

Risk identification.

Preventive efforts should be targeted at those who will benefit the most and systematic risk screening can be easily integrated into routine clinical practice using global risk assessment tools (see 'Concept of total cardiovascular risk and total risk management'). These tools provide a valuable guide for primary care nurses to prioritize and plan prevention management.

Providing a clear understanding of the patient's cardiovascular risk along with potential effects of lifestyle and/or pharmacological interventions is key to fulfilling their active role in shared decision-making. Importance of training staff to overcome challenges of communicating this risk has been highlighted within screening programmes.[197] Considering patients' level of health literacy, avoiding technical terms, and using tailored, and/or interactive decision aids can all enhance the nurse–patient risk discussion. In particular, the ESC HeartScore, an interactive online version of SCORE, is valuable for conveying powerful messages, such as risk age and demonstrating the relative contribution of each risk factor to overall risk.[198] For example, illustrating to a smoker how smoking alone impacts their risk may be more compelling than just words.

Brief and very brief interventions opportunities in primary care

Lifestyle change is a key priority in promoting CVH (see 'Components of prevention and rehabilitation in clinical practice'). Primary care nurses are in an ideal position to offer brief, opportunistic advice about behaviour change during routine encounters with their patients. These 'teachable moments' are a powerful strategy to identify and effectively address unhealthy behaviours, without using additional resources.[199,200] For example, a child's visit for immunization, with a history of repeated otitis media, represents a *teachable moment* to counsel parents regarding the health effects of passive smoking (i.e. doubles the risk of a child having an ear infection).[201] Very brief interventions (<5 minutes), while limited to active behaviour change techniques such as self-monitoring and review of behavioural goals are equally valuable and crucial in a busy primary care setting.

The therapeutic relationship established between primary care nurses and patients through repeated encounters provides a strong foundation to incorporate behavioural strategies and offers a menu of strategies to move patients from the 'why to how'. While these evidence-based approaches are no 'magic bullet', they are useful in time-limited health consultations serving as catalysts for more comprehensive, personalized discussions contributing to healthy lifestyle changes.

Active follow-up is vital to build a relationship, evaluate interventions, and adjust action plans accordingly. As long-term adherence diminishes, primarily with reduced interactions, booster reinforcement sessions are essential. While family and other caregivers add an important source of social support to improve long-term changes, it also increases the reach of preventive care.[57,202]

Health education programmes and self-management support

Patients with chronic conditions interact frequently in primary care and self-management support, a key component of the Chronic Care Model, enhances patient skills and confidence to manage their chronic condition. Nurse-led self-management support interventions have yielded numerous health outcomes in a range of chronic diseases,[203–206] thus, embedding systematic education and supportive interventions (e.g. goal-setting, self-monitoring) into routine practice is now a priority.[207] Employing simple but effective tools can empower patients such as, for example, the 'Guide to Healthy Shopping' card which develops knowledge and skills in understanding food labels and facilitates informed healthy choices.[208] This guide from Ireland uses traffic light colours to facilitate patients to make informed healthier food choices. While some manufacturers use traffic light labelling on prepacked food and drinks, it is inconsistent. Other successful factors include having interactive components such as online tools (e.g. tracking dietary progress) and providing opportunities for peer support (e.g. family/friends, social groups).

Guideline implementation and quality

Nurse-led teams have proven effective in implementing evidence-based guidelines,[20,209–211] which in turn, provide clinical standards for high-quality preventive care and decision support. Systematic monitoring of these activities and outcomes are important drivers of translating evidence into clinical practice with publishable outcomes. This exploration of programme effectiveness enhances good practice, builds an evidence-base for effectiveness to drive service improvement, and improves care.[57]

Clinical community linkage

As a gateway to community prevention resources, primary care should have an established link to a comprehensive network both locally and nationally. This community linkage will facilitate the nurse's role as preventive health navigators, especially for vulnerable patients, providing information and steering them to link with other providers (e.g. community-based support groups).

Options for the future

Primary care has a key role in the frontline management of prevention, treatment, and control across the lifespan with the patient/family as central entities in the process. Nurses working in primary care, as effective champions, are well poised to guide patient care delivery, coordination, and lead interdisciplinary teams to optimize preventive efforts. Risk stratification, driving resource allocation and directing care intensity, accompanied by routine application of behaviour change practices can enhance frequency and quality of preventive care. While competency-based pathways can support expanding roles of these nurses, political activism is vital to influence a higher investment in preventive activities.

Community setting

Internationally, there is a growing need to extend the current provision of CVPR beyond the traditional hospital and primary care settings and develop more innovative, integrated models of high-quality care that will address the challenges that exist around uptake and accessibility of these programmes.

The community is particularly important as a setting for prevention as it offers many opportunities to address the barriers associated with prevention (➤ Box 11.10). It offers greater access to 'hard to reach' population groups including ethnic minorities, women, the elderly, and those with limited social support and low socioeconomic status. Individuals with low socioeconomic status as defined by educational attainment, income level, employment status, and environmental factors, are at increased CVD risk and disproportionately experience poor health outcomes and CVD prognosis. With 80% of the global CVD burden in low- to middle-income countries,[212] translating evidence-based practice to non-conventional community-based healthcare settings offers an alternative way to address the health inequalities associated with CVD. There is increasing evidence to support these non-traditional health promotion approaches to prevention in community settings such as schools, social networks, religious organizations, workplaces, and retail outlets. Data from recent RCTs of blood pressure

Box 11.10 Opportunities to address the barriers to prevention in the community

- Offers greater convenience, overcoming barriers related to access, geography, and transport.
- Promotes greater uptake of prevention and cardiac rehabilitation among underserved populations which include women, heart failure, stroke and peripheral vascular disease patients, and ethnic minority groups.
- Removes the barrier of attending the general practitioner and hospital clinic.
- Promotes long-term maintenance of behaviour change as the individual is empowered to continue making lifestyle changes in their local community where they live, work, and play.

management in black barbershops and community-based lifestyle interventions in churches[213,214] demonstrated improved health outcomes and significantly greater reductions in blood pressure than those in the control group. Furthermore, the Fifty, Fifty study[215] demonstrated the benefits of a comprehensive lifestyle peer group-based programme delivered in the community on cardiovascular risk factors.

Integrated models of community-based cardiovascular disease care

In reorientating health systems to respond effectively to the increasing burden of non-communicable diseases including CVD, global recommendations call for community-based, patient-centred, integrated models of chronic disease management.[216] The MyAction programme[26,209] is an example of one such model, which manages CVD as a single family of diseases and integrates primary and secondary prevention in one community-based service. The programme is nurse led and is based on the EUROACTION study intervention model[208] which demonstrated that an intensive nurse-led programme can achieve effective and substantial improvement of CVD risk factors in high-risk groups of patients in comparison to usual care (see also 'The global imperative'). The key components of this 12–16-week interdisciplinary care model include lifestyle modification (smoking cessation, healthy food choices, and physical activity), medical risk factor management (blood pressure, lipids, and glucose), and the prescription of cardioprotective medication where appropriate. Utilizing specific behavioural change techniques, the programme places a strong emphasis on the promotion of self-management, where patients are empowered to become active participants in their own care. Adopting this multifactorial approach, which addresses six or more risk factors, has been shown to achieve best patient outcomes, reducing myocardial infarction, stroke, cardiovascular, and all-cause mortality.[12]

The MyAction programme has demonstrated effectiveness in a real-world setting,[26,209] among different population cohorts and geographical regions, highlighting its acceptability and transferability as an alternative, model of preventive care. Critical to the success of the programme has been its patient-centred approach ensuring a flexible offering of sessions and involvement of families recognizing that healthy lifestyle change is easier to achieve if the family change together. The outcomes of MyAction emphasize that it is possible to implement prevention guidelines into everyday clinical practice and achieve significant reductions in cardiovascular risk in those with established CVD and asymptomatic high-risk individuals, which are sustained at 1 year follow-up.

Optimizing on the role of the nurse in the community

Lack of access to healthcare providers, is a well-documented barrier to prevention,[212] particularly in low- to middle-income countries. Given the increasing demands and reorientation of health services to primary care, there needs to be an increased focus on task sharing or team-based care models, maximizing the role of nurses working outside hospital and primary care settings and other healthcare professionals working in prevention and chronic disease management. This may involve opportunistic approaches to screening and early detection of CVD, addressing major modifiable risk factors, including tobacco use, hypertension, high blood cholesterol, and diabetes, through comprehensive prevention and rehabilitation programmes and promoting lifelong CVD prevention. While there are various specialities of nurses working in the community, including, but not limited to, public health nurses, community registered nurses, to those working with non-governmental organizations, their roles tend to be more of a generalist nature, with variations in skill set, competencies, and experience in cardiovascular care. Therefore, to truly optimize the role of nurses working in cardiovascular health promotion, prevention, and management, there is a recognized need to build capacity around nursing education and training to ensure that nurses are equipped with the appropriate skills and strategies to deliver evidence-based, high-quality, patient-centred care.[217,218]

The community is one of many settings where comprehensive prevention and cardiac rehabilitation can be successfully delivered; however, due consideration does need to be given to a number of factors in establishing programmes in this setting (➤ Box 11.11). The community offers a modern-day approach to addressing the challenges that exist around implementing evidence-based guidelines and should be considered as part of a menu-based approach that promotes individual choice.

Technology to support prevention and rehabilitation initiatives

While provision of prevention and rehabilitation programmes in the community, closer to people's homes,

Box 11.11 Key considerations for delivering programmes in the community

- There is no 'one-size-fits-all' approach and for optimal impact prevention programmes must be designed with service user input, and shaped accordingly to the cultural needs and literacy levels of the target population.
- There should be close alignment between community-based prevention and rehabilitation programmes and hospital programmes to ensure patient choice is prioritized and supported by one efficient and effective seamless referral system.
- It is imperative that all models of prevention and cardiac rehabilitation service provision, regardless of setting should be underpinned by evidence-based, nationally/internationally accepted key components. This will reduce variability of service provision and ensure standardization of care.
- Appropriate clinical governance and programme protocols with standard operating procedures including inclusion and exclusion criteria, key performance indicators, and policies and procedures should be in place.
- Nurses who work in the community need to be equipped with the appropriate skills and training to deliver evidence-based, high-quality, patient-centred care.

has the potential to improve access and so increase uptake as explained previously (see 'Community setting'), integrating technology may address other barriers to uptake such as, for example, a dislike of group-based programmes and timing in relation to working hours. Technology offers more flexibility and alternative delivery models that may include interventions based in general practice or in the home environment.

Over the past 10 years, there has been a marked increase in the number of health interventions which are delivered digitally. Digital health, or 'telehealth', including mobile apps, Internet-based interventions, and videoconferencing have been shown to be effective in reducing risk factors and improving quality of life. Moreover, these interventions can also be used as an adjunct to traditional CVPR, and provide additive benefit to those who received both interventions. The key challenge exists in understanding the active ingredients of digital health solutions. A recent systematic review[219] of 30 unique trials investigating the effects of telehealth highlighted the complexity of the interventions and the difficulty in understanding which element works for whom. Indeed, among individual trials delivered via mobile apps, only one of them used a single intervention (➤ **Table 11.26**).[220–226] This study, called 'TEXT ME',[220] used a computer to randomly select study participants to receive text messages providing information on lifestyle change semi-tailored to the individual. Although the participants were told that they should not respond to the messages, a number of them did. They associated these computer-provided messages with the research assistant who had recruited them to the study.

This fascinating finding of 'TEXT ME' highlights the importance of personalization in digital health. In future, virtual coaches in the form of avatars may help to increase the sense of personalized support and so reduce the burden on healthcare providers. An avatar is the graphical representation of a healthcare provider in a digital environment. Avatars can be simple, for example, the Apple watch activity app provides a visual representation of the user's daily activity using circles. Avatars also have the capacity to deliver more complex information. Recent work in Australia has highlighted the potential for an avatar to improve understanding of chest pain and timely presentation to healthcare services (➤ **Fig. 11.16**).[227] Of even more importance, avatars can be tailored to be culturally sensitive, to speak multiple languages, and information can be revisited multiple times.

One of the key challenges that exists in delivering digital health is the rapid evolution of technology. Over 6000 apps are released daily in the Google play store. Researchers struggle with the rapid evolution of technology and the slow pace of research funding, ethics approval, and length of time for conducting studies. This means it is critical for us to understand what is likely to be the active ingredient of an app. A review conducted in 2015[228] demonstrated some key features that are likely to be critical in improving cardiovascular health:

1. Simplicity of the app appears to be of great importance in acceptance and use of health-related apps. If the app requires active input from the user, the choices must be clear and unambiguous, and minimal steps must be required to navigate from one part of the app to another.
2. Users want to be assured that the information comes from a credible source, such as the national heart foundation of the country of origin.
3. It is thought that embedding behaviour change concepts will improve use and effectiveness of apps.

Table 11.26 Key components of digital interventions

Blasco et al.[221]	Acute coronary syndrome patients with 1+ cardiovascular risk factor (Spain)	Combination: telephone, Internet, risk factor monitoring by cardiologist, individualized SMS feedback
Chow et al. (TEXT ME)[220]	Patients >18 years with coronary heart disease (Australia)	Text messages, based on American Heart Foundation guidelines, regular semi-personalized messages, individualized risk factor modification
Johnston et al. (SUPPORT)[222]	Myocardial infarction patients prescribed ticagrelor (Sweden)	Combination: smartphone app, self-managed, risk factor monitoring, automated feedback SMS
Karhula et al.[223]	Patients >18 years with coronary heart disease or diabetes (Finland)	Combination: Internet, health coaching, mobile phone coaching to risk factor targets, self-management
Maddison et al. (HEART)[224]	Patients >18 years diagnosed with ischaemic heart disease within past 3–24 months (New Zealand)	Combination: Internet, web-based exercise intervention, self-managed, behaviour change, Internet behaviour monitoring, SMS encouragement
Pfaeffli Dale et al. (Text4Heart)[225]	Coronary heart disease patients with home Internet access (New Zealand)	Combination: text messaging, based on cardiac rehabilitation, patient education, risk factor management, daily messages, Internet support
Varnfield et al. (CAP-CR)[226]	Post-myocardial infarction patients referred to cardiac rehabilitation (Australia)	Combination: smartphone, mentor-managed, motivational/education messages, weekly phone consultation, web monitoring with weekly consultation

4. Being able to track behaviour in real-time is also thought to be very important. For example, wearable technology may improve engagement.
5. Personalized information is particularly important. The ability in the future for patients to hold their own electronic information will increase the possibility for personalized tailored information.
6. Opportunities for social comparison and social support have been shown to improve physical activity compared to apps without these features. In cardiovascular health prevention, there is limited trial evidence about the importance of these features. However, work by an Australian group led by Tashi Dorje (unpublished data) demonstrates the huge

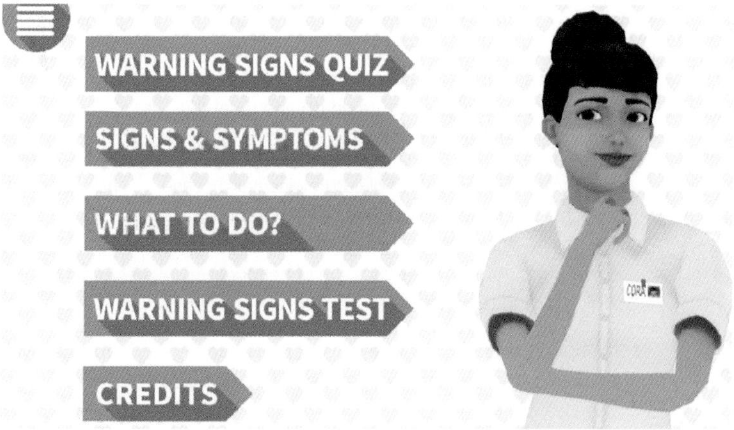

Fig. 11.16 Cora digital avatar provides health information to improve timely presentation with chest pain.

potential of social media sites such as WeChat to reach patients who otherwise have no opportunities to participate in CVPR.

Although critics suggest that digital health may not be suitable for older adults, this is not supported by the available evidence. Smartphone ownership is on the rise among the older generation. Digital technology has been used to successfully improve physical activity and cognitive function in the older adult. There are some considerations for app use in older adults, for example, decreased vision and reduced fine motor skills may make using apps on a smartphone more challenging. Another finding is that older adults are less likely to feel confident navigating apps and may worry that they will break it. Providing older apps with digital resources requires reassurance that the apps cannot be broken.

The potential for digital technology to transform CVPR is vast. Consequently, it is essential that healthcare providers are familiar with technologies and understand what to recommend to improve access to CVPR and give people opportunities to improve their cardiovascular health.

Role of professional societies, associations, and foundations in cardiovascular prevention and rehabilitation

Professional associations and societies play an important role in supporting healthcare providers, patients, and caregivers. It is important for nurses to engage with these organizations to support their continuing professional development (see also Chapter 3). They have the power to influence policy, advocate for professionals and patients, provide educational materials and programmes, publish and disseminate research in journals, offer networking opportunities, patient support groups, and professional development. ➤ **Table 11.27** provides a list of organizations that are concerned with CVPR across the globe.

Table 11.27 The professional association/societies listed focus on cardiovascular disease prevention and management

Name	Mission	Website
ACNAP (Association of Cardiovascular Nursing and Allied Professionals)	Our mission: to reduce the burden of cardiovascular disease	https://www.escardio.org/Sub-specialty-communities/Association-of-Cardiovascular-Nursing-&-Allied-Professions/About
AHA (American Heart Association)	To be a relentless force for a world of longer, healthier lives	https://www.heart.org/en/about-us
AHN (African Heart Network)	The African Heart Network's vision is to play a leading role in the prevention and reduction of the burden related to cardiovascular disease, including heart disease and stroke, so that it will no longer be the major cause of premature death and disability throughout Africa	http://www.ahnetwork.org/about-us/vision-mission
ASPC (American Society for Preventive Cardiology)	To promote the prevention of cardiovascular disease, advocate for the preservation of cardiovascular health, and disseminate high-quality, evidence-based information through the education of healthcare clinicians and their patients	https://www.aspconline.org/
BHF (British Heart Foundation)	To support research into the causes, prevention, diagnosis, and treatment of heart and circulatory diseases	https://www.bhf.org.uk/

Table 11.27 Continued

Name	Mission	Website
BACPR (British Association for Cardiovascular Prevention and Rehabilitation)	To support health professionals in the development, delivery, and assessment of evidence-based, individualized programmes of prevention and rehabilitation which have been appropriately funded and which are accessed both by individuals with established cardiovascular disease and those with significant cardiovascular disease risk factors	https://www.bacpr.com/pages/default.asp
CACPR (Canadian Association of Cardiovascular Prevention and Rehabilitation)	The Canadian Association of Cardiovascular Prevention and Rehabilitation (CACPR) is a national body comprised of interdisciplinary health professionals. Our focus is enhancing knowledge and clinical care, as well as enabling research for those who work in cardiovascular prevention and rehabilitation	https://cacpr.ca/About-Us
CIPRECAR (acronym in Spanish)	The Inter-American Working Committee on Cardiovascular Prevention and Rehabilitation is composed of people interested in the prevention of cardiovascular diseases and the timely and adequate rehabilitation of patients who already suffer from any of these pathologies. Mission: to reduce the burden of cardiovascular disease in Latin America and reduce the morbidity and mortality of patients already affected with cardiovascular diseases	http://www.ciprecar.org/nosotros/
EAPC (European Association of Preventive Cardiology)	Our mission is to promote excellence in research, practice, education, and policy in cardiovascular health, and primary and secondary prevention	https://www.escardio.org/Sub-specialty-communities/European-Association-of-Preventive-Cardiology-(EAPC)
EHN (European Heart Network)	The European Heart Network plays a leading role in the prevention and reduction of cardiovascular diseases, in particular heart disease and stroke, through advocacy, networking, capacity-building, patient support, and research so that they are no longer a major cause of premature death and disability throughout Europe	http://www.ehnheart.org/
HFATW (Heart Friends Around The World)	Heart Friends Around the World (HFATW) is an international organization and an affiliated member of the WHF that promotes cardiovascular disease prevention worldwide through a membership network	http://www.hfatw.org/

(continued)

Table 11.27 Continued

Name	Mission	Website
IACR (Irish Association of Cardiac Rehabilitation)	To facilitate communication and support between cardiac rehabilitation multidisciplinary professionals who wish to promote a greater awareness and understanding of cardiac rehabilitation throughout the healthcare system. To endeavour to provide and improve the standard of professional education within cardiovascular rehabilitation through the promotion of conferences, scientific meetings, publications, and contact with appropriate national and international agencies. To cooperate and fully collaborate with existing national and international organizations working in this field to promote an evidence-based approach to client care within cardiac rehabilitation	https://iacronline.ie/
ICCPR (International Council of Cardiovascular Prevention and Rehabilitation)	The primary goals of the International Council of Cardiovascular Prevention and Rehabilitation (ICCPR) are to: To bring together national associations from around the world, to harmonize efforts in promoting cardiovascular prevention and rehabilitation. To work towards ongoing consensus among national associations globally, regarding the internationally common core elements and standards of cardiovascular disease prevention and rehabilitation. To promote cardiovascular prevention and rehabilitation as an essential, not optional service to ensure broader access to these proven services. To support countries to establish and augment programmes of cardiovascular prevention and rehabilitation, adapted to local needs and conditions. To consider and communicate the emerging evidence base for cardiac rehabilitation	http://globalcardiacrehab.com/
IHF (Irish Heart Foundation)	Our mission is to affect positive change in the lifestyles of Irish people, to achieve better outcomes for those affected by heart disease and stroke, and to challenge when the health of our nation is put at risk. We empower people to live longer, healthier lives	https://irishheart.ie/our-mission/mission-statement/
NIPC (National Institute for Prevention and Cardiovascular Health, Ireland)	To provide leadership through discovery, training, and applied programmes to prevent and control cardiovascular disease for all, promote healthier living, raise the standards of preventive cardiology practice, and prepare leaders to advance preventive healthcare in Ireland	http://www.nipc.ie/about.html

Table 11.27 Continued

Name	Mission	Website
PCNA (Preventive Cardiovascular Nurses Association) and GCNLF (The Global Cardiovascular Nursing Leadership Forum)	PCNA's mission is to promote nurses as leaders in cardiovascular disease prevention and management across the lifespan. The mission of the GCNLF is to engage and mobilize an international community of nurse leaders to promote the prevention of cardiovascular disease and stroke worldwide through research, education, policy, and advocacy	https://pcna.net/about/
NHF (Nigerian Heart Foundation)	To play a leading role in the fight against heart disease and stroke with the aim of reducing the number of Nigerians suffering from premature death and disabilities	http://www.nigerianheart.org/
Russian National Medical Society of Preventive Cardiology	To promote the development of policy, improvement of scientific research, clinical practice and education projects in the field of preventive cardiology in the Russian Federation	http://www.cardioprevent.ru/scientific-society/about/_eng_/default.asp
SBC (Society of Brazilian Cardiology)	Expand and disseminate knowledge in cardiovascular science representing and promoting the development of the cardiologist to carry out actions in favour of cardiovascular health in the country	http://prevencao.cardiol.br/quem_somos.asp
SHA (Saudi Heart Association)	Promote research in cardiovascular medicine through the *Journal of the Saudi Heart Association* where specialists in cardiovascular medicine exchange knowledge	https://saudi-heart.com/
The Global Heart Hub	An international alliance of heart patient organizations established to create a unified global voice for those living with or affected by heart disease	https://www.heartscore.org/
WHF (World Heart Federation)	By 2025, we aim to drive the WHO target for non-communicable disease mortality reduction by reducing premature deaths from cardiovascular disease by at least 25%	https://www.world-heart-federation.org/about-us/

References

1. World Health Organization. Needs and Action Priorities in Cardiac Rehabilitation and Secondary Prevention in Patients with Coronary Heart Disease. Geneva: WHO Regional Office for Europe; 1993.
2. Preventive Cardiovascular Nurses' Association (PCNA) and the Council on Cardiovascular Nursing and Allied Professions (CCNAP). Global cardiovascular disease prevention: a call to action for nursing. Eur J Cardiovasc Nurs. 2011;10(2):S1–S57.
3. Grace SL, Warburton DR, Stone JA, Sanderson BK, Oldridge N, Jones J, et al. International charter on cardiovascular prevention and rehabilitation: a call for action. J Cardiopulm Rehabil Prev. 2013;33(2):128–31.
4. McCullough ML, Patel AV, Kushi LH, Patel R, Willett WC, Doyle C, et al. Following cancer prevention guidelines reduces risk of cancer, cardiovascular disease, and

all-cause mortality. Cancer Epidemiol Biomarkers Prev. 2011;20(6):1089–97.

5. Sandesara PB, Lambert CT, Gordon NF, Fletcher GF, Franklin BA, Wenger NK, et al. Cardiac rehabilitation and risk reduction: time to 'rebrand and reinvigorate'. J Am Coll Cardiol. 2015;65(4):389–95.
6. Kotseva K, De Backer G, De Bacquer D, Rydén L, Hoes A, Grobbee D, et al. Lifestyle and impact on cardiovascular risk factor control in coronary patients across 27 countries: results from the European Society of Cardiology ESC-EORP EUROASPIRE V registry. Eur J Prev Cardiol. 2019;26(8):824–35.
7. Gee PM, Greenwood DA, Paterniti DA, Ward D, Miller LMS. The eHealth enhanced chronic care model: a theory derivation approach. J Med Internet Res. 2015;17(4):e86.
8. Wagner EH. Chronic disease management: what will it take to improve care for chronic illness? Eff Clin Pract. 1998;1(1):2–4.
9. Yusuf S, Hawken S, Ounpuu S, Dans T, Avezum A, Lanas F, et al. Effect of potentially modifiable risk factors associated with myocardial infarction in 52 countries (the INTERHEART study): case-control study. Lancet. 2004;364(9438):937–52.
10. O'Donnell MJ, Chin SL, Rangarajan S, Xavier D, Liu L, Zhang H, et al. Global and regional effects of potentially modifiable risk factors associated with acute stroke in 32 countries (INTERSTROKE): a case-control study. Lancet. 2016;388(10046):761–75.
11. Anderson L, Thompson DR, Oldridge N, Zwisler AD, Rees K, Martin N, et al. Exercise-based cardiac rehabilitation for coronary heart disease. Cochrane Database Syst Rev. 2016;1:CD001800.
12. van Halewijn G, Deckers J, Tay HY, van Domburg R, Kotseva K, Wood D. Lessons from contemporary trials of cardiovascular prevention and rehabilitation: a systematic review and meta-analysis. Int J Cardiol. 2017;232:294–303.
13. Haskell WL, Alderman EL, Fair JM, Maron DJ, Mackey SF, Superko HR, et al. Effects of intensive multiple risk factor reduction on coronary atherosclerosis and clinical cardiac events in men and women with coronary artery disease. The Stanford Coronary Risk Intervention Project (SCRIP). Circulation. 1994;89(3):975–90.
14. DeBusk RF, Miller NH, Superko HR, Dennis CA, Thomas RJ, Lew HT, et al. A case-management system for coronary risk factor modification after acute myocardial infarction. Ann Intern Med. 1994;120(9):721–729.
15. Campbell NC, Ritchie LD, Thain J, Deans HG, Rawles JM, Squair JL. Secondary prevention in coronary heart disease: a randomised trial of nurse led clinics in primary care. Heart. 1998;80(5):447–52.
16. Fonarow GC, Gawlinski A. Rationale and design of the cardiac hospitalization atherosclerosis management program at the University of California Los Angeles. Am J Cardiol. 2000;85(3A):10A–17A.
17. Vale MJ, Jelinek MV, Best JD, Dart AM, Grigg LE, Hare DL, et al. Coaching patients On Achieving Cardiovascular Health (COACH): a multicenter randomized trial in patients with coronary heart disease. Arch Intern Med. 2003;163(22):2775–83.
18. Vale MJ, Sundararajan V, Jelinek MV, Best JD. Four-year follow-up of the multicenter RCT of Coaching patients On Achieving cardiovascular Health (the COACH Study) shows that the COACH program keeps patients out of hospital. Circulation. 2004;110(Suppl):III–801.
19. Boden WE, O'Rourke RA, Teo KK, Hartigan PM, Maron DJ, Kostuk WJ, et al. Optimal medical therapy with or without PCI for stable coronary disease. N Engl J Med. 2007;356(15):1503–16.
20. Wood DA, Kotseva K, Connolly S, Jennings C, Mead A, Jones J, et al. Nurse-coordinated multidisciplinary, family-based cardiovascular disease prevention programme (EUROACTION) for patients with coronary heart disease and asymptomatic individuals at high risk of cardiovascular disease: a paired, cluster-randomised controlled trial. Lancet. 2008;371(9629):1999–2012.
21. Allen JK, Dennison-Himmelfarb CR, Szanton SL, Bone L, Hill MN, Levine DM, et al. Community Outreach and Cardiovascular Health (COACH) trial: a randomized, controlled trial of nurse practitioner/community health worker cardiovascular disease risk reduction in urban community health centers. Circ Cardiovasc Qual Outcomes. 2011;4(6):595–602.
22. Jorstad HT, von Birgelen C, Alings AMW, Liem A, van Dantzig JM, Jaarsma W, et al. Effect of a nurse-coordinated prevention programme on cardiovascular risk after an acute coronary syndrome: main results of the RESPONSE randomised trial. Heart. 2013;99(19):1421–30.
23. Minneboo M, Lachman S, Snaterse M, Jørstad HT, Ter Riet G, Boekholdt SM, et al. Community-based lifestyle intervention in patients with coronary artery disease. J Am Coll Cardiol. 2017;70(3):318–27.
24. Jennings C, Kotseva K, De Bacquer D, Hoes A, de Velasco J, Brusaferro S, et al. Effectiveness of a preventive cardiology programme for high CVD risk persistent smokers: the EUROACTION PLUS varenicline trial. Eur Heart J. 2014;35(21):1411–20.
25. Connolly S, Holden A, Turner E, Fiumicelli G, Stevenson J, Hunjan M, et al. MyAction: an innovative approach to the prevention of cardiovascular disease in the community. Br J Cardiol. 2011;18:171–76.
26. Connolly SB, Kotseva K, Jennings C, Atrey A, Jones J, Brown A, et al. Outcomes of an integrated community-based nurse-led cardiovascular disease prevention programme. Heart. 2017;103(11):840–47.

27. Gibson I, Flaherty G, Cormican S, Jones J, Kerins C, Walsh AM, et al. Translating guidelines to practice: findings from a multidisciplinary preventive cardiology programme in the west of Ireland. Eur J Prev Cardiol. 2014;21(3):366–76.
28. Berra K, Ma J, Klieman L, Hyde S, Monti V, Guardado A, et al. Implementing cardiac risk-factor case management: lessons learned in a county health system. Crit Pathw Cardiol. 2007;6(4):173–79.
29. Salisbury C. Multimorbidity: redesigning health care for people who use it. Lancet. 2012;380(9836):7–9.
30. Al-Mallah MH, Farah I, Al-Madani W, Bdeir B, Al Habib S, Bigelow ML, et al. The impact of nurse-led clinics on the mortality and morbidity of patients with cardiovascular diseases: a systematic review and meta-analysis. J Cardiovasc Nurs. 2016;31(1):89–95.
31. Jennings C, Astin F. A multidisciplinary approach to prevention. Eur J Prev Cardiol. 2017;24(3 Suppl):77–87.
32. Lloyd-Jones DM, Nam BH, D'Agostino RB, Levy D, Murabito JM, Wang TJ, et al. Parental cardiovascular disease as a risk factor for cardiovascular disease in middle-aged adults: a prospective study of parents and offspring. JAMA. 2004;291(18):2204–11.
33. Steinberger J, Daniels SR, Eckel RH, Hayman L, Lustig RH, McCrindle B, et al. Progress and challenges in metabolic syndrome in children and adolescents: a scientific statement from the American Heart Association Atherosclerosis, hypertension, and Obesity in the Young Committee of the Council on Cardiovascular Disease in the Young; Council on Cardiovascular Nursing; and Council on Nutrition, Physical Activity, and Metabolism. Circulation. 2009;119(4):628–47.
34. Nasir K, Budoff MJ, Wong ND, Scheuner M, Herrington D, Arnett DK, et al. Family history of premature coronary heart disease and coronary artery calcification: Multi-Ethnic Study of Atherosclerosis (MESA). Circulation. 2007;116(6):619–26.
35. Muchira JM, Gona PN, Mogos MF, Stuart-Shor E, Leveille SG, Piano MR, Hayman LL. Parental cardiovascular health predicts time to onset of cardiovascular disease in offspring. Eur J Prev Cardiol. 2020;Nov 5:zwaa072.
36. Uijen AA, van de Lisdonk EH. Multimorbidity in primary care: prevalence and trend over the last 20 years. Eur J Gen Pract. 2008;14(Suppl 1):28–32.
37. Tate DF, Wing RR, Winett RA. Using Internet technology to deliver a behavioral weight loss program. JAMA. 2001;285(9):1172–77.
38. Kinn JW, O'Toole MF, Rowley SM, Marek JC, Bufalino VJ, Brown AS. Effectiveness of the electronic medical record in cholesterol management in patients with coronary artery disease (Virtual Lipid Clinic). Am J Cardiol. 2001;88(2):163–65, A5.
39. Tomita MR, Tsai BM, Fisher NM, Kumar NA, Wilding G, Stanton K, Naughton BJ. Effects of multidisciplinary Internet-based program on management of heart failure. J Multidiscip Healthc. 2008;2009(2):13–21.
40. Burke LE, Ma J, Azar KM, Bennett GG, Peterson ED, Zheng Y, et al. Current science on consumer use of mobile health for cardiovascular disease prevention: a scientific statement from the American Heart Association. Circulation. 2015;132(12):1157–213.
41. GBD 2017 Risk Factor Collaborators. Global, regional, and national comparative risk assessment of 84 behavioural, environmental and occupational, and metabolic risks or clusters of risks for 195 countries and territories, 1990–2017: a systematic analysis for the Global Burden of Disease Study 2017. Lancet. 2018;392(10159):1923–94.
42. Strasser T. Reflections on cardiovascular diseases. Interdiscip Sci Rev. 1978;3(3):225–30.
43. Weintraub WS, Daniels SR, Burke LE, Franklin BA, Goff DC, Hayman LL, et al. Value of primordial and primary prevention for cardiovascular disease: a policy statement from the American Heart Association. Circulation. 2011;124(8):967–90.
44. Strong JP, Malcom GT, McMahan CA, Tracy RE, Newman WP, Herderick EE, et al. Prevalence and extent of atherosclerosis in adolescents and young adults: implications for prevention from the pathobiological Determinants of Atherosclerosis in Youth Study. JAMA. 1999;281(8):727–35.
45. Berenson GS, Srinivasan SR, Bao W, Newman WP, 3rd, Tracy RE, Wattigney WA. Association between multiple cardiovascular risk factors and atherosclerosis in children and young adults: the Bogalusa Heart Study. N Engl J Med. 1998;338(23):1650–56.
46. Lloyd-Jones DM, Leip EP, Larson MG, D'Agostino RB, Beiser A, Wilson PW. Prediction of lifetime risk for cardiovascular disease by risk factor burden at 50 years of age. Circulation. 2006;113(6):791–98.
47. Pahkala K, Heitilampi H, Laitinen TT, Viikari JS, Ronnemaa T, Niiinikoski H, et al. Ideal cardiovascular health in adolescence: effect of lifestyle intervention and association with vascular intima-media thickness and elasticity (the Special Turku Coronary InterventionProject for Children [STRIP Study]). Circulation. 2013;127(21):2088–96.
48. Nupponen M, Pahkala K, Juonala M, Magnussen CG, Niinikoski H, Rönnemaa T, et al. Metabolic syndrome from adolescence to early adulthood: effect of infancy-onset dietary counseling of low saturated fat: the Special Turku Coronary Risk factor Intervention Project (STRIP). Circulation. 2015;131(7):605–13.
49. Expert Panel on Integrated Guidelines for Cardiovascular Health and Risk Reduction in Children and Adolescents, National Heart, Lung, and Blood

Institute. Expert panel on integrated guidelines for cardiovascular health and risk reduction in children and adolescents: summary report. Summary report. Pediatrics. 2011;128(Suppl 5):S213–56.

50. Pulkki-Råback L, Elovainio M, Hakulinen C, Lipsanen J, Hintsanen M, Jokela M, et al. Cumulative effect of psychosocial factors in youth on ideal cardiovascular health in adulthood: the Cardiovascular Risk in Young Finns Study. Circulation. 2015;131(3):245–53.
51. Suglia SF, Koenen KC, Boynton-Jarrett R, Chan PS, Clark CJ, Danese A, et al. Childhood and adolescent adversity and cardiometabolic outcomes: a Scientific Statement from the American Heart Association. Circulation. 2018;137(5):e15–28.
52. Hayman LL. Preventive cardiovascular health in schools: current status. Curr Cardiovasc Risk Rep. 2017;11(9):24–29.
53. Unger E, Diez-Roux AV, Lloyd-Jones DM. Association of neighborhood characteristics with cardiovascular health in the Multi-Ethnic Study of Atherosclerosis. Cardiovasc Quality Outcomes. 2014;7(4):524–31.
54. Harper S, Lynch J, Smith GD. Social determinants and the decline of cardiovascular diseases: understanding the links. Annu Rev Public Health. 2011;32:39–69.
55. Kontis V. Cobb LK, Mathers CD, Frieden TR. Ezzati M, Danaei G. Three public health interventions could save 94 million lives in 25 years: global impact assessment analysis. Circulation. 2019;140(9):715–25.
56. World Health Organization. REPLACE trans fat: an action package to eliminate industrially produced trans-fatty acids. https://www.who.int/teams/nutrition-and-food-safety/replace-trans-fat.
57. Visseren FLJ, Mach F, Smulders YM, et al. ESC Scientific Document Group. 2021 ESC Guidelines on cardiovascular disease prevention in clinical practice. Eur Heart J. 2021 Sep 7;42(34):3227–337. doi: 10.1093/eurheartj/ehab484. PMID: 34458905.
58. Mossakowska TJ, Saunders CL, Corbett J, MacLure C, Winpenny EM, Dujso E, et al. Current and future cardiovascular disease risk assessment in the European Union: an international comparative study. Eur J Public Health. 2018;28(4):748–54.
59. Kotseva K, De Backer G, De Bacquer D, Rydén L, Hoes A, Grobbee D, et al. Lifestyle and impact on cardiovascular risk factor control in coronary patients across 27 countries: results from the European Society of Cardiology ESC-EORP EUROASPIRE V registry. Eur J Prev Cardiol. 2019;26(8):824–35.
60. Rossello X, Dorresteijn J, Janesson AN, A, et al. Risk predication tools in cardiovascular disease prevention: a report from the ESC Prevention of CVD Programme led by the European Society of Cardiology in collaboration with the Acute cardiovascular care Association (ACCA) and the Association of Cardiovascular Nursing and Allied Professions (ACNAP). Eur J Prev Cardiol. 2019;26(14):1534–44.
61. Haskell WL, Berra K, Arias E, Christopherson D, Clark A, George J, Hyde S, Klieman L, Myll J. Multifactor cardiovascular disease risk reduction in medically underserved, high-risk patients. Am J Cardiol. 2006 Dec 1;98(11):1472–9. doi:10.1016/j.amjcard.2006.06.049. Epub 2006 Oct 12. PMID: 17126653.
62. Jackson R, Lawes CM, Bennett DA, Milne RJ, Rodgers A. Treatment with drugs to lower blood pressure and blood cholesterol based on an individual's absolute cardiovascular risk. Lancet. 2005;365(9457):434–41.
63. European Society of Cardiology, European Association for Cardiovascular Disease Prevention & Rehabilitation, HeartScore. https://www.heartscore.org/.
64. Williams B, Mancia G, Spiering W, Agabiti Rosei E, Azizi M, Burnier M, et al. ESC Scientific Document Group. ESC/ESH Guidelines for the management of arterial hypertension: the Task Force for the management of arterial hypertension of the European Society of Cardiology (ESC) and the European Society of Hypertension (ESH). Eur Heart J. 2018;39(33):3021–104.
65. Mach F, Baigent C, Catapano AL, Koskinas KC, Casula M, Badimon L, et al. 2019 ESC/EAS Guidelines for the management of dyslipidaemias: lipid modification to reduce cardiovascular risk. Eur Heart J. 2020;41(1):111–88.
66. Cosentino F, Grant PJ, Aboyans V, Bailey CJ, Ceriello A, Delgado V, et al. ESC Guidelines on diabetes, pre-diabetes, and cardiovascular diseases developed in collaboration with the EASD: the Task Force for diabetes, pre-diabetes, and cardiovascular diseases of the European Society of Cardiology (ESC) and the European Association for the Study of Diabetes (EASD). Eur Heart J. 2020;41(2):255–323.
67. Seedhouse D. Health Promotion: Philosophy, Prejudice and Practice (2nd ed). Chichester: Wiley; 2003.
68. Green LW. Editorial. Health Educ Monogr. 1974;2(4):324–25.
69. Bandura A. Self-efficacy mechanism in human agency. Am Psychol. 1982;37(2):122–47.
70. Prochaska JO, DiClemente CC, Norcross JC. In search of how people change: applications to addictive behaviour. Am Psychol. 1992;47(9):1102–14.
71. Michie S, Atkins L, West R. The Behaviour Change Wheel: A Guide to Designing Interventions. London:Silverback Publishing; 2014.
72. Michie S, van Stralen MM, West R. The behaviour change wheel: a new method for characterising and designing behaviour change interventions. Implement Sci. 2011;6:42.

73. Miller WR, Rose GS. Toward a theory of motivational interviewing. Am Psychol. 2009;64(6):527–37.
74. Doll R, Peto R, Boreham J, Sutherland I. Mortality in relation to smoking: 50 years' observations on male British doctors. BMJ. 2004;328(7455):1519.
75. Jha P, Ramasundarahettige C, Landsman V, Rostron B, Thun M, Anderson RN, et al. 21st-century hazards of smoking and benefits of cessation in the United States. N Engl J Med. 2013;368(4):341–50.
76. Critchley JA, Capewell S. Mortality risk reduction associated with smoking cessation in patients with coronary heart disease: a systematic review. JAMA. 2003;290(1):86–97.
77. Chabrol H, Niezborala M, Chastan E, De Leon J. Comparison of the Heavy Smoking Index and of the Fagerstrom Test for Nicotine Dependence in a sample of 749 cigarette smokers. Addict Behav. 2005;30(7):1474–77.
78. Heatherton TF, Kozlowski LT, Frecker RC, Fagerström KO. The Fagerstrom Test for Nicotine Dependence: a revision of the Fagerstrom Tolerance Questionnaire. Br J Addict. 1991;86(9):1119–27.
79. Taylor G, McNeill A, Girling A, Farley A, Lindson-Hawley N, Aveyard P. Change in mental health after smoking cessation: systematic review and meta-analysis. BMJ. 2014;348:g1151.
80. Hajek P. Withdrawal-oriented therapy for smokers. Br J Addict. 1989;84(6):591–98.
81. Gielen S, De Backer G, Piepoli M, Wood D (Eds). *The ESC Textbook of Preventive Cardiology*. Oxford: Oxford University Press; 2015.
82. Jennings C, Graham I, Gielen S (Eds). *The ESC Handbook of Preventive Cardiology: Putting Prevention into Practice*. Oxford: Oxford University Press; 2016.
83. Cahill K, Stevens S, Perera R, Lancaster T. Pharmacological interventions for smoking cessation: an overview and network meta-analysis. Cochrane Database Syst Rev. 2013;5:CD009329.
84. Eisenberg MJ, Windle SB, Roy N, Old W, Grondin FR, Bata I, et al. Varenicline for smoking cessation in hospitalized patients with acute coronary syndrome. Circulation. 2016;133(1):21–30.
85. Rigotti NA, Pipe AL, Benowitz NL, Arteaga C, Garza D, Tonstad S. Efficacy and safety of varenicline for smoking cessation in patients with cardiovascular disease: a randomized trial. Circulation. 2010;121(2):221–29.
86. Anthenelli RM, Benowitz NL, West R, St Aubin L, McRae T, Lawrence D, et al. Neuropsychiatric safety and efficacy of varenicline, bupropion, and nicotine patch in smokers with and without psychiatric disorders (Eagles): a double-blind, randomised, placebo-controlled clinical trial. Lancet. 2016;387(10037):2507–20.
87. Chang PH, Chiang CH, Ho WC, Wu PZ, Tsai JS, Guo FR. Combination therapy of varenicline with nicotine replacement therapy is better than varenicline alone: a systematic review and meta-analysis of randomized controlled trials. BMC Public Health. 2015;15:689.
88. Hajek P, Tønnesen P, Arteaga C, Russ C, Tonstad S. Varenicline in prevention of relapse to smoking: effect of quit pattern on response to extended treatment. Addiction. 2009;104(9):1597–602.
89. Ebbert JO, Hughes JR, West RJ, Rennard SI, Russ C, McRae TD, et al. Effect of varenicline on smoking cessation through smoking reduction: a randomized clinical trial. JAMA. 2015;313(7):687–94.
90. Aubin HJ, Farley A, Lycett D, Lahmek P, Aveyard P. Weight gain in smokers after quitting cigarettes: meta-analysis. BMJ. 2012;345:e4439.
91. Jennings C, Kotseva K, De Bacquer D, Hoes A, De Velasco J, Brusaferro S, et al. Effectiveness of a preventive cardiology programme for high CVD risk persistent smokers: the EUROACTION PLUS varenicline trial. Eur Heart J. 2014;35(21):1411–20.
92. Appel LJ, Moore TJ, Obarzanek E, Vollmer WM, Svetkey LP, Sacks FM, et al. A clinical trial of the effects of dietary patterns on blood pressure. N Engl J Med. 1997;336(16):1117–24.
93. Estruch R, Ros E, Salas-Salvadó J, Covas MI, Corella D, Arós F, et al. Primary prevention of cardiovascular disease with a Mediterranean diet supplemented with extra-virgin olive oil or nuts. N Engl J Med. 2018;378(25):e34.
94. Schröder H, Fitó M, Estruch R, Martínez-González MA, Corella D, Salas-Salvadó J, et al. A short screener is valid for assessing Mediterranean diet adherence among older Spanish men and women. J Nutr. 2011;141(6):1140–45.
95. García-López M, Toledo E, Beunza JJ, Aros F, Estruch R, Salas-Salvadó J, et al. Mediterranean diet and heart rate: the PREDIMED randomised trial. Int J Cardiol. 2014;171(2):299–301.
96. Papadaki A, Johnson L, Toumpakari Z, England C, Rai M, Toms S, et al. Validation of the English version of the 14-item Mediterranean diet adherence screener of the PREDIMED study, in people at high cardiovascular risk in the UK. Nutrients. 2018;10(2):138.
97. Hebestreit K, Yahiaoui-Doktor M, Engel C, Vetter W, Siniatchkin M, Erickson N, et al. Validation of the German version of the Mediterranean Diet Adherence Screener (MEDAS) questionnaire. BMC Cancer. 2017;17(1):341.
98. Gnagnarella P, Dragà D, Misotti AM, Sieri S, Spaggiari L, Cassano E, et al. Validation of a short questionnaire to record adherence to the Mediterranean diet: an Italian experience. Nutr Metab Cardiovasc Dis. 2018;28(11):1140–47.
99. Stefler D, Malyutina S, Kubinova R, Pajak A, Peasey A, Pikhart H, et al. Mediterranean diet score and total and cardiovascular mortality in Eastern Europe: the HAPIEE study. Eur J Nutr. 2017;56(1):421–29.

100. Sofi F, Cesari F, Abbate R, Gensini GF, Casini A. Adherence to Mediterranean diet and health status: meta-analysis. BMJ. 2008;337:a1344.
101. Bhaskaran K, dos-Santos-Silva I, Leon DA, Douglas IJ, Smeeth L. Association of BMI with overall and cause-specific mortality: a population-based cohort study of 3.6 million adults in the UK. Lancet Diabetes Endocrinol. 2018;6(12):944–53.
102. WHO Expert Committee. Appropriate body-mass index for Asian populations and its implications for policy and intervention strategies. Lancet. 2004;363(9403):157–63.
103. Mulligan AA, Lentjes MAH, Luben RN, Wareham NJ, Khaw KT. Changes in waist circumference and risk of all-cause and CVD mortality: results from the European Prospective Investigation into Cancer in Norfolk (EPIC-Norfolk) cohort study. BMC Cardiovasc Disord. 2019;19(1):238.
104. International Diabetes Federation. IDF consensus worldwide definition of the metabolic syndrome. 2006 (updated 2020). https://www.idf.org/component/attachments/attachments.html?id=705&task=download.
105. Seidelmann SB, Claggett B, Cheng S, Henglin M, Shah A, Steffen LM, et al. Dietary carbohydrate intake and mortality: a prospective cohort study and meta-analysis. Lancet Public Health. 2018;3(9):e419–28.
106. Li S, Flint A, Pai JK, Forman JP, Hu FB, Willett WC, et al. Low carbohydrate diet from plant or animal sources and mortality among myocardial infarction survivors. J Am Heart Assoc. 2014;3(5):e001169.
107. Zubrzycki A, Cierpka-Kmiec K, Kmiec Z, Wronska A. The role of low-calorie diets and intermittent fasting in the treatment of obesity and type-2 diabetes. J Physiol Pharmacol. 2018;69(5):663–83.
108. World Health Organization. Global health risks: mortality and burden of disease attributable to selected major risks. 2009. https://www.who.int/healthinfo/global_burden_disease/GlobalHealthRisks_report_full.pdf.
109. Shortreed SM, Peeters A, Forbes AB. Estimating the effect of long-term physical activity on cardiovascular disease and mortality: evidence from the Framingham Heart Study. Heart. 2013;99(9):649–54.
110. Arraiz GA, Wigle DT, Mao Y. Risk assessment of physical activity and physical fitness in the Canada Health Survey mortality follow-up study. J Clin Epidemiol. 1992;45(4):419–28.
111. Statistics Sweden. The Swedish Survey of Living Conditions: Design and Method. 1996. Stockholm: Statistics Sweden.
112. Garcia-Palmieri MR, Costas R Jr, Cruz-Vidal M, Sorlie PD, Havlik RJ. Increased physical activity: a protective factor against heart attacks in Puerto Rico. Am J Cardiol. 1982;50(4):749–55.
113. Aijö M, Heikkinen E, Schroll M, Steen B. Physical activity and mortality of 75-year-old people in three Nordic localities: a five-year follow-up. Aging Clin Exp Res. 2002;14(3 Suppl):83–89.
114. Rockhill B, Willett WC, Manson JE, Leitzmann MF, Stampfer MJ, Hunter DJ, et al. Physical activity and mortality: a prospective study among women. Am J Public Health. 2001;91(4):578–83.
115. Davey Smith G, Shipley MJ, Batty GD, Morris JN, Marmot M. Physical activity and cause-specific mortality in the Whitehall study. Public Health. 2000;114(5):308–15.
116. Nystoriak MA, Bhatnagar A. Cardiovascular effects and benefits of exercise. Front Cardiovasc Med. 2018;5:135.
117. Lee IM, Shiroma EJ, Lobelo F, Puska P, Blair SN, Katzmarzyk PT, Lancet Physical Activity Series Working Group. Effect of physical inactivity on major non-communicable diseases worldwide: an analysis of burden of disease and life expectancy. Lancet. 2012;380(9838):219–29.
118. Franklin BA, Gordon NF. Contemporary Diagnosis and Management in Cardiovascular Exercise (2nd ed). Newtown, PA: Handbooks in Health Care; 2009.
119. Durstine JL, Grandjean PW, Cox CA, Thompson PD. Lipids, lipoproteins, and exercise. J Cardiopulm Rehabil. 2002;22(6):385–98.
120. Leon AS, Sanchez OA. Response of blood lipids and lipoproteins to exercise training alone or combined with dietary intervention. Med Sci Sports Exerc. 2001;33(6 Suppl):S502–15.
121. Kelley GA, Kelley KS, Franklin B. Aerobic exercise and lipids and lipoproteins in patients with cardiovascular disease: a meta-analysis of randomized controlled trials. J Cardiopulm Rehabil. 2006;26(3):131–39.
122. Kelley GA, Kelley KS, Vu Tran ZV. Aerobic exercise, lipids and lipoproteins in overweight and obese adults: a meta-analysis of randomized controlled trials. Int J Obes (Lond). 2005;29(8):881–93.
123. Cornelissen VA, Smart NA. Exercise training for blood pressure: a systematic review and meta-analysis. J Am Heart Assoc. 2013;2(1):e004473.
124. Wagenknecht LE, Mayer EJ, Rewers M, Haffner S, Selby J, Borok GM, et al. The insulin resistance atherosclerosis study (IRAS) objectives, design, and recruitment results. Ann Epidemiol. 1995;5(6):464–72.
125. Fiuza-Luces C, Garatachea N, Berger NA, Lucia A. Exercise is the real polypill. Physiology (Bethesda). 2013;28(5):330–58.
126. Myers J, Nead KT, Chang P, Abella J, Kokkinos P, Leeper NJ. Improved reclassification of mortality risk by assessment of physical activity in patients referred for exercise testing. Am J Med. 2015;128(4):396–402.
127. Thorp AA, Owen N, Neuhaus M, Dunstan DW. Sedentary behaviors and subsequent health outcomes

in adults a systematic review of longitudinal studies, 1996–2011. Am J Prev Med. 2011;41(2):207–15.
128. Katzmarzyk PT, Church TS, Craig CL, Bouchard C. Sitting time and mortality from all causes, cardiovascular disease, and cancer. Med Sci Sports Exerc. 2009;41(5):998–1005.
129. Healy GN, Winkler EA, Owen N, Anuradha S, Dunstan DW. Replacing sitting time with standing or stepping: associations with cardio-metabolic risk biomarkers. Eur Heart J. 2015;36(39):2643–49.
130. Crichton GE, Alkerwi A. Physical activity, sedentary behavior time and lipid levels in the observation of cardiovascular risk factors in Luxembourg study. Lipids Health Dis. 2015;14:87.
131. Sallis RE, Matuszak JM, Baggish AL, Franklin BA, Chodzko-Zajko W, Fletcher BJ, et al. Call to action on making physical activity assessment and prescription a medical standard of care. Curr Sports Med Rep. 2016;15(3):207–14.
132. Sylvia LG, Bernstein EE, Hubbard JL, Keating L, Anderson EJ. Practical guide to measuring physical activity. J Acad Nutr Diet. 2014;114(2):199–208.
133. Gyberg V, De Bacquer D, Kotseva K, De Backer G, Schnell O, Sundvall J, et al. Screening for dysglycaemia in patients with coronary artery disease as reflected by fasting glucose, oral glucose tolerance test, and HbA1c: a report from EUROASPIRE IV—a survey from the European Society of Cardiology. Eur Heart J. 2015;36(19):1171–77.
134. World Health Organization. Consultation. Definition and Diagnosis of Diabetes and Intermediate Hyperglycaemia. Geneva: World Health Organization; 2006. http://www.who.int/diabetes/publications/diagnosis_diabetes2006/en/.
135. World Health Organization. Use of glycated haemoglobin (HbA1c) in the diagnosis of diabetes mellitus: abbreviated report of a WHO consultation. 2011. https://www.who.int/diabetes/publications/report-hba1c_2011.pdf.
136. Thompson DR, Ski CF. Psychosocial interventions in cardiovascular disease—what are they? Eur J Prev Cardiol. 2013;20(6):916–17.
137. Thompson DR, Ski CF, Saner H. Psychosocial assessment and intervention—are we doing enough? Heart Lung. 2018;47(4):278–79.
138. Pogosova N, Saner H, Pedersen SS, et al. Cardiac rehabilitation section of the European Association of Cardiovascular Prevention and Rehabilitation of the European Society of Cardiology. Psychosocial aspects in cardiac rehabilitation: from theory to practice. A position paper from the Cardiac Rehabilitation Section of the European Association of Cardiovascular Prevention and Rehabilitation of the European Society of Cardiology. Eur J Prev Cardiol. 2015;22(10):1290–306.
139. Pedersen SS, von Känel R, Tully PJ, Denollet J. Psychosocial perspectives in cardiovascular disease. Eur J Prev Cardiol. 2017;24(3 Suppl):108–15.
140. Pedersen SS, Andersen CM. Minding the heart: why are we still not closer to treating depression and anxiety in clinical cardiology practice? Eur J Prev Cardiol. 2018;25(3):244–46.
141. Astin F, Lucock M, Jennings CS. Heart and mind: behavioural cardiology demystified for the clinician. Heart. 2019;105(11):881–88.
142. Pogosova N, Kotseva K, De Bacquer D, von Känel R, De Smedt D, Bruthans J, et al. Psychosocial risk factors in relation to other cardiovascular risk factors in coronary heart disease: results from the EUROASPIRE IV survey. A registry from the European Society of Cardiology. Eur J Prev Cardiol. 2017;24(13):1371–80.
143. Norlund F, Lissåker C, Wallert J, Held C, Olsson EM. Factors associated with emotional distress in patients with myocardial infarction: results from the SWEDEHEART registry. Eur J Prev Cardiol. 2018;25(9):910–20.
144. Hare DL, Toukhsati SR, Johansson P, Jaarsma T. Depression and cardiovascular disease: a clinical review. Eur Heart J. 2014;35(21):1365–72.
145. Havranek EP, Mujahid MS, Barr DA, Blair IV, Cohen MS, Cruz-Flores S, et al. Social determinants of risk and outcomes for cardiovascular disease. A scientific statement from the American Heart Association. Circulation 2015;132(9):873–98.
146. Valtorta NK, Kanaan M, Gilbody S, Ronzi S, Hanratty B. Loneliness and social isolation as risk factors for coronary heart disease and stroke: systematic review and meta-analysis of longitudinal observational studies. Heart. 2016;102(13):1009–16.
147. Schultz WM, Kelli HM, Lisko JC, Varghese T, Shen J, Sandesara P, et al. Socioeconomic status and cardiovascular outcomes: challenges and interventions. Circulation. 2018;137(20):2166–78.
148. Jensen MT, Marott JL, Holtermann A, Gyntelberg F. Living alone is associated with all-cause and cardiovascular mortality: 32 years of follow-up in the Copenhagen Male Study. Eur Heart J Qual Care Clin Outcomes. 2019;5(3):208–17.
149. Gariépy G, Honkaniemi H, Quesnel-Vallée A. Social support and protection from depression: systematic review of current findings in Western countries. Br J Psychiatry. 2016;209(4):284–93.
150. Dempster M, Howell D, McCorry NK. Illness perceptions and coping in physical health conditions: a meta-analysis. J Psychosom Res. 2015;79(6):506–13.
151. Le J, Dorstyn DS, Mpofu E, Prior E, Tully PJ. Health-related quality of life in coronary heart disease: a systematic review and meta-analysis mapped against the International Classification of

Functioning, Disability and Health. Qual Life Res. 2018;27(10):2491–503.

152. Coorey GM, Neubeck L, Mulley J, Redfern J. Effectiveness, acceptability and usefulness of mobile applications for cardiovascular disease self-management: systematic review with meta-synthesis of quantitative and qualitative data. Eur J Prev Cardiol. 2018;25(5):505–21.
153. Kroenke K, Spitzer RL, Williams JB. The PHQ-0: validity of a brief depression severity measure. J Gen Intern Med. 2001;16(9):606–13.
154. Spitzer RL, Kroenke K, Williams JB, Löwe B. A brief measure for assessing generalized anxiety disorder: the GAD-7. Arch Intern Med. 2006;166(10):1092–97.
155. Zigmond AS, Snaith RP. The Hospital Anxiety and Depression scale. Acta Psychiatr Scand. 1983;67(6):361–70.
156. Zimet GD, Dahlem NW, Zimet SG, Farley GK. The Multidimensional Scale of Perceived Social Support. J Assess. 1988;52(1):30–41.
157. Broadbent E, Petrie KJ, Main J, Weinman J. The brief illness perception questionnaire. J Psychosom Res. 2006;60(6):631–37.
158. Sararoudi RB, Motmaen M, Maracy MR, Pishghadam E, Kheirabadi GR. Efficacy of illness perception focused intervention on quality of life, anxiety, and depression in patients with myocardial infarction. J Res Med Sci. 2016;21:125.
159. Thompson DR, Ski CF, Garside J, Astin F. A review of health-related quality of life patient-reported outcome measures in cardiovascular nursing. Eur J Cardiovasc Nurs. 2016;15(2):114–25.
160. Ware JE, Snow KK, Kosinski MK, et al. SF-36 Health Survey Manual and Interpretation Guide. Boston, MA: Health Institute; 1993.
161. EuroQol Group. EuroQol—a new facility for the measurement of health-related quality of life. Health Policy. 1990;16(3):199–208.
162. Spertus JA, Winder JA, Dewhurst TA, Deyo RA, Prodzinski J, McDonell M, Fihn SD. Development and evaluation of the Seattle Angina Questionnaire: a new functional status measure for coronary artery disease. J Am Coll Cardiol. 1995;25(2):333–41.
163. Thompson DR, Jenkinson C, Roebuck A, Lewin RJ, Boyle RM, Chandola T. Development and validation of a short measure of health status for individuals with acute myocardial infarction: the myocardial infarction dimensional assessment scale (MIDAS). Qual Life Res. 2002;11(6):535–43.
164. Rector TS, Kubo SH, Cohn JN, et al. Patients' self-assessment of their congestive heart failure, part 2: content, reliability and validity of a new measure, the Minnesota Living with Heart Failure questionnaire. Heart Fail. 1987;3:198–209.
165. Richards SH, Anderson L, Jenkinson CE, Whalley B, Rees K, Davies P, et al. Psychological interventions for coronary heart disease: Cochrane systematic review and meta-analysis. Eur J Prev Cardiol. 2018;25(3):247–59.
166. Cauter JV, Bacquer D, Clays E, Smedt D, Kotseva K, Braeckman L. Return to work and associations with psychosocial well-being and health-related quality of life in coronary heart disease patients: results from EUROASPIRE IV. Eur J Prev Cardiol. 2019;26(13):1386–95.
167. Ski CF, Worrall-Carter L, Cameron J, Castle DJ, Rahman MA, Thompson DR. Depression screening and referral in cardiac wards: a 12-month patient trajectory. Eur J Cardiovasc Nurs. 2017;16(2):157–66.
168. Davidson KW, Bigger JT, Burg MM, Carney RM, Chaplin WF, Czajkowski S, et al. Centralized, stepped, patient preference-based treatment for patients with post-acute coronary syndrome depression: CODIACS vanguard randomized controlled trial. JAMA Intern Med. 2013;173(11):997–1004.
169. Huffman JC, Mastromauro CA, Beach SR, Celano CM, DuBois CM, Healy BC, et al. Collaborative care for depression and anxiety disorders in patients with recent cardiac events: the Management of sadness and Anxiety in Cardiology (MOSAIC) randomized clinical trial. JAMA Intern Med. 2014;174(6):927–35.
170. Arnberg FK, Linton SJ, Hultcrantz M, Heintz E, Jonsson U. Internet-delivered psychological treatments for mood and anxiety disorders: a systematic review of their efficacy, safety, and cost-effectiveness. PLoS One. 2014;9(5):e98118.
171. Cohen BE, Edmondson D, Kronish IM. State of the art review: depression, stress, anxiety, and cardiovascular disease. Am J Hypertens. 2015;28(11):1295–302.
172. Tully PJ, Sardinha A, Nardi AE. A new CBT model of Panic Attack Treatment in Comorbid Heart Diseases (PATCHD): how to calm an anxious heart and mind. Cogn Behav Pract. 2017;24(3):329–41.
173. Richards DA, Ekers D, McMillan D, Taylor RS, Byford S, Warren FC, et al. Cost and outcome of behavioural activation versus cognitive behavioural therapy for depression (COBRA): a randomised, controlled, non-inferiority trial. Lancet. 2016;388(10047):871–80.
174. Corra U. Cardiac rehabilitation and exercise training. In: Camm AJ, Lüscher TF, Maurer G, Serruys PW (Eds), The ESC Textbook of Cardiovascular Medicine (3rd ed). Oxford: Oxford University Press; 2019:882–92.
175. Piepoli MF, Corrà U, Dendale P, Frederix I, Prescott E, Schmid JP, et al. Challenges in secondary prevention after acute myocardial infarction: a call for action. Eur J Prev Cardiol. 2016;23(18):1994–2006.

176. Price KJ, Gordon BA, Bird SR, Benson AC. A review of guidelines for cardiac rehabilitation exercise programmes: is there an international consensus? Eur J Prev Cardiol. 2016;23(16):1715–33.
177. White PD. Heart Disease. London: McMillian Co; 1951.
178. Levine SA, Lown B. Armchair treatment of acute coronary thrombosis. JAMA. 1952;148(16):1365–69.
179. Bethal H. Historical background. In: Coates A, McGee HM, Stokes H, Thompson D, (Eds), BACR Guidelines for Cardiac Rehabilitation. London: Blackwell Science; 1995:1–11.
180. Harrington KA, Smith KH, Schumacher M, Lunsford BR, Watson KL, Selvester RH. Cardiac rehabilitation evaluation and intervention less than six weeks after myocardial infarction. Physical Med Rehabil. 1981;2:151–55.
181. Gottheiner V. Long Range strenuous sports training for cardiac redeconditioning and rehabilitation. Am J Cardiol. 1968;22:462–35.
182. Brunner D. Active exercise for coronary patients. Rehabil Rec. 1968;5:29–31.
183. Naughton J, Bruhn J, Lategola MT, Whitsett T. Rehabilitation following myocardial infarction. Am J Med. 1969;46(5):725–34.
184. Hellerstein HK, Ford AB. Rehabilitation of the cardiac patient. JAMA. 1957;164(3):225–31.
185. Vanhees L, McGee HM, Dugmore LD, Schepers D, van Daele P, Carinex Working Group. A representative study of cardiac rehabilitation activities in European Union Member States: the Carinex survey. J Cardiopulm Rehabil. 2002;22(4):264–72.
186. McCreery C, Cradock K, Fallon N, et al. Cardiac Rehabilitation Guidelines 2013. Dublin: Irish Association of Cardiac Rehabilitation; 2013. http://www.iacr.info/about/guidelines/.
187. Thompson DR. Improving the organisation and delivery of cardiac rehabilitation. Eur J Cardiovasc Nurs. 2003;2(4):245–46.
188. Abreu A, Pesah E, Supervia M, Turk-Adawi K, Bjarnason-Wehrens B, Lopez-Jimenez F. Cardiac rehabilitation availability and delivery in Europe: how does it differ by region and compare with other high-income countries? Endorsed by the European Association of Preventive Cardiology European. Eur J Prev Cardiol. 2019;26(11):1131–46.
189. British Association for Cardiovascular Prevention and Rehabilitation. The BACPR Standards and Core Components for Cardiovascular Disease Prevention and Rehabilitation 2017 (3rd ed). London: British Association for Cardiovascular Prevention and Rehabilitation.
190. Cowie A, Buckley J, Doherty P, Furze G, Hayward J, Hinton S, et al. Standards and core components for cardiovascular disease prevention and rehabilitation. Heart. 2019;105(7):510–15.
191. Bjarnason-Wehrens B, McGee H, Zwisler AD, Piepoli MF, Benzer W, Schmid JP, et al. Cardiac rehabilitation in Europe: results from the European Cardiac Rehabilitation Inventory Survey. Eur J Cardiovasc Prev Rehabil. 2010;17(4):410–18.
192. Yusuf SF, Wood D, Ralston J, Reddy KS. The World Heart Federation's vision for worldwide cardiovascular disease prevention. Lancet. 2015;386(9991):399–402.
193. Kelehera H, Parker R. Health promotion by primary care nurses in Australian general practice. Collegian. 2013;20(4):215–21.
194. Randall S, Crawford T, Currie J, River J, Betihavas V. Impact of community based nurse-led clinics on patient outcomes, patient satisfaction, patient access and cost effectiveness: a systematic review. Int J Nurs Stud. 2017;73:24–33.
195. Bauer L, Bodenheimer T. Expanded roles of registered nurses in primary care delivery of the future. Nurs Outlook. 2017;65(5):624–32.
196. Astin F, Carroll DL, Ruppar T, Uchmanowicz I, Hinterbuchner L, Kletsiou E, et al. A core curriculum for the continuing professional development of nurses: developed by the Education Committee on behalf of the Council on Cardiovascular Nursing and Allied Professions of the ESC. Eur J CardioVasc Nur. 2015;14(3):190–97.
197. Department of Health. Putting Prevention First. NHS Health Check Vascular Risk Assessment and Management. Best Practice Guidance. London: Department of Health; 2009.
198. Conroy RM, Pyörälä K, Fitzgerald AP, Sans S, Menotti A, De Backer G, et al. Estimation of ten-year risk of fatal cardiovascular disease in Europe: the SCORE project. Eur Heart J. 2003;24(11):987–1003.
199. Aveyard P, Begh R, Parsons A, West R. Brief opportunistic smoking cessation interventions: a systematic review and meta-analysis to compare advice to quit and offer of assistance. Addiction. 2012;107(6):1066–73.
200. Aveyard P, Lewis A, Tearne S, Hood K, Christian-Brown A, Adab P, et al. Screening and brief intervention for obesity in primary care: a parallel, two-arm, randomised trial. Lancet. 2016;388(10059):2492–500.
201. Jones LL, Hassanien A, Cook DG, Britton J, Leonardi-Bee J. Parental smoking and the risk of middle ear disease in children: a systematic review and meta-analysis. Arch Pediatr Adolesc Med. 2012;166(1):18–27.
202. Rathert C, Wyrwich MD, Boren SA. Patient-centered care and outcomes: a systematic review of the literature. Med Care Res Rev. 2013;70(4):351–79.

203. Massimi A, De Vito C, Brufola I, Corsaro A, Marzuillo C, Migliara G, et al. Are community-based nurse-led self-management support interventions effective in chronic patients? Results of a systematic review and meta-analysis. PLoS One. 2017;12(3):e0173617.
204. Parlour R, Slater PF. An Evaluation of the Effectiveness of a Self-Management Programme. Dublin: Office of the Nursing and Midwifery Services Director, Health Service Executive; 2011.
205. Jonkman NH, Westland H, Groenwold RH, Ågren S, Atienza F, Blue L, et al. Do self-management interventions work in patients with heart failure? An individual patient data meta-analysis. Circulation. 2016;133(12):1189–98.
206. Pinnock H, Parke HL, Panagioti M, Daines L, Pearce G, Epiphaniou E, et al. Systematic meta-review of supported self-management for asthma: a healthcare perspective. BMC Med. 2017;15(1):64.
207. Riegel B, Moser DK, Buck HG, Dickson VV, Dunbar SB, Lee CS, et al. Self-care for the prevention and management of cardiovascular disease and stroke: a scientific statement for healthcare professionals from the American Heart Association. J Am Heart Assoc. 2017;6(9):e006997
208. Croi. Guide to healthy shopping. https://croi.ie/wp-content/uploads/2019/11/Healthy-Shopping-Card-largerText-85x54mm.pdf.
209. Gibson I, Flaherty G, Cormican S, Jones J, Kerins C, Walsh AM, et al. Translating guidelines to practice: findings from a multidisciplinary preventive cardiology programme in the west of Ireland. Eur J Prev Cardiol. 2014;21(3):366–76.
210. Berra K, Miller NH, Jennings CJ. Nurse-based models for cardiovascular disease prevention: from research to clinical practice. J Cardiovasc Nurs. 2011;26(4 Suppl):S46–55.
211. Berra K. Does nurse case management improve implementation of guidelines for cardiovascular disease risk reduction? J Cardiovasc Nurs. 2011;26(2):145–67.
212. Schultz WM, Kelli HM, Lisko JC, Varghese T, Shen J, Sandesara P, et al. Socioeconomic status and cardiovascular outcomes: challenges and interventions. Circulation. 2018;137(20):2166–78.
213. Victor RG, Lynch K, Li N, Blyler C, Muhammad E, Handler J, et al. A cluster-randomized trial of blood-pressure reduction in black barbershops. N Engl J Med. 2018;378(14):1291–301.
214. Schoenthaler AM, Lancaster KJ, Chaplin W, Butler M, Forsyth J, Ogedegbe G. Cluster randomized clinical trial of FAITH (faith-based approaches in the treatment of hypertension) in blacks. Circ Cardiovasc Qual Outcomes. 2018;11(10):e004691.
215. Gómez-Pardo E, Fernández-Alvira JM, Vilanova M, Haro D, Martínez R, Carvajal I, et al. A comprehensive lifestyle peer group-based intervention on cardiovascular risk factors: the randomized controlled fifty-fifty program. J Am Coll Cardiol. 2016;67(5):476–85.
216. World Health Organization. Hearts technical management for CVD management in primary health care. 2016. https://apps.who.int/iris/handle/10665/252661.
217. Heery S, Gibson I, Dunne D, Flaherty G. The role of public health nurses in risk factor modification within a high-risk cardiovascular disease population in Ireland—a qualitative analysis. Eur J Cardiovasc Nurs. 2019;18(7):584–92.
218. Hayman LL, Berra K, Fletcher BJ, Houston Miller N. The role of nurses in promoting cardiovascular health worldwide: the global cardiovascular nursing leadership forum. J Am Coll Cardiol. 2015;66(7):864–66.
219. Jin K, Khonsari S, Gallagher R, Gallagher P, Clark AM, Freedman B, et al. Telehealth interventions for the secondary prevention of coronary heart disease: a systematic review and meta-analysis. Eur J Cardiovasc Nurs. 2019;18(4):260–71.
220. Chow CK, Redfern J, Hillis GS, Thakkar J, Santo K, Hackett ML, et al. Effect of lifestyle-focused text messaging on risk factor modification in patients with coronary heart disease: a randomized clinical trial. JAMA. 2015;314(12):1255–63.
221. Blasco A, Carmona M, Fernández-Lozano I, Salvador CH, Pascual M, Sagredo PG, et al. Evaluation of a telemedicine service for the secondary prevention of coronary artery disease. J Cardiopulm Rehabil Prev. 2012;32(1):25–31.
222. Johnston N, Bodegard J, Jerström S, Åkesson J, Brorsson H, Alfredsson J, et al. Effects of interactive patient smartphone support app on drug adherence and lifestyle changes in myocardial infarction patients: a randomized study. Am Heart J. 2016;178:85–94.
223. Karhula T, Vuorinen AL. Telemonitoring and mobile phone-based health coaching among Finnish diabetic and heart disease patients: randomized controlled trial 2015;17:e153.
224. Maddison R, Pfaeffli L, Whittaker R, Stewart R, Kerr A, Jiang Y, et al. A mobile phone intervention increases physical activity in people with cardiovascular disease: results from the HEART randomized controlled trial. Eur J Prev Cardiol. 2015;22(6):701–709.
225. Pfaeffli Dale L, Whittaker R, Jiang Y, Stewart R, Rolleston A, Maddison R. Text message and internet support for coronary heart disease self-management: results from the Text4Heart randomized controlled trial. J Med Internet Res. 2015;17(10):e237.

226. Varnfield M, Karunanithi M, Lee CK, Honeyman E, Arnold D, Ding H, et al. Smartphone-based home care model improved use of cardiac rehabilitation in postmyocardial infarction patients: results from a randomised controlled trial. Heart. 2014;100(22):1770–79.
227. Tongpeth J, Du H, Barry T, Clark RA. Effectiveness of an Avatar application for teaching heart attack recognition and response: a pragmatic randomized control trial. J Adv Nurs. 2020;76(1):297–311.
228. Coorey GM, Neubeck L, Mulley J, Redfern J. Effectiveness, acceptability and usefulness of mobile applications for cardiovascular disease self-management: systematic review with meta-synthesis of quantitative and qualitative data. Eur J Prev Cardiol. 2018;25(5):505–21.

12 Pharmacology for cardiovascular nurses

JAN KEENAN, RANI KHATIB, GABRIELLE MCKEE, TODD RUPPAR, AND FRANKI WILSON

CHAPTER CONTENTS

This chapter aims to develop understanding of pharmacology gained from earlier chapters by introducing some of the main drug groups used in cardiovascular care. It describes developments in nurse and allied health professional prescribing, and its potential benefits across the patient pathway. Examples are offered of how non-medical prescribing contributes to good practice in managing medication and the achievement of secondary prevention targets. The concept of medication adherence is explored and applied to the practice of managing medication and individualizing patient care and its importance emphasized in long-term management of the patient with cardiovascular disease.

KEY MESSAGES

1. Pharmacological therapies are the mainstay in management of primary and secondary prevention of cardiovascular disease.

2. Nurses have an important role in medicines management in collaboration with professional colleagues, particularly physicians and pharmacists.
3. Training nurses in advanced practice skills in relation to medications can improve post-acute event care.
4. Approaches to nursing and allied health professional prescribing are described in three different ways, referred to as 'independent', 'supplementary', and 'dependent' prescribing.
5. Up to half of patients prescribed medication for long-term conditions are not adherent to their prescribed regimen.
6. It is important for nurses to identify the reason for non-adherence before attempting to implement strategies to address it.
7. In cases of intentional non-adherence, it is essential to address patients' beliefs or concerns, or advocate for the patient to have the treatment plan modified to an approach that fits the patient's needs.

Introduction

Nurses have an important role to play in the management of their patients' medicines in cardiovascular care in collaboration with other disciplines, in particular physicians and pharmacists. This role covers elements such as coordination of their patients' medicines which is a part of the overall coordination of their care. In both acute and community settings, nurses take a holistic approach to care which involves viewing the big picture of the care that the patient and their family are receiving. Nurses are often responsible for 'joining up the dots' and ensuring integrated care. Nurses may also be involved in prescribing and optimization of drug therapies whether as an independent prescriber or in collaboration with physicians and pharmacists. This varies across countries and depends on education, training, and legislation. In the UK and the US, legislation now allows and facilitates independent prescribing by nurses and pharmacists with appropriate training and specialization. Nurses can also contribute to the reconciliation of medicines process because of their close and frequent contact with their patients which helps to avoid unnecessary polypharmacy and ensures safety and avoidance of adverse events.

In order to maximize adherence with medicines by patients, nurses are also well placed and can initiate educational (see also Chapter 13) and other interventions. In this chapter, we will cover these elements of the nurse's role in more detail and also describe how this role dovetails with that of other health professionals, in particular, physicians and pharmacists.

Management of medication in people with cardiovascular disease

Cardiovascular patients encounter many health professionals across their treatment pathway in primary, secondary, and tertiary care sectors; all those professionals will have an impact or influence on the patient's management, whether in prescribing or monitoring the effects of preventive therapies, and the ongoing identification and management of risk factors such as diabetes, high blood pressure, hyperlipidaemias, and health behaviours. There is nevertheless evidence that a large majority of coronary patients do not achieve guideline standards for secondary prevention[1] with a high prevalence of persistent smoking, unhealthy diets, physical inactivity, and inadequate risk factor control despite high reported use of medications.[1] Ongoing care and management of risk factors remains a challenge.

Cardiovascular medications remain the commonest intervention worldwide for primary and secondary prevention of cardiovascular diseases, yet despite their importance and known benefit, appropriate medication use is a challenge for both patients and for providers of healthcare. Patients frequently do not adhere to medications, resulting in poor clinical outcomes.[2] There is little question that in the management of cardiovascular disease, all health professionals across the patient pathway through presentation, acute treatment, follow-up, prevention, and rehabilitation need to have the ability to proactively influence pharmacological and non-pharmacological approaches to the management of the patient. ➤ Box 12.1 shows an example of how training nurses in advanced practice skills in relation to medications management can improve care following an acute event.

Nursing and allied health professional prescribing

The development of prescribing by nurses and allied health professionals has been driven by the necessity to improve healthcare delivery in an era in which there is a need to improve accessibility to treatment, including medication, at the point of care. The growth of nursing and allied health professional prescribing has been influenced by economic circumstances, a diminishing number of medical providers, the unavailability of adequate healthcare services in rural areas, and growing specialization among the professions.[3] Nurse and pharmacist prescribing is increasing

Box 12.1 Improving risk factor control, patient management, and access to cardiac rehabilitation through advanced nursing

The Oxford University Hospitals NHS Foundation Trust in the UK has invested in the development of members of the cardiac rehabilitation team to enable team members to develop skills in advanced practice, including history taking and physical assessment, and prescribing (see also Chapter 3).

In Oxford, UK, an audit of risk factor modification established that the achievement of targets for lipid lowering and for blood pressure levels was suboptimal. In addition, the uptitration of cardioprotective medication such as angiotensin-converting enzyme inhibitors (ACEIs) was not taking place after patients were discharged from hospital.

Through establishing a programme of early follow-up and early access to cardiovascular prevention and rehabilitation (see also Chapter 11) alongside the development of advanced skills, the nursing team proactively manage risk factors, titrate medication in a timely way, and address early medication concerns. Where people have been offered earlier access (within 2 weeks) to the commencement of the programme, the uptake of the programme has improved, patients have returned to work earlier after myocardial infarction (MI), and smoking cessation rates have improved. Unintended benefits were the early identification of complications of MI, and improvement in referral pathways to primary care or back to secondary care for the management of ongoing symptoms, higher-risk patients, or those in need of specialist advice from, for example, diabetologists or lipid specialists.

Recovery and rehabilitation after an acute coronary syndrome: the Oxford pathway

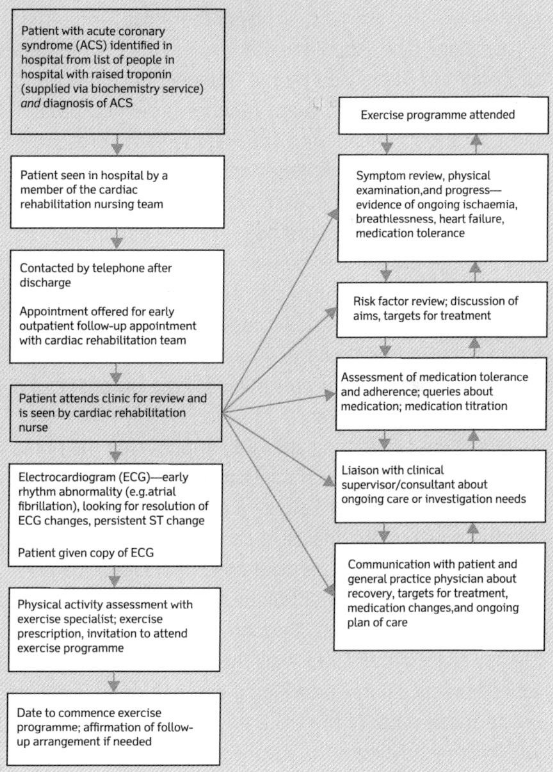

in primary and secondary care settings in the UK and is safe, clinically appropriate, acceptable to patients, and viewed positively by other health professionals.[4] Nursing and allied health professional prescribers as well as physicians have reported that patients accessing prescribing from nurses and allied health professionals receive higher-quality care, with more choice and convenience,[5] greater flexibility, and access to appointments.[6]

Approaches to nursing and allied health professional prescribing

Nursing and allied health professional prescribing was introduced in the UK in 1992. Its development has been influenced by changes in legislation that have led to the development of independent prescribing for nurses, pharmacists, and a range of allied health professionals.[7] While the UK has led the way in introducing nursing and allied health professional prescribing, it is emerging as an integral part of patient care in many Western European countries, the US, Canada, Australia, and New Zealand, although in most areas prescribing authority is restricted only to nurses and pharmacists. However, while the term 'nurse prescribing' suffices as a description of an activity, the practice it refers to varies between countries and internationally.[8] Approaches to nursing and allied health professional prescribing are described in three different ways, referred to as 'independent', 'supplementary', and 'dependent' prescribing.

An independent prescriber is responsible for clinical assessment, diagnosis, decisions about the appropriateness of a medication, and the issuing of a prescription. The independent prescriber has the authority to prescribe medications without the supervision of another health professional. This might be undertaken from a limited formulary that defines the medications that can be prescribed, or from an open formulary.

Supplementary prescribing is a voluntary relationship between an independent prescriber, usually a physician or dentist, and a supplementary prescriber who might be a nurse or pharmacist, or in the UK an allied health professional, for example, a physiotherapist, podiatrist, or dietitian. The supplementary prescriber manages the condition diagnosed by the independent prescriber, within a clinical management plan for a defined patient and condition, agreed with the independent prescriber and the patient, and specifies the medications that might be used to manage a specific condition (e.g. asthma, diabetes, or coronary heart disease) and the circumstances in which the patient will be referred to the independent prescriber for review. In the UK, nurses and pharmacists qualify as both independent and supplementary prescribers, but currently a nurse or pharmacist cannot be the named independent prescriber for the purposes of a clinical management plan.

Dependent prescribing authority implies that the nurse or pharmacist's prescribing authority is delegated by an independent prescriber, usually a physician, on the basis that the nurse or pharmacist is capable of performing the delegated duty.[9] The dependent prescriber shares responsibility for the management of the patient with the shared responsibility described through a collaborative drug therapy management. This was the original model for advanced practice nurse prescribing in the US, and is still in use in those parts of the US that have not implemented full practice privileges for advanced practice nurses (e.g. nurse practitioners).

Interdisciplinary working in medicines reconciliation

Community heart failure care setting

At Leeds Teaching Hospitals in the UK, pharmacists and nurses work together in the care of heart failure patients in the community. This partnership between heart failure nurses and cardiology pharmacists operates as a virtual clinic, whereby the nurse reviews patients in the community and seeks expert advice on heart failure medication from the hospital-based cardiology pharmacist. There is traditionally an emphasis on medicines reconciliation at transfer of care, for example, when a patient is discharged back to the care of the community heart failure nurse following a hospital admission. Here, community heart failure nurses ensure that an accurate list of medication is maintained and may consult with the cardiology pharmacist, via a virtual clinic, to clarify and confirm the rationale for changes made during hospital admission. The ongoing challenge is to ensure that this list of medication is adjusted and optimized to prevent hospital admissions. The heart failure nurse and cardiology pharmacist work together to ensure that medications are assessed when the patient's clinical condition changes.

Heart failure care across acute and community settings

Community and acute services heart failure teams at the Oxford University Hospitals NHS Foundation Trust in the UK meet on a monthly basis to discuss and review cases. The review is undertaken with a consultant cardiologist, a cardiac pharmacist, and the nursing teams working in acute and community settings. This provides an opportunity for clinical supervision and for those involved in the patient's care pathway to discuss management of particularly complex patients. The treatment pathway can be discussed and the evidence supporting the use of novel treatments for heart failure that might benefit the individual patient discussed with review planned for the patient to discuss changes or developments that may have benefit. This multiprofessional approach gives an opportunity for learning, for discussion of how treatment decisions impact the individual, and for individual optimization of medication for heart failure.

Introducing novel treatments in coronary artery disease

In 2019, the European Society of Cardiology asserted that clinical presentations of coronary artery disease can be categorized as either acute or chronic coronary syndrome and updated its guideline for management. Previous guidance is extended to add the use of, for example, sodium–glucose co-transporter 2 inhibitors (e.g. empagliflozin and dapagliflozin) for diabetes and cardiovascular disease, and the use of glucagon-like peptide-1 receptor agonists (e.g. liraglutide) for people with diabetes and cardiovascular disease. There are novel treatments for people with hyperlipidaemias recommended and there is clearer guidance for people taking oral anticoagulation. There is an era rapidly upon us in which individualization of secondary prevention medication is necessary in order to achieve the greatest risk reduction, particularly for high-risk patients with coronary artery disease.

One reaction to this at the Oxford University Hospitals NHS Foundation Trust in the UK has been to develop protocols for the set-up of a new clinic, for people at high risk of recurrent cardiovascular events. People who fulfil the criteria will be identified in hospital by the medical or nursing teams caring for the patient, who will be invited to discuss the management of their individual risk profile with experts in, for example, lipid management, coronary artery disease, diabetes, and hypertension, with a view to optimizing and individualizing medication and communicating long-term management plans with primary care physicians.

Adherence to medication regimens

➤ Box 12.2 provides an evolution of terminology used in relation to medication adherence.[10–13]

Overview of medication adherence in cardiovascular disease

Pharmacotherapy for patients with cardiovascular disease can only be effective if patients are willing and able to take the medications appropriately prescribed for their condition. Unfortunately, up to half of patients prescribed medication for long-term conditions are not adherent to their prescribed regimen.[14,15] Low adherence to cardiovascular medications has been associated with poor clinical outcomes including higher rates of MI, stroke, renal failure, and overall mortality.[16,17] Estimates of the proportion of hospitalizations due to medication non-adherence range from 4.3% to 69%, with cardiovascular conditions having higher rates of non-adherence-related hospitalizations.[18,19]

Medication non-adherence is estimated to cost over €125 billion per year and $105 billion per year in avoidable healthcare costs.[20] Patients who adhere to cardiovascular medication regimens have 15–23% lower healthcare costs than patients who are non-adherent.[21] While pharmacy costs are typically higher for adherent patients, overall healthcare costs are consistently much lower.[22]

The term 'adherence' considers that people choose to take medication and have control over its use. Adherence to medications is defined as the process by which patients take medications as agreed with the prescriber.[13] Successful medication adherence involves multiple behaviours. The prescription must be filled and picked up from the pharmacy and the first dose taken (initiation); doses must be correctly taken as prescribed on a day-to-day basis (implementation); and patients must continue to take the medication for as long as it is indicated (persistence).[13] When addressing non-adherence to medications, the type of non-adherence will contribute to the approach a healthcare provider will take towards helping the patient improve their medication-taking. Further, the patient's reasons for non-adherence will be

Box 12.2 The evolution of medication adherence terminology

Many terms have been used in the literature to describe the process of how patients manage and take medications. The original term, 'compliance', emerged in the 1970s and was defined as 'the extent to which the patient's behaviour coincides with the clinical prescription'. Over time, 'compliance' became viewed as reflecting a paternalistic approach to healthcare delivery, and the term 'adherence' emerged in the 1990s as a concept that acknowledges the shared decision-making by patients and healthcare providers in the prescribing and medication-taking processes. This movement to 'adherence' culminated in a 2003 World Health Organization report that defined adherence as 'the extent to which a person's behaviour—taking medication, following a diet, and/or executing lifestyle changes—corresponds with agreed recommendations from a health care provider'.

During the same time period that 'adherence' emerged, the concept of 'concordance' was developed to describe the process of healthcare providers and patients working together to identify mutually agreeable treatment plans.

The Ascertaining Barriers to Adherence (ABC) Project published an expanded review and taxonomy of medication adherence in 2012, defining adherence to medications as 'the process by which patients take their medications as prescribed, composed of initiation, implementation, and discontinuation':

Initiation is the time point when a patient takes the first dose of medication regimen.

Implementation is the extent to which the patient takes the doses as prescribed, on a daily basis.

Discontinuation is the time point when a patient stops taking a medication, regardless of the reason.

Persistence is then measured as the time between initiation and the last dose of medication.

of great importance. Broadly, a distinction can be made between non-adherence that is unintentional, or intentional. Unintentional non-adherence occurs when a patient wishes to follow a prescribed regimen but is unable to do so due to factors beyond their control, such as poor recall, inability to pay, problems with the treatment, or simply forgetting. Unintentional non-adherence will necessarily require different intervention approaches than would intentional non-adherence, where a patient decides not to take their medication, or modifies their medication regimen. Intentional non-adherence is a far more complex phenomenon that is 'likely better explained with an understanding of beliefs and preferences that influence motivation to start and continue with treatment'.[23]

Influences on medication adherence

There is an array of factors that impact intentional medication adherence, including sociodemographic and psychosocial factors, beliefs about medication, health system factors, and the patient's experience of their illness and recovery. Sociodemographic influences include a higher level of education and increasing age,[24] which have a positive influence on adherence. Cost of medication[25] and unemployment[26] can have a negative impact on adherence, and it has also been established that a lack of information about medication can have a negative impact on adherence, as can the perception of side effects.[24] Psychosocial factors that impact adherence include a low understanding of treatment, with some studies suggesting that very early in starting treatment, there are unmet needs for information about both the disease and the medication.[26,27] Beliefs about medication also influence adherence, specifically concerns about medication and its perceived necessity[28] as does the patient's experience of the health system, including follow-up care,[29] their recovery, and their perception of the illness itself.[30]

Identifying and addressing non-adherence

Addressing medicines non-adherence requires it to be identified first. In line with the National Institute for Health and Care Excellence (NICE) recommendations[23] in its guidance on adherence, the medicines-taking experience of patients should be routinely explored and modifiable barriers to adherence should be addressed. Evidence shows that non-adherence behaviour is often a hidden problem which is under-recognized by prescribers. Most importantly, it is not necessarily disclosed by patients and it can change. Therefore, healthcare professionals should assess, elicit, and explore patients' beliefs and experiences with their medicines to help them make informed choices and address any barriers.

The complexity of non-adherence behaviour was illustrated in a study which explored barriers to adhering to secondary prevention medicines among patients with coronary artery disease.[31] Among those who were non-adherent, over half had non-adherence to only one secondary prevention medicine, indicating that certain patients have 'selective' non-adherence. Barriers to adherence included forgetfulness, worry that medicines will do more harm than good, feeling hassled about medicines taking, feeling worse when taking medicines, and not being convinced of the benefit of medicines. Different factors were often associated with intentional versus unintentional non-adherence.

The recently introduced concept of 'medicines optimization'[32] has these elements at the heart of its definition: 'a person-centred approach to safe and effective medicines use, to ensure people obtain the best possible outcomes from their medicines'. Delivering person-centred medicines optimization requires understanding the patient's experience; this is one of the four pillars of medicines optimization as defined by NICE.[33] In addition, NICE places an emphasis on the importance of adopting a shared decision-making approach in delivering medicines optimization. Shared decision-making is an essential part of evidence-based medicine, seeking to use the best available evidence to guide decisions about the care of the individual patient, taking into account their needs, preferences, and values. This more person-centred approach (see also Chapter 2) is more likely to address barriers to adherence and improve it. Further, when patients have caregivers involved with helping to manage their health conditions, person-centred care may also incorporate caregivers in medication education and discussions, as caregiver involvement has been shown to improve adherence to medications for persons with cardiovascular disease.[34] ➤ **Box 12.3** shows an example of a pharmacist-led intervention to improving medicines optimization and adherence.[35]

The role of the cardiovascular nurse in addressing adherence

Cardiovascular nurses play an important role in helping patients to successfully adhere to medication regimens, and ultimately reduce patients' risk for poor cardiovascular health outcomes. Cardiovascular nurses are likely to spend a greater amount of time with patients and can

Box 12.3 Good practice example: medicines optimization

The use of appropriate self-report tools can assist learning about the patient experience and identify barriers to adherence. A UK-based study[35] which used a locally developed tool, the 'My Experience of Taking Medicines' (MYMEDS), succeeded in giving patients the opportunity to share any barriers they might have to adherence to post-MI secondary prevention medicines. In this model, after completing the MYMEDS questionnaire, patients attended a consultant pharmacist-led medicines optimization clinic. Adopting the principles of medicines optimization, the pharmacist had a better understanding of individual patient's experiences in taking secondary prevention medicines and their needs and barriers to adherence were identified and addressed. This model of working led to substantial improvement in the levels of medicines optimization, patient concerns about their medications were significantly decreased, rates of non-adherence fell, and readmission rates also declined after the service was delivered.

use that time to identify medication-taking behaviour that may be inhibiting the success of therapy, and work with the healthcare team to identify appropriate interventions for each patient.

Assessment

The first step in addressing adherence is to assess patients' adherence to their medication regimen. The simplest approach is to ask patients in a non-judgemental manner whether they have ever missed or skipped any doses of their medication. It is important to phrase questions in a manner that will elicit responses about both unintentional and intentional non-adherence. Self-report of adherence behaviour, however, is subject to recall bias. Patients often think they do better with managing their medications than they actually do. If the patient is not using a type of medication organization system that would provide feedback about missed doses (blister packs, pill organizers, etc.), the patient may be unaware of missed doses. The cardiovascular nurse may suggest that the patient use a pill organizer or keep a medication log for a defined period to monitor their own medication-taking and see if they are missing doses.

Another method for assessing adherence is to look at pharmacy refill data, if it is available. If patients are not refilling prescriptions on time, it is likely that they are not correctly implementing the dosing regimen, and this should be investigated further. However, pharmacy refill data can only reflect adherence behaviour over long periods of time and cannot provide information on specific patterns of medication-taking behaviour that would help to guide selection of interventions. Thus, pharmacy refill data may be useful as a screening tool for potential non-adherence but is less useful for guiding interventions.

Additional technological approaches for assessing adherence are available, such as electronic adherence monitoring caps, but these methods typically involve substantial added cost. The benefit of such methods, however, is detailed, objective information about patients' medication-taking patterns that can be used to identify when doses are missed or skipped, and what factors may be influencing the low adherence.

Side effects are one of the most common reasons that patients report not taking medications as prescribed.[36–38] Cardiovascular nurses should ask patients if they are experiencing any problematic symptoms or side effects. This is an opportunity to educate patients on likely side effects, how to manage problematic side effects, and to reshape thinking about side effects when a patient has misattributed a symptom as a side effect. Part of the cardiovascular nurse's role also includes identifying, advocating, and, where possible, making changes in therapy when problematic side effects are causing distress for patients or are impeding a patient's ability or willingness to adhere to their medication regimen.

Implementing adherence-enhancing strategies

Cardiovascular nurses have available a number of interventions that may help to improve patients' adherence to cardiovascular medications (➤ Table 12.1). Interventions should be chosen based on the assessment of the type of non-adherence and the patient's reasons for non-adherence (e.g. barriers, medication, or health beliefs). For patients who struggle to remember to take medications, the first-line approach is to suggest a medication organizer, pillbox, or blister pack system, if the patient is not already using such an approach.[39] This allows patients to be able to quickly identify which medications should be taken at the time of medication administration, reducing cognitive burden, and allows patients to easily see whether doses have been taken or missed.

After medication organizer systems, the next approach could include a type of a reminder system. This could be done using technology such as a smartphone app or through a simple alarm; however, some patients eventually tire of simple alarms. Many apps are available

Table 12.1 Strategies to enhance medication adherence

Strategies	Type of non-adherence	Description
Medications organizer, pillbox, blister pack	Unintentional	Organization system that separates medications by dose so that patients are able to see whether a particular dose has been taken
Reminder system, e.g. mobile device app, alarm	Unintentional	Reminders or cues that prompt patients to take their medications at the appropriate time
Integrate into daily habits, e.g. tooth brushing	Unintentional	Strategies that link medication-taking with existing daily habits and routines so that medication-taking can, over time, become a habitual behaviour
Educational intervention	Intentional	Education interventions typically focus on content about the specifics of a patient's medication regimen—the names of medications, reasons why medications are needed, doses, frequency, potential side effects, what to do if a dose is missed, etc. These strategies ensure that patients have the information necessary to successfully adhere to their medication regimen
Motivational interviewing	Intentional	Motivational interventions move beyond education to address *why* patients have been prescribed medications. Addresses what medications do, what the consequences might be if medications are discontinued or doses are missed. These interventions typically also address patients' goals, and how medication-taking fits into their health and life goals

[a] See 'Overview of medication adherence in cardiovascular disease' section for definitions.

with different types of reminders or the ability to track medication-taking. It may be more helpful for long-term behaviour change to also counsel the patient to integrate medication-taking into other daily habits and routines. Keeping medications in a visible location next to other objects that are tied to habitual behaviour, such as a toothbrush or coffee equipment, can help patients to link medication-taking with those habits and make the medication-taking a regular habit itself. Habit formation interventions have been shown to be effective at helping to improve unintentional non-adherence.[40]

Sometimes low medication adherence is driven by a low intention to adhere. Patients may be unsure of the efficacy or have concerns about the safety of their prescribed medications or may have made a decision not to take their medication. Cardiovascular nurses can intervene by providing evidence-based education on the specific medications the patient has been prescribed, the reasons why the medication is needed, and the health risks involved in not taking the medication. Motivational interviewing approaches (see also Chapter 11) have been shown to be effective at augmenting standard patient education methods.[41,42] If the patient continues to have concerns, the cardiovascular nurse's role will also involve facilitating communication between the patient and the prescriber, or to intervene as the prescriber where possible, to explore alternative treatment options.

Improving medication adherence is often a gradual process. Several different approaches may need to be attempted or combined to find the strategy that works for a particular patient. Recent studies have shown success at taking a continuous self-improvement approach, similar to the model used for quality improvement in healthcare institutions.[43,44] The cardiovascular nurse helps the patient to assess their reasons for non-adherence, implements a strategy to improve adherence, evaluates the impact of that strategy, and then decides whether additional strategies are needed.

Adherence to cardiovascular medication regimens is key for achieving good clinical outcomes for patients. Whether in an inpatient or outpatient setting, cardiovascular nurses are in an ideal position to influence patients' adherence to medication regimens. Nurses and other professionals such as pharmacists can do this by thoroughly assessing their patients' level of adherence, their medication-taking processes and habits, and suggesting changes in the patients' systems for managing their medications to reduce the likelihood of missed or forgotten doses. For patients who choose to modify or not take their medications, the cardiovascular nurse should assess each patient's reasons for non-adherence and provide interventions designed to address the patient's beliefs or concerns, or advocate for the patient to have the treatment plan modified to an approach that fits the patient's needs.

Introduction to medicines used in cardiovascular care

This section aims to further develop the understanding of the pharmacological treatment of cardiovascular disease outlined in previous chapters. It will introduce some of the commonly used drug groups, the main disorders in which they are used, outline their mode of action, and highlight some of their potential adverse effects. This serves as a useful introduction for nurses working in cardiovascular care to understand the rationale for the prescribing of the different drug groups, and provides a useful adjunct to European Society of Cardiology guidelines for the management of cardiovascular disorders, national pharmacological drug guidelines, and regulatory sites so as to enhance the understanding of treatment strategies. The section covers lipid-lowering therapies, anticoagulants and antiplatelets, antiarrhythmic drugs, drugs affecting tissue perfusion, new diabetes drugs with cardiovascular benefits, and blood pressure-lowering drugs. In addition, a brief introduction is given to drugs used in emergency and cardiogenic shock. This complements the sections on care of the deteriorating patient (see also Chapter 5). ➤ Table 12.2 and ➤ Table 12.3 provide a summary overview of these therapies. Finally, a brief introduction is provided to the science of pharmacogenetics.

Table 12.2 Overview of medicines for cardioprotection used in cardiovascular care

Action	Drug name	Mode of administration	Side effects
Lipid lowering	Statins HMG-CoA reductase inhibitors Simvastatin, fluvastatin, pravastatin, atorvastatin, rosuvastatin	Oral	Myopathy, gastrointestinal disturbance, insomnia, rash, altered liver function tests Rare: rhabdomyolysis, angioedema
	Anion exchange resins (bile acid sequestrants) Colestyramine, colestipol, colesevelam	Oral	Gastrointestinal symptoms: abdominal bloating, discomfort, diarrhoea, constipation
	Fibrates E.g. gemfibrozil, bezafibrate, fenofibrate	Oral	Myositis Rare: severe rhabdomyolysis
	Niacin; nicotinic acid	Oral	Flushing, palpitations, dizziness, gastrointestinal disturbance
	Cholesterol absorption inhibitors Ezetimibe	Oral	Abdominal pain, diarrhoea, headache Rare: liver dysfunction, thrombocytopenia, pancreatitis Very rare: muscle toxicity
	PCSK9 inhibitors Evolocumab, alirocumab	Subcutaneous injection	Flu-like symptoms, injection-site reactions, nausea, rash
	Inclisiran	Subcutaneous injection	None yet seen

Table 12.2 Continued

Action	Drug name	Mode of administration	Side effects
Anticoagulant	Heparin and related drugs Unfractionated heparin (UFH) Low-molecular-weight heparin (LMWH)—dalteparin, enoxaparin, tinzaparin, fondaparinux	Intravenous or subcutaneous injection	Increased haemorrhage risk, hyperkalaemia, heparin-induced thrombocytopenia, osteoporosis
	Vitamin K antagonists Warfarin	Oral	Haemorrhage
	Direct oral anticoagulants (DOACs) Apixaban, edoxaban, rivaroxaban, dabigatran	Oral	Haemorrhage
Antiplatelet	Aspirin	Oral	Aspirin: nausea, heartburn, indigestion, major bleeding Rare: urticaria, rhinitis, bronchoconstriction, respiratory compromise
	ADP inhibitors: clopidogrel, prasugrel, ticagrelor	Oral	Bleeding, dyspnoea
	Glycoprotein IIb/IIIa inhibitors Abciximab, tirofiban, eptifibatide	Intravenous	Bleeding, hypotension, hypersensitivity
Dual pathway inhibition	Low-dose rivaroxaban plus aspirin	Oral	Gastrointestinal bleeding
Antiarrhythmic	Vaughan Williams classification E.g. disopyramide, lidocaine, flecainide, propranolol, amiodarone, verapamil	Oral and intravenous	Bradycardia, rhythm disturbance, fatigue, exercise intolerance, malaise, cold extremities, sexual dysfunction Amiodarone: altered liver and thyroid function, skin discoloration, photosensitivity, pulmonary toxicity, corneal deposits
	Not classified in Vaughan Williams classification E.g. atropine, adrenaline (epinephrine), isoprenaline, digoxin, adenosine, calcium chloride, magnesium chloride		Bradycardia, rhythm disturbance, fatigue, exercise intolerance, malaise, cold extremities, sexual dysfunction Digoxin toxicity: severe bradycardia, diarrhoea, vomiting, dizziness, visual disturbance
New diabetes dugs with cardiovascular benefits	GLP-1RAs E.g. dulaglutide, liraglutide, semaglutide	Subcutaneous injection	Back pain, cystitis, increased infection risk
	SGL2 inhibitors E.g. empagliflozin, dapagliflozin, canagliflozin	Oral	Skin reactions, thirst, urinary disorders, hypoglycaemia Euglycaemic ketoacidosis in patients with diabetes

Table 12.2 Continued

Action	Drug name	Mode of administration	Side effects
Promotion of tissue perfusion	Nitrates Glycerol trinitrate (GTN)	Sublingual	Flushing, dizziness, migraine type headaches, hypotension
Blood pressure lowering	Angiotensin-converting enzyme inhibitors (ACEIs) E.g. ramipril, perindopril, lisinopril	Oral	Cough, headaches, dizziness, rash, postural hypotension, angiodema, acute kidney injury
	Angiotensin II receptor blocker (ARBs) E.g. candesartan, valsartan, losartan	Oral	Headaches, dizziness, postural hypotension, angiodema, acute kidney injury
	Mineralocorticoid receptor antagonists for heart failure Spironolactone, eplerenone	Oral	Hyperkalaemia, gynaecomastia, mastondynia, vaginal bleeding
	Combination ARB plus neprilysin inhibitor for heart failure Sacubitril–valsartan	Oral	Dizziness, postural hypotension, hyperkalaemia, renal impairment, angioedema
	Beta-blockers Atenolol, bisoprolol	Oral	Bradycardia, rhythm disturbance, fatigue, exercise intolerance, malaise, cold extremities, sexual dysfunction
	Calcium channel blockers (two types) Dihydropyridine, e.g. amlodipine, felodipine, and nifedipine More cardioselective, e.g. verapamil, diltiazem	Oral	Headache, flushing, rash, swelling, malaise, constipation Excessive bradycardia, heart block Rare: hepatoxicity, MI, heart failure, hypotension, hypersensitivity

Table 12.3 Vaughan Williams classification of antiarrhythmic agents

Class	Example	Mechanism
Ia	Disopyramide	Sodium channel blockade
Ib	Lidocaine	Sodium channel blockade
Ic	Flecainide	Sodium channel blockade
II	Propranolol	Beta-adrenoceptor blockade
III	Amiodarone, sotalol	Potassium channel blockade
IV	Verapamil	Calcium channel blockade

Lipid-lowering therapies

Atherosclerosis provides a common underlying theme for many cardiovascular diseases, including thrombotic MI, heart failure, and stroke. In addition to hypertension, dyslipidaemia is a significant risk factor for atherosclerosis. Here we describe how various agents target lipid transport systems to reduce low-density lipoprotein cholesterol (LDL-C) and atheroma.

Patients most likely to benefit from lipid-lowering therapy are those with known cardiovascular disease, including coronary artery disease, history of MI and/or stroke, those at high risk of developing cardiovascular disease, and those with familial hypercholesterolaemia.

Statins: HMG-CoA reductase inhibitors

Statins are usually the lipid-lowering agent of first choice, owing to their ability to produce significant reductions in plasma LDL-C, coupled with strong evidence that this leads to a reduction in cardiovascular events and all-cause mortality.[45]

Statins in clinical use are simvastatin, fluvastatin, pravastatin, atorvastatin, and rosuvastatin. The latter two are longer acting and produce the greatest reductions in cholesterol[46] and, from a clinical perspective, are often better tolerated.

Mechanism of action: statins inhibit hepatic cholesterol synthesis, which leads to upregulation of the transport receptors responsible for removing LDL-C from the plasma into the liver.[47] Statins also exhibit a number of 'pleiotropic effects'; that is, they have actions other than those for which they were specifically developed. These include improved endothelial function, reduced vascular inflammation, and stabilization of atherosclerotic plaques, which may also be important in reducing cardiovascular events.[48]

Adverse effects: statins are well tolerated; however, side effects include myopathy, gastrointestinal disturbance, insomnia, rash, and altered liver function tests.[49] More serious adverse effects are rare and include rhabdomyolysis and angioedema.[50] Myopathy is a class effect of statins and other lipid-lowering agents and is more likely to occur in patients with low muscle mass, uncorrected hypothyroidism, or on interacting medications.

Interactions: simvastatin, fluvastatin, and atorvastatin are metabolized by cytochrome P450 enzymes and are affected, in varying degrees, by drugs which induce or inhibit this enzyme system. Rosuvastatin and pravastatin do not undergo extensive metabolism and therefore have fewer metabolic interactions.

Anion exchange resins (bile acid sequestrants)

Colestyramine, colestipol, and colesevelam are not generally recommended for primary and secondary prevention of cardiovascular disease due to a lack of evidence for clinically relevant outcomes, such as reductions in cardiovascular or all-cause mortality.[45] Their main place in therapy is for the treatment of familial hypercholesterolaemia, where they may be added to statin therapy under specialist care.[45] However, their poor adherence due to side effect and interaction profiles makes anion exchange resins unlikely candidates as a second-line cholesterol-lowering agent in statin intolerance.

Mechanism of action: anion exchange resins bind to intestinal bile acids, forming an insoluble complex and increasing their excretion. This leads to an increase in conversion of cholesterol to bile acids and a compensatory upregulation of hepatic LDL-C receptors, with a subsequent reduction in plasma LDL-C. They have little effect on high-density lipoprotein cholesterol (HDL-C) but can elevate triglycerides.

Adverse effects: as anion exchange resins are not absorbed, adverse effects are limited to the gastrointestinal tract. These are often the cause of poor adherence to treatment and include abdominal bloating and discomfort, diarrhoea, and constipation.

Interactions: anion exchange resins can bind to other medications in the gut and prevent their absorption. For this reason, other medications should be taken at least 1 hour prior to or 4 hours after anion exchange resins, to avoid this interaction.[49]

Fibrates

Fibrates (e.g. gemfibrozil, bezafibrate, fenofibrate) are not routinely offered for primary or secondary prevention of cardiovascular disease in the UK or in Europe.[45,46] They elicit a reduction in LDL-C and increase in HDL-C by up to 20%, as well as eliciting up to a 50% reduction in triglycerides.[51] This makes them potentially useful in treating mixed dyslipidaemias. In specialist use they can be combined with statins for patients who meet LDL-C targets but have raised triglycerides.[45]

Mechanism of action: through a complex mechanism of action, fibrates increase transcription of genes encoding proteins involved in lipid and lipoprotein metabolism and increase hepatic uptake of LDL-C to remove it from plasma.[45]

Adverse effects: myositis, rarely including severe rhabdomyolysis, can be caused by fibrates and is more common in alcoholics and patients with renal dysfunction. The risk is increased by concomitant administration of statins. Gemfibrozil is contraindicated alongside a statin; however, other fibrates may be cautiously combined with statins in specialist use.[49]

Interactions: there are a significant number of drug interactions, some theoretical and some having arisen from their use in studies. Particularly of note is the interaction with statins, which is why fibrates should be used under specialist advice in combination therapy; there are also potential interactions with insulins and with ezetimibe.

Niacin or nicotinic acid

Nicotinic acid, or niacin, is rarely used. It is not recommended for primary or secondary prevention of cardiovascular disease, owing to the lack of evidence for mortality reduction[52,53] and its unacceptable side effect profile.

Mechanism of action: nicotinamide, the active form, inhibits the release of very LDL-C in the liver, which results in a reduction in plasma triglycerides and LDL-C, and an increase in HDL-C. The exact mechanism by which this occurs is poorly understood.

Adverse effects: use of nicotinic acid is limited by the frequency of side effects, which include flushing, palpitations, dizziness, and gastrointestinal disturbance. Dose-related adverse effects include impairment of glucose tolerance, increased uric acid, and deranged liver function.[51]

Cholesterol absorption inhibitor (ezetimibe)

Ezetimibe is most effective as add-on therapy for patients who do not meet secondary preventative LDL-C targets on maximum tolerated statin therapy.[54] It can also be combined with a proprotein convertase subtilisin/kexin type 9 (PCSK9) inhibitor or used as monotherapy in true statin intolerance.[45]

Mechanism of action: ezetimibe inhibits duodenal absorption of dietary and biliary cholesterol, increasing excretion. This reduces hepatic cholesterol, which causes upregulation of hepatic LDL-C receptors and, consequently, increased removal of LDL-C from plasma.[55] Ezetimibe alone reduces LDL-C by approximately 20%[56]; however, its synergy with statins means that greater reductions can be seen when combined.

Adverse effects: ezetimibe is usually well tolerated with the most frequent unwanted effects being abdominal pain, diarrhoea, and headache. Rarely, more severe side effects can occur, including liver dysfunction, thrombocytopenia, and pancreatitis. Muscle toxicity is very rare, and the frequency is unlikely to increase on combination with a statin.[57]

PCSK9 inhibitors

PCSK9 inhibitors form a relatively new class of drugs comprising evolocumab and alirocumab. They are monoclonal antibodies, which are administered by subcutaneous injection every 2–4 weeks. Clinical trials have demonstrated significant LDL-C reductions (average 60%) in patients at high risk of CVD (primary or secondary prevention), including those with familial hypercholesterolaemia who are intolerant of statins or fail to meet target LDL-C on the maximum tolerated dose of statin in combination with ezetimibe.[58,59] There is some evidence that this reduction in LDL-C corresponds to a reduction in CV events.[60,61]

Mechanism of action: PCSK9 inhibitors block the targeted degradation of LDL-C receptors in the hepatocellular membrane, thereby reducing plasma LDL-C.[62] The greatest LDL-C reductions are seen when used in combination with a statin, owing to the compensatory increase in PCSK9 caused by statins.

Adverse effects: few side effects were reported in the clinical trials leading to marketing authorization but include flu-like symptoms, injection site reactions, nausea, and rash.[49] Active post-marketing surveillance continues, with patients and healthcare professionals encouraged to report any unwanted effects to the relevant regulatory body.

Inclisiran

Inclisiran is a small interfering RNA (siRNA) which is administered every 6 months by subcutaneous injection. This new, emerging treatment will provide a more convenient alternative to the monoclonal antibody PCSK9 inhibitors, with potential for improved adherence.

Mechanism of action: inclisiran blocks the hepatic production of PCSK9, which reduces the targeted degradation of LDL-C receptors in the hepatocellular membrane and, ultimately, plasma LDL-C.[63] It has been shown to reduce LDL-C by 56% in patients with stable atherosclerotic cardiovascular disease on maximally tolerated statin therapy.[64] Trials investigating the impact of this LDL-C lowering on cardiovascular outcomes are ongoing at the time of writing.

Adverse events: inclisiran has been shown to be safe and tolerable so far, with no detrimental effects on kidneys, liver, muscle, or platelets seen in clinical trials to date.[65]

Anticoagulants and antiplatelet drugs

Anticoagulants inhibit thrombin generation and antiplatelets inhibit platelet activation at various points in their respective cascades. ➤ Fig. 12.1 and ➤ Fig. 12.2

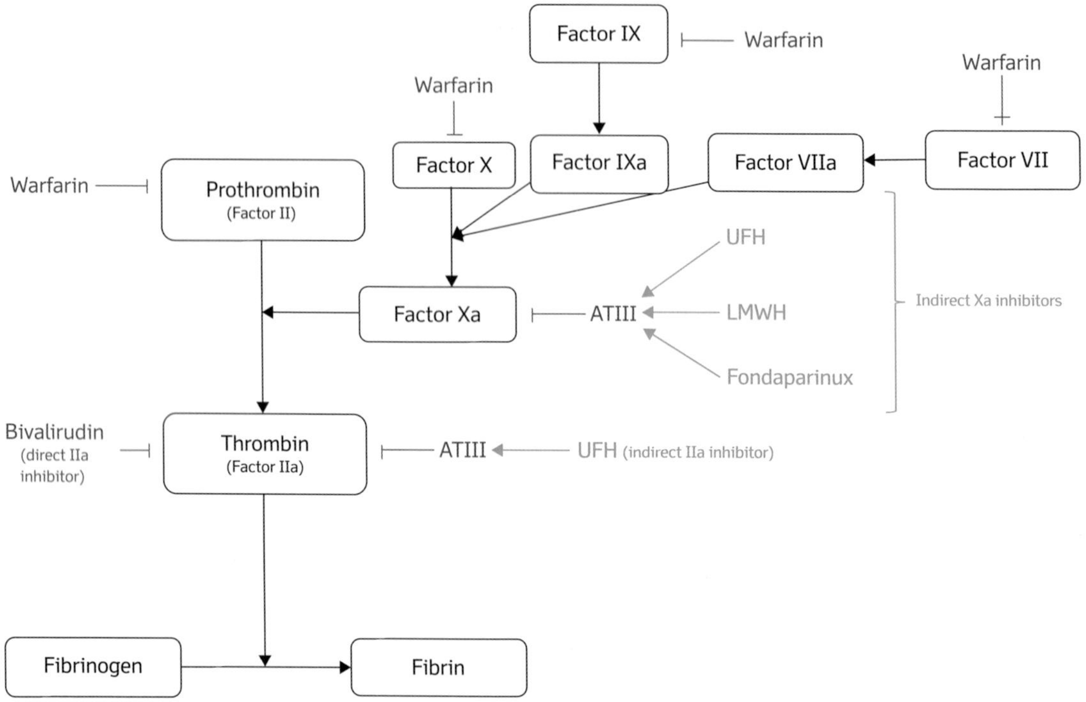

Fig. 12.1 Site(s) of action of anticoagulant agents within the clotting cascade.
ATIII, antithrombin III; LMWH, low-molecular-weight heparin; UFH, unfractionated heparin.

show the sites of action of the anticoagulants and antiplatelets discussed in this chapter, respectively.

Anticoagulants

Heparin and related drugs

Unfractionated heparin (UFH), low-molecular-weight heparins (LMWHs) such as dalteparin, enoxaparin, and tinzaparin, and fondaparinux, a synthetic pentasaccharide, are parenteral anticoagulants. The longer-acting LMWHs have replaced heparin for many indications, including prevention and treatment of venous thromboembolism and treatment of acute coronary syndromes. They can be administered subcutaneously once daily and require no routine monitoring for most patients; the exceptions being extremes of body weight and renal failure, where monitoring anti-factor Xa levels as a surrogate to measure the activity of the drug might be indicated.

UFH is still used when a rapid offset of action is required (e.g. high bleeding risk due to patient or procedural factors) and sometimes in patients with poor renal function. It is usually administered as an intravenous infusion and the dose is adjusted according to activated partial thromboplastin time. It is also commonly used during procedures such as coronary angiography due to its rapid onset and offset as an anticoagulant.

UFH and LMWH are porcine-derived so care should be taken in groups of patients in whom porcine-derived products may not be acceptable, such as practising Jewish and Muslim patients.

Mechanism of action: UFH, LMWH, and fondaparinux inhibit coagulation by preventing thrombin generation (➤ **Fig. 12.1**). They bind to antithrombin III, inducing a conformational change which increases its ability to inhibit clotting factors, primarily factor Xa and thrombin.

Adverse effects: parenteral anticoagulants increase the risk of haemorrhage. As heparin is short acting, ceasing administration may be sufficient to control bleeding. Protamine, a specific antidote, can be injected intravenously to neutralize heparin. It can also be used to partially reverse LMWH-induced bleeding. There is no specific antidote for fondaparinux.

Other unwanted effects of heparins include hyperkalaemia, particularly in patients with diabetes and renal impairment, and heparin-induced thrombocytopenia, which is a potentially devastating immune reaction caused by antibodies that activate platelets in the presence of heparin. Both are less likely to occur with

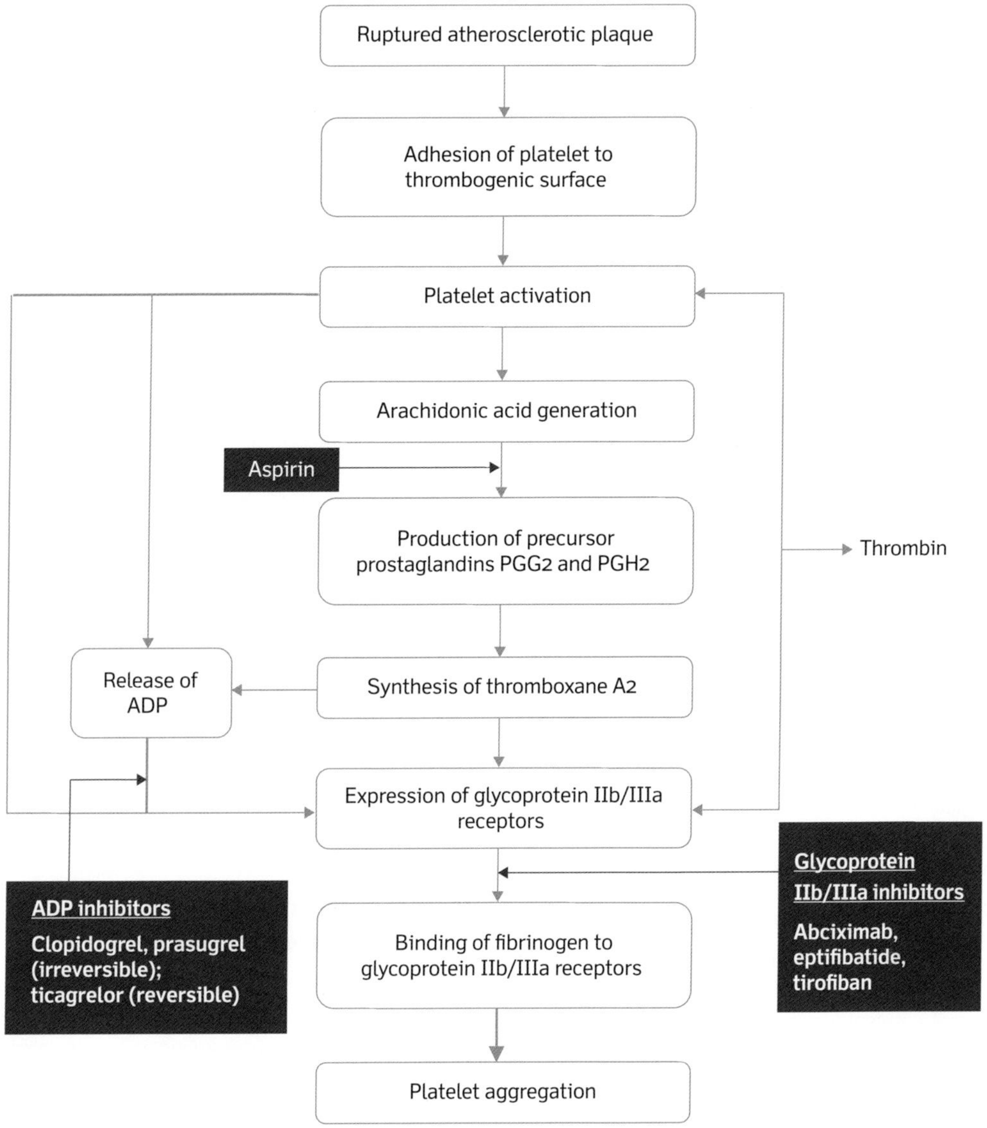

Fig. 12.2 Site of action of antiplatelet agents within the platelet aggregation pathway.

LMWH compared to UFH. Osteoporosis is associated with prolonged use.[48]

Vitamin K antagonists

Warfarin is the most commonly used vitamin K antagonist. The alternatives (phenindione and acenocoumarol) are generally only used in patients who cannot tolerate warfarin. Warfarin is the main stay of anticoagulation for patients with mechanical valve replacements. Its use for atrial fibrillation has diminished since the establishment of direct oral anticoagulants (DOACs), although use continues in some patients, particularly where DOACs are not tolerated or are contraindicated, for example, in severe renal impairment or valvular atrial fibrillation, or where DOACs are not recommended, for example, in people with very high body weight (>120 kg) (see 'Direct oral anticoagulants').

Mechanism of action: warfarin inhibits the synthesis of vitamin K-dependent clotting factors II, VII, IX, and X, which ultimately prevents conversion of fibrinogen to fibrin that is required for clot formation (➤ **Fig. 12.1**). Therapy takes several days to become established, due to the need for natural degradation of existing clotting factors. Its narrow therapeutic window necessitates frequent monitoring of the international normalized ratio (INR). The dose is adjusted to achieve an INR of between 2 and 4, depending on the indication and patient risk factors. However, it is this need for dose adjustment and monitoring, along with its multiple food and drug interactions, that makes warfarin an inconvenient treatment for most patients.

Adverse effects: as with all anticoagulants, haemorrhage is the most common adverse effect, but can be more difficult to manage due to its long duration of action. Treatment of warfarin-induced bleeding ranges from withholding warfarin, for example, for minor bleeds, to administration of vitamin K, fresh frozen plasma, or coagulation factor concentrates for life-threatening haemorrhage.

Interactions: warfarin is subject to multiple drug, food, and disease interactions. Enzyme inducers, for example, rifampicin or carbamazepine, and foods containing vitamin K such as spinach or egg yolk, reduce its effect and will therefore reduce the INR leading to a reduction or even loss of its therapeutic effect. Enzyme inhibitors such as amiodarone or erythromycin increase the effect of warfarin and therefore increase the INR, leading to an increased risk of bleeding. Liver disease can cause impaired levels of clotting factors, leading to prolonged prothrombin time and higher INR, and other disease states such as decompensated heart failure can also alter the effect of warfarin.

Direct oral anticoagulants

DOACs are a convenient alternative to vitamin K antagonists for oral anticoagulation for many patients. They are licensed for treatment and prevention of venous thromboembolism and for prophylaxis of stroke in patients with non-valvular AF.[49] They are also used for the treatment of deep vein thrombosis and pulmonary embolus and prevention of recurrence; they can be used to prevent stroke in patients undergoing cardioversion and ablation, and to treat left ventricular thrombus. The benefits offered by DOACs include faster onset of action, lack of monitoring and dose adjustment, and the ability to dispense in a compliance aid. However, the short duration of action of the DOACs makes adherence to the intended treatment regimen, including accurately spaced dosing in daily or twice-daily DOACs, of paramount importance.

The major trials of DOACs excluded patients with significant mitral stenosis, and their use is therefore currently contraindicated in patients with moderate to severe mitral stenosis due to lack of evidence for their efficacy. In addition, a very low number of patients with bioprosthetic valves were included in trials and recommendations suggest the DOACs should be avoided in the first 3 months following bioprosthetic valve replacement, until more data are available.[66]

Mechanism of action: DOACs are direct inhibitors of factor Xa (apixaban, edoxaban, rivaroxaban) or thrombin (dabigatran). They act at a more specific point in the clotting cascade to prevent generation of fibrin and clots. Specific anti-factor Xa assays can be performed in patients at high risk of thrombosis or haemorrhage, for example, people who are at the extremes of weight or who have renal failure.

Adverse effects: as with other anticoagulants, bleeding is the most important side effect of DOACs. Risk of bleeding is generally lower than with warfarin and their shorter duration of action can mean that minor bleeding is more easily controlled. An early concern about the routine use of DOACs was lack of reversibility, although Praxbind, a specific antidote to dabigatran and Ondexxya, an antidote to rivaroxaban and apixaban, are available' At the time of writing, a specific reversal agent for apixaban and rivaroxaban is in development.

Antiplatelet drugs

Platelet activation pathways are important therapeutic targets in the treatment and prevention of cardiovascular disease.

Platelet inhibitors: aspirin and adenosine diphosphate receptor antagonists (P2Y12 inhibitors)

Aspirin is used in the primary and secondary prevention of cardiovascular disease. Adenosine diphosphate (ADP) inhibitors include clopidogrel, prasugrel, and ticagrelor. They are combined with aspirin following MI and/or percutaneous coronary intervention for 1–12 months depending on their original indication, bleeding risk, stent type, and the need for concomitant anticoagulation (➤ **Fig. 12.3**).

Mechanism of action: aspirin irreversibly inhibits cyclooxygenase-1 (COX-1), which results in decreased thromboxane A2 (TA2) synthesis, and a subsequent reduction in platelet activation and aggregation (➤ **Fig. 12.2**). Since platelets cannot produce more TA2, inhibition occurs for the duration of the cell life cycle, which is 7–10 days.

ADP mediates platelet activation and aggregation by binding to the P2Y12 receptor on the platelet surface. Clopidogrel and prasugrel are prodrugs; this means that they need to be metabolized to form an active drug.

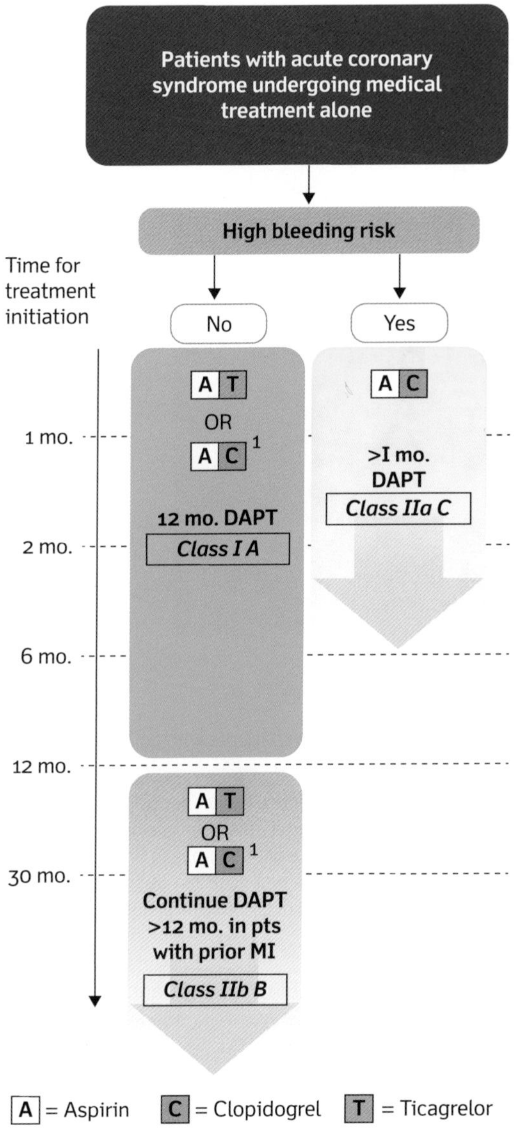

Fig. 12.3 European Society of Cardiology recommendations for duration of antiplatelet agents in acute coronary syndromes.

Valgimigli M, Bueno H, Byrne RA, et al; ESC Scientific Document Group; ESC Committee for Practice Guidelines (CPG); ESC National Cardiac Societies. 2017 ESC focused update on dual antiplatelet therapy in coronary artery disease developed in collaboration with EACTS: The Task Force for dual antiplatelet therapy in coronary artery disease of the European Society of Cardiology (ESC) and of the European Association for Cardio-Thoracic Surgery (EACTS). Eur Heart J. 2018 Jan 14;39(3):213–260. doi: 10.1093/eurheartj/ehx419. © The European Society of Cardiology. Reprinted by permission of Oxford University Press.

Once activated, they bind covalently to P2Y12 receptors, therefore preventing binding of ADP, causing irreversible platelet inhibition.[67] Like with aspirin, platelet activity recovers only when new platelets are generated. Ticagrelor is a reversible inhibitor of ADP, which means platelet function is more rapidly recovered on cessation of therapy, taking approximately 5 days. Ticagrelor is not a prodrug and does not therefore require activation, making it faster acting and more potent than clopidogrel.[68]

Adverse effects: aspirin's dose-related adverse gastrointestinal effects range from minor symptoms (nausea, heartburn, indigestion) to major bleeding.[49] Antisecretory drugs, such as proton pump inhibitors, can be used to reduce the risk of gastrointestinal bleeding. A small proportion of patients suffering with asthma are sensitive to aspirin, which may result in symptoms ranging from urticaria and rhinitis to bronchoconstriction and respiratory compromise.

Of the ADP inhibitors, the bleeding risk is greatest with ticagrelor and prasugrel, owing to their higher potency.[69] Ticagrelor can cause dyspnoea through an adenosine-like reaction[70]; this tends to be harmless and often transient, although it can be an effect that is poorly tolerated.

Interactions: combining antiplatelets with other antiplatelets or anticoagulants has known therapeutic benefits; however, caution is required due to increased bleeding risk. Use with other drugs known to increase the risk of bleeding, such as non-steroidal anti-inflammatory drugs, should be avoided or used with caution. Clopidogrel and ticagrelor are subject to metabolic interactions via cytochrome P450 enzymes. Strong inducers, such as carbamazepine, and strong inhibitors, such as clarithromycin, can decrease or increase the efficacy of ticagrelor, respectively. This effect is thought to be significant enough to warrant a change in therapy. Prasugrel has far fewer clinically relevant interactions.

Dual and triple therapy

In patients with an indication for antiplatelets and an anticoagulant, for example, a patient with atrial fibrillation, or following a mechanical valve replacement who undergo percutaneous coronary intervention, it may be necessary to combine antiplatelet and anticoagulant therapies. The management strategy is individualized, depending on the specific indication, as well as disease severity, past medical history, and bleeding risk (➤ **Fig. 12.4**).

Dual or triple therapy warrants caution due to additive bleeding risk. Compared to anticoagulant therapy alone, the risk of bleeding can increase two- to threefold for patients taking dual antiplatelet therapy with

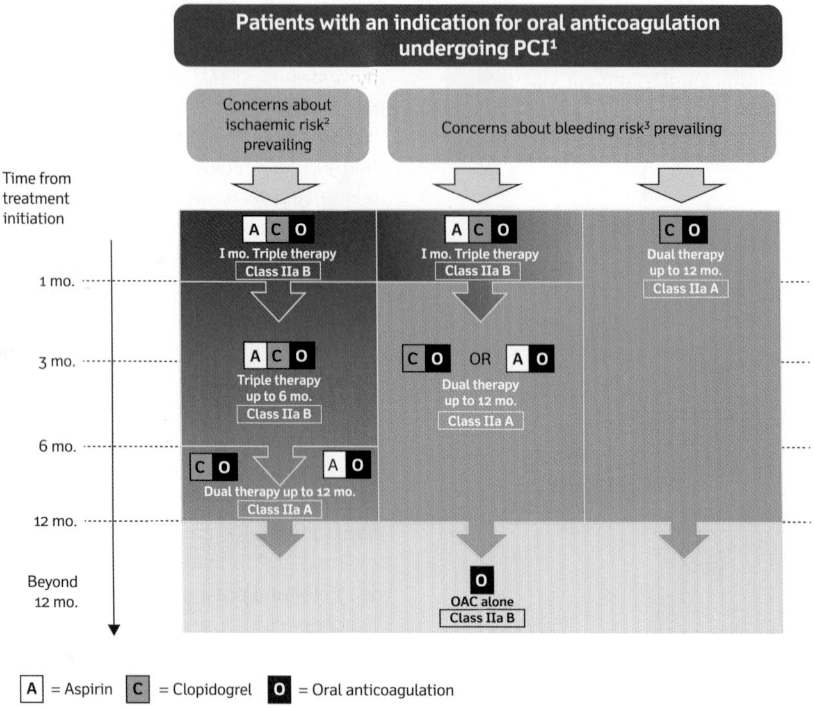

Fig. 12.4 European Society of Cardiology recommendations for antithrombotic strategy in patients with an indication for anticoagulation who undergo percutaneous coronary intervention.

Valgimigli M, Bueno H, Byrne RA, et al; ESC Scientific Document Group; ESC Committee for Practice Guidelines (CPG); ESC National Cardiac Societies. 2017 ESC focused update on dual antiplatelet therapy in coronary artery disease developed in collaboration with EACTS: The Task Force for dual antiplatelet therapy in coronary artery disease of the European Society of Cardiology (ESC) and of the European Association for Cardio-Thoracic Surgery (EACTS). Eur Heart J. 2018 Jan 14;39(3):213–260. doi: 10.1093/eurheartj/ehx419. © The European Society of Cardiology. Reprinted by permission of Oxford University Press.

anticoagulation. Careful management involves close monitoring of INR in patients taking warfarin and consideration of dose reduction of a DOAC where appropriate.

Glycoprotein IIb/IIIa inhibitors

This class of intravenous antiplatelets comprises abciximab, tirofiban, and eptifibatide, which are licensed for use alongside heparin and oral antiplatelets for ST-segment elevation MI and non-ST-segment elevation MI, particularly for patients at risk of a further coronary event who are unable to have percutaneous coronary intervention immediately.

Mechanism of action: glycoprotein IIb/IIIa inhibitors inhibit the binding of pro-aggregatory substances to activated platelets.[71] Because their site of action is near the end of the clotting cascade (➤ Fig. 12.2), they inhibit platelet activation irrespective of the provoking factor.

Adverse effects: combination with antithrombins and oral antiplatelets offers therapeutic benefit; however, the increased bleeding risk warrants caution.[72] Other side effects include hypotension and hypersensitivity, particularly with abciximab which should not be readministered.[72] Dose adjustments may be required in renal impairment.

Dual pathway inhibition (low-dose rivaroxaban plus aspirin)

In patients with stable atherosclerotic cardiovascular disease, adding low-dose rivaroxaban 2.5 mg twice daily to aspirin has been shown to improve cardiovascular outcomes compared with aspirin alone.[73] Its place in therapy is in those with coronary artery disease with additional high-risk factors, such as age greater than 65 years, current smoking, history of diabetes, renal impairment, heart failure, stroke, and/or atherosclerosis in another vascular bed.[73]

Adverse effects: combining low-dose rivaroxaban with aspirin increases the risk of major bleeding into the gastrointestinal tract. An assessment of bleeding risk should be made prior to initiation and dual pathway inhibition should be avoided in patients considered to be high bleeding risk.[73]

Antiarrhythmic drugs

- Vaughan Williams classification.
- Digoxin.

The Vaughan Williams classification broadly categorizes antiarrhythmics into four classes according to mechanism of action; however, there are some clinically useful antiarrhythmics which do not meet these criteria. Examples of antiarrhythmic drugs are summarized in ➤ **Table 12.3** and ➤ **Table 12.4** (see also Chapter 7).

Mechanisms of action

Class I antiarrhythmics block voltage-gated sodium channels and can be further divided into three subcategories: Ia, Ib, and Ic. They have differing mechanisms but share a common characteristic: inhibition of high-frequency myocardial excitation in non-nodal tissue. As such, they suppress tachyarrhythmias caused by abnormal conduction. This effect is achieved through 'use dependent block', that is, the higher the frequency of channel activation, the greater the degree of block.

Class II antiarrhythmics block beta-adrenoceptors. Beta-blockers supress the sympathetic response, increasing the refractory period of the atrioventricular node. As such, they are useful in treating ventricular arrhythmias post-MI, supraventricular tachycardia, and paroxysmal atrial fibrillation.

Class III antiarrhythmics prolong the action potential and refractory period in cardiac cells, primarily through inhibition of potassium channels, although the exact mechanism is not well understood. Amiodarone is usually used when other suitable treatments have failed, owing to its poor side effect profile. Sotalol has both class III and class II activity.

Class IV antiarrhythmics block I type voltage-gated calcium channels to slow conduction in both the sinoatrial and atrioventricular nodes. The main use is to terminate supraventricular tachycardia. They also reduce cardiac contractility and for this reason should not be combined with beta-blockers or quinidine.

Digoxin causes release of acetylcholine, which slows atrioventricular node conduction and reduces ventricular rate. It is used to treat rapid atrial fibrillation and flutter. It requires a loading dose, which can be administered orally or intravenously, depending on severity.

Adverse effects: paradoxically, antiarrhythmics can have a proarrhythmic effect. Specifically, they can increase the duration, frequency, or rate of an existing arrhythmia, or cause a new arrhythmia.[50]

The side effects of beta-blockers can mainly be attributed to reduced heart function and output and include most commonly bradycardia, rhythm disturbance, fatigue, exercise intolerance, malaise, cold extremities, and sexual dysfunction. There are also numerous interactions with other drugs; of particular note are the interactions that occur with other cardiovascular therapies such as calcium channel blockers, clonidine, digitalis, and nifedipine.

Amiodarone has many unpleasant side effects, including altered liver and thyroid function, skin discoloration, photosensitivity, pulmonary toxicity, and corneal deposits.[49] Liver and thyroid function tests, as well as a chest X-ray, are required prior to initiation. It also has many drug interactions which, owing to its long duration of action, may persist for weeks after treatment cessation.

Digoxin has a narrow therapeutic window and is affected by serum potassium, renal function, age, and interacting drugs. Therapeutic drug monitoring is warranted in acute kidney injury, hypokalaemia, and in elderly patients or if an interacting medication is started or stopped. Signs of toxicity include severe bradycardia, diarrhoea, vomiting, dizziness, and visual disturbances.[49] A reversal agent is available for extreme digoxin toxicity.

Table 12.4 Antiarrhythmic drugs not classified in Vaughan Williams classification

Drug	Use
Atropine	Sinus bradycardia
Adrenaline (epinephrine)	Cardiac arrest
Isoprenaline	Heart block
Digoxin	Atrial fibrillation
Adenosine	Supraventricular tachycardia
Calcium chloride	Hyperkalaemia-induced ventricular tachycardia
Magnesium chloride	Ventricular fibrillation

New diabetes drugs with cardiovascular benefits

- Glucagon-like peptide-1 receptor agonists (GLP-1RAs).
- Sodium–glucose co-transporter 2 (SGLT2) inhibitors.

A full description of diabetes management is beyond the scope of this chapter; however, the recent surge in evidence from large randomized controlled trials for cardiovascular benefits of two new classes of oral glucose-lowering agents warrants discussion.

GLP-1RAs and SGLT2 inhibitors confer benefit and should be recommended for patients with type 2 diabetes mellitus who have established cardiovascular disease or high cardiovascular disease risk.[74]

GLP-1RAs (e.g. dulaglutide, liraglutide, and semaglutide) are administered by subcutaneous injection and work by activating GLP-1 receptors to increase insulin secretion, suppress glucagon secretion, and slow gastric emptying. They have been shown in trials to reduce cardiovascular events and there is evidence that liraglutide reduces mortality.[75–78] The cardiovascular benefit is likely due to a reduction in atherosclerotic events. Common side effects include back pain, cystitis, and increased risk of infection.

SGLT2 inhibitors (e.g. empagliflozin, dapagliflozin, and canagliflozin) are administered orally and act by blocking this transporter in the renal proximal convoluted tubule to inhibit glucose reabsorption, thus increasing its excretion in the urine. All have been shown to lower heart failure hospitalizations; furthermore, there is evidence that empagliflozin reduces cardiovascular and overall mortality.[80–82] Common side effects include skin reactions, thirst, urinary disorders, and hypoglycaemia (when combined with insulin or a sulphonylurea). In randomized controlled trials, canagliflozin seemed to have an increased risk in lower limb amputation and fracture.[81]

Drugs used to promote tissue perfusion

Tissue perfusion can be restricted due to the presence of atherosclerotic plaque and/or as a result of hypertension (see Chapter 6). In the treatment and prevention of cardiovascular disease, there are a range of drugs prescribed for patients that enhance perfusion, either locally within the coronary circulation or in the periphery. Four main categories are outlined: nitrates, beta-blockers (beta-adrenergic antagonists), drugs that act on the renin–angiotensin–aldosterone system (RAAS) including ACEIs and angiotensin II receptor blockers (ARBs), and calcium channel blockers.

Nitrates

This class of drugs, mainly used in the prevention of or the acute treatment of angina can also be referred to as organic nitrates, and are peripheral or coronary vasodilators. They are available in several different chemical forms, the most commonly used being glyceryl trinitrate (GTN; nitroglycerine). Many nitrates undergo nearly 100% first-pass metabolism in the liver; this means that, for nitrates, the most common route of administration would be sublingual, transdermal, or intravenous.

Glyceryl trinitrate

Mechanism of action: as mentioned in Chapter 4, nitric oxide is a naturally occurring vasodilator that is present in both arterial and venous vasculature. GTN is converted to nitric oxide in the vascular wall, which triggers reduction of calcium in the smooth muscle, creating a consequential relaxation of the smooth muscles of the blood vessels, leading to vasodilation. This increases blood flow in the coronary vessels to the areas of the heart that generate ischaemic angina discomfort and increases venous dilatation, reducing venous return and, therefore, myocardial workload.

Adverse effects: the adverse effects of GTN arise due to excessive vasodilation within the peripheral circulation. Common adverse effects include flushing, dizziness, migraine-type headaches, and hypotension. Caution is needed when taken with other vasodilators as this may result in significant hypotension, leading to collapse.

Drugs that affect the renin–angiotensin–aldosterone system

Two main drug groups affect the RAAS: ACEIs and ARBs. Either of these can be used in the management of hypertension and coronary artery disease. To understand the mode of action of these drugs, it is useful to briefly explain the RAAS (➤ **Fig. 12.5**).

In the normal non-baroreceptor control of blood pressure, the RAAS is activated by the release of renin from the kidney. The main stimulus for this release is a drop in blood pressure. Renin convents the inactive protein angiotensinogen to angiotensin I. As angiotensin I circulates around the body, particularly to the lungs, it comes into contact with angiotensin I-converting enzyme, produced in the lungs, which converts angiotensin I (ACE) to angiotensin II. Angiotensin II has two main actions: it acts directly on the blood vessels as a potent vasoconstrictor, and it stimulates the release of aldosterone, a hormone that will stimulate the retention

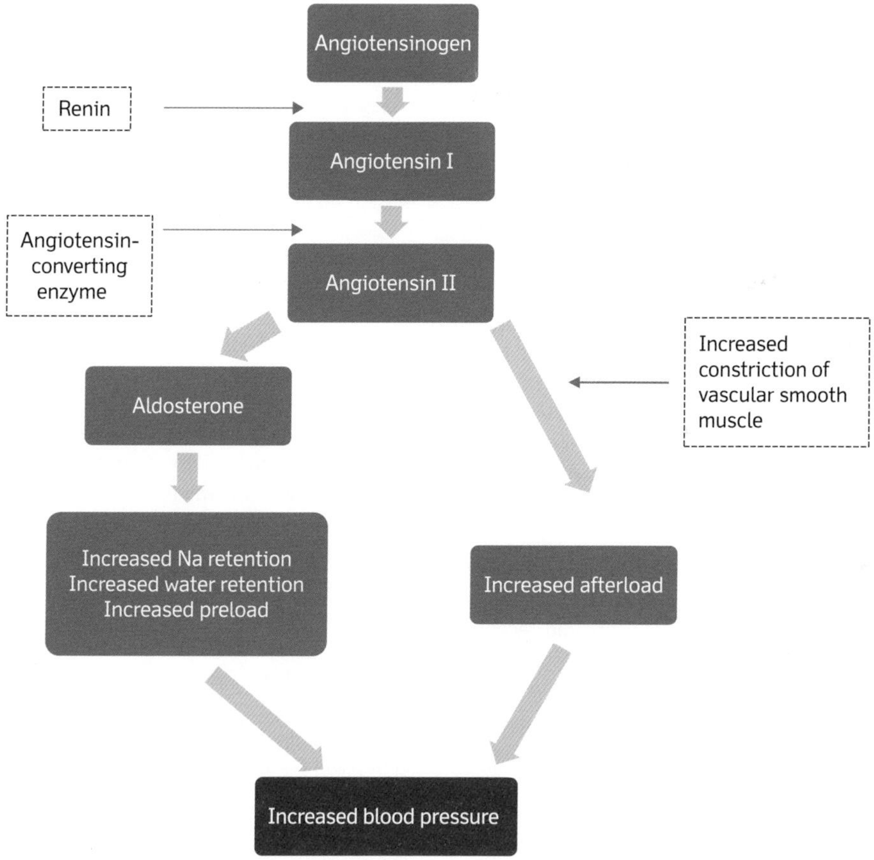

Fig. 12.5 The renin–angiotensin–aldosterone system (RAAS). Na, sodium.

of sodium and consequentially water to increase body fluid volume (➤ **Fig. 12.5**).

Angiotensin-converting enzyme inhibitors

ACEIs are used in the first line of treatment for hypertension and also in heart failure, prevention of stroke, secondary prevention after MI, and in type 1 diabetic nephropathy.

Mechanism of action: ACEIs bind to and inhibit the action of angiotensin-converting enzyme, preventing the production of angiotensin II; in addition, ACEIs prevent the conversion of bradykinin to active metabolites, which has two major effects. First, this action leads to a reduction in vasoconstriction, directly causing a reduction in peripheral resistance and blood pressure. Second, it will reduce sodium retention and consequently blood volume, which proves particularly helpful in the fluid retention associated with heart failure.

Adverse effects: ACEIs are usually well tolerated with transient side effects. As a result of its interference with bradykinin, a cough may develop. The vasodilation that occurs can result in headaches, dizziness, rash, and postural hypotension. Due to aldosterone effects, some patients may develop hyperkalaemia. Serious adverse effects include angioedema and acute kidney injury. For these reasons, the monitoring of serum electrolyte levels and renal function are an important part of initiating, uptitrating, and maintaining therapy.

Angiotensin II receptor blockers

ARBs are also used in the first line of treatment of hypertension, in heart failure, stroke, peripheral vascular disease, and for people with diabetes who have organ failure.

Mechanism of action: ARBs bind to angiotensin II receptors preventing the action of angiotensin II. Its consequences are therefore similar to those of ACEIs in that there is a resultant reduction in vasoconstriction, directly causing a reduction in peripheral resistance and blood pressure, and a reduction in sodium retention, thereby reducing blood volume.

Adverse effects: these are similar to those in ACEIs—headaches, dizziness, postural hypotension, and rash. Due to the aldosterone effects, some patients may develop hyperkalaemia. Serious adverse effects include angioedema, although the incidence is lower than in ACEIs, and acute kidney injury.

Mineralocorticoid receptor antagonists

Mineralocorticoid receptor antagonists, namely spironolactone and eplerenone, are used in the treatment of heart failure with reduced ejection fraction, particularly in patients who continue to have symptoms despite optimal doses of ACEI (or ARB) and beta-blocker. Eplerenone is also licensed in patients who have reduced left ventricular ejection fraction following MI.

Mechanism of action: spironolactone and eplerenone are also termed 'aldosterone antagonists'. They compete with aldosterone to bind to mineralocorticoid receptors, thereby blocking its action.[82] Mineralocorticoid receptor antagonists lower blood pressure by reducing sodium and water reabsorption. Perhaps more importantly, they improve left ventricular function by reducing endothelial dysfunction and collagen overproduction, which contribute to left ventricular remodelling.[83]

Adverse effects: mineralocorticoid receptor antagonists are 'potassium sparing' and can lead to hyperkalaemia. The risk is greater in those with existing renal impairment, diabetes, and those taking other medicines which increase serum potassium. Caution should be exercised in patients with moderate renal impairment, with lower starting doses and more frequent monitoring recommended.

As eplerenone is more selective for mineralocorticoid receptors over other steroid receptors, it is less likely to cause hormone-related side effects such as gynaecomastia, mastodynia, and vaginal bleeding, compared to spironolactone.[82]

Sacubitril–valsartan

Sacubitril–valsartan combines an ARB (valsartan) with a neprilysin inhibitor (sacubitril) for the treatment of heart failure in patients with reduced ejection fraction who remain symptomatic despite optimization of first-line heart failure treatment, such as ACEIs, beta-blockers, and mineralocorticoid receptor antagonists.

Mechanism of action: neprilysin catalyses the degradation of natriuretic peptides, which are responsible for vasodilation, diuresis, and natriuresis, as well as inhibition of renin and aldosterone and improved renal blood flow. Sacubitril inhibits the effect of neprilysin and therefore prolongs the beneficial effect of natriuretic peptides.

Adverse effects: these are similar to ACEIs and ARBs—dizziness, postural hypotension, hyperkalaemia, and renal impairment are often managed with close monitoring and dose adjustment. Again, the incidence of angioedema is lower than with ACEIs.

Beta-blockers (beta-adrenergic antagonists)

Adrenergic antagonists, although now less commonly prescribed than ACEIs or ARBs, continue to be a choice for treatment of hypertension. Beta-blockers are also used in the management of angina, cardiac arrhythmias, in the treatment and prevention of MI, and can also be used in the prevention of migraine.

Mechanism of action: beta-receptors are one of the main types of receptors that are activated by the sympathetic nervous system and are stimulated by adrenaline and noradrenaline. Beta-blockers can be non-selective in that they can block both beta-1 and beta-2 receptors. Beta-1 selective blockers such as atenolol, bisoprolol, metoprolol, and nebivolol are more commonly used as they are better tolerated with fewer people experiencing side effects. Beta-1 receptors are dominant in the heart and the kidney; blocking beta-1 receptors leads to reduced workload of the heart by reducing heart rate and contractility, and consequently cardiac output leading to lower blood pressure. Blocking beta-1 receptors in the kidneys leads to a reduction in renin, resulting in reduction in angiotensin II and thereby causing a reduction in peripheral vasoconstriction and fluid retention, all contributing to reduced blood pressure.

Adverse effects: the side effects were outlined previously, see 'Antiarrhythmic drugs'.

Calcium channel blockers

Calcium channel blockers can be used to treat high blood pressure, angina, and arrhythmias.

Mechanism of action: calcium is an essential element needed in the contraction of all muscle types. Nerve impulses cause the opening of calcium channels in muscle cells to allow calcium to flow into the muscle, causing contraction. There is a wide range of calcium channel blockers that will inhibit this action in cardiac muscle and arterial vessels, which will result in reduced cardiac contractility and vasodilation. Certain types of calcium channel blocker are more effective in the heart than in the blood vessels and vice versa. Dihydropyridine calcium channel blockers such as amlodipine, felodipine, and nifedipine have high vascular selectivity, resulting in systemic vasodilation, reducing blood pressure and also myocardial oxygen demand, which gives rise to their antianginal effect. More cardioselective calcium channel blockers such as verapamil and diltiazem reduce heart rate and therefore myocardial oxygen demand, also making them effective as antianginal agents. These also reduce the firing rate of aberrant pacemaker cells and prolong repolarization, particularly at the atrioventricular node, which makes them useful antiarrhythmic medications.

Adverse effects: adverse effects vary between different types of calcium channel blockers. Common side effects of dihydropyridines include those related to vasodilation such as headache, flushing, rash, and swelling, but malaise and constipation can also occur. The cardioselective calcium channel blockers can cause excessive bradycardia and induce heart blocks and for this reason, are not prescribed alongside other rate-limiting drugs such as beta-blockers. Rare but severe adverse effects with calcium channel blockers include hepatotoxicity, MI, heart failure, hypotension, and some types exhibit hypersensitivity.

Drugs used in emergency and cardiogenic shock

Cardiogenic shock, which involves severely impaired myocardial contractility and circulatory collapse, is the most common cause of mortality in acute MI. The aims of treatment include restoration of adequate blood flow and oxygen delivery to avoid or limit end-organ damage.

A full description of pharmacological management of cardiogenic shock and other emergencies is beyond the scope of this chapter (see also Chapter 5). ➤ Table 12.5 provides a summary of some common emergency medications used in cardiology emergencies. This list is not exhaustive.

How are pharmacodynamics affected by pharmacogenetics and pharmacogenomics?

The influence of genetics on interindividual variability in pharmacodynamics is becoming an increasingly

Table 12.5 Drugs used in emergency and acute care (cardiogenic shock)

Agent	Mechanism	Action
Phenylephrine	Alpha-1 agonist	Vasoconstrictor
Noradrenaline	Alpha (+) and beta (++) agonist	Inotrope Chronotrope Vasoconstrictor
Adrenaline	Alpha (+) and beta (+++) agonist	Inotrope Chronotrope Vasoconstrictor
Dopamine	Alpha, beta, and dopamine agonist (dose dependent)	Inotrope Chronotrope Vasoconstrictor (high doses only)
Dobutamine	Beta agonist	Inotrope Vasodilator (mild)
Vasopressin	Vasopressin-1 agonist	Vasoconstrictor
Milrinone	Phosphodiesterase type 3 inhibitor	Inotrope Vasodilator
Levosimendan	Myocytic calcium sensitizer Potassium channel activator	Inotrope Inodilator

intriguing area. Pharmacogenomics can influence both the degree of response to a medication and the likelihood and severity of side effects. Important drug groups in cardiovascular care include warfarin, clopidogrel, and statins.

Genetic 'resistance' to clopidogrel is seen in approximately 30% of patients,[67] caused by a genetic polymorphism in the gene encoding the enzyme responsible for the conversion of clopidogrel into its active form. This can lead to reduced platelet inhibition and increased risk of cardiovascular events, such as stent thrombosis.

Genetic factors have been demonstrated to have the greatest impact on warfarin dosing variability.[84] A study of 5000 genotyped patients on warfarin showed that patients with genetic polymorphisms which increase sensitivity to warfarin are at higher risk of haemorrhagic events when standard dosing protocols are used.[85] Studies provide conflicting results regarding the clinical application of a pharmacogenetic-guided dosing regimen.[85]

Conclusion

This chapter has reviewed the role of the nurse in adopting pharmacological approaches to the management of cardiovascular disease. It has explored the development of non-medical prescribing and how this might continue to develop, to contribute to the acute and ongoing management of the patient with cardiovascular disease, providing examples of good practice.

In addition, the chapter has addressed the ongoing concern relating to medication adherence in cardiovascular diseases, further exploring the role of the nurse and other health professionals in addressing concerns about medication and the potential for contribution to improving patient adherence to medication regimens.

Resources

Edmunds M. Introduction to Clinical Pharmacology (8th ed). Philadelphia, PA: Elsevier; 2016.

Katzung B. Basic & Clinical Pharmacology (14th ed). New York: McGraw-Hill; 2018.

McGavock H. How Drugs Work: Basic Pharmacology for Health Care Professionals (4th ed). London: Taylor & Francis; 2015.

Ritter J, Flower R, Henderson G, Loke YK, MacEwan D, Rang H. Rang & Dale's Pharmacology (9th ed). Philadelphia, PA: Elsevier; 2020.

For prescribing: British National Formulary. Available from: https://bnf.nice.org.uk/.

References

1. Kotseva K, De Backer G, De Bacquer D, Rydén L, Hoes A, Grobbee D, et al. Lifestyle and impact on cardiovascular risk factor control in coronary patients across 27 countries: results from the European Society of Cardiology ESC-EORP EUROASPIRE V registry. Eur J Prev Cardiol. 2019;26(8):824–35.
2. Bosworth HB, Granger BB, Mendys P, Brindis R, Burkholder R, Czajkowski SM, et al. Medication adherence: a call for action. Am Heart J. 2011;162(3):412–24.
3. Fong J, Buckley T, Cashin A. Nurse practitioner prescribing: an international perspective. Nurs Res Rev. 2015;5:99–108.
4. Latter S, Blenkinsopp A, Smith A, Chapman S, Tinelli M, Gerard K, et al. Evaluation of nurse and pharmacist independent prescribing. Department of Health Policy Research Programme Project 016 0108. University of Southampton; 2010. https://eprints.soton.ac.uk/184777/2/ENPIPexecsummary.pdf.
5. Courtenay M, Berry D. Comparing nurses' and doctors' views of nurse prescribing: a questionnaire survey. Nurs Prescib. 2007;5:205–10.
6. Courtenay M, Carey N, Stenner K, Lawton S, Peters J. Patients' views of nurse prescribing: effects on care, concordance and medicine taking. Br J Dermatol. 2011;164(2):396–401.
7. Cope LC, Abuzour AS, Tully MP. Nonmedical prescribing: where are we now? Ther Adv Drug Saf. 2016;7(4):165–72.
8. Kroezen M, van Dijk L, Groenewegen PP, Francke AL. Nurse prescribing of medicines in Western European and Anglo-Saxon countries: a systematic review of the literature. BMC Health Serv Res. 2011;11:127.
9. Tonna A, Stewart D, McCaig D. An international overview of some pharmacist prescribing models. J Malta Coll Pharm Pract. 2008(14):20–26.
10. Dickinson D, Wilkie P, Harris M. Taking medicines: concordance is not compliance. BMJ. 1999;319(7212):787.
11. Sabate E. Adherence to Long-Term Therapies: Evidence for Action. Geneva: World Health Organization; 2003.
12. Sackett DL, Haynes RB. Compliance with Therapeutic Regimens. Baltimore, MD: Johns Hopkins University Press; 1976.
13. Vrijens B, De Geest S, Hughes DA, Przemyslaw K, Demonceau J, Ruppar T, et al. A new taxonomy for describing and defining adherence to medications. Br J Clin Pharmacol. 2012;73(5):691–705.
14. Ho PM, Bryson CL, Rumsfeld JS. Medication adherence: its importance in cardiovascular outcomes. Circulation. 2009;119(23):3028–35.
15. Navar AM, Roe MT, White JA, Cannon CP, Lokhnygina Y, Newby LK, et al. Medication discontinuation in the IMPROVE-IT trial. Circ Cardiovasc Qual Outcomes. 2019;12(1):e005041.

16. Bansilal S, Castellano JM, Garrido E, Wei HG, Freeman A, Spettell C, et al. Assessing the impact of medication adherence on long-term cardiovascular outcomes. J Am Coll Cardiol. 2016;68(8):789–801.
17. Kim S, Shin DW, Yun JM, Hwang Y, Park SK, Ko YJ, et al. Medication adherence and the risk of cardiovascular mortality and hospitalization among patients with newly prescribed antihypertensive medications. Hypertension. 2016;67(3):506–12.
18. Osterberg L, Blaschke T. Adherence to medication. N Engl J Med. 2005;353(5):487–97.
19. Mongkhon P, Ashcroft DM, Scholfield CN, Kongkaew C. Hospital admissions associated with medication non-adherence: a systematic review of prospective observational studies. BMJ Qual Saf. 2018;27(11):902–14.
20. Khan R, Socha-Dietrich K. Investing in Medication Adherence Improves Health Outcomes and Health System Efficiency. Paris: Organization for Economic Cooperation and Development; 2018.
21. Iuga AO, McGuire MJ. Adherence and health care costs. Risk Manag Healthc Policy. 2014;7:35–44.
22. Cutler RL, Fernandez-Llimos F, Frommer M, Benrimoj C, Garcia-Cardenas V. Economic impact of medication non-adherence by disease groups: a systematic review. BMJ Open. 2018;8(1):e016982.
23. National Institute for Health and Care Excellence. Medicines Adherence: Involving Patients in Decisions about Prescribed Medicines and Supporting Adherence. Clinical guideline (CG76). London: National Institute for Health and Care Excellence; 2009.
24. Johnston N, Weinman J, Ashworth L, Smethurst P, El Khoury J, Moloney C. Systematic reviews: causes of non-adherence to P2Y12 inhibitors in acute coronary syndromes and response to intervention. Open Heart. 2016;3(2):e000479.
25. Chen H, Saczynsky J, Lapane K, Kiefe CI, Goldberg RJ. Adherence to evidence-based secondary prevention pharmacotherapy in patients after an acute coronary syndrome: a systematic review. Heart Lung. 2015;44(4):299–308.
26. Crawshaw J, Auyeung V, Norton S, Weinman J. Identifying psychosocial predictors of medication non-adherence following acute coronary syndrome: a systematic review and meta-analysis. J Psychosom Res. 2016;90:10–32.
27. Rashid MA, Edwards D, Walter FM, Mant J. Medication taking in coronary artery disease: a systematic review and qualitative synthesis. Ann Fam Med. 2014;12(3):224–32.
28. Horne R, Weinman J, Hankins M. The beliefs about medicines questionnaire: the development and evaluation of a new method for assessing the cognitive representation of medication. Psychol Health. 1999;14(1):1–24.
29. Faridi KF, Peterson ED, McCoy LA, Thomas L, Enriquez J, Wang TY. Timing of first postdischarge follow-up and medication adherence after acute myocardial infarction. JAMA Cardiol. 2016;1(2):147–55.
30. Keenan J. Improving adherence to medication for secondary cardiovascular disease prevention. Eur J Prev Cardiol. 2017;24(3 Suppl):29–35.
31. Khatib R, Marshall K, Silcock J, Forrest C, Hall AS. Adherence to coronary artery disease secondary prevention medicines: exploring modifiable barriers. Open Heart. 2019;6(2):e000997.
32. Khatib R, Patel N, Laverty U, Mcgawley G, McLenachan J, Shield S, Hall AS. Re-engineering the post-myocardial infarction medicines optimisation pathway: a retrospective analysis of a joint consultant pharmacist and cardiologist clinic model. Open Heart. 2018;5(2):e000921.
33. National Institute for Health and Care Excellence. Medicines Optimisation: The Safe and Effective Use of Medicines to Enable the Best Possible Outcomes. NICE guideline (NG5). London: National Institute for Health and Care Excellence; 2015.
34. Aggarwal B, Liao M, Mosca L. Medication adherence is associated with having a caregiver among cardiac patients. Ann Behav Med. 2013;46(2):237–42.
35. Khatib R, Patel N, Hall AS. The my experience of taking medicines (MYMEDS) questionnaire for assessing medicines adherence barriers in post-myocardial infarction patients: development and utility. BMC Cardiovasc Disord. 2020;20(1):46.
36. Kardas P, Lewek P, Matyjaszczyk M. Determinants of patient adherence: a review of systematic reviews. Front Pharmacol. 2013;4(91):91.
37. Jarab AS, Alefishat EA, Bani Nasur R, Mukattash TL. Investigation of variables associated with medication nonadherence in patients with hypertension. J Pharm Health Serv Res. 2018;9(4):341–46.
38. Morrison VL, Holmes EA, Parveen S, Plumpton CO, Clyne W, De Geest S, et al. Predictors of self-reported adherence to antihypertensive medicines: a multinational, cross-sectional survey. Value Health. 2015;18(2):206–16.
39. Conn VS, Ruppar TM, Chan KC, Dunbar-Jacob J, Pepper GA, De Geest S. Packaging interventions to increase medication adherence: systematic review and meta-analysis. Curr Med Res Opin. 2015;31(1): 145–60.
40. Conn VS, Ruppar TM. Medication adherence outcomes of 771 intervention trials: systematic review and meta-analysis. Prev Med. 2017;99:269–76.
41. Kini V, Ho PM. Interventions to improve medication adherence: a review. JAMA. 2018;320(23):2461–73.
42. Palacio A, Garay D, Langer B, Taylor J, Wood BA, Tamariz L. Motivational interviewing improves medication

adherence: a systematic review and meta-analysis. J Gen Intern Med. 2016;31(8):929–40.

43. Russell CL, Hathaway D, Remy LM, Aholt D, Clark D, Miller C, et al. Improving medication adherence and outcomes in adult kidney transplant patients using a personal systems approach: SystemCHANGE™ results of the MAGIC randomized clinical trial. Am J Transplant. 2020;20(1):125–36.
44. Russell CL, Ruppar TM, Matteson M. Improving medication adherence: moving from intention and motivation to a personal systems approach. Nurs Clin North Am. 2011;46(3):271–81.
45. Mach F, Baigent C, Capatano AL, Koskinas KC, Casula M, Badimon L, et al. ECS/EAS Guidelines for the management of dyslipidaemias: lipid modification to reduce cardiovascular risk. Eur Heart J. 2020;41(1):111–88.
46. National Institute for Health and Care Excellence. Cardiovascular Disease: Risk Assessment and Reduction, Including Lipid Modification. Clinical guideline (CG181). London: National Institute for Health and Care Excellence; 2014.
47. Knopp RH. Drug treatment of lipid disorders. N Engl J Med. 1999;341(7):498–511.
48. Ferrières J. Effects on coronary atherosclerosis by targeting low-density lipoprotein cholesterol with statins. Am J Cardiovasc Drugs. 2009;9(2):109–15.
49. Joint Formulary Committee. British National Formulary (77th ed). London: BMJ Group and Pharmaceutical Press; 2019.
50. Rosenson RS, Baker SK, Jacobson TA, Kopecky SL, Parker BA, The National Lipid Association's Muscle Safety Expert Panel. An assessment by the statin muscle safety task force: 2014 update. J Clin Lipidol. 2014;8(3 Suppl):S58–71.
51. Chapman MJ, Redfern JS, McGovern ME, Giral P. Niacin and fibrates in atherogenic dyslipidaemia: pharmacotherapy to reduce cardiovascular risk. Pharmacol Ther. 2010;126(3):314–45.
52. AIM-HIGH Investigators, Boden WE, Probstfield JL, Anderson T, Chaitman BR, Desvignes-Nickens P, et al. Niacin in patients with low HDL cholesterol levels receiving intensive statin therapy. N Engl J Med. 2011;365(24):2255–67.
53. HPS2-THRIVE Collaborative Group, Landray MJ, Haynes R, Hopewell JC, Parish S, Aung T, et al. Effects of extended-release niacin with laropiprant in high-risk patients. N Engl J Med. 2014;371(3):203–12.
54. Cannon CP, Blazing MA, Giugliano RP, McCagg A, White JA, Theroux P, et al. Ezetimibe added to statin therapy after acute coronary syndromes. N Engl J Med. 2015;372(25):2387–97.
55. Van Heek M, Davis H. Pharmacology of ezetimibe. Eur Heart J Suppl. 2002;4:J5–8.
56. Bruckert E, Giral P, Tellier P. Perspectives in cholesterol-lowering therapy: the role of ezetimibe, a new selective inhibitor of intestinal cholesterol absorption. Circulation. 2003;107(25):3124–28.
57. Phan BAP, Dayspring TD, Toth PP. Ezetimibe therapy: mechanism of action and clinical update. Vasc Health Risk Manag. 2012;8:415–27.
58. Cannon CP, Cariou B, Blom D, McKenney JM, Lorenzato C, Pordy R, et al. Efficacy and safety of alirocumab in high cardiovascular risk patients with inadequately controlled hypercholesterolaemia on maximally tolerated doses of statins: the Odyssey COMBO II randomized controlled trial. Eur Heart J. 2015;36(19):1186–94.
59. Stroes E, Colquhoun D, Sullivan D, Civeira F, Rosenson RS, Watts GF, et al. Anti-PCSK9 antibody effectively lowers cholesterol in patients with statin intolerance: the GAUSS-2 randomized, placebo-controlled phase 3 clinical trial of evolocumab. J Am Coll Cardiol. 2014;63(23):2541–48.
60. Sabatine MS, Giugliano RP, Keech AC, Honarpour N, Wiviott SD, Murphy SA, et al. Evolocumab and clinical outcomes in patients with cardiovascular disease. N Engl J Med. 2017;376(18):1713–22.
61. Schwartz GG, Steg PG, Szarek M, Bhatt DL, Bittner VA, Diaz R, et al. Alirocumab and cardiovascular outcomes after acute coronary syndrome. N Engl J Med. 2018;379(22):2097–107.
62. Lagace TA. PCSK9 and LDLR degradation: regulatory mechanisms in circulation and in cells. Curr Opin Lipidol. 2014;25(5):387–93.
63. Kosmas CE, Muñoz Estrella AM, Sourlas A, Silverio D, Hilario E, Montan P, Guzman E. Inclisiran: a new promising agent in the management of hypercholesterolemia. Diseases. 2018;6(3):63.
64. Inclisiran for subjects with ASCVD and elevated low-density lipoprotein cholesterol—ORION-10. Presented by R. Scott Wright at the American Heart Association annual scientific sessions (AHA 2019). Philadelphia, PA; 16 November, 2019.
65. ESC Congress News. Substantial LDL-C reductions with the siRNA, inclisiran: results from ORION-11. 2019. https://www.escardio.org/Congresses-&-Events/ESC-Congress/Congress-resources/Congress-news/substantial-ldlc-reductions-with-the-sirna-inclisiran-results-from-orion11.
66. Jan Steffel et al, EP Europace. 2021 European Heart Rhythm Association Practical Guide on the Use of Non-Vitamin K Antagonist Oral Anticoagulants in Patients with Atrial Fibrillation.
67. Kalantzi KI, Tsoumani ME, Goudevenos IA, Tselepis AD. Pharmacodynamic properties of antiplatelet agents: current knowledge and future perspectives. Expert Rev Clin Pharmacol. 2012;5(3):319–36.

68. Gurbel PA, Bliden KP, Butler K, Tantry US, Gesheff T, Wei C, et al. Randomized double-blind assessment of the ONSET and OFFSET of the antiplatelet effects of ticagrelor versus clopidogrel in patients with stable coronary artery disease: the ONSET/OFFSET study. Circulation. 2009;120(25):2577–85.
69. Wiviott SD, Braunwald E, McCabe CH, Montalescot G, Ruzyllo W, Gottlieb S, et al. Prasugrel versus clopidogrel in patients with acute coronary syndromes. N Engl J Med. 2007;357(20):2001–15.
70. Cattaneo M, Schulz R, Nylander S. Adenosine-mediated effects of ticagrelor: evidence and potential clinical relevance. J Am Coll Cardiol. 2014;63(23):2503–509.
71. Stangl PA, Lewis S. Review of currently available GP IIb/IIIa inhibitors and their role in peripheral vascular interventions. Semin Intervent Radiol. 2010;27(4):412–21.
72. Lily. ReoPro 2-mg/ml solution for injection or infusion: summary of product characteristics. Electron Medicines Compendium. https://www.medicines.org.uk/emc/product/11021/smpc#gref.
73. Eikelboom JW, Connolly SJ, Bosch J, Dagenais GR, Hart RG, Shestakovska O, et al. Rivaroxaban with or without aspirin in patients with stable cardiovascular disease. N Engl J Med. 2017;377(14):1319–30.
74. Cosentino F, Grant PJ, Aboyans V, Bailey CJ, Ceriello A, Delgado V, et al. 2019 ESC guidelines on diabetes, pre-diabetes, and cardiovascular diseases developed in collaboration with the EASD. Eur Heart J. 2020;41(2):255–323.
75. Zinman B, Nauck MA, Bosch-Traberg H, Frimer-Larsen H, Ørsted DD, Buse JB, et al. Liraglutide and glycaemic outcomes in the LEADER trial. Diabetes Ther. 2018;9(6):2383–92.
76. Marso SP, Bain SC, Consoli A, Eliaschewitz FG, Jódar E, Leiter LA, et al. Semaglutide and cardiovascular outcomes in patients with type 2 diabetes. N Engl J Med. 2016;375(19):1834–44.
77. Husain M, Birkenfeld AL, Donsmark M, Dungan K, Eliaschewitz FG, Franco DR, et al. Oral semaglutide and cardiovascular outcomes in patients with type 2 diabetes. N Engl J Med. 2019;381(9):841–51.
78. Gerstein HC, Colhoun HM, Dagenais GR, Diaz R, Lakshmanan M, Pais P, et al. Dulaglutide and cardiovascular outcomes in type 2 diabetes (REWIND): a double-blind, randomised placebo-controlled trial. Lancet. 2019;394(10193):121–30.
79. Zinman B, Inzucchi SE, Lachin JM, Wanner C, Ferrari R, Fitchett D, et al. Rationale, design, and baseline characteristics of a randomized, placebo-controlled cardiovascular outcome trial of empagliflozin (EMPA-REG OUTCOME). Cardiovasc Diabetol. 2014;13:102.
80. Wiviott SD, Raz I, Bonaca MP, Mosenzon O, Kato ET, Cahn A, et al. Dapagliflozin and cardiovascular outcomes in type 2 diabetes. N Engl J Med. 2019;380(4):347–57.
81. Neal B, Perkovic V, Mahaffey KW, de Zeeuw D, Fulcher G, Erondu N, et al. Canagliflozin and cardiovascular and renal events in type 2 diabetes. N Engl J Med. 2017;377(7):644–57.
82. Brown NJ. Eplerenone: cardiovascular protection. Circulation. 2003;107(19):2512–18.
83. Fraccarollo D, Galuppo P, Hildemann S, Christ M, Ertl G, Bauersachs J. Additive improvement of left ventricular remodeling and neurohormonal activation by aldosterone receptor blockade with eplerenone and ACE inhibition in rats with myocardial infarction. J Am Coll Cardiol. 2003;42(9):1666–73.
84. Weeke P, Roden DM. Pharmacogenomics and cardiovascular disease. Curr Cardiol Rep. 2013;15(7):376.
85. Mega JL, Walker JR, Ruff CT, Vandell AG, Nordio F, Deenadayalu N, et al. Genetics and the clinical response to warfarin and edoxaban: findings from the randomised, double-blind ENGAGE AF-TIMI 48 trial. Lancet. 2015;385(9984):2280–87.

Section 3: Professional considerations for nurses working in cardiovascular care

13 Patient education and communication

FELICITY ASTIN, EMMA HARRIS, LIS NEUBECK, ROBYN GALLAGHER, AND JENNIFER JONES

CHAPTER CONTENTS

KEY MESSAGES

- Nurses and allied health professionals play a key role in communicating and educating patients and informal carers.
- Comprehensive therapeutic patient education requires planning, delivery, evaluation, and documentation.
- Informal carers should be involved in all aspects of therapeutic education.
- Communication skills training for health professionals can improve patient satisfaction with care.
- Therapeutic education is more likely to be effective if best practice communication and teaching skills are applied in clinical practice which includes a learning needs assessment.
- Single sessions of therapeutic education are less effective than multiple sessions with follow-up.
- Problematic health literacy is a major obstacle to therapeutic patient education.
- Universal health literacy precautions should be implemented to reduce health inequalities.
- Effective therapeutic patient education has the potential to reduce unnecessary health resource use by patients and adverse events.

Introduction

A vital part of the health professional's role is to communicate with patients, and those close to them, in a way that can promote physical and mental health, patient safety, and well-being. Education and communication are important, but rather neglected, aspects of the health professional's role. Education and communication are interrelated; education refers to a process in which knowledge and skills are shared. Communication refers to ways in which information is given, received, or exchanged using spoken and written words as well as body language. Therapeutic patient education goes one step further and is defined as an approach designed to improve patient outcomes in which education is seen as a therapy that is part of overall treatment.[1,2] Successful therapeutic patient education requires a rebalance of the health professional–patient 'power' dynamic to enable the patient to take greater responsibility for their health and well-being, working with the multidisciplinary health and social care team. The aim of therapeutic education is to help patients, and those close to them, to develop competencies to effectively self-manage their health to optimize their quantity and quality of life.[1,2]

This chapter will begin with making a case for the more consistent application of educational theory to underpin educational interventions developed for cardiovascular patients. The section that follows will describe therapeutic patient education and emphasize the importance of involving those close to the patient in educational interventions. We will recap on the principles and practices of effective communication for health professionals and review the characteristics of effective patient education. The next sections of the chapter focus upon the importance of health literacy as a potential barrier to effective therapeutic patient education with concluding comments. The chapter includes case studies to showcase the health education needs of cardiac patients diagnosed with common cardiovascular conditions.

Educational theory and principles of adult learning

All members of the multidisciplinary health and social care team play a role in the education of patients with cardiovascular disease, and those close to them. Effective health education has the potential to improve health outcomes, well-being, and quality of life. There are many stages in the patient journey where effective patient education can improve patient outcomes. The point at which patients are discharged home from hospital is especially important. Hospital readmission within 30 days of discharge is not uncommon among cardiac patients and often for avoidable reasons. Health professionals play an important educational role in the discharge process.

Interestingly the role of 'teacher' is one that health professionals do not always have the opportunity to fully prepare for, or reflect upon. Surprisingly few educational interventions delivered in cardiovascular care settings make any reference to the principles of educational theory. In this context, we refer to theories as simply a set of general rules that can be used to guide the development of an educational intervention. For the purpose of this brief introduction, two key educational theories, or approaches, have been selected for health professionals to integrate into their programme of therapeutic patient and informal carer education.[3]

We will begin with a 'constructivist' approach to teaching. In simple terms this teaching approach recognizes that the adult learner is not a 'blank canvas', but rather a person who will actively decide how, and when, to modify their existing knowledge. Health professionals who use a 'constructivist' teaching approach see their role as a learning 'facilitator', rather than an expert 'informer' who transmits their knowledge to the learner. They involve the patient and informal carer by evaluating their prior knowledge and understanding to identify potential inconsistencies. Participatory teaching and learning techniques are used, such as problem-based learning with time allocated to reflect upon new learning and experiences. In this way, 'new' knowledge is constructed. ➤ **Fig. 13.1** illustrates the difference between a learner/informal carer-centred versus a health professional-centred approach to teaching and learning.

More often than not, health professionals have used the more dated health professional-centred learning approach. Complete the learning activity in ➤ **Box 13.1** to identify your approach to patient education and your perception of the role of 'teacher'.

Experiential learning theory is the second approach we will introduce which focuses upon the process of learning and identifies four steps that occur in a cyclical or spiral sequence:

1. Concrete experience, which refers to 'doing', that is, an event or encounter that has happened to a person in their daily life (e.g. a senior nurse in a coronary care unit instigates a programme of study leave to encourage colleagues to attend an international conference to develop awareness of latest research evidence).

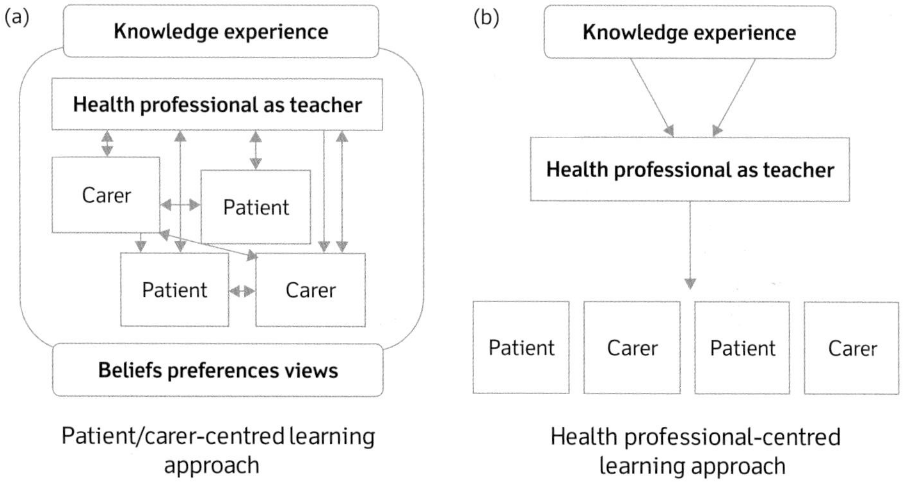

Fig. 13.1 Diagram to compare patient/informal care centred versus health professional-centred education.

2. Reflective observation, a natural 'thinking' process that takes place after a new experience (e.g. the senior nurse thinks about how the colleagues responded differently to this opportunity, develops ideas about why there were differences, and evaluates the impact of them attending the conference).
3. Development of abstract concepts, a 'channelling' process in which new ideas and observations that have evolved from reflecting on the new experience are used as personal feedback that informs future experiences (e.g. the senior nurse talks to other senior colleagues to see if they have had a similar experience with staff attending conferences to understand more generally how different colleagues respond).
4. Testing concepts in a new situation, this step requires the learner to apply the new knowledge to a different situation (e.g. the senior nurse offers a study leave opportunity to allied health professionals to see if there are similar effects on clinical practice).

Box 13.1 What teaching approach do you use?

- Think about a recent discussion with a patient or colleague, in which you were either sharing knowledge or teaching a skill. Write a brief description of what happened.
- Read through your description and note how you felt and what you thought during the interaction.
- Evaluate the overall experience and note what went well and less well.
- Did you use a patient/carer-centred learning approach? Think about why you used the approach that you did.
- What have you learned about your teaching approach and could you have done it differently?
- Would you change anything in a similar situation? If yes, what actions would you consider?

Experiential learning approaches such as apprenticeship, mentorship, and clinical supervision are used in many forms of health professional education. The principles also apply to patient and informal carer education. Many common cardiovascular conditions such as coronary heart disease and heart failure have no cure. Therefore, supporting a patient to develop the necessary knowledge, skills, and confidence to self-manage their own health and care, on a daily basis, is an important approach to maximize patient health and well-being. It is important that health professionals use effective techniques to support patients, and those close to them, to self-manage their lifestyle and adhere to prescribed medications. Interventions designed to optimize health-related quality of life are a priority. For this reason, it is recommended that health professionals draw upon educational theories to inform patient education in clinical practice. The therapeutic value of health education can be realized by assessing patients' learning needs and using a range of teaching and learning approaches to match the health literacy levels of patients and informal carers. Ideas about educational theories and approaches help us to understand the principles of effective teaching.

Involving informal carers in therapeutic patient education

People typically belong to social units and communities. Therefore, there should be an emphasis on how to involve 'informal carers' (defined as family friends or neighbours who provide instrumental or emotional support that is unpaid) anywhere and anytime that healthcare is given.[4] Informal carers can contribute to all aspects of healthcare and also provide emotional and practical support to patients during times of illness. The active involvement of informal carers is pivotal to realizing better health outcomes, both in the individual patient but also in those close to them.[5] The family comprises one of the most immediate contexts of care and family involvement in care can be critical in health outcomes, including the impact on the patient's well-being.[6]

The growing population of older adults living with chronic conditions means that family members play an increasingly essential role in reducing the burden on healthcare systems. The care they provide contributes substantially to tangible benefits, including reduced hospital stay and hospital admissions. Consequently, it is vital for nurses to work in partnership with patients, and those closest to them; the latter are integral members of the healthcare team. It is also important that nurses are aware that informal caregivers often lack support and tend to experience poorer physical and mental health outcomes compared to those without caring responsibilities. Nurses play a vital role in supporting informal carers in maintaining their health and well-being. Finding effective ways to support informal caregivers to provide care to their loved ones is becoming increasingly important as a core part of nurse education, curricula, and practice standards. Regardless of speciality, the proactive involvement of informal carers in promoting health and well-being through prevention or in acute, chronic, or end of life care settings translates into multiple benefits.

High-quality communication is a pivotal part of nursing. How well the nurse communicates with those closest to the patient has a significant impact on not only the individual patient's well-being and outcome but also the quality of the patient and family experience.[2] Providing a good patient experience requires health professionals to work effectively with patients and informal care givers. Communication and relationships are key to the individual nurse–family partnership and important to the provision of coordinated care that extends beyond settings, practitioners, and time.[4]

Health education is more effective when delivered using a family/group-orientated approach, whether this be educating a household to manage a life-limiting condition or supporting a family in wellness and the prevention of cardiovascular disease. Family households, and particularly couples, often share the same lifestyle and risk factors.[7] While a positive family history is an independent risk factor, incidence of cardiovascular disease in families is also a result of the aggregation of major risk factors, for example, raised blood pressure, raised cholesterol, and diabetes, resulting from a shared lifestyle. Consequently, cardiovascular risk is often elevated and partners (spouses) and first-degree relatives of patients with atherosclerotic disease are at a higher risk of developing cardiovascular disease than the general population. For health professionals to deliver optimal care, it is vital to engage patients and their families/informal carers as partners. Informal caregivers are integral members of the healthcare team, contributing substantially to the effective implementation of patient care. There are many health benefits for patients, and those close to them, that can be gained by including them in education-based interventions.[6]

Principles and practices of effective communication

What is effective therapeutic communication?

Effective communication between health professionals, patients, and those close to them is necessary to establish positive and collaborative partnerships which form the foundation of patient-centred care.[8,9] Therapeutic communication occurs as a two-way, interpersonal, interaction in which information, thoughts, and feelings are exchanged and expressed both verbally and non-verbally.[10] Therapeutic communication is central to all aspects of healthcare, such as explanations about diagnoses, shared decision-making about potential treatment options, and the provision of psychological and self-management support, to name a few.[10] Effective communication has a powerful potential influence on patients' physical and psychological health and well-being through multiple mechanisms, including improved access to care, timely and accurate diagnosis and treatment, promoting patients to feel valued, reduction in anxiety levels, and feeling more motivated to self-manage their health and adhere to recommended treatments.[11]

Informal caregivers play an important role in the patient recovery process. Patients' accounts of their recovery experiences provide us with invaluable learning. Mr Brian Boyle, an intensive care unit survivor, described the importance of having his family nearby; 'Having my parents there with me in the hospital meant everything to me. Growing up, they were my role models, my friends, my supporters—and in the hospital, my guardian angels' (p. 5).[12] ➤ Box 13.2 shows Mr Boyle's communication tips for health professionals.

Effective communication between health professionals, patients, and informal care givers is:

- Patient driven: the patient's health and well-being are the main purpose of the interaction. Information should be tailored to each individual.
- Understandable: spoken language should be clear, accurate, and concise. Patients can misinterpret information when medical terminology and complex words are used.
- A reciprocal process: the interaction requires engagement by both parties; it is not a one-way exchange of information. Patients and informal caregivers receive and understand verbal, and non-verbal, information given by healthcare professionals. This prompts a response or reaction by the patient, which allows the health professional to know how well the information was received and understood. The health professional responds appropriately to correct misunderstandings, emphasize key messages, and/or provide further information.[10]
- Supportive and caring: empathic communication helps to build trust and effective relationships with patients. Patients are more engaged with interactions when they feel valued and listened to.

Verbal and non-verbal communication techniques

Verbal communication is the use of spoken language to exchange information during interactions between people. Verbal communication has three important components. First, the literal content of the message including the type of words and sentence structure used. Second, the voice used to convey the message. Third, the non-verbal communication. Health professionals often tend to focus upon the content of a health message. However, the other aspects of communication are equally as important. The vocal aspect of communication is often overlooked (e.g. the volume, tone, pitch, rate, pausing, word emphasis, and use of 'fillers' such as 'OK' and 'um'). Both the content of the message and the characteristics of the voice used to communicate it can influence how well the content is understood. For example, long sentences that are packed with medical jargon, communicated quickly, using a loud voice, can be difficult for a patient to understand.

Non-verbal communication such as body language, eye contact, and facial expressions are important cues that

Box 13.2 Top tips on communication: a patient perspective

Mr Boyle identifies recommendations for health professionals on best practice communication with informal caregivers:

- Identify one person in the social network who will relay information to others.
- Consider using digital approaches, for example, create a website to share information regarding the patient with family and friends (e.g. https://www.caringbridge.org/).
- Recap on key information about hospital procedures, for example, visiting hours, and key contacts and their phone numbers.
- Think about what you are saying but also how you say it.
- Try and use a gentle tone of voice and use the patient's and informal carer's names.
- Try to develop a rapport that will help to promote trust.
- Reflect upon the type of communication that will best match the informal care giver's needs.
- Try to manage expectations so that they are realistic.
- Taking the time to listen is important even if you cannot answer all of their questions.

'Similar to a mechanical system of interlocked gears, the communication between the patient, family, and health care providers is very important throughout the entire recovery process' (p. 5)

Source data from Boyle, Brian (2015). The critical role of family in patient experience. Patient Experience Journal: 2(2), Article 2. Available at: https://pxjournal.org/journal/vol2/iss2/2.

accompany verbal communication and convey thoughts and feelings. Research on non-verbal communication conducted in the 1960s identified that non-verbal communication was more important in the communication process than previously recognized; findings showed that when an inconsistent or mixed message was communicated to a person, they evaluated the message by evaluating non-verbal factors such as voice tone and body language.[13] A communication model developed from this research suggested that in this context, 55% of communication consisted of body language, 38% through the use of one's voice, with only 7% consisting of the literal content of the message. Several techniques can be used to support positive verbal and non-verbal communication which build positive collaborative relationships that are central to patient-centred care.[14]

Active listening

Active listening requires a high degree of concentration to ensure that the health professional focuses completely on the information being communicated by a patient coupled with an appropriate response.[15] If you are already thinking about what you are going to say in response to the dialogue with your patient, then you are probably not actively listening. To actively listen, healthcare professionals must try to minimize any distraction and focus on the patient rather than on their own agenda. It is also important to pay attention to the patients' body language, as well as the types of words they are using to convey their views.

Three approaches that demonstrate active listening are the use of non-verbal cues, verbal prompts, and exploratory questioning techniques. First, non-verbal cues, such as eye contact, head nodding, raising eyebrows, and other facial expressions, are powerful physical demonstrations that can communicate active listening to patients and informal carers. Second, verbal prompts can be used to encourage the patient to continue with their explanations.[10] For example, 'Please tell me more about …' Third, a follow-on question, such as 'Why do you think you are feeling this way?' can be used to help to interpret and clarify patients' 'messages'. ➤ **Table 13.1** shows some examples of verbal and non-verbal communication techniques that can be used in clinical practice.

Demonstrating empathy

Showing empathy is a core skill for all healthcare professionals. Empathy is a way of expressing understanding of a patient's experience and concerns.[15] Showing empathy as part of healthcare helps patients to feel valued, reassured, and comforted. Non-verbal gestures may include sympathetic head nodding, appropriate facial expressions, and leaning forwards.[15] Touching or holding a patient's hand is a powerful emotive gesture, but should only be used in appropriate situations. Empathy can be explicitly conveyed by using specific phrases such as 'I'm very sorry to hear that', 'That must have been difficult for you', and 'I'd like to see you again to find out how you're getting on'.

Table 13.1 Verbal and non-verbal communication techniques

Verbal	Non-verbal
1. Use open-ended questions: 'Can you tell me more about how you're feeling?' √ 'Have you been feeling breathless?' ×	1. Don't interrupt ×
	2. Maintain eye contact to show attentiveness √
	3. Head nodding where appropriate √
2. Summarize what the patient has said: 'In summary, you have told me so far …'√	4. Avoid crossing arms/legs ×
	5. Turn towards the patient √
3. Repeat important information √	6. Avoid completing other tasks such as updating medical records, while the patient is talking ×
4. Avoid complex medical words and abbreviations: 'Your ICD may be deactivated at end of life' ×	7. Use appropriate facial expressions, e.g. concerned frowning, smiling √
5. Speak at a moderate pace: Speaking too fast makes it difficult to understand and retain information ×	8. Use touch when appropriate √ 9. Use silent pauses to encourage patient responses and allow thinking time √
6. Avoid judgemental or confronting language and don't raise the level of your voice People who smoke deserve to get sick ×	
7. Use a tone of voice (i.e. assertive, comforting, persuasive) to match the message √	

Using plain language

Healthcare professionals routinely assess the communication needs of their patients as part of a comprehensive health assessment process. Plain language should be used in all types of communication to help ensure that information is accessible for all patients. Patients and informal carers are more likely to understand the health information you communicate to them the first time they read or hear it if plain language is used. It is important that health-related messages are concise, use simple language, and avoid complex medical terminology and abbreviations. Patients who are not fluent in the language being used should be offered the services of a professional interpreter; this service may be financially costly but the use of professional interpreters reduces adverse events, improves patient outcomes, and increases patient satisfaction.[16] Every effort should be made to avoid using relatives and friends as interpreters as this can cause distress and may compromise the accuracy of the information being conveyed.

Teach-back using 'chunk and check'

It is estimated that between 40% and 80% of health-related information communicated to patients during a consultation is immediately forgotten.[17] Patients may also have difficulty in understanding the information communicated to them. There are many factors that can influence patient comprehension and recall including age, gender, educational level, emotional status, the volume of information presented, perceived importance of the information, and the way that the information is delivered.

Teach-back is an effective communication technique used to evaluate the effectiveness of an educational session; patients are asked to recount the key messages they have learned back to their 'teacher'.[18] The emphasis is upon the skill of the health professional as an educator rather than testing the patient. Teach-back helps to establish whether healthcare professionals have communicated clearly and asks the patient to explain the information in their own words. Teach-back can be applied to any health-related information or skills teaching from diagnosis, prognosis, and shared decision-making about treatment options through to discharge advice and self-management support. Dividing information into shorter sections (chunks) helps patients' understanding. Incorporating the teach-back and 'chunk and check' techniques into clinical practice is an effective way for healthcare professionals to assess patients' comprehension.

The steps involved are shown in ➤ **Fig. 13.2**. Essentially, the technique involves dividing information into shorter

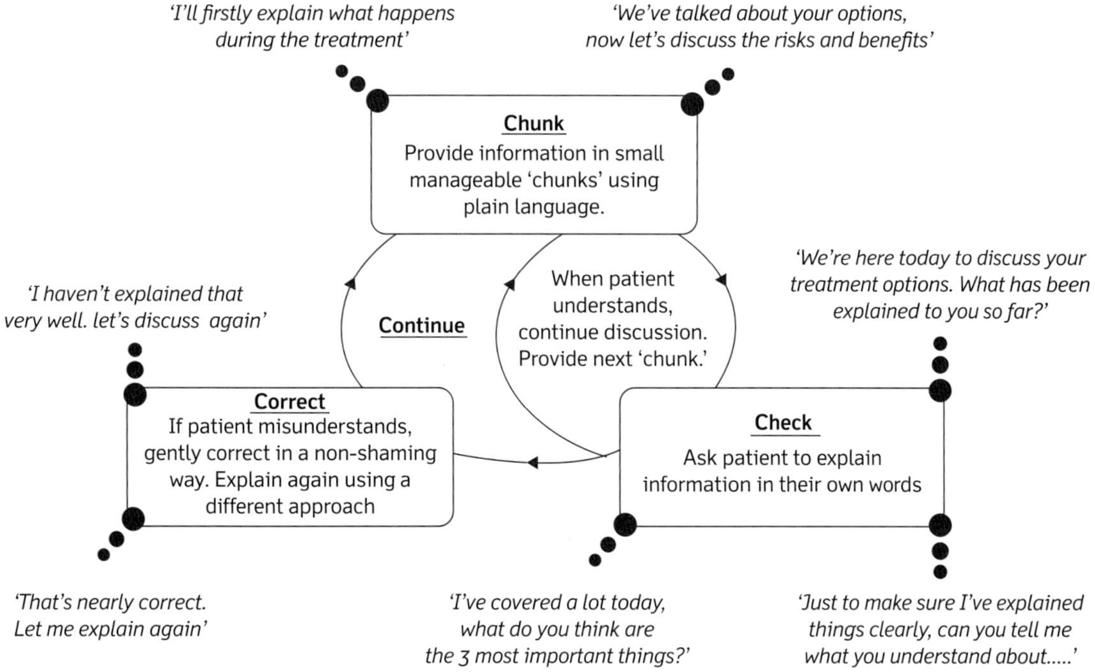

Fig. 13.2 Diagram of Teach-Back technique.

sections (chunks) and getting the patient to 'teach-back' to you, in their own words, after each 'chunk'. In this way, you can check that your teaching has been effective in helping the patients to understand the health information you presented.

This approach can also be applied to skills teaching such as using a glyceryl trinitrate spray (e.g. Nitrolingual® Pumpspray). If the patient is unable to provide an adequate explanation, the healthcare professional can communicate the information again in a different way. The cycle is repeated once or twice until it is clear the patient has understood the health information. This also has a positive effect on patient outcomes. When used correctly, teach-back can result in improved patient self-efficacy (the belief in oneself that a given task can be completed), knowledge of health condition and self-management, as well as reduced hospitalization and readmissions.[18]

In summary, effective communication between health professionals, patients, and informal caregivers is an important skill that contributes to overall care quality and is central to high-quality patient education.

Which patient education strategies are effective?

Systematic reviews bring together primary research to help us to identify which teaching and learning approaches are most likely to be effective in therapeutic patient education for patients with cardiovascular disease and cancer. From this evidence, we can identify some general themes that can be implemented to maximize the positive effects of therapeutic patient education for patients with cardiovascular disease and their informal caregivers.

Top tips in providing quality patient education

Planning patient education

When an educational intervention is planned, it is very important that the health professional considers the educational outcomes and focus upon 'teaching to goal', that is, being very clear about the educational outcomes you wish to achieve which may be changes in knowledge, skills, or behaviours. The learning objectives agreed with the patient should be realistic and match the amount of patient contact time available. Some flexibility is required as depending on the context of care as there may be just a few minutes of patient contact time available or longer. Educational interventions that focus upon skills development to enhance communication, self-care, and problem-solving are known to be more effective in enabling lifestyle change and improving clinical outcomes, compared to interventions that focus upon the provision of information alone.[19] It is important to build in time to assess the patient's learning needs and preferred learning style. This aligns with the constructionist learning theory described at the beginning of the chapter.

The teaching session may start by asking the patient about what they already know about their health condition to establish what their learning needs are. This will also provide an opportunity to correct any misunderstandings. To stimulate patient interest, it is essential to help them to understand why the educational session is important to them. One way to achieve this is to ask about any specific concerns they have about their health.

Asking a patient about whether they learn best by reading or watching a video (please replace 'DVD' with 'video' as I do not think people use DVDs anymore!) will give you information that can be used to tailor educational resources to a preferred learning style. This will also give some indication of the patient's health literacy level (see 'Health literacy as a barrier to effective therapeutic patient education' for more detail). A mismatch between the health literacy level of the patient and the educational resources being used is a major barrier to effective therapeutic patient education. Physical or cognitive impairments can also impact the ability to learn. For example, if a patient is hearing impaired, using visual resources may be more effective than verbal instruction alone. Other factors such as fatigue, distress, anxiety, and depression can blunt the ability of patients to process and retain health-related information. By combining the information gathered in the initial assessment, patient education can be individualized to specific learning needs which is more effective compared to a more generic 'one-size-fits-all' approach.

Teaching tips

The teaching approaches you use will depend upon the amount of patient contact time available but there are some important principles that you can consider.

Single educational sessions are less likely to be effective compared to programmes with scheduled follow-up.[19] To address this challenge, you may integrate different modes of educational delivery to supplement face-to-face education. For example, self-management support for patients with cardiovascular disease can be provided using telehealth approaches such as telephoning, video conferencing, and telemonitoring.[20]

Verbal teaching and discussion are two of the most frequently used teaching strategies, but are the least effective approaches unless used in conjunction with other teaching methods.[21] Think creatively about the educational approaches you use and consider using a combination of audiotapes, videotapes, written materials, and lectures.[21] Some other approaches you may wish to try are the use of posters or charts, checklists, video or DVDs, podcasts, models or props, group sessions, or trained peer educators.

The use of computers as part of a patient education strategy has also been shown to be effective.[21] Digital solutions offer several advantages as potential barriers to patient education can be addressed. Educational content can be needs based and provided in advance of consultations. This frees up health professional time to focus upon discussion of the educational content, rather than on delivery. Educational content can be referred to as many times as desired to boost patient comprehension and recall. The user can also tailor their learning making it individualized and learner centred. The use of multimedia can accommodate different learning styles and health literacy levels as well as promoting patient engagement. High-quality verbal and visual information can be provided at the patient's bedside using videos delivered via a tablet or television. Where possible, encourage patients and informal carers to demonstrate the practical skills you are teaching, such as the use of glyceryl trinitrate spray. Demonstration is proven to be one of the most effective teaching techniques.

Patients frequently need to make important decisions about their care which requires them to choose between different treatment options. As part of making an informed decision, patients need to have comprehensive information about their treatment options provided to them in a way that they understand to help them make choices. This is an important aspect of patient education as, to be fully informed, patients need to be supported to understand the risks and benefits of each treatment option, what alternative treatments are available, and what would happen if they decided to refuse treatment. Research about this process in patients treated with coronary angioplasty has shown that there is room for improvement; patients often underestimate the risks and overestimate the benefits believing that the treatment has 'fixed' their coronary heart disease.[22]

Patient decision aids are effective educational tools that help people to make informed decisions about their healthcare that match their personal preferences and personal values. Patient decision aids help to support a shared decision-making process between patients, those close to them, and health professionals. There are a range of high-quality tools available that can complement the discussions that take place between a patient and health professional about treatment options (https://decisionaid.ohri.ca/implement.html). Digital resources can be used to support shared decision-making and provide another example of the potential benefit of using technology in the context of patient education.

The integration of a patient decision aids into the patient pathway can lead to several improvements in patients' understanding and recall of health information. Patients tend to be more involved in the overall decision-making process and are better informed, clearer about their values and preferences, and have a more realistic understanding of treatment risks.[23] See ➤ **Box 13.3** for some other examples of other digital approaches that can be used to support patients with cardiovascular disease.[24,25]

As well as using digital aids to enhance patient education, it is also important to spend some time refining your communication skills and techniques (see 'Principles and practices of effective communication') to maximize the effectiveness of your therapeutic patient education.

When designing written resources, it is important to ensure that materials are of a suitable reading age for the general population and that the content is culturally appropriate and available in different languages.[21] Ensure that any written information resources are reviewed by the target patient group to improve the accessibility of the information.

Your educational interventions are much more likely to be effective if you involve those people close to the patients who may be either family or friends (see 'Involving informal caregivers in therapeutic patient education').

To ensure there is continuity in the provision of patient education it is important to document the details of your teaching in the patient records. Key aspects to document include a brief description of the goal of the teaching session, any barriers to learning, a list of the resources you supplied or 'sign-posted' the patient to and techniques you used to evaluate what the patients had learnt, for example, Teach-back (see 'Teach-back using 'chunk and check'). Documenting this information will enhance the continuity of care for your patients and enable other members of the multidisciplinary team to build upon the educational sessions you have delivered.

Finally, an important part of patient education is to regularly evaluate your teaching. As a health professional, you will be familiar with the process of self-reflection in which you evaluate your performance. This can be readily applied to your role as a 'teacher' (see 'Educational theory and principles of adult learning'). It is also helpful to ask patients and those close to them to give you informal feedback about what they liked about the educational session and what could be improved. Other potential evaluation questions

Box 13.3 Examples of the use of digital technology to enhance cardiovascular care

Digital interventions to improve adherence to lipid-lowering medication

What did the systematic review show?

Lowering elevated lipid levels reduces the risk of cardiovascular events. Only about one in four patients take this medicine as prescribed. As part of this review, 35 studies, with over 925,000 adult participants prescribed lipid-lowering therapy, were evaluated.[24] The authors concluded that there was high-quality evidence to support 'intensified care' interventions that led to better medication adherence rates in the short (≤6 months) and long (≥6 months) term, when compared to usual care. Moreover, the changes in medication adherence rates led to measurable improvements in total cholesterol levels in the intervention group.

Which interventions worked in the 'intensification' interventions?

The types of interventions that were most effective, compared to usual care, were telephone reminders, calendar reminders, integrated multidisciplinary educational activities, and pharmacist-led interventions. Effective educational interventions used a variety of approaches including educative text messages, videotapes, information booklets, freephone patient helplines, websites, tailored medication labels, personalized letters, and phone calls.

Take-home message

A combination of strategies including information, reminders, adherence reinforcement techniques, and an understanding of the patient perspective are likely to improve adherence to lipid-lowering medications.

Mobile phone text messaging and app-based interventions for smoking cessation

What did the systematic review show?

Tobacco smoking is an addiction that causes avoidable premature death. Not everybody attempting to quit wants face-to-face support. Mobile phone-based smoking cessation support (mCessation) is an alternative. As part of this review, 26 studies, with over 33,000 adult participants, attempting to quit tobacco smoking were evaluated.[25] The authors concluded that there was moderate-quality evidence that automated text message-based smoking cessation interventions resulted in quit rates 50–60% greater than minimal smoking cessation support. The evidence to support smartphone apps was of low certainty and more research is required.

Which interventions worked?

The text message interventions varied in duration and ran from 1 week to 6 months. Some text messages were individualized and/or contained interactive components while others were not. The frequency of text messaging varied across studies from 1 to 35 texts per week. Additional analysis indicated that the intensity of the intervention did not influence abstinence rates.

Take-home message

Text messages are an effective addition and increase quit rates when added to minimal smoking cessation support interventions.

may focus upon your communication techniques, content and organization of the subject matter, and appropriateness of learning objectives/teaching goals. Feedback can be used to inform a cycle of continuous improvement.

Health literacy as a barrier to effective therapeutic patient education

Health professionals communicate with a diverse range of people in their day-to-day work. Some people may not have had the opportunity to experience ongoing education. This will influence how well they can understand verbal communication and written information. This means that they may have difficulties in understanding medication prescriptions, food labels, and health information leaflets. Tailoring health information to an individual's health literacy level helps to make it accessible to everyone.

The concept of health literacy first appeared in academic literature in 1974, but the more modern interpretation did not appear until the 1990s. Several definitions of health literacy exist; the European Health Literacy Study Consortium integrated 17 health literacy definitions to produce the comprehensive version shown here[26]:

> **"Health literacy is linked to literacy and entails people's knowledge, motivation and competences to *access*, *understand*, *appraise*, and *apply* health information in order to make judgments and take decisions in everyday life concerning healthcare,**

disease prevention and health promotion to maintain or improve quality of life during the life course". (p. 3)

In simple terms, health literacy is the ability to read and understand health information and successfully use it to undertake activities that are beneficial to one's health. Health literacy can be categorized into three levels: functional, interactive, and critical, as described in ➤ Table 13.2.[27]

Prevalence and impact of inadequate health literacy

In adults, an inadequate level of health literacy refers to those with a US/international sixth grade reading level or lower, which equates to the reading level of an average 11–12-year-old child. A survey of 7795 people from the general population of eight European countries showed that 47.6% of the sample had a limited (i.e. inadequate or problematic) health literacy level.[28] Other studies focusing on patients with cardiovascular disease have reported that 30–40% of heart failure and coronary artery disease patients have low health literacy levels respectively.[29,30]

To put this into context, about half of the patients you see in practice are likely to have a below-average level of functional health literacy. As a result, many patients will have difficulties with a variety of health-related activities and tasks. Patients with low levels of health literacy are more likely to be older (>65 years), non-white, or have a lower socioeconomic status, income, or level of education.[28,30] In cardiovascular patients, low health literacy is independently associated with increased healthcare use.[31]

It is important to provide support for patients with low health literacy levels as these patients are more likely to experience poorer health outcomes. For example, in patients with chronic cardiac conditions, low health literacy levels are associated with poorer self-care, quality of life, cardiac knowledge, and adherence to medications and increased hospitalization.[29,30] Therefore, differences in health literacy levels are powerful determinants that can widen existing health inequalities.[32] Improving health literacy and ensuring that health services are accessible for everyone is advocated by the World Health Organization and included within country-specific health policies.[32]

As a healthcare professional, there are two key things to think about with regard to health literacy:

1. Identifying patients with low health literacy levels.
2. Ensuring communication is accessible to all patients (see ' Which patient education strategies are effective?').

It can be challenging to identify patients who have low levels of health literacy in the busy environment of a

Table 13.2 Levels of health literacy

Classification	Description	Example
Functional health literacy	Attained basic literacy and numeracy skills required to access and understand relevant health information related to one's self. Able to relate to the communication of information about health risks and health services	A 55-year-old man receives information about referral to cardiac rehabilitation following acute myocardial infarction. After reading the information he decides to attend the programme
Interactive health literacy	Attained a level of functional health literacy plus additional personal skills that enable oneself to respond to health information from different sources. Involves motivational skills and self-confidence	As above plus: during cardiac rehabilitation, the patient asks questions relevant to his own health and lifestyle. He follows the advice given and sets lifestyle change goals to self-manage his health condition
Critical health literacy	Attained advanced cognitive and social skills that lead to personal and community empowerment. Involves critically analysing information and using initiative to respond to changes in personal, social, and economic circumstances	As above plus: the patient knows that he will need further support to help him maintain a healthier lifestyle. To do this he thinks about what will help him. He joins a heart support group. The patient understands the barriers that prevents people like him from attending cardiac rehabilitation. He initiates a walking group at his local community general practice

hospital or clinic. Many patients will feel embarrassed by their level of ability and will try to hide this from others. Although factors such as older age and ethnicity are associated with low health literacy, these are generalizations and do not apply to every individual. Therefore, it is important not to make judgements about health literacy levels based on a patient's appearance or demographics alone. However, there are several signs that may indicate that a patient has a limited level of health literacy[33]:

- Patient uses excuses when asked to read written text. For example, 'I've forgotten my glasses'.
- Forms (e.g. consent forms) are filled out incompletely or inaccurately.
- Appointments are often missed or referral appointments not booked.
- Health and lifestyle advice are not followed.
- Poor medication adherence or patient identifies tablets from their appearance and does not refer to their name.
- Lack of engagement during consultations with few questions asked.

Another way of assessing patients' health literacy levels is by using specific validated screening tools. A variety of different instruments have been used to assess the health literacy of patients with cardiovascular disease and several are available in different languages.[34] Among the most commonly used are the short version of the Test of Functional Health Literacy in Adults (s-TOFHLA), Rapid Estimate of Adult Literacy in Medicine (REALM), and the Three-item Brief Health Literacy Screen (3-item BHLS).[34] The characteristics of each instrument are provided in ➤ Table 13.3.

However, in routine clinical practice it may not be feasible to administer these instruments. Studies have shown that asking patients a simple screening question can effectively identify those with low levels of health literacy[33] such as 'How confident are you filling out medical forms by yourself?' (responses range from '5', extremely, to '1', not at all).

Free toolkits are available that have been designed to support healthcare professionals to implement health literacy universal precautions in practice (e.g. from the Agency for Healthcare Research and Quality (https://www.ahrq.gov/health-literacy/improve/precautions/index.html) and the Health Literacy Centre for Europe (http://healthliteracycentre.eu/)). By adopting health literacy universal precautions, health professionals can work towards ensuring that all health-related communication for patients is simplified. Using this universal approach means that health literacy screening is no longer necessary and the risk of miscommunication reduced. Adapting all aspects of health communication to reflect health literacy universal precautions is an effective way to improve care quality and the health outcomes of your patients and informal carers.

Table 13.3 Comparison of commonly used health literacy screening instruments in patients with cardiovascular disease

Instrument	Number of items	Advantages and disadvantages
s-TOFHLA	36 items	+ Objective measure of functional health literacy + Completed by the patient, therefore less likely to cause embarrassment – Time-consuming to complete (15 minutes) – Requires a level of writing ability and visual acuity – Not specific to cardiovascular disease
REALM	66 words	+ Objective measure of functional health literacy + Quick to complete (<3 minutes) – Administered by a clinician – Requires a level of writing ability and visual acuity – Not specific to cardiovascular disease
3-item BHLS	3 questions	+ Quick to complete (1–2 minutes) + Feasible for use in clinical settings + Not performance based so less likely to cause the patient embarrassment – Administered by a clinician – Subjective measure of confidence in health-related tasks – Difficult to equate to a specific health literacy level – Not specific to cardiovascular disease

Health educational needs of patients with cardiovascular disease

Cardiovascular disease once diagnosed is a lifelong condition that is primarily managed by the patient. The effectiveness of current treatment guidelines depends on the patient being appropriately informed and engaged in their treatment plan. The aim of patient education for all cardiac patients is to improve health outcomes, avoid complications, and implement long-term secondary prevention behaviours. However, in an era of short hospital stays, therapeutic patient education must be targeted, effective, and efficient with a seamless transition to post-discharge education and support.

Cardiac patients need sufficient information about their disease process, tests, and treatments so that they understand how their treatments work and can recognize any side effects or complications and seek medical help when required. Patients also need to know about follow-up appointments, medication dosage and frequency, how to manage symptoms including anxiety and depression, and how best to implement lifestyle behaviours such as physical activity and dietary changes.[20] Health information needs will vary according to the specific cardiac condition and patient circumstances. For instance, heart failure patients often manage multiple symptoms and the stress of having a chronic condition as well as complex medication regimens in the context of a declining disease trajectory, whereas patients diagnosed with acute coronary syndrome often have treatments including percutaneous coronary intervention (PCI) or coronary artery bypass graft surgery. These interventions aim to improve coronary blood flow but have quite different recovery trajectories.

Education of the patient living with heart failure

After hospitalization for an acute heart failure event, patients require substantial support, even when they are considered to be fit for discharge. Transition to home marks a period of time where patients move from having the continuous support of healthcare professionals to being their own primary caregiver.[35] During this time, patients remain at high risk for rehospitalization and death. In fact, the risk of mortality is greater in the immediate discharge phase for up to 3 months, than it was during the inpatient stay. Therefore, every patient who is discharged from hospital should have a personalized discharge and patient education plan, which emphasizes the need for follow-up appointments with their healthcare professionals.[36]

A multidisciplinary approach is essential, and where possible the pharmacist and heart failure nurse should be included. The pharmacist is needed because the majority of people living with heart failure have comorbid disease, for example, one-third of heart failure patients have diabetes, and one-quarter have atrial fibrillation, making medication regimens complex.[37] The pharmacist and heart failure nurse can work effectively to provide tailored patient education concerning self-care and medication management to ensure a smooth transition to specialist services at home. Patients are likely to have complex ongoing learning needs. This emphasizes the importance of working within a multidisciplinary team in liaison with either heart failure management, or cardiac rehabilitation programmes, to ensure that individual patient needs are met. Eligible patients who are able to access comprehensive heart failure management programmes, which include an exercise component, demonstrate clinical improvements in health-related quality of life and a reduced risk of hospitalization.[38] The evidence for the benefit of programmes for patients diagnosed with heart failure with preserved ejection fraction are less clear due to a lack of studies.

As heart failure is both progressive and lifelong, the information provided to patients needs to focus on the long-term management of the condition. Individualized management focuses on maximizing physical capacity, preventing disease progression, and reducing likelihood of relapse.[36] In particular, psychosocial needs are highlighted by patients as being the most pressing concerns they have. In order to achieve these goals, regular consultations will be necessary to assess symptoms, make adjustments to medication, and determine whether a patient would require further treatment.

The patient education plan may need to include topics about potential ongoing treatments and therapies such as the need for the implantation of cardiac resynchronization therapy devices, left ventricular assist devices, or consideration of heart transplantation where warranted. As described in earlier sections, the principles of effective communication and patient education should be fully integrated into care; understanding an individual's health literacy level and their cognitive status will help to tailor the individualized patient education strategy. Importantly, patient education should be individualized to the patient, taking into account their clinical and personal circumstances, and ensuring that the patient's wishes and preferences are discussed.[39]

Self-management in heart failure is essential (see Chapter 10). Self-care education and support should commence during the hospital admission and continue after discharge. Because patients do not live in isolation, it is essential to include family members and informal caregivers in self-care education to ensure retention of health-related information.[40] People living with heart failure need both clinical and psychosocial support, but effective support for self-management is crucial to ensure that heart failure symptoms are minimized.

Assessing patients' learning needs and any obstacles to patient education such as low health literacy or cognitive impairment should be considered in the development of the educational plan. The educational content should include sessions on dietary restrictions, information on key symptoms that flag deterioration, as well as medicines management. It is important to help patients and informal caregivers to develop the knowledge and skills to monitor key signs and symptoms including weight, oedema, and shortness of breath. Support is needed to develop an action plan about how to seek help when signs of clinical deterioration occur. As the ability to self-manage is linked to life circumstances, social support, and individual levels of motivation, the patient education plan should discuss these elements. It may be necessary to make lifestyle changes in order to maintain health. For example, exercise has been shown to improve quality of life, reduce hospitalizations, and decrease mortality in people with heart failure. However, adopting exercise may be difficult for somebody who has previously been inactive.

Developing a therapeutic relationship with patients and their families assists the patient education process. When patients are partners with healthcare providers in their treatment and long-term management plans, there is improved likelihood of effective self-management.[41] As previously discussed, didactic models of education are less likely to engage the individuals and support effective self-care behaviour. Techniques of motivational interviewing can also be useful to improve patient engagement and self-management (see Chapter 11).

See ➤ **Table 13.4** for a case study in heart failure.

Table 13.4 Case study 2: heart failure

Mrs Maria Verdi is a 76-year-old female, admitted with heart failure. She lives with her daughter, having emigrated from her home country 10 years ago and has some difficulty with the local language. She has had type 2 diabetes diagnosed 7 years ago. She does not drink alcohol, but does have the occasional cigarette. Her body mass index is 31. On this admission, her electrocardiogram showed atrial fibrillation and she was started on an oral anticoagulant. She also takes aspirin, metformin, bisoprolol, ramipril, and atorvastatin. She lives in a house with stairs which she seldom leaves. She is being discharged from hospital today and you need to provide her with discharge advice. (Strategies described throughout this chapter would be applied in this case study, such as a learning needs assessment and identification of potential preferences for, and obstacles to, learning, e.g. low health literacy level and cognitive impairments)

Essential topics in patient education	Nursing action
Definition and aetiology of heart failure	Provide Mrs Verdi with information she can understand about her health condition. To be effective, verbal instruction should be reinforced with 'easy to read' written information. Cognitive impairment is common in patients with heart failure and recall is likely to be affected. Comprehensive health information can be accessed from national heart foundations, e.g. British Heart Foundation (https://www.bhf.org.uk/). Mrs Verdi may need information translated in to her first language. Having a family member present is important and Mrs Verdi's daughter can play an important role in helping her mother to understand the health information. However, family members should not be routinely used as translators, as they may not wish to pass on difficult information and professional interpreters should be used
Signs and symptoms of heart failure	Mrs Verdi needs to be able to recognize when her condition is deteriorating. She should demonstrate how she will record her daily weight and demonstrate her understanding about the significance of weight gain as a symptom of clinical deterioration. Mrs Verdi will need to know how and when to notify her healthcare provider; you can work together to develop a written action plan. In discussion with Mrs Verdi, it may also be appropriate to initiate a flexible diuretic therapy programme
Pharmacological treatment	Mrs Verdi is on multiple medications and has commenced a new medication during this hospital admission. Using teach-back (see 'Teach-back using 'chunk and check'') will help you to evaluate how effective your teaching has been in helping Mrs Verdi to understand the dose, mode of action, and common side effects of her prescribed medications. It is also important that she understands when to take any 'as-needed' medicines and what to do when she is unwell. In particular, it is important to discuss over-the-counter drugs with Mrs Verdi to ensure that she knows not to take anti-inflammatory drugs, which may increase the risk of bleeding. If available, bilingual staff can provide support or a professional interpreter. Consultation time needs to be allocated to facilitate the necessary time for teach-back and questions

(continued)

Table 13.4 Continued

Risk factor modification	Although Mrs Verdi reports smoking tobacco only occasionally, it is important to recommend that she stops. Her smoking status should be discussed including her readiness to quit and sources of support she might consider. Mrs Verdi should be having her blood pressure checked regularly. She may be able to do this at home, through a telemetry monitoring programme and at regular visits with the heart failure nurse and her home physician. Check Mrs Verdi's understanding of her diabetes and ensure that she can explain and demonstrate how to monitor and manage her diabetes. Mrs Verdi is obese and weight reduction should be considered using a sensitive approach
Dietary recommendations	Sodium restriction may be prescribed by Mrs Verdi's cardiologist, if so, then she needs to be given 'easy-to-read' information on reducing sodium intake. Clear and specific instructions need to be given to Mrs Verdi concerning the avoidance of excessive fluid intake; however, fluid restriction is not usually necessary. Loss of appetite could be of concern and unintentional weight loss can be a predictor of morbidity and mortality. However, Mrs Verdi may benefit from a referral to a dietician to discuss how to manage her diabetes and concurrently lose weight to improve her overall health
Exercise recommendations	Regular physical activity is important to improve the symptoms of heart failure. Lack of confidence is common in people diagnosed with heart failure and tailored individual advice is important. Specific instructions and a written action plan are recommended. Participation in cardiac rehabilitation where available will help Mrs Verdi to improve her confidence to exercise through experiential learning and peer support
Sexual activity	Although Mrs Verdi does not mention having a current partner, it is still important to offer her the opportunity to discuss sexual activity
Immunization	Mrs Verdi needs to be advised about the need to have annual vaccinations against infections such as influenza and pneumococcal disease and signposted to where she can access services
Sleep and breathing disorders	Mrs Verdi may prefer to sleep more upright. It is important for her to understand that weight loss, and smoking cessation, may improve her breathing, sleep quantity, and quality
Adherence	Non-adherence to medications is common in people diagnosed with heart failure. Ensure that Mrs Verdi understands the key details about her medications; the importance of taking these regularly and for life; and an action plan for strategies she can use to support concordance, such as the use of a dosette/medication organizer. As mentioned earlier, it is important to assess Mrs Verdi's cognitive state as even mild cognitive impairment can affect adherence
Psychosocial aspects	Depressive symptoms are common in patients diagnosed with heart failure and all patients should be screened for depression and referred on for additional support if required. It is important to understand how well Mrs Verdi copes at home while respecting her own goals, values, and preferences
Prognosis	Mrs Verdi needs to understand the lifelong nature of heart failure, the likelihood of deterioration, and the need for further interventions or palliation. It is important to initiate sensitive discussions about Mrs Verdi's prognosis and establish how much she wants to be told. In this way, the amount of information provided will match her preference. Ideally, care should be planned in advance to support her preferences around end of life care

For additional information, please refer to Chapters 10–12.

Education of patients recovering from myocardial infarction and coronary interventions

For many patients diagnosed with acute myocardial infarction (AMI), it is their first cardiac diagnosis and they often experience the stress of acute and life-threatening symptoms and urgent hospitalization. Complications, such as dysrhythmias, are not uncommon and additional interventions including PCI and coronary artery bypass grafting often occur within a short time frame following hospital admission. While clinically ready for discharge, 11–14% of myocardial infarction patients are readmitted within 30 days[42] indicating the need for comprehensive discharge planning, patient education, and follow-up. The goals of patient education are to support the transition home, optimize recovery and adjustment, and ensure secondary prevention behaviours are initiated. Many patients will have coexisting conditions that are both cardiac (heart failure) and non-cardiac (diabetes, kidney disease) that they must also manage with support from the multidisciplinary team.[43]

Post AMI, patients must primarily self-manage, which means dealing with all that AMI and associated treatments, recovery, and secondary prevention of coronary heart disease entails. Optimal self-management is promoted by effective patient education that includes information provision and about coronary heart disease, treatments, and consequences, but also skills concerning symptom management and medicines management. Problem-solving skills need to be developed around which health resources are needed, particularly around care transitions and how to best optimize physical and emotional health.[44] The support of informal caregivers, particularly partners, is vital. Partners may have similar diagnoses and are likely to share lifestyle behaviours, so a collaborative effort must be adopted and informal carers involved in the patient education process.

Discharge planning is essential to safe, coordinated care post AMI, even more so when the length of stay is short.[45] A multidisciplinary effort is required that includes information about coronary heart disease, medications, heart attack warning signs with a related action plan, and a structured physical activity plan that incorporates all aspects of activity including driving, return to work, and sexual activity. Physiotherapists and exercise professionals have an important role in AMI patient education and can accurately assess, prescribe, and provide education for a graduated exercise plan rehabilitation. Additional written advice on sternal precautions if a sternal split has occurred, ongoing exercise and activity, and referral to cardiac rehabilitation is important for short-term safety and long-term success. Similarly, pharmacists should be involved as multiple medications are required long-term. Initial motivation to take medications, spurred by the emergency myocardial infarction event, decreases over time, sometimes due to the occurrence of side effects and widespread misinformation. Many patients diagnosed with AMI stop taking statin medications at 6 months.[24] Medicine information must include information about medication action, common side effects and the importance of concordance. Patients should be advised not to cease any medication without consulting their physician. Their pharmacist will also be able to provide medicines information.

For patients who have wound/s either from the PCI access site or following coronary artery bypass graft surgery, specific guidance is required on how to manage their wound during recovery. Patients must receive guidance on care of the wound during bathing and activity and be made aware of the specific signs and symptoms that warrant seeking health professional advice, such as increased oozing, heat and swelling, and any wound breakdown. Application of thromboembolic prevention stockings and wound observation often requires informal caregiver support in early recovery so they should be involved in education sessions.

Psychosocial adjustment to a coronary heart disease diagnosis with the associated lifelong medications and prevention strategies takes time. Many patients experience depression and/or anxiety and it is important that negative mood states are recognized and treated, especially because depression is associated with increased mortality and morbidity[46] and has pervasive effects on patients. Informal caregivers should be included in patient education regarding psychosocial adjustment as they may be the first to notice signs of depression and have an important role to play in supporting the recovery process including when to seek professional help. Spouses of AMI patients often experience comparable levels of mental distress as their affected partner.

Patients with coronary heart disease benefit from exercise-based cardiac rehabilitation as cardiovascular mortality and hospitalization is reduced.[47]

The case studies in ➤ **Table 13.4** (Mrs Verdi diagnosed with heart failure) and ➤ **Table 13.5** (Mr King diagnosed with acute ST-segment elevation myocardial infarction). provide the reader with an overview of the key topics that should be covered as part of therapeutic patient and family focused health education. Cardiovascular disease is a condition of ageing. Populations have the opportunity to slow the progression of atherosclerosis by making healthy lifestyle changes and taking medicines as

Table 13.5 Case study 2: acute ST-segment elevation myocardial infarction

Mr Robert King is a 62-year-old male, admitted with acute ST-segment elevation myocardial infarction (STEMI) followed by primary PCI and two stents deployed to the left anterior descending artery. He owns and manages a small employment agency, which employs five people and his role requires regular driving. He lives with his wife, two adult daughters, and grandson. He has hypertension controlled by ramipril and type 2 diabetes diagnosed 2 years ago, for which he takes metformin. He drinks 4 units of alcohol four or five times/week, and does not smoke cigarettes. His body mass index is 32 and he walks for 30 minutes every second day. During this admission he has been commenced on clopidogrel, aspirin, atorvastatin, and Nitrolingual® Pumpspray as needed. He is being discharged this afternoon and his wife and oldest daughter are present. (Strategies described earlier sections of this chapter would be applied in this case study, such as a learning needs assessment and identification of preferences for and potential obstacles to learning, e.g. low health literacy level and cognitive impairments)	
Essential topics in patient education	**Nursing action**
Definition and aetiology of coronary heart disease and heart attack; explanation of PCI	Provide Mr King with information about his condition that he can understand. Ensure verbal information is supplemented by written information. It is important to explain that distress in response to a life-threatening event is normal. As a result, health-related information provided during hospitalization may not be fully understood or remembered. Health information from national heart foundations can be used to supplement discussions
Signs and symptoms of heart attack	Mr King needs to be able to recognize when chest symptoms are serious and potentially indicative of a heart attack. He needs to understand and follow an action plan for how he will recognize and respond to a recurrence of symptoms, should they occur, including the appropriate use of Nitrolingual® Pumpspray and seeking help from emergency services
Pharmacological treatment	Mr King is on multiple medications, four of which have been newly prescribed during this hospital admission. Mr King needs to recognize the actions and common side effects of his drugs and understand the importance of using the correct dose and frequency. He must understand the need to persist with these medications even when his cholesterol levels, for instance, return to normal. Using a teach-back technique (see 'Teach-back using 'chunk and check') will help the health professional to be sure that their teaching has been effective and that Mr King understands how to manage his medications. The potential for over-the-counter drugs to interact with dual antiplatelet therapy should also be discussed. Signpost Mr King to the best online websites for information
Psychosocial aspects	Depressive symptoms are common following a heart attack and all patients should be screened for depression given the potential impact on survival and risk factor modification. It is important to provide advice on how Mr King might expect to feel during the process of psychosocial adjustment. It is important to involve informal caregivers as an important source of social support. They may play a role in noticing signs of depression and supporting help-seeking and management strategies should they be required. Cardiac rehabilitation attendance also provides an opportunity to receive social support from peers
Return to work	Mr King owns and manages his own business and is likely to be concerned about when he can resume his work. Temporary restrictions may be placed on driving, which are country specific and must be adhered to. A supportive discussion with Mr King about his specific work demands is essential and a tailored return to work plan including referral to an occupational therapist may be beneficial

(continued)

Table 13.5 Continued

Risk factor modification	Mr King should monitor his blood pressure regularly, which he may be able to do himself at home and track on an App. This will enable him to manage his health and discuss readings with his physician during regular follow-up visits. Check Mr King's understanding of his diabetes and ensure that he knows how to monitor and manage his condition. Mr King drinks 16–20 units of alcohol per week which is above recommendations (14 units per week). It is important to explore his understanding about the impact of this level of alcohol intake on his health and potential interaction with prescribed medications. He should be advised to decrease his alcohol intake
Diet recommendation	Mr King is obese and has type 2 diabetes. He may benefit from referral to a dietician to get support to help him to manage his diabetes and lose weight to improve his health
Exercise recommendations	Regular physical activity is important to improve cardiovascular health, functional capacity, and manage depression post heart attack. Participation in cardiac rehabilitation, where available, will help Mr King to improve his confidence in participating in exercise. While Mr King has regular exercise through walking, he may experience a lack of confidence during recovery and tailored individual advice is important in safely increasing exercise duration, frequency, and intensity
Sexual activity	Mr King is married and sexually active and it is essential that he has the opportunity to discuss resumption of sexual activity, including any safety concerns or medication side effects he may experience
Adherence	Non-adherence to medications and lifestyle changes is common in people with cardiovascular disease. Mr King needs to understand the lifelong nature of coronary heart disease and that the PCI procedure is not a 'fix'. He needs to understand that the PCI treatment has treated culprit lesions but that other narrowings may develop. Making healthy lifestyle changes can improve the health of his heart vessels. Ensure that Mr King understands his medications and the importance of taking them regularly and for life, as well as the need for regular check-ups and discussion of any side effects with his physician

prescribed. Therapeutic patient and family focused health education is the foundation of prevention.

Conclusion

Nurses and allied health professionals play a vital role in the therapeutic education process for patients with cardiovascular disease. To improve patient outcomes, communication and teaching skills need to be fully integrated into educational curricula and continuing professional development. Support is needed for health professionals to consolidate their skills to enable them to plan, deliver, evaluate, and document educational sessions. Universal health literacy precautions should be applied to all health information resources and educational interventions to reduce the health inequalities that currently exist. Opportunities for the integration of digital technologies to enhance patient communication and education should be the focus of future research. Effective therapeutic patient education using appropriate strategies has the potential to reduce unnecessary health resource use by patients and avoidable adverse events.

References

1. Lagger G, Pataky Z, Golay A. Efficacy of therapeutic patient education in chronic diseases and obesity. Patient Educ Couns. 2010;79(3):283–86.
2. World Health Organization. Therapeutic patient education continuing education programmes for health care providers in the field of prevention of chronic diseases. Report of a WHO Working Group. 1998. http://www.euro.who.int/__data/assets/pdf_file/0007/145294/E63674.pdf.

3. Jennings C, Graham I, Gielen S (Eds). Putting educational strategies into practice. In: The ESC Handbook of Preventive Cardiology: Putting Prevention into Practice. Oxford: Oxford University Press; 2016:167–79.
4. Denham S, Eggenberger S, Krumwiede N, Young P. Family-Focused Nursing Care. Philadelphia, PA: FA Davis; 2015.
5. Kynoch K, Chang A, Coyer F, McArdle A. The effectiveness of interventions to meet family needs of critically ill patients in an adult intensive care unit: a systematic review update. JBI Database System Rev Implement Rep. 2016;14(3):181–234.
6. Goodridge D, McDonald M, New L, Scharf M, Harrison E, Rotter T, et al. Building patient capacity to participate in care during hospitalisation: a scoping review. BMJ Open. 2019;9(7):e026551.
7. Han SH, Kim K, Burr JA. Social support and preventive healthcare behaviors among couples in later life. Gerontologist. 2019;59(6):1162–70.
8. Scholl I, Zill JM, Härter M, Dirmaier J. An integrative model of patient-centeredness—a systematic review and concept analysis. PLoS One. 2014;9(9):e107828.
9. World Health Organization. Framework on Integrated, People-Centred Health Services. Report by the Secretariat. Geneva: World Health Organization; 2016.
10. Hugman B. Healthcare Communication. London: Pharmaceutical Press; 2009.
11. Street RL Jr, Makoul G, Arora NK, Epstein RM. How does communication heal? Pathways linking clinician-patient communication to health outcomes. Patient Educ Couns. 2009;74(3):295–301.
12. Boyle B. The critical role of family in patient experience. Patient Experience J. 2015;2(2):Art. 2.
13. Mehrabian A. Silent Messages: Implicit Communication of Emotions and Attitudes. Belmont, CA: Wadsworth Publishing; 1971.
14. Hashim MJ. Patient-centered communication: basic skills. Am Fam Physician. 2017;95(1):29–34.
15. Robertson K. Active listening: more than just paying attention. Aust Fam Physician. 2005;34(12):1053–55.
16. Juckett G, Unger K. Appropriate use of medical interpreters. Am Fam Physician. 2014;90(7):476–80.
17. Kessels RPC. Patients' memory for medical information. J R Soc Med. 2003;96(5):219–22.
18. Ha Dinh TT, Bonner A, Clark R, Ramsbotham J, Hines S. The effectiveness of the teach-back method on adherence and self-management in health education for people with chronic disease: a systematic review. JBI Database System Rev Implement Rep. 2016;14(1):210–47.
19. Commodore-Mensah Y, Himmelfarb CR. Patient education strategies for hospitalized cardiovascular patients: a systematic review. J Cardiovasc Nurs. 2012;27(2):154–74.
20. Barnason S, White-Williams C, Rossi LP, Centeno M, Crabbe DL, Lee KS, et al. Evidence for therapeutic patient education interventions to promote cardiovascular patient self-management: a scientific statement for healthcare professionals from the American Heart Association. Cardiovasc Qual Outcomes. 2017;10:e000025.
21. Friedman AJ, Cosby R, Boyko S, Hatton-Bauer J, Turnbull G. Effective teaching strategies and methods of delivery for patient education: a systematic review and practice guideline recommendations. J Cancer Educ. 2011;26(1):12–21.
22. Astin F, Stephenson J, Probyn J, Holt J, Marshall K, Conway D. Cardiologists' and patients' views about the informed consent process and their understanding of the anticipated treatment benefits of coronary angioplasty: a survey study. Eur J Cardiovasc Nurs. 2020;19(3):260–68.
23. Stacey D, Légaré F, Lewis K, Barry MJ, Bennett CL, Eden KB et al. Decision aids for people facing health treatment or screening decisions. Cochrane Database Syst Rev. 2017;4:CD001431.
24. van Driel ML, Morledge MD, Ulep R, Shaffer JP, Davies P, Deichmann R. Interventions to improve adherence to lipid-lowering medication. Cochrane Database Syst Rev. 2016;12:CD004371.
25. Whittaker R, McRobbie H, Bullen C, Rodgers A, Gu Y, Dobson R. Mobile phone text messaging and app-based interventions for smoking cessation. Cochrane Database Syst Rev. 2019;10:CD006611.
26. Sørensen K, Van den Broucke S, Fullam J, Doyle G, Pelikan J, Slonska Z, et al. Health literacy and public health: a systematic review and integration of definitions and models. BMC Public Health. 2012;12:80.
27. Nutbeam D. Health literacy as a public health goal: a challenge for contemporary health education and communication strategies into the 21st century. Health Promot Int. 2000;15(3):259–67.
28. Sørensen K, Pelikan JM, Röthlin F, Ganahl K, Slonska Z, Doyle G, et al. Health literacy in Europe: comparative results of the European health literacy survey (HLS-EU). Eur J Public Health. 2015;25(6):1053–58.
29. Cajita MI, Cajita TR, Han HR. Health literacy and heart failure: a systematic review. J Cardiovasc Nurs. 2016;31(2):121–30.
30. Ghisi GLM, Chaves GSDS, Britto RR, Oh P. Health literacy and coronary artery disease: a systematic review. Patient Educ Couns. 2018;101(2):177–84.
31. Diederichs C, Jordan S, Domanska O, Neuhauser H. Health literacy in men and women with cardiovascular diseases and its association with the use of health care services—results from the population-based GEDA2014/2015-EHIS survey in Germany. PLoS One. 2018;13(12):e0208303.

32. World Health Organization. Health Literacy: The Solid Facts. Copenhagen: World Health Organization Regional Office for Europe; 2013.
33. Cornett S. Assessing and addressing health literacy. Online J Issues Nurs. 2009;14:3.
34. Elbashir M, Awaisu A, El Hajj MS, Rainkie DC. Measurement of health literacy in patients with cardiovascular diseases: a systematic review. Res Social Adm Pharm. 2019;15(12):1395–405.
35. Säfström E, Jaarsma T, Strömberg A. Continuity and utilization of health and community care in elderly patients with heart failure before and after hospitalization. BMC Geriatr. 2018;18(1):177.
36. Ponikowski P, Voors AA, Anker SD, Bueno H, Cleland JGF, Coats AJS, et al. 2016 ESC Guidelines for the diagnosis and treatment of acute and chronic heart failure: the Task Force for the diagnosis and treatment of acute and chronic heart failure of the European Society of Cardiology (ESC). Developed with the special contribution of the Heart Failure Association (HFA) of the ESC. Eur Heart J. 2016;37(27):2129–200.
37. Kang JE, Han NY, Oh JM, Jin HK, Kim HA, Son IJ, et al. Pharmacist-involved care for patients with heart failure and acute coronary syndrome: a systematic review with qualitative and quantitative meta-analysis. J Clin Pharm Ther. 2016;41(2):145–57.
38. Long L, Mordi IR, Bridges C, Sagar VA, Davies EJ, Coats AJS, et al. Exercise-based cardiac rehabilitation for adults with heart failure. Cochrane Database Syst Rev. 2019;1:CD003331.
39. Ross A, Ohlsson U, Blomberg K, Gustafsson M. Evaluation of an intervention to individualise patient education at a nurse-led heart failure clinic: a mixed-method study. J Clin Nurs. 2015;24(11–12):1594–602.
40. Jonkman NH, Westland H, Groenwold RH, Ågren S, Anguita M, Blue L, et al. What are effective program characteristics of self-management interventions in patients with heart failure? An individual patient data meta-analysis. J Card Fail. 2016;22(11):861–71.
41. Mirzad F, Cramm JM, Nieboer AP. Cross-sectional research conducted in the Netherlands to identify relationships among the actual level of patient-centred care, the care gap (ideal vs actual care delivery) and satisfaction with care. BMJ Open. 2019;9(1):e025147.
42. Wang H, Zhao T, Wei X, Lu H, Lin X. The prevalence of 30-day readmission after acute myocardial infarction: a systematic review and meta-analysis. Clin Cardiol. 2019;42(10):889–98.
43. Fålun N, Fridlund B, Schaufel MA, Schei E, Norekvål TM. Patients' goals, resources, and barriers to future change: a qualitative study of patient reflections at hospital discharge after myocardial infarction. Eur J Cardiovasc Nurs. 2016;15(7):495–503.
44. Ory MG, Ahn S, Jiang L, Lorig K, Ritter P, Laurent DD, et al. National study of chronic disease self-management: six-month outcome findings. J Aging Health. 2013;25(7):1258–74.
45. Gonçalves-Bradley DC, Lannin NA, Clemson LM, Cameron ID, Shepperd S. Discharge planning from hospital. Cochrane Database Syst Rev. 2016;1:CD000313.
46. Smolderen KG, Buchanan DM, Gosch K, Whooley M, Chan PS, Vaccarino V et al. Depression treatment and 1-year mortality after acute myocardial infarction: insights from the TRIUMPH registry (translational research investigating underlying disparities in acute myocardial infarction patients' health status). Circulation. 2017;135(18):1681–89.
47. Anderson L, Thompson DR, Oldridge N, Zwisler AD, Rees K, Martin N, Taylor RS. Exercise-based cardiac rehabilitation for coronary heart disease. Cochrane Database Syst Rev. 2016;1:CD001800.

14 Addressing the current challenges for the delivery of holistic care

DAVID R. THOMPSON, MARTHA KYRIAKOU, IZABELLA UCHMANOWICZ, JAN KEENAN, RANI KHATIB, LOREENA HILL, LIS NEUBECK, EKATERINI LAMBRINOU, AND ABIGAIL BARROWCLIFF

CHAPTER CONTENTS

KEY MESSAGES

- Contemporary challenges for holistic care include frailty and ageing, multimorbidity, polypharmacy, caregiver involvement, palliative and supportive care, and cultural and socioeconomic issues.
- Frailty is a growing health problem among older people, especially women, and in the very old, linked with an increased risk in mortality, disability, and cognitive decline.
- Patients with cardiovascular disease often present with other conditions—multimorbidity—such as diabetes, obesity, cancer, depression, arthritis, frailty, and cognitive

impairment, which require a more nuanced approach to care than the usual focus on a single condition.

- Polypharmacy, the concurrent use of multiple medications by a person, is a growing issue, especially among older people with multimorbidity, and requires regular review.
- Many patients with advanced cardiovascular disease and serious symptoms now require palliative and supportive care which should be integrated early in cardiovascular management, preferably following diagnosis.
- Cultural and socioeconomic issues are increasingly being recognized as important determinants of the cause and outcome of cardiovascular disease and should be considered in any intervention, such as health behaviour change, when holistically assessing a patient with cardiovascular disease and when developing a person-centred nursing care plan.
- Females with cardiovascular disease should be provided with equal access to care, a prompt diagnosis, and treatments based on the guidelines and recommendations at the same rate and intensity as their male counterparts.

Outlining the challenges

In this chapter, the contemporary challenges for holistic care will be described and solutions proposed on how they can be addressed (➤ **Fig. 14.1**). Challenges include a frail and ageing population with multimorbidity and environmental, psychosocial, and cultural issues. This patient population is often prescribed a multitude of medications causing problems associated with polypharmacy, they have both formal and informal caregiver involvement, require palliative and supportive care, and often have cultural and socioeconomic issues. Women often bear a major burden in relation to all of these factors, further to the fact they still face gender discriminations in terms of diagnosis and care.

Frailty and ageing

Introduction

Frailty is a syndrome (FS) considered to be a major health problem for older people (see also Chapter 8). The

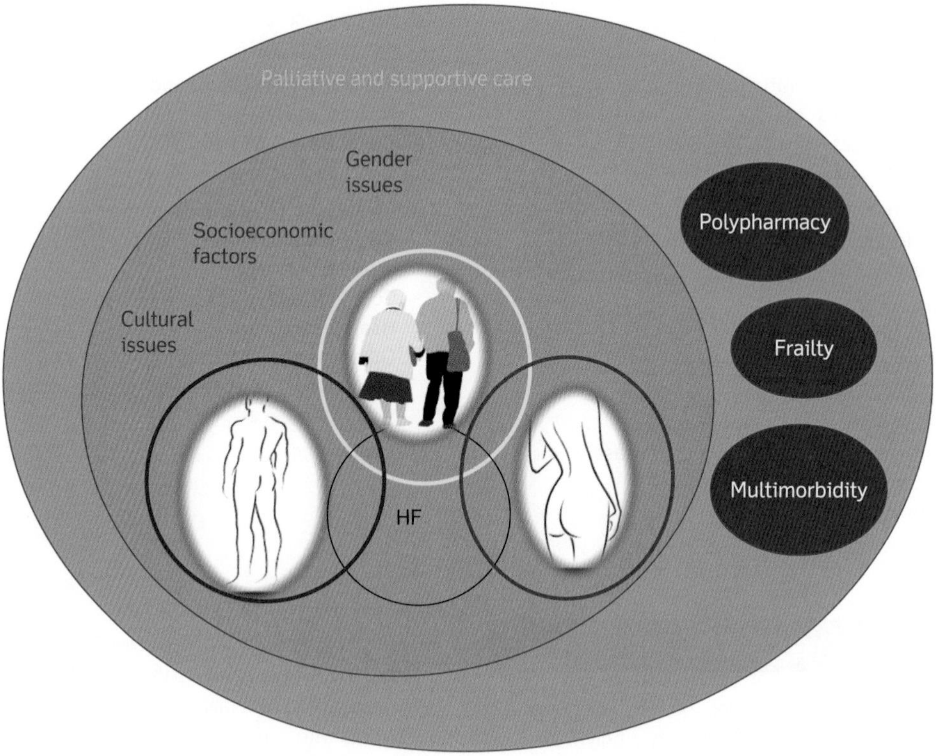

Fig. 14.1 The contemporary challenges to the delivery of holistic cardiovascular care.

prevalence of FS is variable and depends on the type of assessment criteria used and the age group. The prevalence of FS increases with age, so with the current tendency towards higher life expectancy, an increase in the number of people with FS is expected.[1] The overall prevalence of FS in the US population over 65 years of age ranges from 7% to 12%; the incidence of FS increases with age and the FS rate is 3.9% in the 65–74 years of age group, and in the 85+ years of age group it is 25%. It occurs more frequently in women than in men (8% versus 5%).[1]

In very elderly people (80+ years of age), frailty is significantly associated with an increased risk of mortality, disability, and cognitive decline.[2] Moreover, in people aged 65 years and over, the biological age was significantly more related to death than the chronological age.[3] The occurrence of FS is associated with a worse perception of one's health condition, an increase in the number of coexisting diseases, and social isolation.[4]

Definition and recognition criteria

At present, there is insufficient evidence to adopt a single universal definition of FS[5] or explain the relationship between FS and ageing, disability, and chronic diseases.[6] There is a lack of consensus on a uniform definition of FS and a lack of uniform criteria for screening,[7] and the debate continues on whether FS should be defined solely in terms of biomedical factors, or whether it should also include psychosocial and cognitive factors.[8] The Clinical Consortium on Healthy Ageing within the World Health Organization introduced in 2016 the concept of intrinsic capacity which is defined as the composite of all physical and mental capacities that an individual can draw upon during his/her life. Frailty and intrinsic capacity are two constructs stemming from the same need of overcoming traditional medical paradigms that negatively impact the correct way clinical and research practice should be conducted in older people.[9]

Considered in the context of disability, FS is an important forecast measure of the need for care and treatment. Furthermore, the correct delineation of the boundary between FS and disability allows for the implementation of measures to reverse or prevent the progress of current changes.[5,7,10]

FS is an exponent of advanced biological age and an important risk factor for the development of complications in elderly as well as in chronically ill people. The published consensus[11] recommends the introduction of screening for FS in clinical practice. It is proposed that the clinical manifestations of FS are related to the intensification of the negative energy balance cycle, sarcopenia, or reduced effort tolerance[1] and that there are five markers of FS[11]:

- Unintentional weight loss of 10 pounds (4.5 kg) in the last year or up to 10% of age 60 weight.
- Weakness of muscle strength—tested by weakness grip strength.
- Slow walking speed.
- Self-reported exhaustion.
- Low physical activity.

There are at least three diagnostic criteria for the diagnosis of FS: the presence of one or two criteria is referred to as pre-frailty, thus identifying individuals with a high probability of developing FS in the future.[12] However, it is recognized that cognitive function, mood, or even social support are equally important in the assessment.[13–15] The Canadian Initiative on Frailty and Aging[5] indicates that FS should be considered in the context of biological, psychological, and socioenvironmental factors that affect every phase of human life and can be influenced effectively.

Thus, there are currently two approaches that correlate with each other: the biomedical (physical) and the biopsychosocial.[16]

Assessment tools

An important problem in identifying FS is the effective distinction between coexisting diseases or disabilities and FS. Understanding the causes of FS is essential for the early identification of people at risk and for the implementation of preventive measures to reverse the disrupted homeostasis of individual systems that may be potentially reversible. This is why the ability to detect preclinically any symptoms leading to FS is so important.[12]

Tools to evaluate FS can be divided into two groups—the first is based on the physical aspect of FS,[1,16] and the second is based on the biopsychosocial aspect.[14,17,18]

The five markers of FS[1] are based on a narrow definition of FS, which allows the identification of 'physically fragile' individuals.[19] Tools that take into account the broader definition of FS in their assessment are usually more comprehensive and include physical, psychosocial, and/or environmental factors. Tools that can be used in a comprehensive evaluation of FS include the Edmonton Frail Scale[13] and the Canadian Study Health and Aging Frailty Index[17] and others with a more specific focus.[20–25] Other tools are referenced in Chapter 8.

The use of appropriate assessment tools will make it possible to assess and identify individuals with or at risk of developing FS. This, in turn, will allow for preventive action and specific interventions to delay the onset of FS or significantly reduce disability and its negative consequences.[26]

FS is considered an important risk factor for cardiovascular disease (CVD) and a more important predictor of treatment outcome than the chronological age of the patient. Early identification of FS creates a chance for an individually selected and effective treatment and targeted healthcare. Prevention of complications as a strategic health issue should be a priority in therapeutic decision-making based on clinical trials in the elderly. Identification of a frail person or early identification of a pre-frail person can be an important element in preventing the consequences of FS. The prospect of benefits from CVD treatment in the elderly population should be based on identifying potential benefits and risks and of identifying FS. A proper diagnosis of people with FS will identify groups with worse prognosis and a higher risk of occurrence of adverse effects in relation to the treatment being conducted.[27,28]

Conclusion

FS is a growing problem and clinical teams may implement their own strategies to take care of elderly frail patients. FS can be challenging; however, it should be remembered that the proper diagnosis of FS will allow the identification of patients who require intensified care and intervention, to avoid complications of medical treatment and hospitalization.[29] Nursing interventions are outlined in ➤ Box 14.1 based on those outlined in a recent practice update.[29] This requires collaborative skills on the part of the healthcare professionals and also demands a willingness from them to look beyond the borders of their own disciplines.

Box 14.1 Nursing interventions to identify and address frailty

- Maintain a healthy nutritional status.
- Avoid harmful polypharmacy which is linked to multimorbidity and falls (see later in this chapter).
- Improve adherence to treatment (see Chapter 12).
- Prevent falls (risk assessment and appropriate intervention).
- Encourage multicomponent exercise (take into account physical and functional fitness, gait, balance, strength, cognitive function, mood, and overall well-being).
- Improve mood and cognitive function (screen, stimulate, external memory aids, episodic memory such as list recall and face–name association, and self-assertiveness training).

Source data from Uchmanowicz I, Jankowska-Polańska B, Wleklik M, Lisiak M, Gobbens R. Frailty Syndrome: Nursing Interventions. SAGE Open Nurs. 2018;4:1–11.

Multimorbidity

Introduction

Although life expectancy is improving markedly, the proportion of people with two or more health conditions simultaneously is rising steadily.[30] Multimorbidity, commonly defined as the presence of two or more chronic medical conditions in an individual, is increasingly common among older people, the socioeconomically deprived, younger people with congenital or acquired impairments, and those with serious mental illness. Globally, around one in three of all adults suffer from multiple chronic conditions.[31] Patients with comorbidities are characterized by increased mortality, impaired health-related quality of life, and increased use of healthcare services compared to patients without any comorbidity.[32] Patients with CVD are at increased risk for comorbidities[33,34] making the management of the disease more complex. The degree of physical or mental disability, the number of hospitalizations, the number of drugs, the average length of stay, and in-hospital mortality is significantly higher in patients with multiple comorbidities.[35] This impacts healthcare delivery and expenditure and imposes a burden on patients and carers that includes impaired quality of life, polypharmacy, and inability to work, and at the same time, a burden on healthcare services.

More than 70% of adults develop CVD by 70 years of age, two-thirds of whom also develop non-CVD comorbidities.[36] Many people with CVD also have diabetes or chronic pulmonary disease, and older people may also have frailty or cognitive impairment. For example, it is not uncommon for men with CVD to also have depression or another mental health condition.[37] Perhaps surprisingly, common comorbidities include arthritis and mental illness.[38] Patients with heart failure (HF) have two or more non-cardiac comorbidities at 86% and more than 25% have six or more comorbidities.[39] For many older adults with multimorbidity, CVD is not necessarily experienced as the most important of their health or healthcare concerns,[36] even though in older people, isolated cardiovascular multimorbidity is associated with loss of physical mobility, whereas neuropsychiatric multimorbidity is associated with declines in mobility and independence.[40] Non-cardiovascular comorbidities are associated with a higher overall symptom burden and more severe symptoms than cardiovascular comorbidities, and the latter are more likely to be associated with pain and anxiety than shortness of breath and fatigue.[41]

Nowadays, the typical person with CVD is aged older than 65 years and has multiple diseases,[36,38] and the proportion of people with CVD and higher numbers of comorbidities is increasing,[42] and those with a higher burden of multimorbidity are at substantially increased risk of death several years after the acute event.[43] Thus, healthcare professionals must always consider for those comorbid conditions in patients with CVD, and monitor these patients closely in an effort to prevent comorbidities or slow down disease progression over time, resulting in better quality of life and decreased mortality.[32] These days, telemedicine provides solutions and opportunities for close monitoring via telemonitoring (see also Chapter 15).

Caring for people with multimorbidity

Caring for people with multimorbidity is complicated because of the complex interaction between different conditions and their treatments. Conventional care delivery is often based around individual conditions rather than around the person as a whole and, as a consequence, care is often fragmented. Typical priorities among older adults include physical and cognitive functioning, symptom control, reduced burden of therapy, health-related quality of life, maintenance of independence, and overall well-being.[44] These priorities and concerns should serve to inform clinical care.[45]

Guiding principles for the care of older adults with multimorbidity include (1) eliciting and incorporating patient preferences into decision-making; (2) applying evidence but acknowledging the limitations of the evidence base; (3) framing care decisions in a context of risks, burdens, benefits, and prognosis; (4) assessing care complexity and feasibility; and (5) choosing interventions that optimize benefit, minimize harm, and enhance quality of life.[46] A person-centred care approach, incorporating patients' preferences and values and empowering them to work as partners in decision-making with their interdisciplinary teams is advocated.[46–48] This requires the application of good clinical skills, time, and thought, and being cautious of the temptation to intervene and move on.

A tailored 'person-centred' holistic approach using skilled clinical judgement and good communication is likely to be much more effective than merely focusing on the conditions themselves. A person-centred care approach should aim to empower self-management and draw upon a range of resources, including informal carers, friends, and family, who often provide considerable support to people with multimorbidity. Focusing on the patient and not on the disease, better management of the disease, along with patient satisfaction can be achieved through individual empowerment of patients to become knowledgeable and more informed about their diagnosis, successfully manage their symptoms, and engage in self-care behaviours.[49,50] In this context, person-centred care is effective regarding a patient's self-efficacy, improving health-related quality of life and reducing healthcare utilization for a number of CVDs[51] (see also Chapter 2 and Chapter 8).

By optimizing care, the aim is to reduce care burden, adverse events, polypharmacy, multiple appointments, and unplanned care, and improve quality of life and care coordination by promoting shared decision-making based on what is important to each patient in terms of care, health priorities, lifestyle, goals, and values.[48] This involves agreeing on an individualized care plan with the patient that incorporates goals and plans for future care (including advance care planning), and identifies who is responsible for care coordination and how this is communicated to all healthcare professionals and services involved (such as mental health or social services). Ideally, this plan of care is offered through a multidisciplinary team. A multidisciplinary team offering adequate care to CVD patients includes physicians, nurses, pharmacists, dieticians, physiotherapists, psychologists, social workers, and other allied professionals.[52,53] No single profession can provide the knowledge, skills, and resources to meet the requirements of today's patient with complex health needs, so contributions from each multidisciplinary team member are important.[54,55] Efficient team-based care is crucial to effective management of CVD conditions; however, since goals have been agreed and action plans developed, the patient and their family have to integrate the new behaviours into their everyday lives in order to manage the lifestyle recommendations and medication regimens.[55] Especially for HF patients, there is a variety of different management programmes[56,57] all aiming to provide evidence-based diagnosis and therapy to these patients and to educate patients and their caregivers.[58] The implementation of the management programme begins with discharge planning, involving the patient and their family[59] (see also Chapter 10). It should specify the timing of follow-up and how to access urgent care if needed, recognizing that many people with multimorbidity are forced to navigate complex and fragmented healthcare systems. To do this well requires listening to people and asking what matters to them, their carers, and their family, including their outcomes and experiences through continuous assessment of the patient's needs. Continuing individualized assessment gives both to the patients and the healthcare professionals the capacity of early recognition and action to meet patients' needs.[60]

Conclusion

Healthcare professionals need to rise to the challenge of multimorbidity and change the care approach to better respond to it. This should focus on goal-oriented outcomes and emphasize communication and collaboration across healthcare professionals and care settings. It is important to acknowledge that so-called mental and physical illnesses frequently coexist and that this conceptual distinction between them is artificial and highly questionable. Person-centred care, regular reassessment of patients' needs, and adapting of tailored therapy accordingly, gives the opportunity of a holistic approach and care. Multidisciplinary teams could offer more comprehensive care as each profession discipline offers 'different' knowledge and skills management programmes. We must be able to respond to this growing problem and recognize that the pattern of health and disease and care delivery in our population is changing. ➤ **Box 14.2** summarizes the nursing priorities in caring for adults with comorbidities.

Polypharmacy

Introduction

Polypharmacy refers to the concurrent use of multiple medications by one individual. This may be considered appropriate or problematic. It is important to distinguish between the two as in some scenarios the combination of at least two or three drugs can be beneficial to the patient.[61]

Polypharmacy is becoming increasingly common. In the UK, the number of items prescribed per patient increased from 11.9 to 18.3 between 2001 and 2011. Contributing factors include the increase in prescribing of preventive medication, and the ageing population and the subsequent increase in chronic disease prevalence resulting in comorbidity and multimorbidity.[62]

Box 14.2 Nursing priorities in caring for adults with multimorbidity

- Identify comorbidities when assessing patients with cardiovascular problems (e.g. arthritis and mental illness).
- Adopt a holistic person/patient-centred approach taking into account patient preferences and values in shared decision-making.
- Empower patients to self-manage.
- Draw on family and other social support.
- Ensure care is well coordinated, joined up, and integrated between various disciplines.

Appropriate polypharmacy

The number of medicines appropriate for a patient depends on their conditions, functional status, life expectancy, and drug-taking preferences.[61] In patients with complex comorbidities, there are cases where prescribing several medicines is the best management for the patient.[62] Polypharmacy can be considered appropriate when each medicine is prescribed to achieve a specific, achievable benefit and they have been optimized in order to reduce the risk of adverse drug events.[61] The emphasis needs to be on a person-centred approach (see also Chapter 2) which involves collaborating with the patient to identify an appropriate combination of drugs. Patients should be involved in this decision and be motivated and capable of taking the medicines as prescribed. The objective of polypharmacy in this scenario is to maintain quality of life, improve longevity, and minimize harm.[61]

Problematic polypharmacy

Problematic polypharmacy is the inappropriate prescribing of several medications. This is either when the intended benefits of medicines are not realized or the patient is unable to cope with the demands of taking all the medication.[61] The importance of discussions with the patient cannot be overstated. Other examples of inappropriate problematic pharmacy occur when risks of adverse drug reactions (ADRs) outweigh benefits or if one or more medicines are no longer required.[61] It can also arise when medicines are prescribed to combat the side effects of other drugs (incremental prescribing).[61]

There are several reasons for problematic polypharmacy and they include hesitation from prescribers to add in extra medication with a strong evidence base due to 'pill burden', failure to frequently assess medications for their continued benefit and appropriateness, and prescribing of medication to overcome side effects where an alternative solution is available.

Why polypharmacy is an issue

Although sometimes appropriate, polypharmacy can pose challenges for healthcare professionals and patients:

1. *Polypharmacy increases the risk of ADRs.* ADRs are unwanted reactions after taking a drug under normal clinical conditions and may result in harm to the patient. Two types have been reported. Type A reactions are a predictable, exaggerated reaction based on the known pharmacology (i.e. bradycardia in patients taking a beta-blocker) and have a high morbidity and low mortality; type B reactions are unpredictable and idiosyncratic reactions to a medication (i.e. anaphylaxis after taking a penicillin) and have a low morbidity and high mortality. One study found that over four non-consecutive weeks, the incidence of hospital admissions due to ADRs was 8.37 per 100 admissions. The number of drugs taken was listed as one of the most important factors associated with ADRs.[63]
2. *Polypharmacy increases the risk of drug–drug interactions.* Drug–drug interactions occur when the effect of a drug is altered by the presence of another. This may result in reduced effectiveness of one or more medications, or even harm to the patient from toxicity. A comparison of drugs recommended by the UK National Institute for Health and Care Excellence (NICE) for HF, depression, and type 2 diabetes against 11 other comorbidities seen among patients with these three conditions identified 111, 89, and 133 potentially serious drug–drug interactions, respectively.[64] The study highlighted the importance of considering drug–drug interactions in the context of polypharmacy and when prescribing a new medication in those patients with comorbidities, even when recommended by clinical guidelines.
3. *Polypharmacy can be associated with unwanted drug–disease interaction.* Unwanted drug–disease interaction is an adverse outcome resulting from a drug exacerbating a chronic disease.[65] A study identified 32 potentially serious drug–disease interactions between drugs recommended in the NICE guidelines for managing type 2 diabetes and 11 other common comorbidities. There were ten potentially serious drug–disease interactions for drugs recommended in the guideline for HF. Of these drug–disease interactions, 27 (84%) in the type 2 diabetes guidelines and all of those in the HF guidelines were between the recommended drug and chronic kidney disease.[64] In the context of CVD, one study found that the two most common drug–disease interactions were use of first-generation calcium channel blockers in patients with congestive HF and use of aspirin in patients with peptic ulcer disease (both, 3.7%).[65]
4. *Polypharmacy can impact medicines adherence* (see also Chapter 12). Polypharmacy can lead to suboptimal adherence. Adherence to medicines is defined as the extent to which a patient's drug-taking behaviour matches the agreement between them and the prescriber, based on the prescriber's recommendations.[66] This may be unintentional, where the patient wants to follow treatment recommendations but is unable (forgetting, difficulty understanding, problems with using the treatment, inability to pay), or intentional, where the patient decides not to follow recommended treatment (beliefs, preferences).[66]

Polypharmacy and cardiovascular disease

Polypharmacy is a particular issue in those patients with established CVD or at high risk of developing it.[67,68] CVD is highly preventable, and many more asymptomatic patients are being treated with preventive medication.[69] As well as lifestyle changes, six conditions are associated with a high risk of causing CVD events[69]—high blood pressure, high cholesterol, atrial fibrillation (AF), chronic kidney disease, pre-diabetes, and diabetes—recommendations for the management of which are associated with use of drugs and therefore lead to polypharmacy.

In addition to the hypoglycaemic medicine required for adequate treatment of diabetes to prevent the microvascular complications, patients with diabetes are all recognized as at least moderate risk of developing CVD.[70] As well as lifestyle factors, the following are recommended to help prevent CVD: tight blood pressure control (drug therapy often necessary); lower target for LDL cholesterol in patients with a moderate risk of CVD and combination therapy with statin and ezetimibe recommended if statin therapy alone is insufficient; and in high/very high risk patients aspirin can be considered as primary prevention plus a proton pump inhibitor (PPI) to prevent gastrointestinal bleeding. Thus, it is easy to see how the number of medications in patients with diabetes can add up, simply for primary prevention of CVD. Also, an unhealthy lifestyle can impact the control of modifiable cardiovascular risk and subsequently contribute to polypharmacy, leading to poor management of blood pressure and cholesterol. This can increase the risk of cardiovascular events and the number of medications required for secondary prevention or optimizing control.[67]

As the aetiology of CVD is multifactorial, patients with this condition are usually prescribed multiple medicines to manage lipids and blood pressure, for example, often based on the recommendations of various evidence-based guidelines. In addition, more than one cardiovascular condition could be present which requires multiple therapies for each of those conditions. Among those with post-acute coronary syndrome, the following medications are recommended: aspirin (plus a second antiplatelet for a year), beta-blockers, angiotensin converting enzyme inhibitors/ angiotensin receptor blockers and statins. Similar prescribing of multiple medicines occurs in patients with HF. A study reported that the prevalence of polypharmacy (ten or more drugs) among the 848 hospitalizations for HF, in patients over 65 years old, was 47%. At discharge, the number of medications was increased and the prevalence of polypharmacy was 58%.[71] Patients with atrial fibrillation are often managed with prophylactic anticoagulants and rate and/or rhythm control medications. These are high-risk medications and can result in ADRs and harm for the patient. Also, atrial fibrillation rarely occurs in isolation and is known to coexist with multiple other conditions (most commonly, hypertension, HF, diabetes, stroke, and myocardial infarction) and therefore polypharmacy has high prevalence among patients with atrial fibrillation, as high as 76.5%.[72]

With an estimated fourfold increase in people aged 75 years or older by 2050,[67] and increases in the prevalence of comorbid conditions and CVD as well, the number of relative medications required for their treatment (cardiovascular and non-cardiovascular drugs) will also increase.[67]

What can we do?

Awareness of polypharmacy, particularly in relation to CVD, has increased. Polypharmacy can be associated with harm, as the number of drugs prescribed increases so does the risk of prescribing errors and ADRs.[61] Further research is required to examine medicines management in polypharmacy as well as better education around multimorbidity and polypharmacy. In the meantime, we can examine patient preferences with regard to medicines taking, review how we manage multimorbidity, and consider appropriate deprescribing (see Chapter 12). A study of multimorbidity in older people and their desired processes of care found that they wanted convenient access to healthcare, individualized care plans, support from one care coordinator, continuity of relationships with healthcare professionals, and healthcare professionals who were caring and listened, appreciating that their needs were unique.[73]

To best understand issues around adherence, ADRs, and other medicines-related harm, it is important to ask patients about their medicines and listen to any concerns. This is part of the medicines optimization process (see also Chapter 12). As multimorbidity can lead to polypharmacy when the management of each condition is considered in isolation, this may necessitate longer consultation times, 'generalist' clinicians managing several conditions simultaneously, reviewing single condition clinics, and moving towards patients having all their conditions managed in one visit.[62] This involves careful consideration of skill mixes and clearly defined roles for all healthcare professionals, of clinical pharmacists having a bigger role in overseeing complicated drug treatments, and of healthcare professionals working in a community setting having an important role in identifying those patients on multiple medicines. Deprescribing is the gradual withdrawal and cessation of medications by a healthcare professional after discussions and agreement with the patient, the objective being to cease inappropriate medications and improve outcomes relating to polypharmacy.[74] Deprescribing can be considered in the following scenarios[61,62]: no indication; change in condition; the patient is no longer benefiting; change in evidence/guidelines; if the drug is being used to treat an iatrogenic condition; and patient choice. Especially in older people, the goals of treatments should be reviewed regularly. If a patient has a life-limiting illness, the value of some preventive medications should be considered.

Conclusion

Improvements in the management of CVD are contributing to an ageing population with several multimorbidities which require multiple therapies. In addition, guidelines are increasingly recommending preventive medications. All of this can lead to polypharmacy. Improving awareness of the issues surrounding both appropriate and problematic polypharmacy means that we can offer patients with CVD or those who are at risk of CVD better options to maximize their benefits from prescribed medicines, reduce their harm, and improve their quality of life. Thus, healthcare professionals should ensure that any polypharmacy is appropriate and address problematic polypharmacy. To do that, we must ensure that care is person-centred and medicines are optimized regularly to meet the patient's needs. We should also remember that appropriate deprescribing is part of the medicines

Box 14.3 Nursing considerations regarding polypharmacy

- Ensure a holistic integrated approach is adopted.
- Ensure a clear definition of roles/appropriate skill mix.
- Ensure access to medicines optimization and deprescribing.

optimization process. ➤ Box 14.3 summarizes the key consideration for avoiding harmful polypharmacy.

Palliative and supportive care

Introduction

Individuals with cardiovascular conditions struggle with deteriorating health, symptom burden, or permanent disabilities facing palliative needs. Palliative care according to the World Health Organization (2009)[75] has the scope to 'improve the quality of life of patients and their families facing problems that are associated with life-threatening illness, through the prevention and relief of suffering by means of early identification and impeccable assessment and treatment of pain and other problems, physical, psychosocial and spiritual'.

The need of palliative care in CVD, especially in patients with HF, has been recognized in a more holistic approach, delivered to patients along with other treatments from the initial diagnosis to the end of life.[76,77] Palliative care for HF patients has a dual role: treating symptoms and ensuring that patients' treatment plans match their and family's values and needs.[76]

But is palliative care enough to meet patients' needs? Patients with CVD have unmet supportive care needs,[78,79] particularly HF patients, as they have higher needs than patients with other cardiovascular disorders regarding daily living.[79] The terms 'palliative' and 'supportive' care often cause confusion; however, there are different definitions for these two terms. A common goal is to improve the health-related quality of life of patients who have a serious or life-threatening disease and provide them with support.[77]

Supportive care is multidisciplinary holistic care provided to the patient and his/her family, from the time of diagnosis and throughout treatment with the aim of prolonging life expectancy and improving health-related quality of life, and into end of life care.[79,80] It is essential to clarify that palliative care is an important part of supportive care, mainly concerning the internal and psychosocial components of supportive care.[80] Supportive care includes modifying interventions in an effort to manage symptoms, and psychosocial or existential distress, and to identify strategies in order to cope with HF.[79,81] Supportive care is composed of four components: communication and decision-making; education; symptom management; and psychological and spiritual issues.[81]

It is important to highlight that patients require support and individualized care based on their preferences and values[81] beginning from the time of the diagnosis.[82,83] Typically, HF is characterized by acute events and followed by periods of stabilization, making prognosis challenging.[59,79,83]

There is recognition for the benefits of supportive and palliative care for patients with CVD as this is referred to guidelines,[59,82] although there is no available systematic design of supportive interventions that might be comparable with each other.[79] The challenge for healthcare professionals in CVD caring is to identify this design and this may occur through continuous assessment of the patient's and the family's needs and therefore advance care planning. Advance care planning is 'a process that enables individuals to define goals and preferences for future medical treatment and care, to discuss these goals and preferences with family and healthcare providers, and to record and review these preferences if appropriate'.[84] Advance care planning is an essential component of palliative care; it increases the completion of advance directives, discussion of end of life preferences, and improves the concordance between preferred and received care.[52]

Advance care planning as a supportive care approach may enhance patient–clinician communication, creating a relationship between them and allowing health professionals to assess the patient's level of understanding regarding his or her condition.[84] Following the disease trajectory, health professionals have to explain the disease process to the patient and discuss the implications of advanced heart disease, ensuring that the patient has an adequate understanding of the disease process.[77,79,82] Both the patient and family member should be provided with honest, up-to-date information concerning the prognosis, to enable an open discussion with shared realistic expectations and decisions to inform future management. Many professionals are reluctant to engage in prognostic discussions or make end of life decisions for fear of provoking unnecessary anxiety and removal of hope,[85–87] but studies[88–90] demonstrate the value of integrating a palliative HF approach, with involvement of the specialist palliative care team as necessary, in terms of better communication, reduced anxiety, and improved quality of life. Practical tools are available[91] to prompt the patient to raise conversations which may be challenging, but which the patient or family member would prefer to discuss when given the opportunity. Furthermore, during the coronavirus 2019 pandemic, a range of online resources in the form of communication scripts and conversation videos are available for professionals to access and provide support to initiate these conversations more readily.[92]

Communications about end of life issues are also very important aspects of supportive and palliative care. Discussions about healthcare proxy, resuscitation, and potentially implantable cardioverter defibrillator/ventricular assist device deactivation have to be addressed with the patient and their family.[83] Once discussed and when an agreement is reached, it is vital that decisions are clearly documented and communicated with the rest of the multidisciplinary team (see also Chapter 7 and Chapter 10).

In conclusion, early implementation of supportive and palliative care is necessary for patients with CVD in order to ameliorate symptoms, carry out the expressed wishes of patients, and provide emotional support for their loved ones.

Conclusion

Supportive and palliative care must be offered to CVD patients from diagnosis to the end of life, aiming to improve patients' quality of life and provide them with support. Supportive care is a multidisciplinary holistic care approach compromised of interventions to help patients manage chronic conditions such as CVD. Through continuing assessment, healthcare professionals are willing to identify patient's needs, preferences, and values of care, offering them modifying interventions to meet those needs. This process compromises advance care planning—the development of a therapeutic relationship between healthcare professionals and patients throughout the disease trajectory. An important part of the disease trajectory is the end of life stage. End of life issues are part of palliative care and thereafter supportive care. Healthcare professionals need to have the skills and competencies to discuss and plan end of life issues according to patients' wishes. ➤ Box 14.4 summarizes the key consideration of supportive and palliative care.

Box 14.4 Nursing priorities for delivering palliative care

- Be aware of triggers for the planning of palliative care (e.g. referral for device).
- Ensure patient and family are given honest up-to-date information about prognosis.
- Use communication skills to open up conversation and discussion (see also Chapter 13).
- Ensure clear communication within the interdisciplinary care team (e.g. 'do not attempt resuscitation' orders).
- Advocate for high-quality end of life care.
- Advance care planning implementation requires regular reassessment to follow the patient's needs, preferences, and values.

Cultural and gender issues and socioeconomic factors

Introduction

Cultural norms, such as socioeconomic status, contribute to behaviours associated with risk factors for chronic diseases including CVD[93] (see also Chapter 1). Convincing evidence has shown that there is an independent association between socioeconomic factors and mortality which is comparable to the traditional major risk factors.[94] The increased burden of CVD in individuals with low socioeconomic status is due to several factors including biological, behavioural, and psychosocial factors that are more prevalent to the particular population.[95] Four aspects of socioeconomic status are found to be linked with CVD in high-income countries; income level, educational level, employment status, and environmental factors.[94,95]

The World Health Organization reports that CVD deaths are especially prevalent in low-income and middle-income countries due to unequal living conditions, maldistribution of healthcare services, and poor social policies.[96] The explanation of this phenomenon is multifactorial.[93,95] Mortality differences may be driven by disparities in standards of care including accessibility to healthcare including screening for prevention,[97] percutaneous coronary interventions when presenting with acute myocardial infarction[98] or guideline-recommended medications such as statin therapy after acute myocardial infarction,[99] and cardiovascular prevention and rehabilitation which has been found to improve outcomes.[100]

The same inverse relation applies for education level. Education affects multiple conditions from childhood onwards, including exposures to community-level factors (such as living or working in healthier environments), and better access to health and social resources. Educational reforms can lead to reductions in cardiovascular and non-cardiovascular-related mortality.[101] Individuals with a low educational level, independently of sociodemographic factors,[102] face a higher risk of CVD, higher incidence of cardiovascular events, and higher cardiovascular mortality. Individuals with a low education level tend to have an increased number of CVD risk factors[101]; a potential contribution to CVD risk is the strong correlation between education and health literacy (see also Chapter 13).[103,104] Individuals with a low educational level are less likely to adhere to medical recommendations; they are less physically active and adopt unhealthy lifestyle habits.[105] While higher education is associated with increased alcohol consumption, it is inversely related to smoking, high blood pressure, cholesterol levels, and diabetes.[95] Also, the epidemic of obesity is found to affect persons with lower educational level more.[105,106]

Environmental and social circumstances influence exposure to risk factors and health. Furthermore, social isolation and a lack of social support are linked to increased CVD risk. Exposure to social risk factors starts at birth. The environment that someone is born into, and their lifestyle during childhood and adulthood, influence health status in later life. Socioeconomic differences in neighbourhood characteristics may impact the availability of resources and influence the promotion or maintenance of a healthy lifestyle.[107] It has been shown that individuals living in a disadvantaged environment have a higher risk of CVD, compared with individuals who live in a facilitated environment with easier access to physical activity and healthy food. This results in a lower prevalence of obesity and lower incidence of diabetes.[95] Adding to that, differences in health by race and ethnicity are a major public health concern.[102] Furthermore, sharp shifts in demographic patterns and lifestyles have resulted from urbanization and industrialization, the globalization of the twentieth century that drove countries, communities, and non-Western cultures into the worldwide epidemic of CVD. The change reflects both a demographic shift towards increasing life expectancy and a shift in nutrition. People who live longer have greater exposure to cardiovascular risk factors, Westernized diets (e.g. higher animal products and fat), and patterns of physical inactivity resulting in elevations in blood pressure, body weight, blood glucose levels, and lipid concentrations.[106] Ambient air pollution is also found to be associated with a higher risk of CVD, while household air pollution is strongly associated with a higher risk of death.[101]

Psychosocial factors, including stress and depression, are strongly associated with adverse CVD outcomes, such as cardiac death, arrhythmia, and changes in heart function. Growing evidence suggests that such factors may disparately affect individuals with low socioeconomic status.[101] Psychosocial stress is recognized as a non-traditional risk factor for CVD and is strictly correlated with culture[108] and race discrimination. Race-related stress may also increase the tendency to follow negative health behaviours that impact the management of several CVD factors.[109] Furthermore, there is a greater burden of CVD in low- and middle-income countries where there may be cultural barriers, reduced accessibility to healthcare, and lower-quality healthcare services.[106] One global study that was undertaken in the US, Europe, Australasia, and South America investigated self-care behaviours in HF and found low adherence across countries in all behaviours except self-reported medication adherence. Patients from some cultures may use herbal or other traditional medication in addition to their prescribed pharmacotherapy. Furthermore, in some countries, people may have beliefs that pharmacotherapy is a 'Western medication' made of chemical ingredients which result in many side effects.[110]

Women are over-represented among those living in poverty. Reviews have shown that being older, being a woman, and being unemployed are factors associated with accessibility to healthcare. In more detail, restricted accessibility includes screening for cardiovascular prevention guideline-recommended interventions, medications, and non-participation in cardiovascular prevention and rehabilitation.[100] Gender differences, which are influenced by ethnicity, culture, and socioeconomic environment, are intimately involved in risk factors and risk behaviours (e.g. psychosocial risk factors, physical inactivity, participation in cardiovascular prevention and rehabilitation, obesity, and tobacco use). Those factors play a far greater role in outcomes among women with coronary heart disease than biological sex differences (see 'Cardiovascular disease in women and sex disparities'). A woman's ethnicity or cultural background creates complex norms and expectations that affect all aspects of life (e.g. marital status, childbearing, caregiving roles, food preparation, educational level, job choices, wage rates, health beliefs/practices, amount of political power, and degree of social influence).[111] These differences affect the mechanism and expression of CVD between the sexes. Data from registries and studies demonstrate discrepant results with respect to access to healthcare, the use of evidence-based therapy, and clinical outcomes between men and women presenting with acute coronary syndrome[112–117] (see 'Coronary heart disease in women'). Even though much success has been achieved in reducing the components of delay once a patient enters the healthcare system, little has changed in treatment-seeking delay times for women. Women are less likely to be assessed for cardiac symptoms, but when assessment is performed, sex- and gender-based differences exist.

Risk factors have changed in recent years as evidenced by one review[118] which found an important change in HF demography with HF occurring at an older age but with less traditional cardiovascular risk factors (e.g. smoking and blood pressure). Diabetes mellitus, obesity, hypertension, chronic kidney disease, and cancer comorbidities at HF onset are increasing, and these factors may be associated with the increasing prevalence of HF with preserved ejection fraction.[119,120] Also, risk factors leading to CVD seem to have changed in the last decade making individual approaches necessary. HF prevention and treatment should be tailored to individual risk profiles to respond better to the individual's needs and have the best possible outcomes.[118]

It is vital that healthcare providers accurately use cardiovascular risk assessment tools and effectively treat cardiovascular risk using recommended guidelines. It is equally vital that healthcare providers teach all patients about their cardiovascular risk in simple terms they can understand and provide lifestyle management counselling (see Chapter 13). Reducing any kind of disparities in health requires a multilevel and collaborative approach with a focus on identifying individuals and communities at greatest risk and putting more resources towards these groups, improving access to quality healthcare, increasing cultural competence, and revamping education of nurses and health professionals in general. Through the use of existing cohesive networks such as healthcare facilities, schools, religious organizations, worksites, social networks, media networks, e-health, and virtual communities, physicians, policymakers, and activists can develop a more effective platform to engage and intervene in communities at a grassroots level.

The relationship of patient and provider is crucial, as it may promote or discourage patient and family engagement in self-management of chronic conditions and adherence to therapy. A negative experience may reduce a patient's use of healthcare services and have a negative impact on patient adherence and satisfaction.[109] It is very important to take into consideration cultural issues and socioeconomic factors when holistically assessing a patient with CVD and when developing a person-centred nursing care plan. It will result in the development of enhanced trust between patients, families, and health professionals aiming for the same goals and health outcomes.

Conclusion

Culture, gender, psychosocial, and socioeconomic status are associated with risk factors leading to CVD. Several factors including low educational level, health literacy, social isolation, and lack of social support are linked with higher cardiovascular events and mortality. Also, socioeconomic differences may impact availability of resources or create barriers to maintain a healthy lifestyle. In addition, there is a complex relationship between gender differences, ethnicity, culture, and socioeconomic environment. Healthcare professionals must take into account differences regarding culture and socioeconomic status when they develop a plan of healthcare. Disparities in cardiovascular care could be addressed by identifying individuals at greatest risk, improving access to quality healthcare, increasing cultural competence, and revamping education of nurses and health professionals. ➤ **Box 14.5** summarizes the key factors relating to socioeconomic status and culture important to the awareness of nurses.

Box 14.5 Key factors relating to socioeconomic status and culture important for the awareness of nurses

- Low socioeconomic status is associated with low income, low educational level, employment status, and the environment.
- Individuals with low socioeconomic status are more at risk of CVD because of a higher prevalence of adverse health behaviours and cardiovascular risk factors.
- Race and culture are associated with increased cardiovascular risk because of a complex interrelationship with financial, educational, occupational, and environmental factors.
- Nurses should be aware of all of these factors when caring for their patients to avoid discrimination.
- Psychosocial factors are strongly associated with adverse CVD outcomes.
- Gender disparities do exist in cardiovascular care. Disparities in cardiovascular care could be addressed by identifying individuals at greatest risk, improving access to quality healthcare, increasing cultural competence, tailoring healthcare provided, and following clinical recommendations and guidelines for all patients with cardiovascular needs.

Cardiovascular disease in women and sex disparities

Introduction

CVD is the leading cause of death in women worldwide. In Europe, more women (51%) died from CVD compared with men (42%). However, the misconception of CVD as a man's disease and breast cancer as the greatest threat to women is still prevalent. Awareness of CVD as the primary cause of mortality in women has been slowly increasing; however, recent data suggest stagnation in the improvements in incidence and mortality of coronary heart disease, specifically among younger women (<55 years).[121] In fact, CVD causes over 50% of death compared to 3% of death caused by breast cancer in women.[122] Women have a higher prevalence of persistent chest pain, rehospitalization, and mortality from ischaemic heart disease than men, along with higher direct costs.[123,124] Women also have greater patient-related delays, and these have remained unchanged for more than a decade.[123,125,126] Despite the substantial risk of heart disease, women are less likely to receive guideline-directed care and counselling on their risk reduction from their clinicians than men. Importantly, once a diagnosis is correctly made, women with heart disease respond well to symptoms after prescription of cardiac medication.[124,127] This evidence highlights the important gap in risk assessment, diagnosis, management, and prevention of heart disease in women.

Biological variances among women and men are called sex differences and are frequently reproducible. Sex differences in the cardiovascular system are due to differences in gene expression from the sex chromosomes, which may be further modified by sex differences in hormones resulting in sex-unique gene expression and function. These differences result in variations in prevalence and presentation of cardiovascular conditions, including those associated with autonomic regulation, hypertension, diabetes, and vascular and cardiac remodelling. The existence of crucial sex/gender-related differences in the prevalence, presentation, management, and outcomes of different CVDs, is related to differences in fat tissue distribution and different hormonal profiles and fluctuations.[121] The key role of sex hormones in protecting women from CVD during the premenopausal state, providing an advantage over men, is lost when the hormonal profile changes at menopause transition. This hormonal-dependent shift of sex-related CVD risk strongly affects CVD epidemiology and CVD prevention/treatment, particularly in light of the ageing of the overall population. In contrast, gender differences are unique to the human and arise from sociocultural practices (e.g. behaviours, environment)[121,127,128] (see later sections in this chapter).

Coronary heart disease in women

Coronary heart disease in women includes not only atherosclerotic obstructive coronary artery disease, but also an expanded spectrum of coronary disease, including coronary microvascular dysfunction, endothelial dysfunction, vasomotor abnormalities, spontaneous coronary artery dissection, and stress-induced cardiomyopathy.[121,127,129] The three most important characteristics of coronary heart disease in women are that they have (1) a higher prevalence of angina, (2) a lower burden of obstructive coronary heart disease on angiography, and (3) a poorer prognosis in comparison to men.[121] Compared with men, women more commonly present with non-ST-segment elevation myocardial infarction. Women are also more likely to have unusual pathophysiological mechanisms of coronary artery disease such as spontaneous coronary artery dissection or coronary artery spasm.[121,130] Women are more likely to show ischaemia with no obstructive coronary arteries, although they report more chest pain compared to men.[121,125] However, sex differences may also have a different impact on traditional CVD risk factors. Diabetes is associated with higher ischaemic heart disease in women compared to men, even if risk factors are exclusive to women (e.g. pregnancy-related complications) or they mainly disadvantage women (e.g. depression).[123,125] After an acute coronary syndrome or coronary revascularization, women will spend longer in hospital, have higher in-hospital mortality, experience more bleeding complications, and have up to 30% more readmissions within 30 days after the index event compared to men.[123,125,128] Sex and gender disparities in acute coronary syndrome are presented in ➤ **Table 14.1**.

Heart failure

Chronic HF (see also Chapter 10) predominantly affects the elderly; its incidence doubles in men and triples in women with each decade after the age of 65 years.[130] Registries and studies indicate women are around 5 years older than men at the time of HF diagnosis[118,131] and more symptomatic, as indicated by a greater proportion of New York Heart Association class III or IV symptoms, present with more symptom burden, including more dyspnoea, bronchitis-like symptoms, oedema, fatigue, and worse health-related quality of life, despite similar clinical presentations and better left ventricular ejection fraction.[131,132]

Table 14.1 Sex and gender disparities in Acute Coronary Syndromes

MALE	Risk factors	FEMALE
Prior MI or stroke (more common) (123,125)	Age (121,125,127)	Age (older than men) (123,125,127)
Younger men have higher BMI, prior MI, increased incidence of dyslipidemia and more likely to smoke, drink alcohol (125)	hypertension, dyslipidemia, abdominal obesity, high risk diet diabetes, lack of regular physical activity, psychosocial factors, alcohol consumption (121,125,127)	**Increased correlation with coronary artery events** (125,127) Smoking Diabetes Psychosocial Factors
		Women Specific Cardiovascular Risk Factors (125,127) Contraceptive Induced Hypertension Gestational Diabetes Hypertensive pregnancy disorders (gestational Hypertension, pre-eclampsia) Persistence of weight gain after pregnancy Prophylactic salpingo-oophorectomy and Menopause Autoimmune diseases (e.g. rheumatoid arthritis and systematic lupus erythematosus) are more common. Radiation and chemotherapy for breast cancer.
		More comorbidities: diabetes, anemia, hypertension, renal impairment, heart Failure, CVD, COPD (125,127)
	Symptoms	
Chest pain is more intense. Fatigue, weakness described as "aching", "burning" or "dull" (125)	Chest pain (most common in both sexes) (127)	Back, neck, jaw pain, palpitations Chest Pain described as "crushing", "burning", "squeezing" or "tightness" (125)
	ECG	
Younger men (n≤55years old): anterior ST-segment depression (more common) (129)		N-STEMI (more common) Younger women (n≤55years old): anterior negative T waves (more common) (129)
	MINOCA	
		More common (121,125,130)
	DELAYS IN MEDICAL CARE	
		Longer delay in seeking emergency care (125)
	GUIDELINES BASED MANAGEMENT	
		Less likely to receive evidence-based treatment (125)

Table 14.1 Continued

MALE	Risk factors	FEMALE
	CORONARY INTERVENTIONS	
		Less likely to be referred to PCI
		Less likely to be referred to CABG
		Low risk women have better outcomes with a more conservative strategy
		Non-obstructive coronary artery disease (more frequent) More calcified lesions, smaller Vessel sizes Bleeding after PCI (more frequent in younger women) More complications after PCI (123,125)
		Higher all cause mortality after PCI for coronary artery disease (123,125)
		Higher readmission within 30 days after PCI due to cardiac reasons (123,125,128)

Some HF aetiologies are singular to women, such as peripartum cardiomyopathy, which can present up to 6 months after delivery and be confused with the early demands of an infant on the mother. Stress cardiomyopathy is also more common in women and comprises approximately 90% of cases and 80% of patients who present with spontaneous coronary artery dissection are female, and this should be considered in perimenopausal patients with chest pain.[132]

The complex comorbid profile of women with HF with increasing hypertension and obesity may partly explain the higher proportion of women diagnosed first in hospital, compared with men, and highlights an emerging trend for primary prevention that will require novel approaches to improve prognosis and health.[118] Also, the frequency of depression in HF in female patients is found to be more than double than in male patients.[131] Nevertheless, women are under-represented in most of the registries and trials[131–133] and the reasons remain unresolved. Possible explanations include women's or doctors' underestimation of cardiovascular symptoms in female patients and sociocultural difficulties faced by women in participating in clinical trials or registries. This discrepancy may be relevant in the applicability of evidence-based therapies to both sexes. For that reason, HF prevention and treatment need to be tailored to individual risk profiles and be person-centred based.

Heart failure with preserved ejection fraction

Women with HF who present tend to be older than men[43,131] and are approximately two times more likely than men to develop heart failure with preserved ejection fraction (HFpEF). The HFpEF phenotype is heterogeneous, encompassing various degrees of left ventricular systolic and diastolic function, pulmonary hypertension, and comorbid conditions. Specific risk factors for developing HFpEF include hypertension, obesity, and atrial fibrillation and common risk factors are ageing, adiposity, hypertension, and metabolic stress with impairments in cardiac, vascular, and peripheral reserve.[132] There is no single diagnostic test with adequate predictive characteristics for the diagnosis of HFpEF. Symptoms of HFpEF are often nonspecific, and thus, diagnosis is often supported with the addition of biomarkers, echocardiography, and right heart invasive catheterization. As this poorly understood entity disproportionately affects women, and particularly older women, it is in dire need of an individualized, person-centred, and holistic approach and care.

Peripartum cardiomyopathy

Peripartum is an idiopathic myocardial failure with onset in the puerperium and in the postpartum period[134] and is also known as pregnancy-associated cardiomyopathy.[135] Peripartum cardiomyopathy (PPCM) is defined as HF with unknown aetiology, with onset of symptoms in a period comprising the last month of pregnancy and the first 5 months postpartum,[134,136] although there are several risk factors associated with PPCM including multiple pregnancies, increasing parity, advanced maternal age, chronic hypertension, obesity, smoking, and genetics.[134]

Early signs and symptoms of PPCM may often mimic normal physiological findings of pregnancy such as pedal oedema, dyspnoea on exertion, orthopnoea, paroxysmal nocturnal dyspnoea, and persistent cough. Specific symptoms of PPCM are abdominal discomfort secondary to hepatic congestion, dizziness, precordial pain, and palpitations and in the later stages, postural hypotension. PPCM is a diagnosis of exclusion, thus all patients should have to undergo an investigation to identify any alternative aetiology of HF, considering all cardiac and non-cardiac causes of symptoms.[134]

The majority of women demonstrate a partial or complete recovery within 2–6 months after the diagnosis of PPCM and the treatment is the same as in acute HF.[127,134] Patients should be managed by a multidisciplinary team including cardiologists, obstetricians, neonatologists, nurses, and midwives.[134]

Other vascular diseases in women

Stroke

Stroke incidence, prevalence, and mortality are higher in men than women in developing countries, except in Arab countries in the Middle East and North Africa, where the stroke mortality is higher in women. In Israel, women have a higher stroke mortality than men, and in western Europe, the stroke incidence is higher or similar in women compared with men.[137] Nevertheless, studies are showing differences in incidence when comparing different groups of age; a higher incidence of all stroke in men compared with women up to age 74 years, but a higher incidence in women older than 74 years.[138–141] Individualized person-centred approach prevention is an important approach that focuses not only on genetics but also clinical data, environmental exposures, and lifestyle choices. Knowledge of differential susceptibility to risk factors informs the clinical management of patients to prevent the incidence and reduce the burden of stroke. The larger influence of both diabetes and heart disease on white women than for men, suggests that, compared with white men[138] additional clinical attention should be focused on these factors in white women to reduce their stroke risk. While the findings for systolic blood pressure and use of antihypertensive medications are complex, the larger magnitude of association for systolic blood pressure suggests that increased attention to achieving blood pressure control in white women may also be particularly important.[140]

Peripheral arterial disease

Peripheral arterial disease is a term used to describe atherosclerotic narrowing in arteries, other than coronary arteries and the aorta.[142] It is associated with equal morbidity and mortality to coronary artery disease and stroke and is associated with significantly reduced quality of life, increased functional disability, myocardial infarction, stroke, and death from cardiovascular and non-cardiovascular causes.[143] Females tend to be older and suffer from different or even atypical symptoms at the time of presentation compared with their male counterparts.[142,144] Intermittent claudication has been considered the hallmark feature of peripheral arterial disease, although women may often be asymptomatic, or present with atypical symptoms.[142,143] Women compared with men are also shown to be associated with increased risk of depression and cardiovascular mortality.[143] Thorough clinical history and physical examination are key steps in peripheral arterial disease management. The non-invasive ankle–brachial index can diagnose lower extremity peripheral arterial disease and is also a strong marker for cardiovascular events. The management of peripheral arterial disease includes all interventions to address specific arterial symptoms and general cardiovascular risk prevention.[142]

Abdominal aortic aneurysms

Abdominal aortic aneurysm is a condition characterized by dilatation of the abdominal aorta. It is the result of continues degradation of the structural components of the arterial wall. It is more common in men, develops later in women, but when established, appears to be more detrimental in women, who experience a higher risk of aneurysm rapture and a worse outcome after surgery than men. Nurses and other health professionals need to be aware that even though women are less likely to develop an abdominal aortic aneurysm, those who do fare worse than men.[145]

Management of women with cardiovascular diseases

New therapeutic treatments useful to men have not led to a significant decrease in CVD fatality rates in women, supporting the key role of sex/gender differences in determining CVD risk, diagnosis, and prognosis and explaining the existing gap in the progress achieved to treat CVD in women compared to men. Although milestone studies in the last few decades have allowed the development/optimization of actual standard care in the context of CVD by taking advantage of more accurate clinical tests that have allowed a better definition of the risks and benefits of effective prevention/therapies, the majority of these studies did not appropriately consider women.[125,146] Thus, much of the actual standard care available to test, prevent, and treat CVD in women can be considered a mere translation of the findings of studies conducted predominantly on middle-aged men, an approach that is inappropriate and risky given the emerging role of sex/gender differences in CVD pathophysiology.[147] Particular attention should also be paid to the transgender population. In light of the use of sex hormone treatments, this population needs careful consideration in order to address the real impact of therapies on metabolic profile, CVD risk, and other pathological conditions, such as diabetes, as well as to establish how tailored physical activity may decrease disease risk.[148]

The 'gap' of disparities in knowledge regarding CVD in women over men can be overcome through a sex/gender-based 'holistic' approach to disease pathophysiology, spanning from clinical signs and manifestations up to risk establishment, diagnosis definition, and dedicated person-centred approach treatment with the close collaboration of a broader interdisciplinary team including nurses, midwives, gynaecologists (who often is the first medical doctor or health professional a woman visits), general practitioners, cardiologists, and allied professionals. A focus on primary prevention of CVD is necessary to reduce CVD mortality and the overall CVD burden. Also, the development of clinical recommendations and sex-specific therapeutic strategies for CVD based on ad hoc and ad personam physical exercise approaches will contribute to a more focused approach on sex/gender disparities.[125,127,146]

Conclusion

CVD is the leading cause of death in women worldwide, even though it is not considered to be the greatest threat to women. Sex differences result in variations in prevalence and presentation of cardiovascular conditions, including those associated with autonomic regulation, hypertension, diabetes, and vascular and cardiac remodelling. The existence of crucial sex/gender-related differences in the prevalence, presentation, management, and outcomes of different CVDs means that women are less likely to receive guideline-directed care and counselling. The 'gap' of disparities in knowledge regarding CVD in women over men can be overcome through a sex/gender-based 'holistic' tailored approach by the interdisciplinary team including cardiology specialists, gynaecologists, and midwives. ➤ Box 14.6 summarizes the key factors on sex disparities.

Box 14.6 Key factors relating to women and sex disparities important for the awareness of nurses

- There are crucial sex/gender-related differences in the prevalence, presentation, management, and outcomes of different CVDs.
- A sex/gender-based 'holistic' approach by the interdisciplinary team focusing on primary prevention of CVD may be the key to reduce CVD mortality and the overall CVD burden.
- Biological variances result in variations in prevalence and presentation of cardiovascular conditions and also in the management and outcomes of different cardiovascular conditions.
- Women are more commonly presented with non-ST-segment elevation myocardial infarction, have ischaemia with no obstructive coronary arteries, and more often are underdiagnosed with HF due to the more complex multimorbidity profile—they are more likely to have heart failure with preserved ejection fraction.
- Existing therapies are controversial regarding their effectiveness in women. A more 'holistic' individual approach is needed in the context of an interdisciplinary team including midwives, gynaecologists, as well as the cardiology specialists.
- The need of primary prevention of CVD, focusing on sex-specific therapeutic strategies.

Conclusion

In this chapter we have explored some of the challenges that nurses and other professionals face in delivering high-quality holistic care to their patients. These were identified as frailty, multimorbidity, polypharmacy, the need for palliative and supportive care, and inequalities associated with sex and gender, social, and cultural factors. Much of this challenge arises from the presence of increasingly ageing populations living with non-communicable diseases. Principles for delivering holistic care in response to the challenges are as follows:

1. Care should be integrated, joined up, and well coordinated.
2. Care should be person/patient centred.
3. Care should strive to empower patients to self-manage with the support of their families and other carers.
4. Care should be organized around the convenience of patients, families, and other carers.
5. Every effort should be made to avoid discrimination in relation to culture and special circumstances.
6. Care should be offered to patients through an interdisciplinary team in an effort to meet all patients' needs.
7. Care must include continuing assessment through regular follow-ups or even more often depending on each patient in an effort to meet patients' needs, preferences, and values.
8. Taking care of women must always consider the sex- and gender-related differences and in some cases the interdisciplinary team must include midwives and gynaecologists.

References

1. Fried LP, Tangen CM, Walston J, Newman AB, Hirsch C, Gottdiener J, et al. Frailty in older adults: evidence for a phenotype. J Gerontol A Biol Sci Med Sci. 2001;56(3):M146–56.
2. Rockwood K, Abeysundera MJ, Mitnitski A. How should we grade frailty in nursing home patients? J Am Med Dir Assoc. 2007;8(9):595–603.
3. Mitnitski AB, Graham JE, Mogilner AJ, Rockwood K. Frailty, fitness and late-life mortality in relation to chronological and biological age. BMC Geriatr. 2002;2(1):1–8.
4. Abate M, Di Iorio A, Di Renzo D, Paganelli R, Saggini R, Abate G. Frailty in the elderly: the physical dimension. Eura Medicophys. 2007;43(3):407–15.
5. Hogan D, MacKnight C, Bergman H, Steering Committee, Canadian Initiative on Frailty and Aging. Models, definitions, and criteria of frailty. Aging Clin Exp Res. 2003;15(3 Suppl):1–29.
6. Grundy E. Ageing and vulnerable elderly people: European perspectives. Ageing Soc. 2006;26(1):105–34.
7. Aminzadeh F, Dalziel WB, Molnar FJ. Targeting frail older adults for outpatient comprehensive geriatric assessment and management services: an overview of concepts and criteria. Rev Clin Gerontol. 2002;12(1):82–92.
8. Lally F, Crome P. Understanding frailty. Postgrad Med J. 2007;83(975):16–20.
9. WHO Clinical Consortium on Healthy Ageing. Report of Consortium Meeting 1–2 December 2016 in Geneva, Switzerland. Geneva: World Health Organization; 2017.
10. Hallberg IR, Kristensson J. Preventive home care of frail older people: a review of recent case management studies. J Clin Nurs. 2004;13(6B):112–20.
11. Morley JE, Vellas B, Abellan van Kan G, Anker SD, Bauer JM, Bernabei R, et al. Frailty consensus: a call to action. J Am Med Dir Assoc. 2013;14(6):392–97.
12. Xue QL. The frailty syndrome: definition and natural history. Clin Geriatr Med. 2011;27(1):1–15.
13. Woo J, Goggins W, Sham A, Ho SC. Social determinants of frailty. Gerontology. 2005;51(6):402–408.
14. Rolfson DB, Majumdar SR, Tsuyuki RT, Tahir A, Rockwood K. Validity and reliability of the Edmonton Frail Scale. Age Ageing. 2006;35(5):526–29.
15. Ostir GV, Ottenbacher KJ, Markides KS. Onset of frailty in older adults and the protective role of positive affect. Psychol Aging. 2004;19(3):402–408.
16. Whitson HE, Purser JL, Cohen HJ. Frailty thy name is ... Phrailty? J Gerontol A Biol Sci Med Sci. 2007;62(7):728–30.
17. Rockwood K, Song X, MacKnight C, Bergman H, Hogan DB, McDowell I, et al. A global clinical measure of fitness and frailty in elderly people. CMAJ. 2005;173(5):489–95.
18. Slaets JPJ. Vulnerability in the elderly: frailty. Med Clin North Am. 2006;90(4):593–601.
19. Syddall H, Cooper C, Martin F, Briggs R, Sayer AA. Is grip strength a useful single marker of frailty? Age Ageing. 2003;32(6):650–56.
20. Dendukuri N, McCusker J, Belzile E. The Identification of Seniors At Risk Screening Tool: further evidence of concurrent and predictive validity. J Am Geriatr Soc. 2004;52(2):290–96.
21. Matthews M, Lucas A, Boland R, Hirth V, Odenheimer G, Wieland D, et al. Use of a questionnaire to screen for frailty in the elderly: an exploratory study. Aging Clin Exp Res. 2004;16(1):34–40.
22. Sager MA, Rudberg MA, Jalaluddin M, Franke T, Inouye SK, Seth Landefeld C, et al. Hospital Admission Risk Profile (HARP): identifying older patients at risk for functional decline following acute medical illness and hospitalization. J Am Geriatr Soc. 1996;44(3):251–57.
23. Min LC, Elliott MN, Wenger NS, Saliba D. Higher vulnerable elders survey scores predict death and functional decline in vulnerable older people. J Am Geriatr Soc. 2006;54(3):507–11.

24. Hébert R, Bravo G, Korner-Bitensky N, Voyer L. Predictive validity of a postal questionnaire for screening community-dwelling elderly individuals at risk of functional decline. Age Ageing. 1996;25(2):159–67.
25. Fan J, Worster A, Fernandes CMB. Predictive validity of the Triage Risk Screening Tool for elderly patients in a Canadian emergency department. Am J Emerg Med. 2006;24(5):540–44.
26. Uchmanowicz I, Lisiak M, Wontor R, Łoboz-Rudnicka M, Jankowska-Polańska B, Łoboz-Grudzień K, et al. Frailty syndrome in cardiovascular disease: clinical significance and research tools. Eur J Cardiovasc Nurs. 2015;14(4):303–309.
27. Uchmanowicz I, Nessler J, Gobbens R, Gackowski A, Kurpas D, Straburzynska-Migaj E, et al. Coexisting frailty with heart failure. Front Physiol. 2019;10:791.
28. Uchmanowicz I, Młynarska A, Lisiak M, Kałuzna-Oleksy M, Wleklik M, Chudiak A, et al. Heart failure and problems with frailty syndrome: why it is time to care about frailty syndrome in heart failure. Card Fail Rev. 2019;5(1):37–43.
29. Uchmanowicz I, Jankowska-Polańska B, Wleklik M, Lisiak M, Gobbens R. Frailty syndrome: nursing interventions. SAGE Open Nurs. 2018;4:1–11.
30. Whitty CJM, MacEwen C, Goddard A, Alderson D, Marshall M, Calderwood C, et al. Rising to the challenge of multimorbidity. BMJ. 2020;368:l6964.
31. Hajat C, Stein E. The global burden of multiple chronic conditions: a narrative review. Prev Med Reports. 2018;12:284–93.
32. Kendir C, van den Akker M, Vos R, Metsemakers J. Cardiovascular disease patients have increased risk for comorbidity: a cross-sectional study in the Netherlands. Eur J Gen Pract. 2018;24(1):45–50.
33. Bruce DG, Davis WA, Dragovic M, Davis TME, Starkstein SE. Comorbid anxiety and depression and their impact on cardiovascular disease in type 2 diabetes: the Fremantle Diabetes Study Phase II. Depress Anxiety. 2016;33(10):960–66.
34. Tripathy JP, Thakur JS, Jeet G, Jain S. Prevalence and determinants of comorbid diabetes and hypertension: evidence from non communicable disease risk factor STEPS survey, India. Diabetes Metab Syndr Clin Res Rev. 2017;11(S1):S459–65.
35. Ruiz-Laiglesia FJ, Sánchez-Marteles M, Pérez-Calvo JI, Formiga F, Bartolomé-Satué JA, Armengou-Arxé A, et al. Comorbidity in heart failure. Results of the Spanish RICA registry. QJM. 2014;107(12):989–94.
36. Tinetti ME, Fried TR, Boyd CM. Designing health care for the most common chronic condition—multimorbidity. JAMA. 2012;307(23):2493–94.
37. Thompson DR, Ski CF. Cardiovascular disease and mental health in men. In: Castle DJ, Coghill D (Eds), Comprehensive Men's Mental Health. Cambridge: Cambridge University Press; 2020:222–31.
38. Rahimi K, Lam CSP, Steinhubl S. Cardiovascular disease and multimorbidity: a call for interdisciplinary research and personalized cardiovascular care. PLoS Med. 2018;15(3):e1002545.
39. Murad K, Goff DC, Morgan TM, Burke GL, Bartz TM, Kizer JR, et al. Burden of comorbidities and functional and cognitive impairments in elderly patients at the initial diagnosis of heart failure and their impact on total mortality. The Cardiovascular Health Study. JACC Heart Fail. 2015;3(7):542–50.
40. Hall M, Dondo TB, Yan AT, Mamas MA, Timmis AD, Deanfield JE, et al. Multimorbidity and survival for patients with acute myocardial infarction in England and Wales: latent class analysis of a nationwide population-based cohort. PLoS Med. 2018;15(3):e1002501.
41. Vetrano DL, Rizzuto D, Calderón-Larrañaga A, Onder G, Welmer AK, Bernabei R, et al. Trajectories of functional decline in older adults with neuropsychiatric and cardiovascular multimorbidity: a Swedish cohort study. PLoS Med. 2018;15(3):e1002503.
42. Tran J, Norton R, Conrad N, Rahimian F, Canoy D, Nazarzadeh M, et al. Patterns and temporal trends of comorbidity among adult patients with incident cardiovascular disease in the UK between 2000 and 2014: a population-based cohort study. PLoS Med. 2018;15(3):e1002513.
43. Lawson CA, Solis-Trapala I, Dahlstrom U, Mamas M, Jaarsma T, Kadam UT, et al. Comorbidity health pathways in heart failure patients: a sequences-of-regressions analysis using cross-sectional data from 10,575 patients in the Swedish Heart Failure Registry. PLoS Med. 2018;15(3):e1002540.
44. Working Group on Health Outcomes for Older Persons with Multiple Chronic Conditions. Universal health outcome measures for older persons with multiple chronic conditions. J Am Geriatr Soc. 2012;60(12):2333–41.
45. Bennett WL, Robbins CW, Bayliss EA, Wilson R, Tabano H, Mularski RA, et al. Engaging stakeholders to inform clinical practice guidelines that address multiple chronic conditions. J Gen Intern Med. 2017;32(8):883–90.
46. American Geriatrics Society Expert Panel on the Care of Older Adults with Multimorbidity. Guiding principles for the care of older adults with multimorbidity: an approach for clinicians. J Am Geriatr Soc. 2012;60(10):E1–25.
47. Forman DE, Maurer MS, Boyd C, Brindis R, Salive ME, Horne FMF, et al. Multimorbidity in older adults with cardiovascular disease. J Am Coll Cardiol. 2018;71(19):2149–61.
48. National Institute for Health and Care Excellence. Multimorbidity: Clinical Assessment and Management.

NICE guidelines (NG56). London: National Institute for Health and Care Excellence; 2016.
49. Casimir YE, Williams MM, Liang MY, Pitakmongkolkul S, Slyer JT. The effectiveness of patient-centered self-care education for adults with heart failure on knowledge, self-care behaviors, quality of life, and readmissions: a systematic review. JBI Database Syst Rev Implement Rep. 2014;12(2):188–262.
50. Ekman I, Swedberg K, Taft C, Lindseth A, Norberg A, Brink E, et al. Person-centered care—ready for prime time. Eur J Cardiovasc Nurs. 2011;10(4):248–51.
51. Pirhonen L, Bolin K, Olofsson EH, Fors A, Ekman I, Swedberg K, et al. Person-centred care in patients with acute coronary syndrome: cost-effectiveness analysis alongside a randomised controlled trial. Pharmacoecon Open. 2019;3(4):495–504.
52. Sobanski PZ, Alt-Epping B, Currow DC, Goodlin SJ, Grodzicki T, Hogg K, et al. Palliative care for people living with heart failure: European Association for Palliative Care Task Force expert position statement. Cardiovasc Res. 2020;116(1):12–27.
53. Slawnych M. New dimensions in palliative care cardiology. Can J Cardiol. 2018;34(7):914–24.
54. Arnett DK, Blumenthal RS, Albert MA, Buroker AB, Goldberger ZD, Hahn EJ, et al. 2019 ACC/AHA guideline on the primary prevention of cardiovascular disease: a report of the American College of Cardiology/American Heart Association Task Force on Clinical Practice Guidelines. Circulation. 2019;74(10):1376–414.
55. Jennings C, Astin F. A multidisciplinary approach to prevention. Eur J Prev Cardiol. 2017;23(3 Suppl):77–87.
56. Leventhal ME, Denhaerynck K, Brunner-La Rocca HP, Burnand B, Conca A, Bernasconi AT, et al. Swiss Interdisciplinary Management programme for Heart Failure (SWIM-HF): a randomised controlled trial study of an outpatient inter-professional management programme for heart failure patients in Switzerland. Swiss Med Wkly. 2011;141:w13171.
57. Feltner C, Jones CD, Cené CW, Zheng ZJ, Sueta CA, Coker-Schwimmer EJL, et al. Transitional care interventions to prevent readmissions for persons with heart failure: a systematic review and meta-analysis. Ann Intern Med. 2014;160(11):774–84.
58. Moertl D, Altenberger J, Bauer N, Berent R, Berger R, Boehmer A, et al. Disease management programs in chronic heart failure: position statement of the Heart Failure Working Group and the Working Group of the Cardiological Assistance and Care Personnel of the Austrian Society of Cardiology. Wien Klin Wochenschr. 2017;129(23–24):869–78.
59. Ponikowski P, Voors AA, Anker SD, Bueno H, Cleland JGF, Coats AJS, et al. 2016 ESC Guidelines for the diagnosis and treatment of acute and chronic heart failure: the Task Force for the diagnosis and treatment of acute and chronic heart failure of the European Society of Cardiology (ESC). Developed with the special contribution of the Heart Failure Association (HFA) of the ESC. Eur J Heart Fail. 2016;37(27):2129–200.
60. Buck HG, Hoyt Zambroski C. Upstreaming palliative care for patients with heart failure. J Cardiovasc Nurs. 2012;27(2):147–53.
61. Kaufman G. Polypharmacy: the challenge for nurses. Nurs Stand. 2016;30(39):52–58.
62. Duerden M, Avery T, Payne R. Polypharmacy and medicines optimisation: making it safe and sound. The King's Fund; 2013. https://www.kingsfund.org.uk/publications/polypharmacy-and-medicines-optimisation.
63. Olivier P, Bertrand L, Tubery M, Lauque D, Montastruc JL, Lapeyre-Mestre M. Hospitalizations because of adverse drug reactions in elderly patients admitted through the emergency department: a prospective survey. Drugs Aging. 2009;26(6):475–82.
64. Dumbreck S, Flynn A, Nairn M, Wilson M, Treweek S, Mercer SW, et al. Drug-disease and drug-drug interactions: systematic examination of recommendations in 12 UK national clinical guidelines. BMJ. 2015;350:h949.
65. Lindblad CI, Hanlon JT, Gross CR, Sloane RJ, Pieper CF, Hajjar ER, et al. Clinically important drug-disease interactions and their prevalence in older adults. Clin Ther. 2006;28(8):1133–43.
66. National Institute for Health and Care Excellence. Medicines Adherence: Involving Patients in Decisions About Prescribed Medicines and Supporting Adherence. Clinical guidelines (CG76). London: National Institute for Health and Care Excellence; 2009.
67. Volpe M, Chin D, Paneni F. The challenge of polypharmacy in cardiovascular medicine. Fundam Clin Pharmacol. 2010;24(1):9–17.
68. World Health Organization. Cardiovascular diseases. 2017. https://www.who.int/health-topics/cardiovascular-diseases/#tab=tab_1.
69. National Institute for Health and Care Excellence. NICE impact: cardiovascular disease prevention. 2018. https://www.nice.org.uk/media/default/about/what-we-do/into-practice/measuring-uptake/nice-impact-cardiovascular-disease-prevention.pdf.
70. Cosentino F, Grant PJ, Aboyans V, Bailey CJ, Ceriello A, Delgado V, et al. 2019 ESC Guidelines on diabetes, pre-diabetes, and cardiovascular diseases developed in collaboration with the EASD. Eur Heart J. 2020;41(2):255–323.
71. Unlu O, Dharamdasani T, Archambault A, Diaz I, Chen L, Levitan E, et al. Polypharmacy increases in prevalence and severity following a heart failure hospitalization. J Am Coll Cardiol. 2019;73(9S1):789.

72. Shaikh F, Pasch LB, Newton PJ, Bajorek BV, Ferguson C. Addressing multimorbidity and polypharmacy in individuals with atrial fibrillation. Curr Cardiol Rep. 2018;20(5):32.
73. Bayliss EA, Edwards AE, Steiner JF, Main DS. Processes of care desired by elderly patients with multimorbidities. Fam Pract. 2008;25(4):287–93.
74. Ulley J, Harrop D, Ali A, Alton S, Fowler Davis S. Deprescribing interventions and their impact on medication adherence in community-dwelling older adults with polypharmacy: a systematic review. BMC Geriatr. 2019;19(1):15.
75. World Health Organization. WHO definition of palliative care. 2009. http://www.who.int/cancer/palliative/en/.
76. Hupcey JE. The state of palliative care and heart failure. Heart Lung J Acute Crit Care. 2012;41(6):529–30.
77. Fitzsimons D, Mullan D, Wilson JS, Conway B, Corcoran B, Dempster M, et al. The challenge of patients' unmet palliative care needs in the final stages of chronic illness. Palliat Med. 2007;21(4):313–22.
78. Howlett JG. Palliative care in heart failure: addressing the largest care gap. Curr Opin Cardiol. 2011;26(2):144–48.
79. Kyriakou M, Middleton N, Ktisti S, Philippou K, Lambrinou E. Supportive care interventions to promote health-related quality of life in patients living with heart failure: a systematic review and meta-analysis. Heart Lung Circ. 2020;29(11):1633–47.
80. Klastersky J, Libert I, Michel B, Obiols M, Lossignol D. Supportive/palliative care in cancer patients: quo vadis? Support Care Cancer. 2016;24(4):1883–88.
81. Goodlin SJ, Hauptman PJ, Arnold R, Grady K, Hershberger RE, Kutner J, et al. Consensus statement: palliative and supportive care in advanced heart failure. J Card Fail. 2004;10(3):200–209.
82. Jaarsma T, Beattie JM, Ryder M, Rutten FH, McDonagh T, Mohacsi P, et al. Palliative care in heart failure: a position statement from the palliative care workshop of the Heart Failure Association of the European Society of Cardiology. Eur J Heart Fail. 2009;11(5):433–43.
83. Kavalieratos D, Gelfman LP, Tycon LE, Riegel B, Bekelman DB, Ikejiani DZ, et al. Palliative care in heart failure: rationale, evidence, and future priorities. J Am Coll Cardiol. 2017;70(15):1919–30.
84. Rietjens JAC, Sudore RL, Connolly M, van Delden JJ, Drickamer MA, Droger M, et al. Definition and recommendations for advance care planning: an international consensus supported by the European Association for Palliative Care. Lancet Oncol. 2017;18(9):e543–51.
85. Marinskis G, Van Erven L. Deactivation of implanted cardioverter-defibrillators at the end of life: results of the EHRA survey. Europace. 2010;12(8):1176–77.
86. Caldwell PH, Arthur HM, Demers C. Preferences of patients with heart failure for prognosis communication. Can J Cardiol. 2007;23(10):791–96.
87. Hill L, McIlfatrick S, Taylor BJ, Jaarsma T, Moser D, Slater P, et al. Patient and professional factors that impact the perceived likelihood and confidence of healthcare professionals to discuss implantable cardioverter defibrillator deactivation in advanced heart failure. J Cardiovasc Nurs. 2018;33(6):527–35.
88. Brännström M, Boman K. Effects of person-centred and integrated chronic heart failure and palliative home care. PREFER: a randomized controlled study. Eur J Heart Fail. 2014;16(10):1142–51.
89. Rogers JG, Patel CB, Mentz RJ, Granger BB, Steinhauser KE, Fiuzat M, et al. Palliative care in heart failure: the PAL-HF randomized, controlled clinical trial. J Am Coll Cardiol. 2017;70(3):331–41.
90. O'Donnell AE, Schaefer KG, Stevenson LW, Devoe K, Walsh K, Mehra MR, et al. Social worker-aided palliative care intervention in high-risk patients with heart failure (SWAP-HF). A pilot randomized clinical trial. JAMA Cardiol. 2018;3(6):516–19.
91. Hjelmfors L, Strömberg A, Friedrichsen M, Sandgren A, Mårtensson J, Jaarsma T. Using co-design to develop an intervention to improve communication about the heart failure trajectory and end-of-life care. BMC Palliat Care. 2018;17(1):85.
92. Center to Advance Palliative Care. CAPC COVID-19 response resources. http://www.capc.org/toolkits/covid-19-response-resources.
93. Callander EJ, McDermott R. Measuring the effects of CVD interventions and studies across socioeconomic groups: a brief review. Int J Cardiol. 2017;227:635–43.
94. Stringhini S, Carmeli C, Jokela M, Avendaño M, Muennig P, Guida F, et al. LIFEPATH consortium. Socioeconomic status and the 25 × 25 risk factors as determinants of premature mortality: a multicohort study and meta-analysis of 1.7 million men and women. Lancet. 2017;389(10075):1229–37.
95. Schultz WM, Kelli HM, Lisko JC, Varghese T, Shen J, Sandesara P, et al. Socioeconomic status and cardiovascular outcomes: challenges and interventions. Circulation. 2018;137:2166–78.
96. Marmot M, Friel S, Bell R, Houweling TA, Taylor S. Closing the gap in a generation: health equity through action on the social determinants of health. Lancet. 2008;372(9650):1661–69.
97. Parikh PB, Yang J, Leigh S, Dorjee K, Parikh R, Sakellarios N, et al. The impact of financial barriers on access to care, quality of care and vascular morbidity among patients with diabetes and coronary heart disease. J Gen Intern Med. 2014;29(1):76–81.
98. Yong CM, Abnousi F, Asch SM, Heidenreich PA. Socioeconomic inequalities in quality of care and

outcomes among patients with acute coronary syndrome in the modern era of drug eluting stents. J Am Heart Assoc. 2014;3(6):e001029.
99. Hanley GE, Morgan S, Reid RJ. Income-related inequity in initiation of evidence-based therapies among patients with acute myocardial infarction. J Gen Intern Med. 2011;26(11):1329–35.
100. Resurrección DM, Moreno-Peral P, Gómez-Herranz M, Rubio-Valera M, Pastor L, Caldas de Almeida JM, et al. Factors associated with non-participation in and dropout from cardiac rehabilitation programmes: a systematic review of prospective cohort studies. Eur J Cardiovasc Nurs. 2019;18(1):38–47.
101. Yusuf S, Joseph P, Rangarajan S, Islam S, Mente A, Hystad P, et al. Modifiable risk factors, cardiovascular disease, and mortality in 155 722 individuals from 21 high-income, middle-income, and low-income countries (PURE): a prospective cohort study. Lancet. 2020;395(10226):795–808.
102. Havranek EP, Mujahid MS, Barr DA, Blair I V, Cohen MS, Cruz-Flores S, et al. Social determinants of risk and outcomes for cardiovascular disease: a scientific statement from the American Heart Association. Circulation. 2015;132(9):873–98.
103. Cajita MI, Cajita TR, Han HR. Health literacy and heart failure a systematic review. J Cardiovasc Nurs. 2016;31(2):121–30.
104. Ghisi GL de M, Chaves GS da S, Britto RR, Oh P. Health literacy and coronary artery disease: a systematic review. Patient Educ Couns. 2018;101(2):177–84.
105. Bruthans J, Mayer O, De Bacquer D, De Smedt D, Reiner Z, Kotseva K, et al. Educational level and risk profile and risk control in patients with coronary heart disease. Eur J Prev Cardiol. 2016;23(8):881–90.
106. Kreatsoulas C, Anand SS. The impact of social determinants on cardiovascular disease. Can J Cardiol. 2010;26:8C–13C.
107. Kollia N, Panagiotakos DB, Georgousopoulou E, Chrysohoou C, Tousoulis D, Stefanadis C, et al. Exploring the association between low socioeconomic status and cardiovascular disease risk in healthy Greeks, in the years of financial crisis (2002–2012): the ATTICA study. Int J Cardiol. 2016;223:758–63.
108. Protopapas A, Lambrinou E. Cultural factors and the circadian rhythm of ST elevation myocardial infarction in patients in a Mediterranean island. Eur J Cardiovasc Nurs. 2019;18(7):562–68.
109. Brewer LPC, Cooper LA. Race, discrimination, and cardiovascular disease. Virtual Mentor. 2014;16(6):455–60.
110. Jaarsma T, Strömberg A, Ben Gal T, Cameron J, Driscoll A, Duengen HD, et al. Comparison of self-care behaviors of heart failure patients in 15 countries worldwide. Patient Educ Couns. 2013;92(1):114–20.
111. Benson J, Maldari T, Williams J, Hanifi H. The impact of culture and ethnicity on women's perceived role in society and their attendant health beliefs. InnovAiT Educ Inspir Gen Pract. 2010;3:358–65.
112. Rashid M, Fischman DL, Gulati M, Tamman K, Potts J, Kwok CS, et al. Temporal trends and inequalities in coronary angiography utilization in the management of non-ST-elevation acute coronary syndromes in the U.S. Sci Rep. 2019;9(1):1–4.
113. Gudnadottir GS, Andersen K, Thrainsdottir IS, James SK, Lagerqvist B, Gudnason T. Gender differences in coronary angiography, subsequent interventions, and outcomes among patients with acute coronary syndromes. Am Heart J. 2017;191:65–74.
114. Gargiulo G, Ariotti S, Santucci A, Piccolo R, Baldo A, Franzone A, et al. Impact of sex on 2-year clinical outcomes in patients treated with 6-month or 24-month dual-antiplatelet therapy duration: a pre-specified analysis from the PRODIGY Trial. JACC Cardiovasc Interv. 2016;9(17):1780–89.
115. Araújo C, Pereira M, Laszczyńska O, Dias P, Azevedo A. Sex-related inequalities in management of patients with acute coronary syndrome—results from the EURHOBOP study. Int J Clin Pract. 2018;72(1):e13049.
116. Alabas OA, Gale CP, Hall M, Rutherford MJ, Szummer K, Lawesson SS, et al. Sex differences in treatments, relative survival, and excess mortality following acute myocardial infarction: national cohort study using the SWEDEHEART registry. J Am Heart Assoc. 2017;6(12):e007123.
117. Wilkinson C, Bebb O, Dondo TB, Munyombwe T, Casadei B, Clarke S, et al. Sex differences in quality indicator attainment for myocardial infarction: a nationwide cohort study. Heart. 2019;105(7):516–23.
118. Lawson CA, Zaccardi F, Squire I, Okhai H, Davies M, Huang W, et al. Risk factors for heart failure: 20-year population-based trends by sex, socioeconomic status, and ethnicity. Circ Heart Fail. 2020;13(2):e006472.
119. Canto JG, Rogers WJ, Goldberg RJ, Peterson ED, Wenger NK, Vaccarino V, et al. Association of age and sex with myocardial infarction symptom presentation and in-hospital mortality. JAMA. 2012;307(8):813–22.
120. Steinberg BA, Zhao X, Heidenreich PA, Peterson ED, Bhatt DL, Cannon CP, et al. Trends in patients hospitalized with heart failure and preserved left ventricular ejection fraction: prevalence, therapies, and outcomes. Circulation. 2012;126(1):65–75.
121. Vaccarezza M, Papa V, Milani D, Gonelli A, Secchiero P, Zauli G, et al. Sex/gender-specific imbalance in CVD: could physical activity help to improve clinical outcome targeting CVD molecular mechanisms in women? Int J Mol Sci. 2020;21(4):1477.
122. European Society of Cardiology. Cardiovascular disease kills 51% of women in Europe and breast

cancer kills 3%. 2015. https://www.escardio.org/The-ESC/Press-Office/Press-releases/Cardiovascular-disease-kills-51-of-women-in-Europe-and-breast-cancer-kills-3.

123. Ma Q, Wang J, Jin J, Gao M, Liu F, Zhou S, et al. Clinical characteristics and prognosis of acute coronary syndrome in young women and men: a systematic review and meta-analysis of prospective studies. Int J Cardiol. 2017;228:837–43.
124. Safdar B, Nagurney JT, Anise A, Devon HA, D'Onofrio G, Hess EP, et al. Gender-specific research for emergency diagnosis and management of ischemic heart disease: proceedings from the 2014 academic emergency medicine consensus conference cardiovascular research workgroup. Acad Emerg Med. 2014;21(12):1350–60.
125. Davis E, Gorog DA, Rihal C, Prasad A, Srinivasan M. "Mind the gap" acute coronary syndrome in women: a contemporary review of current clinical evidence. Int J Cardiol. 2017;227:840–49.
126. Meyer MR, Bernheim AM, Kurz DJ, O'Sullivan CJ, Tüller D, Zbinden R, et al. Gender differences in patient and system delay for primary percutaneous coronary intervention: current trends in a Swiss ST-segment elevation myocardial infarction population. Eur Heart J Acute Cardiovasc Care. 2019;8(3):283–90.
127. Garcia M, Mulvagh SL, Merz CNB, Buring JE, Manson JAE. Cardiovascular disease in women: clinical perspectives. Circ Res. 2016;118(8):1273–93.
128. Mehta LS, Beckie TM, DeVon HA, Grines CL, Krumholz HM, Johnson MN, et al. Acute myocardial infarction in women a scientific statement from the American Heart Association. Circulation. 2016;133(9):916–47.
129. Barrabés JA, Gupta A, Porta-Sánchez A, Strait KM, Acosta-Vélez JG, D'Onofrio G, et al. Comparison of electrocardiographic characteristics in men versus women ≤ 55 years with acute myocardial infarction (a Variation in Recovery: Role of Gender on Outcomes of Young Acute Myocardial Infarction Patients substudy). Am J Cardiol. 2017;120(10):1727–33.
130. Vaccarino V, Badimon L, Corti R, De Wit C, Dorobantu M, Hall A, et al. Ischaemic heart disease in women: are there sex differences in pathophysiology and risk factors? Position Paper from the Working Group on Coronary Pathophysiology and Microcirculation of the European Society of Cardiology. Cardiovasc Res. 2011;90(1):9–17.
131. Lainšcak M, Milinkovic I, Polovina M, Crespo-Leiro MG, Lund LH, Anker S, et al. Sex- and age-related differences in the management and outcomes of chronic heart failure: an analysis of patients from the ESC HFA EORP Heart Failure Long-Term Registry. Eur J Heart Fail. 2020;22(1):92–102.
132. Eisenberg E, Di Palo KE, Piña IL. Sex differences in heart failure. Clin Cardiol. 2018;41(2):211–16.
133. Martínez-Sellés M, Doughty RN, Poppe K, Whalley GA, Earle N, Tribouilloy C, et al. Gender and survival in patients with heart failure: Interactions with diabetes and aetiology. Results from the MAGGIC individual patient meta-analysis. Eur J Heart Fail. 2012;14(5):473–79.
134. Azibani F, Sliwa K. Peripartum cardiomyopathy: an update. Curr Heart Fail Rep. 2018;15(5):297–306.
135. Elkayam U, Akhter MW, Singh H, Khan S, Bitar F, Hameed A, et al. Pregnancy-associated cardiomyopathy: clinical characteristics and a comparison between early and late presentation. Circulation. 2005;111(16):2050–55.
136. Pearson GD, Veille JC, Rahimtoola S, Hsia J, Oakley CM, Hosenpud JD, et al. Peripartum cardiomyopathy: National Heart, Lung, and Blood Institute and Office of Rare Diseases (National Institutes of Health) workshop recommendations and review. JAMA. 2000;283(9):1183–88.
137. Christensen H, Bushnell C. Stroke in women. Contin Lifelong Learn Neurol. 2020;26(2):363–85.
138. Aboyans V, Ricco JB, Bartelink MLEL, Björck M, Brodmann M, Cohnert T, et al. 2017 ESC Guidelines on the diagnosis and treatment of peripheral arterial diseases, in collaboration with the European Society for Vascular Surgery (ESVS). Eur Heart J. 2018;39(9):763–816.
139. Howard VJ, Madsen TE, Kleindorfer DO, Judd SE, Rhodes JD, Soliman EZ, et al. Sex and race differences in the association of incident ischemic stroke with risk factors. JAMA Neurol. 2019;76(2):179–86.
140. Madsen TE, Khoury J, Alwell K, Moomaw CJ, Rademacher E, Flaherty ML, et al. Sex-specific stroke incidence over time in the Greater Cincinnati/Northern Kentucky Stroke Study. Neurology. 2017;89(10):990–96.
141. Petrea RE, Beiser AS, Seshadri S, Kelly-Hayes M, Kase CS, Wolf PA. Gender differences in stroke incidence and poststroke disability in the Framingham Heart Study. Stroke. 2009;40(4):1032–37.
142. Sacco RL, Boden-Albala B, Gan R, Chen X, Kargman DE, Shea S, et al. Stroke incidence among white, black, and Hispanic residents of an urban community: the Northern Manhattan Stroke Study. Am J Epidemiol. 1998;147(3):259–68.
143. Patel T, Baydoun H, Patel NK, Tripathi B, Nanavaty S, Savani S, et al. Peripheral arterial disease in women: the gender effect. Cardiovasc Revascularization Med. 2020;21(3):404–408.
144. Behrendt CA, Bischoff MS, Schwaneberg T, Hohnhold R, Diener H, Debus ES, et al. Population based analysis of gender disparities in 23,715 percutaneous

endovascular revascularisations in the Metropolitan Area of Hamburg. Eur J Vasc Endovasc Surg. 2019;57(5):658–65.
145. Desai M, Choke E, Sayers RD, Nath M, Bown MJ. Sex-related trends in mortality after elective abdominal aortic aneurysm surgery between 2002 and 2013 at National Health Service hospitals in England: Less benefit for women compared with men. Eur Heart J. 2016;37(46):3452–60.
146. Collet JP, Thiele H, Barbato E, Barthélémy O, Bauersachs J, Bhatt DL, et al. 2020 ESC Guidelines for the management of acute coronary syndromes in patients presenting without persistent ST-segment elevation. Eur Heart J. 2021;42(14):1289–367.
147. Brown HL, Warner JJ, Gianos E, Gulati M, Hill AJ, Hollier LM, et al. Promoting risk identification and reduction of cardiovascular disease in women through collaboration with obstetricians and gynecologists: a presidential advisory from the American Heart Association and the American College of Obstetricians and Gynecologists. Circulation. 2018;137(24):e843–52.
148. O'Neil A, Scovelle AJ, Milner AJ, Kavanagh A. Gender/sex as a social determinant of cardiovascular risk. Circulation. 2018;137(8):854–64.

15 Looking forward: the future of cardiovascular care

DAVID R. THOMPSON, LIS NEUBECK, AND ROBYN GALLAGHER

CHAPTER CONTENTS

KEY MESSAGES

- Cardiovascular care is evolving rapidly in an era of unprecedented demand.
- Nurses are caring for a growing number of people who are older, present with multiple chronic conditions, and are socially isolated.
- There is public, political, economic, and professional pressure to work effectively and efficiently, ensuring value for money, and better patient outcomes and experience.
- Health services aim to keep people out of hospital; reduce waiting times and hospital stays; speed up, shorten, and avoid duplication of diagnostics, treatments, and clinic visits; and ensure care is patient centred and coordinated.
- Healthcare should be responsive and patient driven with staff thinking creatively, working smartly, and exploiting technology and other resources appropriately, taking account of patient and family needs, values, choices, and preferences.

Introduction

The cardiovascular care landscape is changing rapidly, more so now than at any other time. This is typified by quicker and shorter diagnosis, access, treatment, and aftercare due to a host of factors including increased knowledge, expectations, and demands among the public and health professionals, and rapid advances in science and technology. The patient journey, experience, and outcome nowadays are vastly different from even 10–20 years ago. For example, patient and health professional access to information is immediate, though the validity of some of this information may be questionable, so patients and families need to be pointed to reliable sources. This is even more pressing when patients are living longer and also presenting with more than one chronic health condition. It is not uncommon nowadays to see a patient with cardiovascular disease (CVD) also present with diabetes, a respiratory disease, or a mental illness. This presents many challenges to nurses working in cardiovascular care, an environment that is changing rapidly and is characterized by complexity, uncertainty, and unpredictability. Thus, nurses are being expected to work smartly and be more responsive, flexible, lean, and agile.

If nurses are to provide the best care, it is important that they keep abreast of developments in their own field and those of the social, behavioural, mathematical, engineering, and clinical sciences, recognizing their potential application to cardiovascular care (from CVD prevention, management, rehabilitation, and aftercare to palliative care). For instance, in terms of the social and behavioural sciences, nurses need to learn how better to engage and communicate with patients, families, and the public about their risks for CVD and the options for preventing and managing it, including how to tackle misconceptions and fear and avoid stigmatization. Rapid developments in science and technology are enabling a shift in cardiovascular care towards a more predictive, preventive, and personalized approach, where patients are truly leading their care, supported by nurses and easily accessible online applications that take advantage of artificial intelligence (AI).

Technology and digital health

Technology is being used across the whole spectrum of cardiovascular care including detection, monitoring, and treatment. Smartphone apps are rapidly being developed and applied for lifestyle modifications in CVD such as addressing obesity, physical inactivity, poor diet, and smoking.[1] These technologies can be quite simple, such as involving simple mobile text messaging, through tracking activities and measuring data such as the number of steps walked, heart rate, and quality of sleep, and using smartwatches to monitor heart rhythm, take an electrocardiogram, and detect atrial fibrillation.[2] Indeed, they can be used to detect acute coronary occlusion.[3] Whatever type of technology is used, its purpose, benefits, and potential harms need to be explained to the patient and their family.

The evidence base for using technology to enhance care is large, complex, and growing rapidly. Despite concerns that technology might supplant humans, this is unlikely in the foreseeable future. Rather, technology should be embraced as an adjunct to human interaction between the nurse and patient and an aid to the nurse providing care. Care is increasingly delivered in the home and technology is being used for social connectivity, independence, and emotional support. Wearable technologies combined with video encounters with nurses create new, convenient, and more realistic points of care. This approach particularly lends itself to certain clinical scenarios such as cardiac rehabilitation and secondary prevention programmes and heart failure management clinics.

Often the most important drivers for successful long-term behavioural change are a strong relationship between the patient and nurse together with collaborative eHealth tools.[4]

eHealth—health services and information delivered or enhanced through the Internet and related technologies[5]—encompasses the provision of health-related services, hardware devices, and software such as use of the Internet, Bluetooth devices, remote monitoring devices, wearable devices, text messages, and smartphone apps.[6]

Such tools are likely to be most effective if they facilitate one-to-one consultations, personalized lifestyle plans, coaching, self-monitoring and tracking, peer-to-peer support, and reminders and notifications. The combined effect of convenient, powerful digital technology and the motivation of frequent human-to-human interaction is likely to be more effective than either of these components alone.

Recent eHealth interventions have been shown to support positive behaviour and lifestyle change in reducing CVD such as increasing physical activity[7] and reducing weight,[8] and appear to have the potential to improve cardiovascular risk profiles.[9]

eHealth interventions offer tremendous potential for patient engagement and to support CVD care and can overcome the barriers of distance, capacity, and resources while being simple and meaningful.[10] An added appeal of using eHealth approaches is to support the partner (who is often the informal carer) who may have similar or more distress than the patient. Poor partner health may compromise their ability to carry out their carer role and partners may lack information about CVD and the expectations of their role, which can lead to worry and uncertainty. Targeting both the patient and partner ensures that they receive the same information and support, thus maximizing retention and minimizing possible misinterpretation; facilitates sharing the emotional burden; and provides social support, bolsters confidence, instils hope, and encourages the patient to seek healthcare, attend cardiac rehabilitation, and adhere to lifestyle plans and medications.

However, although these technologies have much to offer, they are often not used optimally and may provide information that appears redundant or of limited relevance to nurses; thus, nurses need to know what type of information is required and how and when to use it. Also, mobile health technologies (mHealth) can deliver interventions to prevent and manage CVD, but despite the high prevalence of smartphone ownership, mHealth uptake among those with or at risk of CVD is unclear.[11] ➤ **Box 15.1** includes a case study of a patient after an acute cardiac event which outlines the care pathway and the role that technology could play.

Artificial intelligence

AI is the simulation of human intelligence processes by machines, especially computers. It is a rapidly evolving field and is revolutionizing health, including cardiovascular care, especially in terms of risk prediction and

Box 15.1 The role of technology in cardiovascular care—the future is now: a case study

Alex is a cardiac nurse coordinator working in the near future. He meets Dora, his new patient, via his personal device. Dora is a 51-year-old woman whose wearable tracker picked up that her heart rate was a bit fast. Dora was experiencing what she thought was indigestion. She sat down and rested and noticed that her discomfort was increasing. She sent an instant message to emergency services. Alex began receiving information when the emergency services data system recognized that her symptoms, electrocardiogram, vital signs as recorded by a fitted sensing fabric, and troponin elevation as noted by point-of-care testing provided a high-risk diagnosis of acute coronary syndrome. Alex approved the system to trigger Dora's rapid access to the cardiac catheterization laboratory (cath lab) for diagnostic angiograms and potential angioplasty and stent. He was also able to approve a trigger to the cath lab to transmit data which provided the size of the catheter and risks that would have to be managed specific to Dora.

Alex then notified the cardiology consultant via his personal device. The consultant then began a preliminary real-time discussion with Dora via video link about the potential procedure and consent processes while she was in transit. Alex also ensured that the consultant was linked to immediate family to discuss their concerns regarding Dora's diagnosis and treatment. Once the family was comfortable with the information that was provided, Alex discussed future care needs so that he could plan for Dora's discharge.

Emergency services signalled their arrival via location mapping of their imminent arrival to the cath lab rapid entrance. Bed management systems were alerted to ensure that beds and staffing were also available. Simultaneously, the cardiac nursing team were alerted and a care plan was generated that was personally tailored for Dora based on her data.

During the cath lab angiogram and intervention, as data were generated an individualized medical treatment plan was created. Genomic data was also collected which enabled identification of medication effects that were personalized to Dora's profile so that dosing was individually tailored and accommodated Dora's existing hypertension and type 2 diabetes. This enabled the pharmacists to ensure that appropriate medications were dispensed.

On the ward, Alex was able to prepare the staff for Dora's arrival. A smart bed was provided that would monitor Dora's vital signs and any signs of distress to enable Alex to ensure that Dora's care was matched to the most appropriate times for her sleep and would minimize disturbance from routine monitoring. Cardiovascular prevention and rehabilitation was alerted to enable development of a tailored personalized programme for Dora. Nurses recorded voice notes after providing Dora's personal care, which helped create a more individual picture of Dora's personal situation so that when the multidisciplinary team met with Dora, a very effective personally appropriate plan could be determined for discharge. In addition, Dora's medications in hospital were stored in a secure bedside unit that could track when medication should be dispensed and the dose required, and record when the medications had been appropriately taken. Dora and her nurse had a discussion about whether Dora would like to be responsible for her medications herself or whether she would prefer the nursing staff to support her. The locker holding the medications was enabled with facial recognition and fingerprint confirmation so that only authorized people, either Dora, her nurse, or the pharmacist, could access the locker.

(continued)

Box 15.1 Continued

In discussion with Dora, Alex noted that she was having difficulty managing her type 2 diabetes. Alex recommended a wearable tracker with individualized sensing of blood glucose levels to help Dora understand the effect of her diet on her diabetes. This data would be transferred to Dora's diabetes educator who will arrange a transition plan to support her diabetes management. In addition, the genomic information helped to identify the effects of different types of nutrition on Dora's health, enabling the dietitian to help Dora tailor a personalized nutrition plan. The system generated a flag that reminded her consultant to discuss genetic risk with Dora's family. In preparation for discharge, Dora's information was shared electronically with the community pharmacist, her general practitioner, and other important members of the social care team who will be supporting Dora with her long-term management.

At the centre of this technology, data systems, and healthcare professional's work was Dora (➤ Fig. 15.1). Her records were personally controlled and she was able to make the decision about access to her data at every point of her care. Like many others, Dora was willing to share health data as long as her privacy was ensured and her data was used to improve her health. This meant that Alex had to be aware of the cyber security risks of using large datasets and ensure that appropriate measures were taken to protect Dora's data at every stage of her journey.

When Dora was ready to go home, Alex arranged for the cardiovascular prevention and rehabilitation team to have a virtual meeting with Dora. Dora was provided with a mobile app that integrated information from her wearable device and provided her with personally tailored multidisciplinary support. Dora was offered a menu-based suite of options for cardiovascular prevention and rehabilitation. Because she did not feel confident exercising, Dora decided to go to a women-only cardiac dance programme which was supported with an online and social networking site. The social networking included support from healthcare professionals and Dora's peers. Dora's family were able to participate in every aspect of her care as and when Dora enabled access and were strongly encouraged to attend the integrated multimorbidity cardiovascular prevention and rehabilitation programme with her. In wrapping up Dora's treatment and clinical journey, her data including

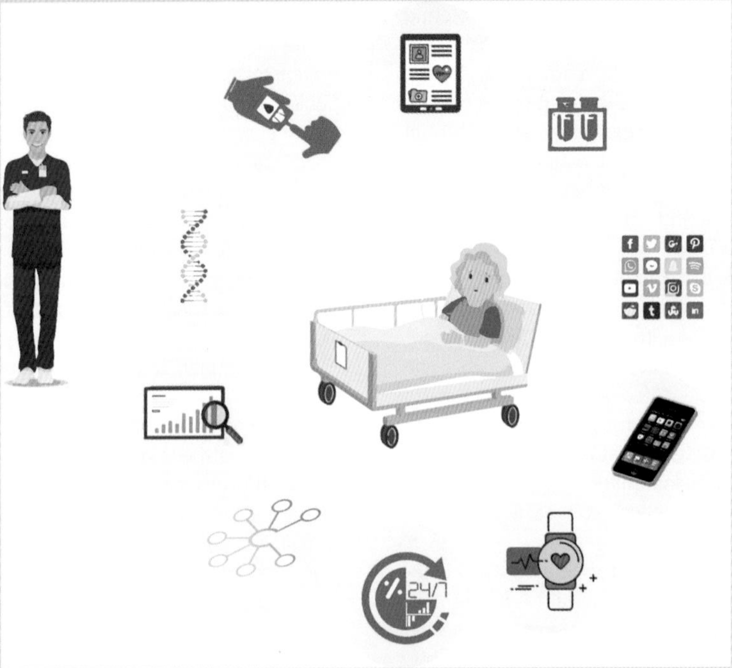

Fig. 15.1 Digital health with the patient at the centre.

Box 15.1 Continued

genomics are safely shared for personal and family health prediction and integrated into public health data for research and health services improvement.

In the very near future, Alex and the nurses involved in this realistic scenario will require training in a range of areas related to delivery of digital health (➤ Fig. 15.2).

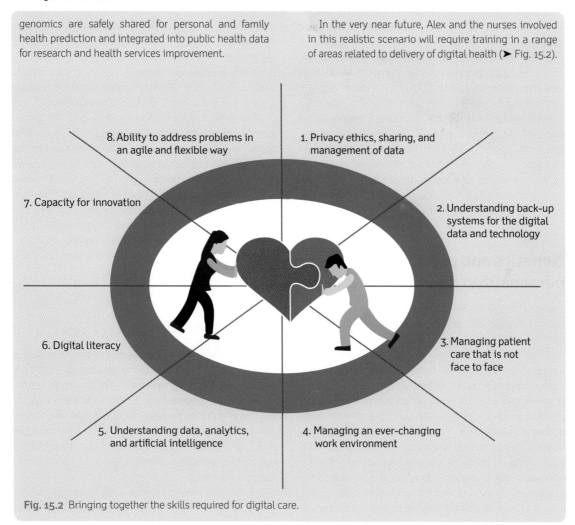

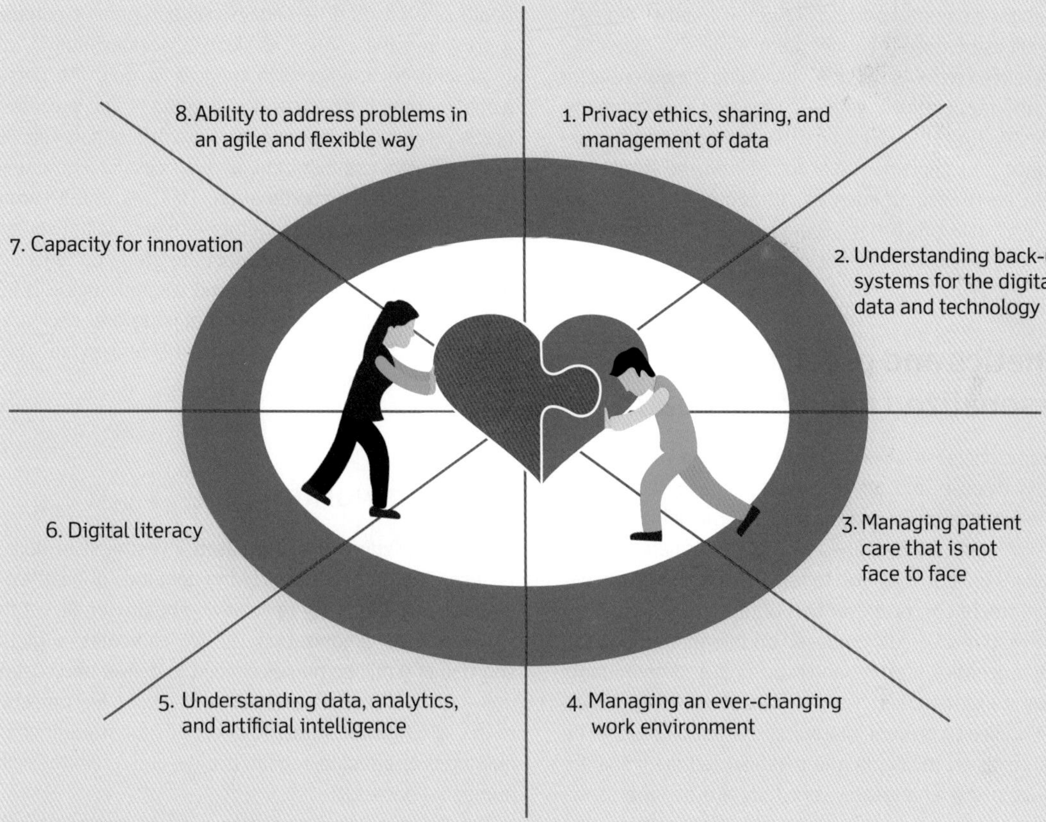

Fig. 15.2 Bringing together the skills required for digital care.

stratification, diagnostics, precision medicine, workflows, and efficiency.[12] AI does this by interpreting and finding meaning in vast sets of data, faster and more effectively than the human brain.[13] Thus, with the exponential growth in all sorts of patient health data, AI offers great potential.

An example of its application is in heart failure with the aim of developing a virtual 'doctor at home' system.14 Being able to pool datasets smartly and extrapolate relevance at an individual level offers huge potential for reducing clinician burden, improving clinical efficacy, and enhancing patient experience and outcomes.[14]

The application of AI in cardiovascular care offers immense advantages for patients and nurses, such as improving clinical decision-making, patient and nurse interactions, and overall patient experience, and reducing the risk of adverse events, patient waiting times, and costs. It is envisaged that AI will make unambiguous decisions and direct advice to patients, leaving more complex or ambiguous decisions to nurses and other healthcare professionals. The expected 'added value' of AI is assisting healthcare professionals in the delivery of care and interrogating 'big data'. Big data refers to extremely large data sets that can be analysed computationally to reveal patterns, trends, and associations. For example, patient health data sets need to be collected, analysed, and incorporated into clinical guidelines. Registries collect and provide data on patients' demographic characteristics, clinical profiles, management or care processes, and outcomes, and serve an important role in quality assurance, in developing research hypotheses, and as a resource for information about patients receiving care outside of clinical trials. They provide standardized data collection with definitions and reporting, rapid feedback, centralized data compilation, and statistical analysis, as well as transparent reporting. However, whether big data can fulfil its promise is a moot point.[15]

There are concerns about AI, including the potential for error and fraud, ethics, data security, and accountability. The legal, ethical, and societal issues regarding the acceptance and implementation of AI into the healthcare system are profound, such as discrimination, transparency, and data protection. Therefore, standard reporting guidelines for AI and machine learning are needed.

Genetics and precision/personalized medicine/health

The rapid increase in understanding of the role of genetics in disease and advancement in gene sequencing technology has given rise to precision medicine in CVD. Precision medicine is defined as using information about a person's genetic make-up to tailor strategies for the detection, treatment, or prevention of disease.[16] It is an integrative form of medicine based on information about a person's genetics, lifestyle, and exposures as determinants of their cardiovascular health and disease phenotypes, which is used to prevent, diagnose, or treat disease.[17] The terms precision medicine and personalized medicine are often used interchangeably, but they are not the same, though they do overlap. Precision medicine identifies the unique aspects of a person related to health and disease to select appropriate therapy, whereas personalized medicine refers to implementation of these data into a person-specific treatment plan.[17]

Precision medicine strives to delineate disease using multiple sources (including genomics and digital health metrics) to be more precise and accurate in diagnoses, definitions, and treatments of disease subtypes.[17] However, despite some spectacular success in cardiovascular genetics research, there has been little evidence of personalizing treatment for CVD on the basis of an individual patient's genetic make-up or biomarkers. Indeed, there is scepticism about the promises made by proponents of precision medicine, which are yet to be realized, and the amount of money invested in it.[18] For instance, there is little recognition of the inherent limits of prediction for individuals or the limits of approaches to prevention that rely on individual agency. There also appears to be undue emphasis placed on individuals' genes and their 'big data' at the expense of their own preferences for a particular treatment.

Precision health—a more appealing and appropriate term in cardiovascular nursing—refers to personalized healthcare based on a person's unique genetic composition within the context of lifestyle, socioeconomic, cultural, and environmental influences to help the person achieve optimal health and well-being.[19] The success of precision health depends on interdisciplinary clinical and research collaboration and successful community outreach and care coordination. This will entail cardiovascular nurses working together with data scientists, epidemiologists, and basic scientists to study patients and populations in clinical setting and communities.[20] It is a relatively recent development in nursing and efforts are needed to inform nurses of its potential and engage them in its possible application.

Nursing workforce

It is acknowledged that increased investment in nurses is necessary to meet the growing demands of healthcare globally. Nursing is key to achieving health for all, yet the World Health Organization (WHO) estimates a global shortfall of 9 million nurses needed to deliver and sustain universal health coverage by 2030.[21] Thus, a key objective of the WHO global strategic directions for strengthening nursing is to educate, recruit, deploy, and retain the right number of nurses.[21]

The 'Nursing Now' campaign aims to improve health and healthcare globally by raising the status and profile of nursing worldwide.[22] The campaign has several ambitious objectives, one of which is more nurses in education and employment.

The recent WHO report 'The State of the World's Nursing 2020' illustrates how nurses are critical to the delivery of healthcare and central to strengthening the health system, though the WHO notes that nursing is primarily a female-dominated profession.[23] Indeed, nursing is still perceived in many quarters as 'women's work'. Men continue to comprise only a small percentage—about 10%—of the global nursing workforce, even though men comprise roughly half of the population.[23]

An important aspect of any profession is to accurately reflect the make-up of the general population, and to do this nursing needs to diversify and attract men to ultimately improve the patient experience. The numbers of men in nursing remain low despite efforts to attract them into the profession. Addressing this disparity is important if the healthcare workforce is to reflect the diversity of the general population issue, especially in the context of today's changing sociocultural and healthcare landscapes.[24]

Compounding the shortage of nurses is the fact that the nursing workforce is ageing and this is evident not just among clinicians but also educators. This dearth in educators impacts the education and preparation of the next generation of nurses. Regardless of gender, age, or ethnicity, there is a growing recognition of the need to attract and retain more nurses. Recruitment drives include a positive rebranding of nursing at a national level that is gender-neutral and education beginning early (preschool and in primary schools). However, there is an urgent need for a concerted effort to examine the reasons why so many nurses are leaving the profession. Efforts to reward, regrade, or rebrand nurses may help in the short term but are not long-term corrective measures.

Today, patients require increasingly complex care and many nurses feel overburdened. Optimizing skill mix so that the more highly qualified staff focus on tasks only they are qualified to undertake, can lead to lower costs, improved staff satisfaction, and better patient outcomes. Higher staff satisfaction often lowers staff turnover which benefits patients because of the increased time spent with them which, in turn, results in additional cost savings. However, it is important to acknowledge that a good proportion of activities, such as assisting patients with activities of daily living or transportation, can be safely performed by non-professional staff. This is why there has been a surge in the employment of healthcare assistants in hospitals, clinics, and the community.

The shift towards a patient-led, preventative health system will necessitate reshaping the healthcare workforce, and nowhere is this more apparent than in nursing. Nursing roles and responsibilities are changing rapidly but this should be done taking a systematic approach, taking account of training and development needs and ensuring sustainability.[25] Currently, there is a mix of skill flexibility (role substitution or delegation), skill development (role enhancement or enlargement), and new roles in nursing. But there is often a lack of role clarity and of national competence frameworks and regulation, which can result in a fragmentation of care and dissatisfaction among nurses.

Having sufficient and appropriately qualified (graduate) nurses impacts patient safety.[26] Also, when experienced specialist cardiac nurses are not allocated to patients requiring their expertise, they often report lower work satisfaction and self-esteem.[27] Thus, nurses need to be better resourced, equipped, and prepared to address many of the new challenges they face.

An important consideration for the workforce is the issue of professional identity: the core beliefs, attitudes, values, motives, and experiences through which a person defines themselves. These core values and perspectives are integral to the art and science of nursing and become evident as the nurse learns, gains experience, and reflects.

Advanced practice

Nurses continue to be creative and make innovative and transformative actions in developing new roles to provide high-quality and safe care to patients, families, and communities. One area in which this is most apparent is advanced practice.

Surprisingly, there is no standard, accepted definition of advanced practice and its core competencies even though a plethora of specialist roles exist, including the clinical nurse specialist, nurse practitioner, advanced nurse practitioner, consultant nurse, and nurse case manager. However, many of these roles are unclear and their remit varies markedly. This is compounded, for instance, by the different preparation, education, registration, competencies, and autonomy of nurses in each country across Europe. The International Council of Nurses defines an advanced practice nurse (APN) as 'a registered nurse who has acquired the expert knowledge base, complex decision-making skills and clinical competencies for expanded practice, the characteristics of which are shaped by the context and/or country in which s/he is credentialed to practice. A master's degree is recommended for entry level'.[28] Though generally APN roles comprise clinical, educational, research, and management components, there is no common understanding or universal agreement about the APN role and wide variation in its regulation, licensure, and credentialing, as well as opposition from vested interests, including physicians.[29] In the US, the American College of Cardiology in its mission to transform cardiovascular care and improve heart health notes the importance of cardiovascular team-based care and collaborative care models. The American College of Cardiology exhorts team members to optimize their education, training, experience, and talent and recommends developing residency training programmes and other educational opportunities for advanced practice providers, including APNs.[30] Unfortunately, there appear to be few postgraduate programmes for nurses in cardiovascular care to address workforce needs.[31]

Opportunities

Nurses are key, indeed, central, members of the cardiovascular care team by virtue of spending more time with the patient and family and having greater opportunity to instigate health promotion, risk reduction, and disease prevention, as well as management and rehabilitation. Nurses have made, and continue to make, significant—in some cases pioneering—contributions to key areas of cardiovascular care, such as cardiac rehabilitation,[32] heart failure management,[33] and palliative and supportive care.[34] They have also led the way in examining the experiences and needs of patients, carers, and family members as well as developing novel interventions to address their needs and outcome measures to evaluate them.[35]

In order to address the increasing demands of patients and healthcare systems, nurses have also been innovative in introducing new roles, and extending and expanding these and their scope of practice, and models and systems of care, including transitional care between the hospital and home or community setting. While these developments are all welcome, there are opportunities for nurses and nursing to better articulate, introduce, evaluate, and implement some of these developments and be more adroit at persuading opinion leaders and stakeholders and influencing policymaking. For instance, there has been a tendency to develop new initiatives and introduce them with little thought to rigorous and systematic evaluation and replication. Also, many initiatives which are essentially nurse led, such as cardiac rehabilitation or heart failure management, are undoubtedly effective but their evaluation has tended to be simplistic with questions posed such as 'What works?' Yet most of the clinical scenarios that nurses operate in and the interventions they deliver are complex; moreover, each patient is unique, with different experiences, needs, preferences, expectations, and outcome. Thus, nurses operate in a healthcare system that is 'messy', an environment typified by complexity, uncertainty, and unpredictability. A 'one-size-fits-all' approach to patient care is no longer tenable: the key question is to examine whether interventions that nurses design and deliver are beneficial or harmful to patients and/or families.[33]

Nurses should focus on 'What works for whom, when, and why?'[33] For example, although cardiac rehabilitation is effective in reducing mortality and morbidity and improving quality of life, many of the programmes are standardized with little consideration given to choice of delivery and preferred outcomes[32]; likewise with heart failure management and other nurse-led interventions.[33] Patient outcomes are rarely shaped by a single factor such as age, sex, race, and class but rather a combination of various factors such as middle-class, male, older adult of Asian origin who is an immigrant to the UK.[36] It is through adopting such approaches that we can help identify factors such as the crucial characteristics of a programme and determinants of issues such as self-care as well as context, settings, and possible mechanisms by which health outcomes are improved.

Finally, consideration of other important patient and family issues such as satisfaction with and experiences of their care is essential. It is all too easy for nurses to still adopt a 'we know what's best' attitude when in fact the patient is the expert in their disease and its management.

Conclusion

Looking forward, cardiovascular care is evolving at a rapid pace and likely to present many challenges which, if grasped, will prove exciting and present cardiovascular nurses with the opportunity to think creatively and work nimbly. To optimize their potential to better meet the challenges they face, cardiovascular nurses need to be well prepared, equipped, supported, and led. Strong leadership is vital but so too is individual professional responsibility and accountability to ensure that nurses do the right thing, for the right person, at the right time, and in the right place. This depends on preparing staff with a sound education and training, equipping them with sufficient resources, encouraging them to make decisions and take risks in a supportive environment, fostering an ethos of thinking big and being bold and unafraid to challenge, while mindful of working collaboratively and keeping the patient at the centre of care. To deal with contemporary and ever-changing scenarios, nurses need support in the form of coaching, mentoring, and supervision as well as investment in research and development, education, and clinical skills training.[37] Good leadership should be about maximizing human capabilities: stirring curiosity, imagination, intuition, creativity, and empathy, but above all humility and compassion. Nursing needs to acknowledge and celebrate the vast array of talent among cardiovascular nurses and ensure it is harnessed to the betterment of our patients and society, who deserve nothing less. The future of cardiovascular nursing is bright.

References

1. Wongvibulsin S, Martin SS, Steinhubl SR, Muse ED. Connected health technology for cardiovascular disease prevention and management. Curr Treat Options Cardiovasc Med. 2019;21(6):29.
2. Perez MV, Mahaffey KW, Hedlin H, Rumsfeld JS, Garcia A, Ferris T, et al. Large-scale assessment of a smartwatch to identify atrial fibrillation. N Eng J Med. 2019;381(20):1909–17.
3. Van Heuverswyn F, De Buyzere M, Coeman M, De Pooter J, Drieghe B, Duytschaever M, et al. Feasibility and performance of a device for automatic self-detection of symptomatic acute coronary artery occlusion in outpatients with coronary artery disease: a multicentre observational study. Lancet Digital Health. 2019;1:e90–99.
4. Brandt CJ, Clemensen J, Neilsen JB, Søndergaard J. Drivers for successful long-term lifestyle change, the role of e-health: a qualitative interview study. BMJ Open. 2018;8(3):e017466.
5. Eysenbach G. What is e-health? J Med Internet Res. 2001;3:e20.
6. Redfern J, Neubeck L. e-Health in cardiovascular medicine. Med Sci. 2019;7:72.
7. Duff OM, Walsh DM, Furlong BA, O'Connor NE, Moran KA, Woods CB. Behavior change techniques in physical activity eHealth interventions for people with cardiovascular disease: systematic review. J Med Internet Res. 2017;19(8):e281.
8. Maddison R, Rawstorn JC, Shariful Islam SM, Ball K, Tighe S, Grant N, et al. mHealth interventions for exercise and risk factor modification in cardiovascular disease. Exerc Sport Sci Rev. 2019;47(2):86–90.
9. Beishuizen CR, Stephan BC, van Gool WA, Brayne C, Peters RJ, Andrieu S, et al. Web-based interventions targeting cardiovascular risk factors in middle-aged and older people: a systematic review and meta-analysis. J Med Internet Res. 2016;18(3):e55.
10. Coorey GM, Neubeck L, Mulley J, Redfern J. Effectiveness, acceptability and usefulness of mobile applications for cardiovascular disease self-management: systematic review with meta-synthesis of quantitative and qualitative data. Eur J Prev Cardiol. 2018;25:505–21.
11. Shan R, Ding J, Plante TB, Martin SS. Mobile health access and use among individuals with or at risk for cardiovascular disease: 2018 Health Information National Trends Survey (HINTS). J Am Heart Assoc. 2019;8(24):e014390.
12. Krittanawong C, Zhang H, Wang Z, Aydar M, Kitai T. Artificial intelligence in precision cardiovascular medicine. J Am Coll Cardiol. 2017;69(21):2657–64.
13. Johnson KW, Soto JT, Glicksberg BS, Shameer K, Miotto R, Ali M, et al. Artificial intelligence in cardiology. J Am Coll Cardiol. 2018;71(23):2668–79.
14. Barrett M, Boyne J, Brandts J, Brunner-La Rocca HP, De Maesschalck L, De Wit K, et al. Artificial intelligence supported patient self-care in chronic heart failure: a paradigm shift from reactive to predictive, preventive and personalised care. EPMA J. 2019;10(4):445–64.
15. Groeneveld PW, Rumsfeld JS. Can big data fulfil its promise? Circ CV Qual Outcomes. 2016;9(6):679–82.
16. Collins FS, Varmus H. A new initiative on precision medicine. N Engl J Med. 2015;372(9):793–95.
17. Leopold JA, Loscalzo J. Emerging role of prevision medicine in cardiovascular disease. Cir Res. 2018;122(9):1302–15.
18. Joyner MJ. Precision medicine, cardiovascular disease and hunting elephants. Prog Cardiovasc Dis. 2016;58(6):651–60.
19. Fu MR, Kurnat-Thoma E, Starkweather A, Anderson WA, Cashion AK, Williams JK, et al. Precision health: a nursing perspective. Int J Nurs Sci. 2020;7(1):5–12.
20. Musunuru K, Arora P, Cooke JP, Ferguson JF, Hershberger RE, Hickey KT, et al. Interdisciplinary models for research and clinical endeavors in genomic medicine. a scientific statement from the American Heart Association. Circ Genom Precis Med. 2018;11(6):e000046.
21. World Health Organization. Global Strategic Directions for Strengthening Nursing and Midwifery 2016–2020. Geneva: World Health Organization; 2016.
22. Crisp N. Nursing now—why nurses and midwives will be even more important and influential in the future. Int Nurs Rev. 2018;65(2):145–47.
23. World Health Organization. State of the World's Nursing 2020: Investing in Education, Jobs and Leadership. Geneva: World Health Organization; 2020.
24. Thompson DR, Quinn B, Watson R. Getting more men into nursing: an urgent priority (too little, too late). J Nurs Manag. 2020;28(7):1463–64.
25. Imison C, Castle Clarke S, Watson R. Reshaping the Workforce to Deliver the Care Patients Need. London: Nuffield Trust; 2016.
26. Aiken LH, Sloane DM, Bruyneel L, Van den Heede K, Griffiths P, Busse R, et al. Nurse staffing and education and hospital mortality in nine European countries: a retrospective observational study. Lancet. 2014;383(9931):1824–30.
27. Currey J, Sprogis SK, Orellana L, Chander A, Meagher S, Kennedy R, et al. Specialty cardiac nurses' work satisfaction is influenced by the type of coronary care unit: a mixed methods study. BMC Nurs. 2019;18:42.
28. International Council of Nurses. Definition and Characteristics of the Role. ICN Nurse Practitioner/

Advanced Practice Network. Geneva: International Council of Nurses; 2018.
29. Thompson DR, Astin F. Education for advanced nursing practice worldwide—is it fit for purpose? Heart Lung. 2019;48(3):176–78.
30. Brush JE, Handberg EM, Biga C, Birtcher KK, Bove AA, Casale PN, et al. 2015 health policy statement on cardiovascular team-based care and the role of advanced practice providers. J Am Coll Cardiol. 2015;65(19):2118–36.
31. Currey J, White K, Rolley J, Oldland E, Driscoll A. Development of a postgraduate interventional cardiac nursing curriculum. Aust Crit Care. 2015;28(4):184–88.
32. Thompson DR, Ski CF, Clark AM. Cardiac rehabilitation and secondary prevention: wrong terms, aims, models and outcomes? Eur J Prev Cardiol. 2019;26(9):995–97.
33. Thompson DR, Clark AM. Heart failure disease management interventions: time for a reappraisal. Eur J Heart Fail. 2020;22(4):578–80.
34. McConnell T, Diffin J, Fitzsimons D, Harrison C, Stone C, Reid J. Palliative care and heart failure: can implementation science help where the evidence alone has failed? Eur J Cardiovasc Nurs. 19(3):190–91.
35. Berg SK, Faerch J, Cromhout PF, Tewes M, Pedersen PU, Rasmussen TB, et al. Questionnaire measuring patient participation in health care: scale development and psychometric evaluation. Eur J Cardiovasc Nurs. 2020;19(7):600–608.
36. Allana S, Thompson DR, Ski CF, Clark AM. Intersectionality in heart failure self-care. Ignorance is not an option. J Cardiovasc Nurs. 2020;35(3):231–33.
37. Thompson DR, Darbyshire P. Nightingale's year of nursing: rising to the challenges of the Covid-19 era. BMJ. 2020;380:m2721.

Index

Tables, figures and boxes are indicated by *t*, *f* and *b* following the page number.

Abbreviations used in the index
CAD - coronary artery disease
CVD - cardiovascular disease
CVPR - cardiovascular disease prevention & rehabilitation
DALYs - disability-adjusted life years
ECG - electrocardiography

A

S